Treatment Interventions in Human Sexuality

CRITICAL ISSUES IN PSYCHIATRY
An Educational Series for Residents and Clinicians

Series Editor: Sherwyn M. Woods, M.D., Ph.D.
University of Southern California School of Medicine
Los Angeles, California

A RESIDENT'S GUIDE TO PSYCHIATRIC EDUCATION
Edited by Michael G. G. Thompson, M.D.

STATES OF MIND: Analysis of Change in Psychotherapy
Mardi J. Horowitz, M.D.

DRUG AND ALCOHOL ABUSE: A Clinical Guide to
Diagnosis and Treatment
Marc A. Schuckit, M.D.

THE INTERFACE BETWEEN THE PSYCHODYNAMIC AND
BEHAVIORAL THERAPIES
Edited by Judd Marmor, M.D., and Sherwyn M. Woods, M.D., Ph.D.

LAW IN THE PRACTICE OF PSYCHIATRY
Seymour L. Halleck, M.D.

NEUROPSYCHIATRIC FEATURES OF MEDICAL DISORDERS
James W. Jefferson, M.D., and John R. Marshall, M.D.

ADULT DEVELOPMENT: A New Dimension in Psychodynamic Theory
and Practice
Calvin A. Colarusso, M.D., and Robert A. Nemiroff, M.D.

SCHIZOPHRENIA
John S. Strauss, M.D., and William T. Carpenter, Jr., M.D.

EXTRAORDINARY DISORDERS OF HUMAN BEHAVIOR
Edited by Claude T. H. Friedmann, M.D., and Robert A. Faguet, M.D.

MARITAL THERAPY: A Combined Psychodynamic–Behavioral Approach
R. Taylor Segraves, M.D., Ph.D.

TREATMENT INTERVENTIONS IN HUMAN SEXUALITY
Edited by Carol C. Nadelson, M.D., and David B. Marcotte, M.D.

A Continuation Order Plan is available for this series. A continuation order will bring
delivery of each new volume immediately upon publication. Volumes are billed only
upon actual shipment. For further information please contact the publisher.

Treatment Interventions in Human Sexuality

Edited by

CAROL C. NADELSON, M.D.
Tufts—New England Medical Center
Boston, Massachusetts

and

DAVID B. MARCOTTE, M.D.
Mandala Center
Winston–Salem, North Carolina

PLENUM PRESS • NEW YORK AND LONDON

Library of Congress Cataloging in Publication Data

Main entry under title:

Treatment interventions in human sexuality.

(Critical issues in psychiatry)
Includes bibliographical references and index.
1. Sex therapy. 2. Psychosexual disorders. 3. Sexual disorders. I. Nadelson, Carol C.
II. Marcotte, David B. III. Series. [DNLM: 1. Sex. 2. Sex behavior. 3. Sex disorders —
Therapy. WM 611 T784]
RC556.T73 1983   616.6′906   83-4078
ISBN 0-306-41082-6

©1983 Plenum Press, New York
A Division of Plenum Publishing Corporation
233 Spring Street, New York, N.Y. 10013

Printed in the United States of America

Contributors

Roberta J. Apfel, M.D. • Department of Psychiatry, Beth Israel Hospital, Boston, Massachusetts

Oliver Bjorksten, M.D. • Department of Psychiatry, Medical University of South Carolina, Charleston, South Carolina

Eugene M. Dagon, M.D. • Department of Psychiatry, College of Medicine, University of South Florida, Tampa, Florida

Howard Dichter, M.D. • Rochester University Medical College, Rochester, New York

Nanette Gartrell, M.D. • Department of Psychiatry, Beth Israel Hospital, Boston, and Harvard University, Cambridge, Massachusetts

Ernest R. Griffith, M.D. • Institute for Rehabilitation Medicine, Good Samaritan Medical Center, Phoenix, Arizona

James W. Grover, M.D. • Department of Obstetrics and Gynecology, Lutheran General Hospital, Park Ridge, Illinois

Eugenia L. Gullick, Ph.D. • Salem Psychiatric Associates, Winston-Salem, North Carolina

James P. Held, B.Che. • Department of Physiology Research, University of Minnesota, Minneapolis, Minnesota

Rona Klein, M.D. • Stone Center for Developmental Services and Studies, Wellesley College, Wellesley, Massachusetts

Noel R. Larson, Ph.D., A.C.S.W. • Meta Resources, Psychotherapy and Training Institute, St. Paul, Minnesota

James W. Maddock, Ph.D. • Meta Resources, P. A.; Department of Family and Social Science and School of Public Health, University of Minnesota, St. Paul, Minnesota

David B. Marcotte, M.D. • Salem Psychiatric Association, Winston-Salem, North Carolina

Carol C. Nadelson, M.D. • Department of Psychiatry, Tufts-New England Medical Center, Boston, Massachusetts

Malkah T. Notman, M.D. • Department of Psychiatry, New England Medical Center, Tufts University School of Medicine, Boston, Massachusetts

Alvin M. Poussaint, M.D. • Department of Psychiatry, Harvard Medical School, Boston, Massachusetts

Esther Shapiro, Ph.D. • *Department of Psychiatry, Beth Israel Hospital, Boston, Massachusetts*

Daniel C. Silverman, M.D. • *Department of Psychiatry, Beth Israel Hospital, Boston, Massachusetts*

Elizabeth C. Small, M.D. • *Department of Psychiatry, University of Nevada Medical School, Reno, Nevada*

Toni E. Svéchin Greatrex, M.D. • *Brookline, Massachusetts*

Roberta B. Trieschmann, Ph.D. • *Psychiatric Consultant, Phoenix, Arizona*

Joseph Westermeyer, M.D. • *Department of Psychiatry, University of Minnesota Hospital, Minneapolis, Minnesota*

Adela G. Wilkeson, M.D. • *Harvard University School of Medicine, Boston; McLean Hospital, Belmont, Massachusetts*

Sherwyn M. Woods, M.D. • *Department of Psychiatry, University of Southern California, Los Angeles, California*

Alayne Yates, M.D. • *Department of Psychiatry, University of Arizona Health Sciences Center, Tucson, Arizona*

Foreword

Despite much progress in the past ten years, American medical schools have woefully inadequate sex education curricula. While some have a reasonable amount of lecture time, few have clinical opportunities for students to develop practical skills in working with patients who are struggling with sexual problems. It is my impression that the same is true in medical and gynecological residencies, as well as in graduate schools of psychology, counseling and social work. This book was specifically written to help fill that gap.

This is a book for clinicians, and it will provide a wealth of practical clinical knowledge and skills in dealing with the gamut of patient's sexual concerns, problems and dilemmas. Twenty-four experts have contributed eighteen chapters which address both the common and unusual sexual issues encountered in practice. These include sexual concerns from childhood to old age; gender identity and sexual preference; sexual dysfunction, including that of the physically ill and disabled; counseling with students, premarital, marital, and divorced patients; fertility and infertility; and chapters dealing with rape, incest and other sexual contacts between adults and children. Of particular importance are chapters on human sexuality in American minority populations, a chapter on alcohol, medication and other drugs, and a chapter on medical management of sexual problems in the gay population, a subject long-ignored by the profession.

The focus on practical intervention and skill development is amplified by the concluding four appendixes devoted to patient management problems. These provide an opportunity to "conduct" the clinical care of common sexual problems.

There have been many books published on human sexuality, but few have addressed themselves as broadly and thoroughly to the sexual problems encountered by psychiatrists and physicians of all specialties, as well as by all mental health practitioners. Still fewer have provided the consistent focus on the development of practical clinical skills and interventions.

Sherwyn M. Woods, M.D., Ph.D.
Series Editor

Contents

Chapter from:
TREATMENT INTERVENTIONS IN
HUMAN SEXUALITY

Edited by: Carol C. Nadelson
David B. Marcotte

1

Sexual History Taking

David B. Marcotte

Introduction

Perhaps the most neglected area of medical education today involves a lack of support in assisting clinicians to develop comfort while inquiring about the personal details of their patients' lives. When required to ask about the color, quantity, and consistency of both stools and sputum, the beginning physician quickly adapts those questions into a routine part of a review of systems and would not delete them from the history. Unless questions about patients' sexual activity, finances, religion, marital relationships, drug use, and conflicts with legal authorities are explored in depth, important information will be omitted from the data base with which the clinician works. The sexual history must become a part of the routine of the health-care provider's complete work-up. Just as one does not inquire about urine color to a patient brought into an emergency room with a massive laceration to the head until the bleeding is stemmed, sexual information must be woven into the routine questions that a clinician asks.

Unfortunately, education programs for the resident in almost every specialty fail to emphasize the importance of sexual functioning. Psychiatrists are expected to be knowledgeable about sexual behavior, yet frequently they too are ill-prepared to obtain information from patients about their sexual activities. Clinicians in each specialty turn to psychiatric consultants for assistance in helping to elucidate sexual concerns in patients if they suspect that there is concern. A consultant can be of enormous assistance to the patient and consultee if prepared to help other clinicians obtain highly personal information while taking a sexual history. Usually, however, a clinician rationalizes his or her failure to obtain a sexual history and to perform a genital exam. Several reasons are advanced:

1. "The patient will become uncomfortable." Upon closer examination, it is actually the clinician who becomes uncomfortable, thinking of himself as being forward, intrusive, or even lascivious. Patients readily talk about sexual function when

---

David B. Marcotte • *Salem Psychiatric Associates, Winston-Salem, North Carolina.*

given permission in a nondefensive manner by the clinician. If a patient has difficulty in providing information about their sexual concerns, an underlying attitudinal conflict should be suspected, which can be approached during the history taking or in a subsequent visit.

2. "Life-threatening situations are important. I will deal with these first before inquiring about sexual function." Levy (1973a, 1973b) and Cole (1975), in fact, have found that patients threatened with life-threatening illnesses usually wish that the clinician bring up current concerns about sexual functioning at a time when the acute crisis has diminished in severity.

3. Other rationales are: "I'm not equipped to do this," and "Others (sexologists, social workers, nurses, etc.) are better equipped to handle the sexual concerns of the patients." According to Lief (1970, 1973), in 1960 only two medical schools in the United States taught a formal sex-education program, whereas Holden (1974) states that 95% of medical schools in the United States have a formal course and the public expects clinicians to be knowledgeable about sexual functions. The California Licensing Board (1978) mandated that sex education was a necessary prerequisite for licensure. The clinician's own discomfort in these areas and lack of information are well documented in the literature. Therefore, the clinician has a special burden; without a support system to help him inquire about the body's function, he is left on his own to learn by the trial-and-error method about taking a sexual history. At times, the skill of sexual history taking will even be omitted entirely from the clinician's expected goals. Uncomfortable, ill at ease, and fearing the consequences of questions about patients' sexual function, he usually asks questions when half out the door, or questions are phrased in such a way that they are met with a reassuring yes or no on the part of the patient. Frequently, beginning efforts of the clinician are stated with a vague question, such as "How's your sex life?" Yet, the same clinician would never think of asking about the patient's coronary life or urinary life. Because the beginning clinician has no framework in which to collect and order the data, he cannot be expected to give a complete, detailed sexual history on each patient.

4. Other special difficulties arise when the clinician obtains sexual information from a patient. Children may offer a special challenge, especially when we consider parents' rights. We feel we are being intrusive into parents' rights when we give sex information or education to children—especially if it is in front of the parents. Children are interested in sexuality and obtain their information from peers outside of the home. Sexuality is usually not broached by most parents at all or by some at specific times of puberty or when rites of passage into adolescence are experienced. So it can become our task to assist parents to acquire and provide accurate sex information for their children. Clinicians may be too uncomfortable to acknowledge that adolescents are sexually active. Frequently, a sexually active teenager can promote fears in the clinician who has children in a similar age group. These hesitancies can operate to inhibit the interviewer from considering sexual thoughts or behaviors as a source of concern for adolescents.

5. Married individuals present an additional problem for the clinician in that we frequently do not inquire of married people the personal details of how they feel about one another.

6. Finally, the clinician finds difficulty with the concept that older people remain sexually active throughout their lives. He or she may imagine that their own parents were not sexually active and find special difficulties in broaching sexual questions to people who approximate his or her own parents' or grandparents' ages.

What are the remedies now for this situation? How can the clinician become as proficient in taking a sexual history and performing a genital exam as they would doing a venipuncture or inquiring about occipital pain? Perhaps the only way in which the clinician will gain comfort and ease in obtaining a sex history and performing a general examination is by practice. Each patient, each different age group, and each gender present their own challenge to the clinician. Inquiries into the sexual functioning of someone of the clinician's own age might be found to be very easy, whereas examining and obtaining information from an older person will evoke marked feelings of anxiety.

Several important factors lead to obtaining accurate information with a minimum of discomfort. First, questions should be prefaced by the importance of the data and its influence on a person. For example, clinicians recently have come to recognize the importance of sexual functioning on self-esteem and satisfaction. Sexual function is intimately associated with states of well-being and frequently can result from physical illnesses as well as cause physical illness. Phrased appropriately, a question asked of a patient will usually elicit a response. For example, "Most well-adjusted persons have concerns and expect to have some experience with sexual dysfunction during their lives. Could you tell me some of your own experiences with this?"

Another statement that might be posed to an early adolescent would be: "Many adolescents feel awkward and uncomfortable about discussing sexuality. They frequently assume that self-stimulation, masturbation, or other sexual activity is bad or forbidden, and they may have concerns that this means they are unusual or perhaps even ill. What have been your thoughts about this?"

Second, the clinician can introduce concerns about sex early in the review of systems instead of waiting until the end of the interview. Frequently hospital forms for write-ups relegate a very small space to information about habits, alcohol, tobacco, and sex. The clinician must not feel constrained by the limitations suggested on such forms. There is no specific outline for a sexual history or review of systems, therefore, the clinician can easily omit obtaining this information if they follow the outline for histories and physicals.

In general, historical information, such as family history and social history (including marital, vocational, and sexual functioning), are easily obtained in a spontaneous manner. If a review of systems proceeds from head to trunk, it is easy to ask, in regard to sexual functioning, whether a person has had specific difficulties from time to time with erection or sexual function.

Third, one should develop specific open-ended questions prefaced by educational comments, such as "Most people are concerned about self-stimulation or masturbation at some time in their lives, can you tell me about your experience with self-stimulation? Usually attitudes influence the way we feel about masturbation. What has been your experience with that?" Women commonly do not identify with the term *masturbation* but more frequently identify with *self-pleasuring* or *self-stimulation*.

An outline for a review of systems should cover the following basic categories during the history taking:

1. Self-stimulation and attitudes about it.
2. Concerns about sexual fantasies.
3. Concerns about sexual functioning with one's regular partner or others.
4. Information should be obtained about the most pleasing and displeasing aspects of sexual behavior currently practiced.
5. The most pleasing aspects of one's body and the most displeasing.
6. What the person would like to change about their sexual behavior and what they would not like to change.

By using this outline, information can be obtained in a relatively short period of time to enable the health professional to decide whether to amplify the sexual history.

When to Amplify the Sexual History

Now that we have seen that a sexual history can be a part of the general history taking, we begin to amplify the sexual history when cognitive dissonance or splitting occur. In other words, the reaction that the patient has to the data being discussed is overdetermined by an emotional response. Usually this occurs when the patient introduces sexual information. They may be inquiring about the use of birth control, but do so in a demanding manner by stating, "Just give me the pills," and "I don't want to talk about it." Others may be embarrassed and ask in a quiet, shy voice at the close of the interview. Usually this information signals to the clinician that there is some discomfort with sexual functioning or behavior, and time is required to deal with attitudes and information about the patient's value system.

Also, we amplify the sexual history when there is a marked change in terms of embarrassment, anxiety, or hostility associated with the data and when the clinician inquires of the patient's sexual functioning and the response is a hostile tirade about how the clinician does not need to know anything about that. Usually, the clinician can note and explore the data later with the patient. Additionally, comments the clinician can make that are helpful in these situations are: "Sexual functioning is important to the clinician's knowledge base about the patient, and it is understood that some people have some concern and anxiety in this area." When the patient wishes to discuss sexual thoughts or behavior, the clinician will be ready to do so.

Another example might be the patient who looks down, wrinkles his face, and avoids the clinician's gaze when asked about self-stimulation. Usually a conflict exists in that the behavior practiced by the patient may not fit the cognitive value system. Frequently, the clinician may be the object of projections, and the patient may wish to maintain a stance of morality that avoids certain sexual behaviors because the patient fears the clinician will think ill of him. Educational statements used to combat such potential projections are: "Most well-adjusted persons engage in self-stimulation throughout their lives. Can you tell me about your own functioning in this area?"

During amplification of the sexual history, the patient may avoid or redirect the data away from sexual concerns or information. The patient may suddenly talk about an unrelated subject when giving a sexual history. Usually the data that they were talking about just prior to redirecting the information is the conflict area and can be explored.

Other occasions for amplification of the sexual history are when the patient data suggest a lack of information about sexuality, and when vague answers are given to the clinician inquiring about specific sexual functioning.

General Guidelines for Taking a Sexual History

1. The clinician should proceed from the least taboo topic to the most taboo topic. Starting the sexual history with inquiry about incest or animal sexual contact usually produces quite a bit of anxiety in the patient and very little information. One of the best ways of proceeding is to inquire about sex education in the home or where the patient obtained sexual information, and then proceed on to thoughts about fantasies or early sexual experiences.

2. A sex history can be organized around the developmental model by proceeding from sex education in the home and the climate of sexual activity, specific information obtained from peers, family members, church, and other organizations and specific sets of behavior engaged in at varying periods of time during infancy, childhood, adolescence, and adulthood.

3. Questions asked about sexual variations should be prefaced by the commonness of such behavior, and educational statements about that behavior, such as "Same-sex sexual contact is quite common for males and females at some time in their lives. Can you tell me your experiences with same-sex sexual contact?" Similar questions can be asked about sadomasochistic sexual activity, fetishism, or incest.

4. Observe the patient's use of language and maintenance of eye contact and listen for signs of voice hesitancy. Each time the clinician takes a sexual history, some discomforting moments in the history will come to light. One can observe them best by tape-recording an interview and noting hesitancy or failure to find the right word, or better yet by videotaping such activities. Differences will also be noted in the clinician especially when interviewing persons of differing gender and age and whether or not one or more persons are in the room. All these situations have an influence on the comfort of the clinician and will not be overcome until practiced sufficiently to minimize discomfort. Practice interviewing might be similar to the knowledge that anxiety will diminish when the clinician draws blood for the one-hundredth time rather than the anxious experience of the first such occasion.

5. When the clinician is speaking of specific sexual behavior, he or she can avoid euphemisms by using a vocabulary with which he or she is comfortable while making sure that the patient understands the words used. To be stating, for example, that the patient engages in cunnilingus may take an explanation in terms of oral/genital contact or "going down" on another person. Before proceeding with the history, make sure you and the patient have a shared meaning of terms being used.

6. Move from very general, open-ended questions like "Many people during

adolescence have sexual experiences with both males and females. What has been your experience with same-sex contact?'' to very specific ones, such as the duration of sexual contact, what was enjoyable about the sexual activity, what was discomforting, and even inquiring in more specific detail. At the close of the interview, ask close-ended questions, such as ''Is my impression accurate that you have some sexual experience with another person weekly?'' Closure questions plus a summation of the salient features of the interview, followed by offering the patient an opportunity to disagree, add or delete information are several interview techniques that assist the clinician taking a sexual history.

7. Preface questions with ubiquitous statements, such as ''What was your experience with masturbation?'' These will help to indicate the commonness of sexual behavior as well as to expect that the patient has engaged in such activity.

Taking a Sexual History

One of the questions that emerges from the clinician on the front line of medical care is how much information should be gathered in a routine office visit? Many clinicians perceive it to be intrusive to ask questions detailing their concerns about sexuality. In reality, patients are frequently greatly relieved when the clinician introduces the subject of their sexual concerns and inquires as to their sexual functioning in a manner that expects patient cooperation and communication. The psychiatric consultant can help to provide the physician with both an opportunity to explore anticipated patient responses as well as emphasizing the importance of the data obtained to the patient's well-being. The consultant can also help to decide, like any of the review-of-systems questions, what specific questions about sexuality and current functioning will bring to the surface the patient's concerns. A brief outline for a review-of-systems questions that will elicit most patients' concerns is the following with an adult patient:

1. Questions and concern on the clinician's part should be directed at self-stimulation currently practiced, the frequency of self-stimulation, satisfaction, and attitudes about it. A large number of patients, both male and female, are greatly concerned about self-stimulation especially as they leave adolescence and become adults. The interviewer can introduce this by saying, ''Many persons have concerns about self-stimulation and solitary sexuality. Can you tell me some of your concerns about self-stimulation?''

2. Most people have concerns about fantasies or thoughts they have had about sexual objects or behavior. The clinician can introduce these concerns by stating, ''Most people have at some time considered their own thoughts to be somewhat unusual or different from other peoples'. Yet as we understand more about sexuality, frequently peoples' fantasies are quite common. Can you tell me some of your concerns about your sexual fantasies and also some of the behaviors based on these fantasies that you have carried out?'' These first two questions are very important and stimulate discussion of usual areas of concern to patients.

3. Patients should be asked about their current sexual functioning, frequency and

degree of pleasure derived from current sexual behaviors, and whether they are moderately satisfied or dissatisfied with both the function and variety of the current sexual practices. This can be amplified to include sex outside of a primary relationship with both males and females.

4. Another review-of-systems question that is most helpful is to ask the patient to identify the most displeasing and pleasing aspects of their current sexual functioning.

5. A review of systems can elicit concerns about a patient's body image. For example, patients can be asked to describe aspects of their bodies that are pleasing to them and those aspects that are displeasing to them. What is their level of comfort when the body is exposed to other people?

6. Finally, in a review of systems, do they have any goals for changing any of the functions to improve or enhance both the variety and pleasure derived from their sexual contact?

Once these brief review-of-systems questions are asked of patients, the data can be further explored if potential areas of conflict are found by the interviewer. Each patient who is getting a general medical history that includes a review of systems should be asked questions, specifically as we have outlined.

Detailed Sexual History

Once concerns about sexuality have surfaced and goals are set with the patient to explore or delineate areas of concern that they wish to work on, a detailed sexual history is in order. It may be accomplished in a second visit or a time set aside for specific information where comfort and time are paramount to the clinician's interaction.

Childhood Sexuality

Information can be obtained about the following categories of sex information:

1. The family's attitudes about sex information and behavior
2. Sexual information gathered from the home or outside of the home
3. Childhood sex activity both in and out of the home
4. Contact with older children or adults during childhood
5. Perception of bodily prepubescent functions
6. Perceptions and cognitive information available about procreation

Onset of Adolescence

Preparation for menstruation and self-stimulation in females and preparation for masturbation and orgasm in males.

Sexual Behavior during Adolescence, Including Orgasmic Experiences

1. Self-stimulation and masturbation.
2. Sexual play with same-sex and opposite-sex children.
3. Oral sexuality, intercourse, contact with older adults, family members, and friends.
4. Questions about their sense of male or femaleness as well as questions about role identity or feelings of fitting the stereotyped role behaviors of males and females.
5. Dating behavior—What was the nature and pattern of dating behaviors? What was the frequency of contact with the dating partner, and what concerns did the patient experience?
6. Sexual behaviors and attitudes during engagement or committed relationships, number and pattern of committed relationships or engagements.

Marriage or Committed-Partner Relationships

1. Fantasies, specific behavior, and variety of behavior.
2. Does the patient wish to change or not change certain behaviors?
3. Pleasure derived from specific sexual behaviors and/or sexual behaviors that are unpleasant.
4. Questions about extramarital sexual contact for both genders outside of the marriage.

Postmarital Sexual Activity

1. Behavior and fantasies following divorce or death of spouse
2. Different behaviors and/or sexual dysfunctions

With this general outline as a guide we will explore, throughout this volume, methods of intervention with persons of different ages and with special concerns. We have organized the book around a life-cycle model with special attention to specific application of skills and knowledge which the clinician will use to intervene in the treatment of sexually dysfunctional and concerned patients.

References

California Licensing Board, 1978, Senate Bill No. 80, Section 2192.3, Business and Professional Code.
Cole, T. M. Sexuality and physical disabilities. *Archives of Sexual Behavior*, 1975, *4*, 389–403.
Holden, C. Sex therapy: Making it as a science and industry. *Science*, 1974, *186*, 330–334.

Levy, N. B. The psychology and care of the maintenance hemodialysis patient. *Heart and Lung*, 1973, *2*, 400–405. (a)

Levy, N. B. Sexual adjustment to maintenance hemodialysis and renal transplantation: National survey by questionnaire, preliminary report. *American Society of Artificial Internal Organs Transactions*, 1973, *19*, 138–143. (b)

Lief, H. I. Sex education in medical school. *Journal of Medical Education*, 1970, *45*, 1025–1031.

Lief, H. I. Obstacles to the ideal and complete sex education of the medical student and physician. In J. Zubin and J. Money (Eds.), *Contemporary sexual behavior: Critical issues in the 1970's*. Johns Hopkins Univ. Press, Baltimore & London: 1973. Chap. 22, pp. 441–453.

Problems in Sexual Functioning

Carol C. Nadelson

People are increasingly recognizing and seeking treatment for sexual problems. They are often seen initially by primary physicians, medical specialists, and other clinicians, because they believe that there is an organic etiology for their symptomatology. Consultation and referral may be sought when an organic etiology is not found or when there is a psychogenic component regardless of the etiology of the symptoms.

Sexual symptoms deriving from sexual inhibition or lack of sexual interest can be distinguished from those specific dysfunctional problems that occur in individuals who are sexually interested and involved but for whom a specific symptom, e.g., impotence or anorgasmia, interferes with performance. Those problems related to lack of interest in sexuality are most often psychogenic or interpersonal in etiology. They are generally best treated by psychotherapeutic techniques, including individual, group, and couples therapy, or by a change in partner.

Sexual dysfunctions are specific disorders for which physical and/or psychogenic factors may be etiological. The sexual dysfunctions may respond to organic treatment, to specific behavioral techniques, and/or to psychotherapy. In this chapter, specific sexual dysfunctions rather than problems with sexual interest or desire will be addressed.

Evaluation

In order to evaluate a patient who presents with a sexual dysfunction symptom, a history and physical examination are a necessary beginning in order to rule out possible organic causes. This requires that the clinician have a thorough knowledge of those potential organic factors that cause sexual symptoms and the skill to elicit a complete developmental, family, and sexual history.

Carol C. Nadelson • Department of Psychiatry, New England Medical Center, Tufts University School of Medicine, Boston, Massachusetts.

The etiology of sexual dysfunction symptoms, although often multifactoral, can be divided into three basic groups:

1. Those with a primarily organic etiology
2. Those with primarily psychogenic etiology
3. Those in which an organic problem results in symptoms related to psychological issues

Physical Causes of Sexual Dysfunction

This group reportedly accounts for between 3 and 20% of sexual dysfunctions seen by clinicians (Kaplan, 1974). There is a wide range of incidence figures, because the population base often varies depending upon the specialty and referral source of the clinician. Thus, selective referral makes it more likely that the gynecologist or endocrinologist will see organic problems and the psychiatrist will see problems that are thought to be clearly psychogenic. Each may overrate the incidence of problems in the category with which they have most expertise and underestimate the other. Furthermore, definitions of dysfunction vary, and patients may be more or less comfortable about reporting certain symptoms.

The physical causes of sexual dysfunction can be grouped in a number of ways. One convenient way of conceptualizing them is to group them according to the mechanism of the dysfunction (Table 1):

1. Dysfunctions related to biochemical/physiological processes produce sexual symptoms related to systemic effects. These include cardiopulmonary, hepatic, renal, endocrine, and degenerative diseases, as well as systemic infections and malignancies. The effect on functioning may be to decrease libido and impair sexual arousal in women or potency in men. The mechanisms of action may be to cause general debilitation, pain, or depression; or the action may be specific, resulting from changes in hormones, such as estrogens or androgens.

2. Dysfunctions related to specific infections (mumps, tuberculosis), tumors, or invasive processes may have direct effects on the testes or ovaries. Certain tumors may also invade specific structures, in addition to the systemic symptoms they produce, which affect libido or arousal.

TABLE 1 Physical Causes of Sexual Dysfunctions

1. Biochemical/physiological disorders
2. Tumor, infection, and invasive process
3. Anatomic or mechanical interference
4. Postsurgery with neurological or vascular damage
5. Neurological disorders
6. Vascular disorders
7. Endocrine disorders
8. Genetic or congenital disorders
9. Drugs and medication

3. Dysfunctions caused by anatomic or mechanical interference primarily with local genital or adjacent structures. These include disorders producing pain, damage, or irritability, such as infection (urethritis, prostatitis, endometritis, vaginitis, and pelvic inflammatory diseases) or trauma. In addition, conditions like priapism, phimosis, and clitoral adhesions produce local discomfort; and chordee, hypospadias, imperforate hymen, or allergic or radiation reactions make intromission difficult. At times, pregnancy produces mechanical interference and requires changes in position or technique for coitus to be comfortable.

4. Dysfunctions may occur after surgical procedures that damage genitals directly or interfere with their nerve or vascular supply. Included in this group are problems related to prostatectomy (especially radical perineal), abdominal perineal resections, lumbar sympathectomies, abdominal aortic surgery, obstetrical trauma, or complications of procedures, such as hysterectomy. Pain, a patulous introitus, or ejaculatory disturbance related to nerve damage may interfere with sexual response.

5. Neurologically related dysfunctions constitute another group. These include disorders where there is damage to higher centers, such as occurs with temporal or frontal lobe damage, or in disorders, such as amyotrophic lateral sclerosis, spina bifida, multiple sclerosis, surgery or trauma to the sacral or lumbar cord, tabes dorsalis, or combined systems disease. In the case of higher center damage, the primary effect is an increase or decrease in libido. With spinal damage, libido is generally not affected, but erection or ejaculation, or orgasm in females, may be.

6. Local vascular disorders may produce an impairment of erectile functioning in males by interfering with penile blood supply [thrombosis of penile veins, arteries, or aortic bifurcation thrombosis (Leriche syndrome), leukemia, sickle cell disease].

7. Endocrine disorders may directly depress libido or erectile response by decreasing effective androgen levels. Pituitary, adrenal, or gonadal diseases, such as tumors, may be etiological.

8. Dysfunctions related to genetic/congenital disorders, such as Klinefelter's syndrome, may result in impotence in males. Other disorders including bladder exstrophy, hypospadius, and undescended testicles also cause dysfunctions. In the female, imperforate hymen and congenital defects of the internal and external genitalia may be responsible for sexual symptoms.

9. Another major category of physical causes of sexual dysfunction include the ingestion of a variety of drugs and medications. Drugs or medications can affect sexual responses directly or indirectly. They may act primarily centrally and change libidinal responses, or they may interfere with peripheral mechanisms via the autonomic nervous system or the alteration of blood flow or muscular activity. The effects of drugs on the male have been better investigated than for the female, therefore, more specific information is available.

At times, drug effects are difficult to specifically assess since mood, personality, and perception may affect the reporting of symptoms or effects. This occurs especially with hallucinogens like LSD, and marijuana.

I.   Centrally acting drugs

   A. Stimulants
        Aphrodisiacs are often said to exist, but this is more fantasy than reality. Currently, there is no drug that can be considered to be a specific aphrodisiac.

Some hallucinogens, as well as drugs like cannabis (marijuana), have been said to increase libido and sexual response. However, this appears to be more related to alterations in perception and cognition than to specific sexual effects.

Alcohol and barbiturates, although usually considered depressants, in small amounts reduce anxiety and inhibition and, thus, increase sexual responsiveness. Amphetamines and cocaine may have a stimulant effect and improve confidence as well as performance, in small amounts. This effect is generally not found in those with addictions.

Androgens, on the other hand, have been reported to alter sexual drive. They act both centrally and peripherally. If no deficiency has been demonstrated, however, the intake of androgens does not have a predictable effect. When a deficiency is demonstrated, these drugs increase potency and libido. In women, they produce side effects, such as hirsutism and acne. In men, side effects may include exacerbation of prostatic carcinoma.

A number of experimental drugs, such as cyclozine, L-DOPA, and PCPA, have been reported to be sexual stimulants. Documentation of consistent responses in humans is not yet available.

B. Depressants

High doses of any drug that causes psychomotor retardation, including alcohol and sedatives, produce central nervous system depression. Narcotics may specifically reduce the sexual drive. Alcohol is perhaps the most frequently used and consistent cause of problems in sexual functioning. It causes impotence as well as ejaculatory disturbance.

II. Peripherally acting drugs

A. Stimulants

Androgens promote growth and sensitivity of the male genitals and the clitoris. Estrogens cause growth of female genitalia and breasts. Although evidence about specific effects of estrogens on libido is unclear, androgens do appear to increase libido.

Cantharides (e.g., Spanish fly) increase sexual excitement, because they increase local tissue irritability. In the male, they produce priapism, which increases excitation. Amyl nitrate acts as a vasodilator and may, thus, heighten the vascular responses in the genitals.

B. Depressants

Anticholinergics affect the parasympathetic nervous system and, thus, penile blood flow, inhibiting full erection. Since these drugs are used frequently in people with gastrointestinal disturbances, complaints of potency problems may be related to prescribed medication.

Anti-adrenergics interfere with the sympathetic nervous system activity and, thus, in the male, may cause difficulties with ejaculation. Since these drugs are used for the management of hypertension, symptoms in men who are on antihypertensives may be drug-related. In addition, ganglionic blocking agents, which are now used extensively for the treatment of hypertension and other disorders, may act on both sympathetic and/or parasympathetic nervous systems.

Drugs that have indirect effects on sexual behavior include psychotropic medications, which may improve sexual behavior because of reduction of anxiety or depression but may also have other effects, i.e., thioridazine produces "dry ejaculation" (retrograde ejaculation into the bladder). Many phenothiazines have been reported to produce potency disturbances. On the other hand, lithium may be seen, by patients using it, to depress sexual functioning because it diminishes elation.

Sexual Dysfunction with Major Psychogenic Components

Symptoms of sexual dysfunction are generally nonspecific, that is, a particular physical or psychological disorder does not cause a specific sexual disorder. The same symptom in different people may well have a different, even opposite, etiology.

Since sexual responses are a complex series of autonomically mediated reflexes, the person who is relaxed, not distracted, and well functioning psychologically is likely to be more sexually responsive. To function well sexually, the person must be able to abandon him/herself to erotic experiences and give up control, and some degree of cognitive contact, with his/her environment. Thus, problems in sexual functioning may arise from long-standing intrapsychic factors, or they may be related to situational or interpersonal disturbances.

Sexual dysfunctional symptoms with psychogenic components derive from a number of sources including (Nadelson, 1979; see Table 2):

1. Early sexual attitudes and experiences. These include a past history of a traumatic sexual experience (rape or incest), guilt about sexuality related to childhood communication (such as "sex is bad or dirty"), or early homosexual experiences that produced anxiety about sexual preference.

2. Lack of information, which may result in ignorance of technique, fears of pregnancy or venereal disease, unrealistic expectations (such as simultaneous orgasm), or the persistence of myths (such as "men are always interested in having sex, but women are not").

3. Situational factors, including acute family or work stress, marital problems, which may be precipitated at specific times, or life-stage differences between partners.

TABLE 2 Sexual Dysfunctions with Psychogenic Causes

1. Early sexual attitudes and experiences
2. Lack of sexual information
3. Situational stress
4. Difficulties in communication
5. Intrapsychic or interpersonal factors

4. Major communication problems in a relationship are often expressed in sexual symptoms. These, however, may merely be the tip of the iceberg. Some couples insist on sexual therapy because they want to believe that the problem is specifically sexual. In this way, they sometimes can avoid facing underlying issues. Often the couple fails initially, for whatever reason, to recognize the source or extent of the problems.

A few attempts at sexual therapy with no results, or the recognition that engagement in sexual therapy, although desired, is not possible, may enable the couple to recognize that there are many problems other than specific sexual symptoms. This occurs because sexual therapy produces pressure for communication and arouses anxiety, which may have been masked by the symptoms. Thus, a man who at 40 begins to feel that he is on the road downhill may search for a younger woman to buoy his flagging self-esteem. The woman who has been at home may find her life ''boring'' when her children leave. She may displace her conflict and complain about her marriage and her husband's lack of sexual attention. They may, in fact, be anxious about the future as each redefines life goals. As we will discuss, individual or marital, rather than sexual therapy may be more helpful with these problems.

5. Intrapsychic and interpersonal issues ranging from performance anxiety (especially when there has been a previous history of failure in sexual functioning) to serious depression may occur and produce symptoms.

Depression is the most serious problem. There can be a number of etiological factors which masquerade as a specific sexual dysfunction. It is critical that depression be completely evaluated so that appropriate treatment is instituted before any attempt is made to provide therapy for the sexual dysfunction. It is necessary to distinguish between depression caused by a sexual dysfunction and depression that produces sexual symptoms. It is important to remember that sexual symptoms may be an expression of an underlying depression or a way of obtaining help when consciously or deliberately acknowledging an emotional problem is even more threatening to the individual or couple than acknowledging the existence of a sexual problem.

Control issues are frequently the conflict areas around which treatment is sought. Since erotic feelings result in potential loss of control, a person who is made anxious by loss of control may be sexually unresponsive. Often these individuals describe that they ''go through the motions'' of sexual interaction but that they are unable to experience sexual feelings. They find themselves ''spectatoring'' or developing obsessional and unrelated thoughts that serve to diminish their sexual pleasure. An example of this is the woman who reported that she often wondered what the fly on the ceiling thought while she was having sexual intercourse.

Problems with low self-esteem may manifest themselves in fears of failure, fear of rejection, performance anxiety, or concerns about sexual identity. At times, this may be experienced directly as sexual anxiety, or it may be displaced or projected and presented as anger at the spouse for failing to perform.

In a relationship where both partners are primarily concerned with satisfying their wishes for gratification of needs for dependency and caretaking, sexual activity may be minimal but mutually satisfactory. However, when one partner becomes dissatisfied, or changes in his/her desire, the balance between the partners may be disrupted, and symptoms may result. Treatment oriented specifically toward relief of symptoms might not be effective, since the underlying needs for gratification of dependency wishes would not be addressed.

Where expectations of the relationship are transference based and depend upon fantasies and past experiences of relationships, the reality of who the current partner is may not meet the fantasy of who is desired, and the relationship will not seem to be satisfying. In this situation, the person may find him/herself unable to perform sexually and may not be consciously aware of the reasons. He/she may not report prior sexual problems and may not have difficulty performing with other partners. This symptom is often first seen after a pregnancy, when the wife or husband becomes a mother or father, thus reviving earlier experiences with or feelings about the opposite-sexed parent. This may interfere with the perception or ability to interact with the partner.

Sexual Problems of Mixed Etiology

The interaction of organic and psychogenic components in producing sexual symptoms is both complex and frequent. Symptoms may emerge after an acute illness or injury because of the requirement for a change in sexual pattern or technique; or long-standing or progressive symptoms may, after many years, bring people into treatment for a variety of reasons. The man with a penile or spinal cord injury who no longer has the same full erection may find sexual intercourse difficult and may become anxious, depressed, feel inadequate, avoid sexual interaction, or even become hostile and angry and blame his partner. His partner may also experience similar symptoms and feelings, and the couple may then be unable to utilize whatever erectile potential exists. The therapist must be cognizant of the dynamics of the interaction between partners and not succumb to seeing one as the damaged and the other as the healthy partner or collude in the hopelessness of the couple. Support, education, and/or therapy may be important to help the couple make necessary changes. For example, a couple who has always had sexual intercourse in the male superior position may need to learn to change to the female superior position when the husband has reduced erectile ability because of diabetes, since this will most likely facilitate successful coitus. They may need support and understanding and even a referral for further therapy if they find the change too difficult. On the other hand, the woman with chronic dyspareunia, because of endometriosis, may decide, as she approaches midlife, that she has missed sexual experiences and seek treatment. The relief of the physical symptoms may not automatically cause her sexual problem to disappear. She may continue to be anxious and/or her partner may even respond negatively. The fact that they did not seek treatment for many years may indicate that it served a purpose in the relationship. In this case, couples therapy rather than focused sexual therapy may be indicated.

Among the most important aspects of sexual functioning involving both physical and psychogenic components are the issues of self-image and body image. The adolescent girl who is fearful of sexuality may unconsciously develop anorexia to "look like and be a boy," and the woman who has had a mastectomy may avoid sexuality because "my body is so ugly." Likewise the paunchy middle-aged man may see himself as sexually repulsive because his physique has changed, and the man with a recent coronary may develop sexual symptoms related to anxiety about cardiac damage and/or a sense of inadequacy.

In each situation, the therapist must understand all of the facets of the problem. This includes the individual issues, as well as how a couple relates to each other. Those whose sexual problems prevent them from seeking a partner may need therapy directed at their self-esteem before they can risk involvement in a relationship. Individual psychotherapy or group therapy may be very effective in this situation.

Classification of Sexual Dysfunctions

A knowledge of the specific phases of the sexual response cycle is critical to the understanding of dysfunctions, regardless of their etiology. As has been noted, the factors that initiate symptoms can be organic and/or psychogenic. The physiological response, however, is the same regardless of the etiology (Masters and Johnson, 1966).

The cycles of both female and male can be divided into four phases involving genital vasocongestion and involuntary smooth, as well as striated muscle responses (Figs. 1 and 2). The responses are summarized as:

1. The *excitement* phase is characterized by increasing pelvic and penile vasocongestion. In the male, erection occurs, and, in the female, labial, vulvar, and perivaginal vasocongestion cause vaginal lubrication and genital swelling. This is mediated by the parasympathetic nervous system. In addition, there are changes in the position of pelvic organs and ballooning of the vagina.

2. *Plateau* occurs when there is the maximal enlargement and congestion of pelvic organs. These organs may shift positions. In the female, vaginal swelling, called the *orgasmic platform,* occurs, and the uterus elevates. In the male, secretions from Cowper's gland occur at this time. This is important clinically since this secretion contains semen, and it may be responsible for impregnation, despite the fact that ejaculation has not occurred.

Immediately prior to ejaculation in the male, there is a period called *ejaculatory*

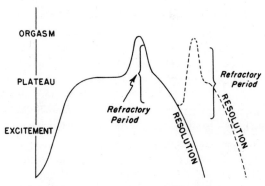

Figure 1 The male sexual response cycle. (Reprinted with permission from Masters and Johnson, 1966, p. 5.)

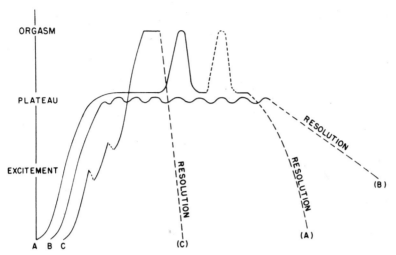

Figure 2 The female sexual response cycle: three representative response patterns. (Reprinted with permission from Masters and Johnson, 1966, p. 5.)

inevitability. At this time, it is no longer possible for the male to voluntarily inhibit ejaculation. There is no comparable period for the female.

3. *Orgasm*—Ejaculation, under sympathetic and somatic motor nervous system control, consists of involuntary contractions at 0.8-sec intervals of the striated muscles surrounding the base of the penis and the smooth muscles of the penile urethra. The female response is similar with both striated and smooth perineal and adjacent musculature contracting at the same rate.

4. *Resolution* consists of an abatement of local vasocongestion and a return to the basal state. For the male, there is a refractory period during which time the excitation phase cannot recur. This period of time varies and tends to increase as an individual becomes older. There is, however, considerable individual variation. For the female, the absence of this phase means that multiple orgasms can occur in rapid succession.

Evidence from studies of the male indicate that there is a biphasic response, based on nervous system mediation. As noted earlier, erection is primarily mediated by the parasympathetic nervous system, and the emission phase of ejaculation, by the sympathetic nervous system and somatic nerves. Clinical evidence from dysfunctional syndromes in females suggests that similar neurological mediation exists. Sexual unresponsiveness in the female can be considered to be related to failure of excitation and is analogous to impotence in the male. Anorgasmia in the female is approximately equivalent to the phase in which ejaculatory disorders occur in males.

Major Coital Problems

Dysfunctional syndromes can be considered primary or secondary, depending upon whether the individual has ever been asymptomatic. Thus, the man with primary impotence has never had the ability to achieve and to maintain an erection for sufficient time to accomplish coitus at any time in his life, whereas the man with secondary impotence has had past success but recent or situational failure. The importance of making this distinction relates to prognosis and treatment. Those with primary disorders are more difficult to treat, and the prognosis is less optimistic, since the etiology is often more complex and multidetermined, and congenital organic factors may play a more prominent role.

It is important to emphasize that there is no specific individual or family dynamic constellation that produces a specific dysfunctional syndrome, although predisposing factors are contributory, e.g., sexual inhibitions in a person raised with negative attitudes toward sexuality because of religious or other values. In addition, since the interpretation of retrospectively remembered data is difficult to assess, we must view with caution interpretations based on these memories. For instance, we cannot say that individuals with "weak" fathers and "dominant" mothers are likely to be impotent, because we are ignoring other data, e.g., that many people with these families do not have sexual difficulty, other factors may be etiological, or the individual may remember this time selectively or inaccurately. A rather complex series of communications and interactions produces this perception and contributes to symptom formation. Thus, oversimplified formulations must be avoided.

Male Sexual Dysfunction

There are two basic categories of male dysfunction that correspond with the phases described earlier. These are disorders of potency and ejaculation. *Impotence* or erectile dysfunction is defined as the inability to achieve and/or maintain an erection. Primary impotence is rare and occurs in approximately 1% of men under 35. Secondary impotence is said to occur if potency is insufficient for coitus in 25% of attempts. It is far more frequent than primary impotence, occurring in 25% of males over 70 (Masters and Johnson, 1970).

In addition to some specific organic etiologic factors, such as diabetes, debilitating illnesses, alcoholism, and endocrinopathies, the erectile mechanism may not function during acute illness, life-threatening situations, psychic trauma, or even when the partner is not physically attractive.

There is also some evidence that the attainment of an erection may proceed more slowly as a man ages, although once an erection occurs, it can be maintained longer in an older man. The anxiety generated by this symptom often intensifies the symptom. Thus, if a man perceives some decrease in erectile capacity and becomes anxious as he grows older, the symptom may become worse because he has become so anxious.

Kaplan considers impotence to be a physiological concomitant of anxiety rather than a defense against the emergence of anxiety, resulting from the reawakening of Oedipal feelings and fantasies or other intrapsychic factors (Kaplan, 1974). Thus, she proposes a psychosomatic model, implying a relationship between stress and symptom. It does appear, however, that the symptom may, at times, be defensive. In this situation, one might expect that if the symptom is relieved with treatment, another symptom might substitute. This does, in fact, sometimes occur.

Premature ejaculation is seen in a wide variety of men and does not appear to be linked with specific sexual conflicts or psychopathologic syndromes. It also occurs in people who report that they have good relationships with partners.

It is difficult to define premature ejaculation out of context since there is no specific time interval after intromission that is "normal." Thus, an accurate description of the symptom should include a partner. Definitions have ranged from consideration of the number of thrusts that occur prior to orgasm to time intervals (ranging from 30 sec to 2 min after intromission) when a partner is orgasmic. Premature ejaculation, according to Masters and Johnson, occurs when a man cannot control his ejaculatory process for sufficient length of time during intravaginal containment to satisfy his partner in at least 50% of their coital attempts (Masters and Johnson, 1970). A crucial concept is the absence of the perception that voluntary control is possible, once an intense level of sexual excitement is attained. Thus, the plateau phase cannot be prolonged. Often this lack of control is accompanied by diminished genital sensation.

Although physical causes for premature ejaculation are rare, this possibility should be considered, especially when the symptom is secondary. Local disorders, like prostatitis, can cause premature ejaculation, and neurological problems, such as multiple sclerosis, can first present as premature ejaculation, although this is extremely rare.

As with other sexual dysfunctions, the experience of sexual inadequacy may result in other problems, either interpersonal or intrapsychic. These compound the initial symptoms. Men with premature ejaculation may also become impotent, and their partners may become anorgasmic when the problem is long-standing. The presenting problem may, thus, be impotence rather than premature ejaculation.

There are a multitude of theoretical formulations about etiology, none of which is specific. Anxiety is a prominent component. It may cause the problem or be secondary to it. There is evidence that fear of discovery, guilt, and performance anxiety occur in a majority of men with this disorder. Very frequently, they give a past history of strong religious upbringing and/or early sexual encounters in forbidden or illicit settings.

Retarded ejaculation or ejaculatory incompetence is defined as the inability of the erect penis to ejaculate. It has been reported in less than 5% of men, most often in those who are younger and less sexually experienced (Masters and Johnson, 1970). In its mildest form, it may occur only in specific anxiety-provoking situations. It may, however, be severe enough to prevent ejaculation entirely. The physical causes of this disorder are rare, but its occurrence may be related to drugs or neurological disorders. As noted, dry ejaculation, i.e., without seminal fluid, has been reported in people who have taken thioridazine.

Other factors that may be important in the etiology of this symptom are strong religious background with guilt about sexuality, fear of impregnating the partner, and anxiety about contamination. Often, men with this symptom are described as rigid and compulsive.

Female Sexual Dysfunction

There is considerable confusion in the classification of female sexual dysfunctions because of the use of the term *frigidity*. This term has been used to describe a variety of symptoms including the failure to be erotically stimulated, ''sexual anaesthesia,'' and/ or inability to achieve orgasm when the woman is sexually excited. When frigidity is the presenting symptom, specific details are necessary in the history to understand what the patient may define as frigidity.

Inhibited sexual desire is the term used by Kaplan that most closely approximates the more common usage of the term *frigidity* (Kaplan, 1979). Psychologically, the woman experiences an inhibition of sexual desire or arousal. Physiologically, she suffers from an impairment of the vasocongestive part of the cycle so that she does not have sufficient vaginal lubrication or change in vaginal size to facilitate coitus. The symptom is generally intrapsychic or interpersonal in etiology. Kaplan describes intense sexual anxiety and/or hostility toward partners, which may be greater than those in patients with other sexual dysfunctions. Cultural factors and negative attitudes toward men are also important.

Orgasmic dysfunction occurs in a woman who is sexually responsive but does not reach orgasm when aroused. She often reports that she enjoys sexual activity despite the lack of orgasm. Although Kaplan considers this the most frequent female complaint, the actual incidence is difficult to ascertain because of the variability of patient populations from which data are derived and the failure of those evaluating the problem to obtain specific descriptions in order to make the diagnosis (Kaplan, 1974). This problem is unlikely to have an organic basis. Cultural and psychological factors are important determinants of this symptom.

Orgasmic dysfunction often occurs in women with fear or anxiety about loss of control or unrealistic expectations about sexual performance, i.e., if the woman feels that simultaneous orgasm(s) only via coitus constitutes adequate performance, she may believe that she or her partner is inadequate. In these women, anxiety appears to be mobilized at the moment of impending orgasm with resultant involuntary inhibition of the reflex.

Vaginismus is defined as the involuntary spastic contraction of the outer one-third of the vagina, including the vaginal and anal sphincter muscles (Masters and Johnson, 1970). Severe vaginismus may entirely prevent intercourse. The woman may avoid any attempt at coitus because of dyspareunia (pain on intercourse). This problem also may be associated with varying degrees of general sexual inhibition or intrapsychic conflict. A definite diagnosis can only be made on physical exam.

This disorder can be uncomfortable, frightening, and humiliating. The partners of women with this symptom are often angry, frustrated, or even rejecting, because they perceive the symptom as voluntary. Often the partners of these women develop secondary impotence.

Since vaginismus may occur because of vaginal or pelvic pain, organic etiologies must be ruled out. The physical causes include any disorder of pelvic organs that make penile entry painful or difficult. This includes a rigid hymen, endometriosis, pelvic inflammatory disease, tumors, vaginitis, and injuries related to obstetrical trauma. When related to psychological factors, vaginismus can be considered a conditioned response, rather than a hysterical conversion reaction. It may or may not be related to psychopathology, and it may have psychosocial determinants including religious restriction, previous sexual trauma (rape or incest), as well as sexual guilt or fear of pregnancy.

Dyspareunia or pain with sexual intercourse may be physiological or psychological in origin. The physical causes are the same as those described for vaginismus, since vaginismus occurs reflexively if intercourse is painful. It is important to differentiate pain near the vaginal entry, which may be due to vaginitis, lacerations, or an unhealed episiotomy, from pain that is deep in the vagina and may signify pelvic pathology, such as endometriosis, pelvic inflammatory disease, or tumor. Pain may also occur after intercourse due to pelvic congestion or uterine spasm. The psychogenic causes are often similar to those producing vaginismus and may relate to anxiety about sexuality because of unconscious conflict, previous sexual trauma, or fear of injury.

Referral Considerations

For all of these symptoms, therapeutic outcome ultimately depends on understanding etiological factors and assessing the maturation of the individual or couple to engage in therapy to relieve the symptom. The clinician who does not have specific training in sexual therapy and/or psychotherapy will generally be most successful in treating those couples and individuals who most likely to require an educational approach or specific suggestions about technique. Referral to those with specific training or experience in evaluating and treating sexual dysfunction should be considered when the following problems are seen:

1. Clinical depression underlying the sexual complaint
2. Significant past psychiatric history
3. Problems complicated by homosexual conflict or gender confusion, overt or latent
4. Patients who present with marked personality or character disorders
5. Primary sexual dysfunctions
6. Lack of commitment to the relationship by one or both partners
7. Lack of commitment to therapy by one or both partners
8. Significant secrets, such as ongoing infidelities, kept by one partner
9. Major reality concerns, such as family or work problems, at the time therapy is sought
10. Major difficulties in a relationship with a partner

Treatment of Sexual Dysfunctions

There is a great deal of confusion concerning the indications for treatment and the prognosis for different symptoms with different techniques of treatment. In discussing prognosis, one must take into account the population being considered, the type(s) of treatment offered, the adequacy of the evaluation, and the motivation for symptom relief.

Motivation is perhaps the most significant variable in outcome. Specific diagnoses do not necessarily carry specific treatment protocols or prognoses. What is most important is that appropriate treatment is offered by a therapist who is flexible and skilled, so that if a particular treatment approach is ineffective, another can be used.

Since people frequently request treatment for a sexual problem when it is apparent that there are more serious underlying problems or when treatment cannot be successful because of the degree of acrimony in the relationship, it is necessary for the evaluator to be aware of the many causes of sexual symptoms, as well as the resistance to acknowledging that all of the problems of an individual or couple are not sexually related. At times, a trial of treatment may be necessary because the couple insists that specific sexual therapy is indicated, regardless of the outcome of the evaluation. It may be more advantageous to attempt therapy, after discussing reservations about its success, rather than to engage in a struggle that frequently results in cessation of productive therapeutic work and therapy shopping and intensification of underlying problems (Nadelson, 1979).

Although there are a number of ways of treating sexual dysfunctions, we will consider in detail the methods based on the pioneer work of Masters and Johnson (1966, 1970) and modified by Kaplan (1979) and others. We will not describe more traditional forms of individual, couples, and group therapy, since treatment of sexual dysfunctions utilizing these modalities does not differ substantially from treatment for other disorders.

The ''new sex therapy'' is predicated on a relationship between a couple, where both parties will participate in the therapy program. If the problem is that the individual is unable to become involved in a meaningful relationship or if the sexual symptom, e.g., impotence, is so disturbing that the man will not risk the humiliation of failure, individual psychotherapy, group psychotherapy, and/or behavior modification techniques may be helpful. In other situations, the partner cannot or will not be involved in the treatment plan. This may require modification of technique or alternative approaches.

We will begin with a basic conceptualization of the therapeutic rationale and then consider specific interventions. The so-called ''new sex therapies'' involve treatment procedures for specific dysfunctional syndromes not for orientation or gender identity problems. The most successful model of treatment involves a synthesis of theory and procedures from psychodynamic systems and behavioral perspectives. An attempt is made to modify the immediate antecedents of the couple's sexual difficulty, recognizing that deeper roots exist (Kaplan, 1974). Resolution is fostered at a more superficial level in order to achieve symptom relief.

Learning theory principles are brought to bear in the process of identifying the mechanisms by which transactions are maintained and reinforced in order to provide appropriate behavioral modifications. The symptoms are considered the disorder rather than a manifestation of an underlying disorder. The interweaving of some of the perspectives derived from the role theory is also useful in understanding and working with the complex interactions that derive from long-standing role definitions and expectations.

Although these approaches do not initially appear to be consistent with psychodynamic understanding, this latter perspective is essential to keep in mind, because individual as well as system contributions often result in subtle resistances to treatment and limit the effectiveness of a primarily behavioral approach. In addition, it has become apparent from clinical work that only a limited number of people can be treated with a specific behavioral approach.

Kaplan has proposed a psychodynamically based model of sex therapy that utilizes behavior modification and other aspects of nondynamically oriented therapies by a therapist who has a psychodynamic understanding of developmental issues and clinical experiences in this area. The presenting problem can be viewed from a transactional perspective. Thus, the relationship, not each individual, is seen as the problem, and the treatment involves the clarification and resolution, as far as possible, of the reciprocal dynamics of the disorder. The analogy that most clearly captures the concept is the treatment of a highly contagious disease, which is only effective if all family members are treated, not the single individual with the infection. Thus, both partners must be evaluated with regard to motivation for therapy, ego resources, coping mechanisms, and psychopathology.

If one of the partners cannot tolerate change and responds with anger, withdrawal, or extreme demands, treatment by a more directive, behaviorally oriented approach will not succeed. In this situation, anxiety may become very intense, and, since performance anxiety is a major feature of all sexual dysfunctions, it must be reduced for treatment to be effective. The intensification of performance anxiety is counterproductive to the goals and process of therapy.

Because the treatment approach described requires that both partners participate, recommendations for treating individuals who are not involved in a relationship or those whose partners do not wish to be included differ. In those situations, as noted earlier, individual psychotherapy or group therapy is recommended. At times, behavior modification techniques may also be employed for individuals.

One must remember that the goals of the new sex therapy are more limited in scope than those of traditional psychotherapy or psychoanalysis. The attempt is to relieve dysfunctional symptoms rather than effect personality change or marital harmony. Kaplan and others report that individuals and couples frequently seek psychotherapy after successful sexual therapy, because other conflicts often emerge and continue to be troublesome even after they have been treated.

In any form of sexual therapy, the goal is to enable people to abandon themselves to their sexual feelings and to free themselves of conscious control. The new sex therapies are directed toward discovering and modifying the specific, immediately operating obstacles to such sexual abandon, regardless of the underlying causes of the sexual dysfunction. The therapist must attempt to foster a sense of security in sexual functioning, facilitate trust in the partner, and relieve excessive judgment, criticism, and anxiety about performance. Guilt must be allayed, and restrictive attitudes and other barriers must be removed. Since the treatment itself involves placing the patient in an anxiety-producing situation, the therapist must be able to help patients tolerate this discomfort and foster the kind of trust that will enable treatment to progress.

The plan requires that the therapist assume a more authoritative position in the treatment in order to prevent conflict between the partners about who is in charge. The therapist must facilitate progress toward the goal of recognizing that each partner must assume responsibility for his/her own feelings and behaviors and not those of the partner. Partners are encouraged to communicate what they each feel and to respect their individual differences. Thus, a husband who is angry with his wife for being too demanding, and blames his impotence on her behavior, may begin to see that she may not be as demanding as he perceives her to be, and, instead of being provocative or withdrawing, he may be encouraged to understand his contribution to the interaction. He hopefully will be able to come to see her as his friend, who has her own style and manner, but who is not an adversary. Although it may be possible to treat a couple without extensive exploration of unconscious issues, these factors must be recognized as contributing to the problem. The couple may be able to learn to understand and appreciate each other's past history and reexplore their relationship in the context of empathy rather than demand and expectation.

There are several basic principles involved in this approach to the treatment of sexual dysfunction:

1. The responsibility for treatment is shared by both partners, regardless of the specific etiology of the disorder. Thus, one cannot place blame or focus specifically on one partner. A husband cannot blame his wife for his premature ejaculation, nor can a wife state that she does not have orgasms because her husband intimidates her. One partner is not seen as "at fault" and, therefore, the "sick" one who should be treated. Both partners are expected to participate in the treatment. They are encouraged to see the solution as a mutual effort, regardless of the original etiology.

2. The therapist provides an atmosphere of acceptance of sexuality and permission for sexual enjoyment and validates the symptom by treating it as a problem and offering help.

3. The partners are encouraged to view sexual activity as a way of relaxing and sharing, not as a "performance" that occurs only at defined times and places. Emphasis is placed on enjoyment of sensuality without requiring a culmination in orgasm for each sexual encounter. Pressure to perform repeatedly is, thus, minimized.

4. There is an emphasis on verbal and physical communication. Partners are encouraged to understand and accept each other's values, preferences, and differences as normal. The communication of motives to the other partner is interdicted. Thus, a partner cannot say "you are rejecting me" but rather "I feel that I am being rejected." This enables them to explore their feelings openly, and it prevents mutual accusation.

There are two areas that have evoked considerable discussion and disagreement among those who define themselves as sex therapists. These are the concepts of a specific time limit and the use of cotherapists. Theoretically, setting a time limit optimizes the pressure to progress and prevents the evolution of a pattern of prolonged resistance. The temptation to become involved in more complex dynamic issues is also limited by this approach. On occasion, more extensive uncovering work may prove to be counterproductive to the goal of producing behavioral change, because it may take a prolonged period of time for a result to be obtained or it may enable the couple to avoid change by talking without acting. On the other hand, a time limit may increase the sense of performance pressure, and a less intensive approach may fail, because it is too superficial to tackle the underlying determinants of the problem. Perhaps what is most important is to reevaluate progress during the course of treatment in order to make necessary modifications in technique.

The indications for conjoint or cotherapy with a male–female therapy team has been a much debated issue. Masters and Johnson (1970) have emphasized the importance of cotherapists, believing that the support of a partner of the same sex is necessary. They also feel that this team approach decreases the intensity of the transference. Others believe that the opposite occurs and that a male–female team intensifies parental transference responses. Kaplan's experience is that mixed-gender cotherapists are not essential to the success of treatment. She states that "when a therapist is sensitive, well trained, and experienced, and when he or she is specifically sensitized to the erotic responses and reactions of the opposite gender, then he or she can effectively conduct sex therapy on a solo basis" (Kaplan, 1974, p. 239). Further, an experienced therapist of either sex is suitable provided that the therapist is well trained in both traditional therapies and in direct sex therapy.

At times, patients express preferences about the sex of the therapist or the use of cotherapists. In the author's experience, the major indication for making a choice on the basis of the sex of the therapist or any other characteristic is the feeling on the part of one or both partners that they cannot work with a specific therapist. It may be helpful to have cotherapists when one of the partners demonstrates more extensive psychopathology, the modification of treatment may take the form of individual meetings, or a partner has a strong preference and may not become engaged in therapy if this request is not respected. Another indication relates to the experience of the therapist. A less experienced therapist is more likely to fail to notice nonverbal interactions or consider alternative ways of understanding or interpreting material. A cotherapist, particularly one who is more experienced, may offer an important opportunity for developing perspective, comfort, and skill. Furthermore, the ability of the therapy team to work together and resolve differences is a useful model for a couple in treatment.

Among the problems that arise with the use of cotherapists involves the choice of who the members of the cotherapy team are. If the therapy team contains partners who differ in strength and ability, they may compete rather than complement each other, or they may inadvertently provide a model that reinforces the problem of the couple. In addition, reality factors, like cost and scheduling, must also be considered.

The practice of using surrogates as therapists has evoked considerable controversy, especially because of the ethical implications of this practice. Further, the efficacy of this form of treatment is questionable, since it does not deal with the context of the relationship and the individual involved may be unable to translate this interaction to an ongoing relationship. The individual who has serious interpersonal or intrapsychic problems may also be unduly stressed when a surrogate is provided.

The Treatment Program

As with many clinical problems, there are, at times, differences of opinion between the clinician and the patient about the etiology of the problem, the goals and methods of treatment, and expectations of therapy. Thus, concerns about whether the disorder is organic or functional and who is "at fault" are frequent. At times, goals differ, and it may be difficult to come to an agreement between partners or between therapist(s) and patient(s). A couple with long-standing marital problems may present with a specific sexual symptom, hoping, even unconsiously, that the therapist will "cure" the marital problem. The therapist must clarify what seems reasonable and realistic. This includes alternative treatment approaches. A discussion of alternatives may facilitate the development of trust and build an alliance. This can potentially improve the chances of success for therapy. Often, a lack of motivation, differences in priorities, or unwillingness to pursue certain suggestions emerge as resistances. These should be clarified early. A discussion of goals, expectations, and techniques, as well as a sharing of information and answering direct questions, will reinforce confidence in the therapist and the therapy and diminish some of the resistances that interfere with progress during the course of therapy.

The basic therapy format proposed by Masters and Johnson involves 2 weeks away from home and work, devoted totally to the treatment. Although they report great therapeutic success, this approach cannot easily be generalized to outpatient clinics or to most private-practice situations. It is expensive and time-consuming for both patients and therapists. Masters and Johnson are also very careful in screening patients and require referrals from therapists or counsellors, as well as other data, which make it less likely that those with serious psychopathology or questionable motivation will commit themselves to this treatment plan.

Thus, not everyone with a sexual problem can benefit from this approach. The preselection factor may account in part for the success reported by Masters and Johnson, as well as other "sex" therapists who treat selective populations. The same results may not be generalizable. It is important then to be cautious about interpretation of results until data on comparable populations are available.

The treatment of specific sexual dysfunction symptoms have common features. These include:

1. An initial period of coital abstinence to reduce performance anxiety and facilitate communication
2. A focus on the substitution of giving and receiving pleasure for the exclusive goal of orgasm, which involves systematic tactile stimulation and exploration in "sensate focus" exercises
3. Sequencing and varying sexual techniques, which facilitates and reinforces success
4. Specific suggestions and directions that meet the needs of the couple, i.e., nondemand coital position for a nonorgasmic female or squeeze technique for the man with premature ejaculation (see p. 43)

In order to clarify the way in which the treatment proceeds, a sample program will provide a guideline. Modifications can be made depending upon the circumstances. Adaptations to the approach and style of the therapist and the couple are often necessary.

Session 1: Interview of each partner by the therapist(s). During this time, in addition to the specifics of the history, important impressions are gained about individual attitudes and values, the quality of interpersonal relationships, ego strengths, and the commitment to the relationship.

If a cotherapy team is used, both the same- and opposite-sexed therapists meet with the partners individually. Discrepancies in history or impressions, as well as differences in the way each partner relates to each therapist, can be assessed.

In addition, the treatment process can be explained, and expectations can be discussed. Guidelines can be clarified about the use of confidential material from each partner, e.g., if there are "secrets," such as one partner having an affair, some clarification of how that is to be handled is necessary. Some therapists insist on disclosure, others are willing to proceed without disclosure. Clinically, if one partner is involved in a sexual affair, it is less likely that he/she is as committed to therapy as is the other partner. In addition, that person is often less available and cooperative, thus, diminishing his/her participation and the chances of success. From an interactional perspective, the secret shared with the therapist(s) creates an imbalance in the therapeutic situation and allows one partner to have a special relationship with the therapist(s).

Session 2: The couple is seen together. In this session, the therapist(s) has the opportunity to observe how the couple interacts with each other and to assess the level of communication, as well as the response to the therapist(s). Questions are answered, and plans are negotiated. This meeting is extremely important in its impact on the course of the therapy. A therapeutic alliance can develop during this time.

During this session, the therapist may recapitulate the history and formulate the etiology with the couple. The therapist must emphasize dual responsibility in making changes and also reinforce the necessity to refrain from mutual blame. The focus of the therapy is on problem solving. This involves the avoidance of predictions or global statements, like "you always" or "I never." The couple begins to work toward understanding and accepting the differences between them.

A frequent problem, usually apparent very early in the evaluation, is that partners tend to deal with each other by using accusations, like "you don't love me" or "you are rejecting me," instead of recognizing that these are statements of perception or interpretation. The therapist should encourage the use of statements that claim responsibility for feelings. Thus, "I feel unloved" or "I feel rejected" is used. In addition, each partner must communicate wishes and preferences directly and not expect that the partner will know or understand automatically. This is an area where couples frequently have difficulty. One often hears a partner exclaim, "Why should I tell him/her what to do, he/she should know what I like by now."

In this session, the couple generally is also asked to refrain from coitus until the therapist tells them to resume. The primary reason for this is to reduce performance anxiety. This relieves the partners from the responsibility of handling the anxiety generated when they are expected to perform sexually. It also enables the therapist to direct the course of the therapy and make appropriate interventions.

Transference responses are clearly elicited although not necessarily explicitly interpreted. On occasion, however, it is useful to clarify the nature of the transference. For example, in one therapy situation, a young man with premature ejaculation, who had always had difficulty in relationships with authority figures, became angry with the therapist for making a demand. When the transference aspects were pointed out, his partner expressed relief at being able to understand some of his "irrational" responses, and he began to be able to work more effectively in treatment.

The *sensate focus exercise* is explained during this meeting. It begins with an emphasis on nonverbal and then on verbal communication. The couple is encouraged to find a mutually agreed upon time and place to focus on their sexual interaction without distraction. This is surprisingly difficult for many people who may have used interferences, such as the telephone and lack of privacy, to sustain a particular kind of interaction. They may be uncomfortable about changing their patterns of behavior. They may be asked to go away for a weekend or a few days to facilitate their engagement in the treatment process, if there are unalterable distractions at home.

They are encouraged to spend time together, every night if possible, and to talk, engage in nongenital stimulation, and verbalize about how they experience the stimulation and what preferences they have. Both partners are asked to remove clothing and to take turns touching and fondling each other only for pleasure, not to achieve orgasm. Either may stop by saying, "I would like to stop," rather than phrasing the remark in a defensive or adversarial fashion, like "Have you had enough?" They are instructed not to press anything that is physically or psychologically uncomfortable for the partner.

Most couples report that this time together is remarkably revealing and gratifying. They may never have engaged in activity of this kind, and they usually report being surprised and delighted by the improvement in communication and the reinforcement of positive feelings toward each other.

Session 3: At the next conjoint session, each partner is asked to talk about the experiences and feelings evoked since the time of the previous meeting. The ability to give and receive pleasure is stressed, as well as the development of increasing comfort with body feelings. When the couple have not done the exercises or when they report some discomfort or difficulty, this is explored.

With this therapeutic technique, resistances to treatment can be major problems. Most often they present as complaints about the availability of time to do the exercises, anger at the partner or therapist, or attempts to sabotage the treatment by withdrawing, somatizing, or developing other symptoms. Complaints that the exercises are mechanical are also frequent. Since resistances appear when anxiety is aroused, the firm support of the therapist is important. The period when resistance is great may represent a critical turning point in treatment. The couple must sustain their work together despite the anxiety generated when they are faced with giving up a symptom. An exploration of the resistances is often helpful. At times, deeper problems are uncovered which may require some therapeutic modification or referral for other treatment modalities.

Subsequent Sessions

As therapy progresses, the therapist makes additional suggestions. Breast and genital stimulation are added, and the couple is encouraged to find verbal and/or nonverbal ways of communicating preferences or responses. They are repeatedly encouraged to consider the comments of their partner as suggestions and not as criticism or demands.

In subsequent sessions the partners continue physical and verbal exploration and communication. They are instructed in a variety of nondemand sexual activities, and then they progress toward coitus. Alternative positions and techniques are suggested. Often couples have not previously felt free to explore these techniques. As resistances emerge, they are dealt with. Rest periods are sometimes suggested to diminish the sense of pressure and/or to heighten sexual tension.

Often obsessive thoughts, particularly about success or failure, distract people. They may "spectator" (maintain control over reactions by continually being aware of and observing them) in order to diminish anxiety. This may become a major resistance, and it is actively discouraged. A sense of humor on the part of the therapist may help.

One expression of this problem is an overconcern with the feelings of the partner. People will worry about how much their partner is enjoying the sexual activity or what he/she thinks of the chances of success or failure. It is important to reinforce the need for the person to open up his/her own awareness and allow him/herself to feel entitled to the time when he/she is pleasured. For some people, taking turns at sexual pleasuring must be specifically permitted and even required in order to begin to relieve anxiety and permit more opened sexual expression.

During the course of the therapy couples often "cheat," i.e., attempt intercourse when it is not permitted. Frequently their attempts are successful, and they achieve coitus. This proves to be a reinforcing experience and can facilitate future success. These attempts at intercourse, even when not specifically permitted, are often good prognostic signs, since those couples who tend to be flexible, defiant, motivated, and able to follow through on suggestions are most likely to cheat.

A brief description of some of the specific treatment issues for the disorders discussed earlier follows. It is important to note that although the attempt is to make this therapy short term and focused, it may not be possible to define the specific number of sessions that will be required. Generally, from 8 to 20 sessions are reported to be necessary. This figure varies because of the many other issues that often emerge when this approach is attempted.

Male Dysfunctions

Erectile Dysfunction

The basic premise of the therapy for this disorder is that anxiety disrupts the erectile response. The objective of the treatment is to diminish this anxiety sufficiently to prevent the symptom from appearing. The patient must be confident enough to be willing to attempt coitus. Since a successful coital experience is highly reinforcing, the treatment aims at enhancing the chances of success.

The treatment begins with a period of ejaculatory abstinence, during which time there is erotic stimulation but no pressure to perform. Erectile confidence gradually builds as the therapist and partner remain sensitive to the appearance of impediments to progress. Because there is no specific strategy or procedure with proven effectiveness, there is considerable variability in the technique that produces a successful outcome. The basic format includes a focus on pleasuring without demand for the first four to eight sessions. Coitus and ejaculation are generally prohibited, and the couple explores a variety of stimulation techniques, first nongenital and then genital. The emphasis is on enjoyment, and the presence or absence of an erection is deemphasized.

It is often important for the man to become comfortable with the idea that erections come and go and are not reflections of his ''masculinity.'' Some authors recommend the squeeze technique (see Premature Ejaculation) to reinforce the idea that waxing and waning of an erection is normal and that if an erection is lost, it can return later.

Generally after several sessions, enough confidence is restored so that the couple can resume coitus. This is a difficult time requiring individual modifications of instructions. A change from a usual position for intercourse may also be helpful. The woman may be encouraged to attempt to take a more active role and to take the female superior position. She may gently move onto the man's penis, withdraw, and attempt to repeat this pattern, while the man attempts to prevent ejaculation. Vaginal containment can, thus, lose its demand quality.

There are couples who have difficulty changing patterns or positions. Pressure imposed by the therapist to do this may be destructive. If it is not counter to the values of the individual or the couple, it may be helpful to support the ''normality'' of fantasy. It is important to remember, however, that although it is helpful to encourage fantasy, it is not helpful if it induces guilt or anxiety.

Another problem can arise when the female partner feels ''there is nothing in it for me.'' She may react negatively and even undermine the treatment. It is important for the therapist to understand the difficulty she faces in taking an active role, often without gratification, for a long period of time.

Couples frequently raise questions about the efficacy of using testosterone to increase libido and performance. Results with this treatment are variable and difficult to document. Positive results using hormones may be as much related to the pharmacologic effect of the drugs as to the psychological effect of enhanced confidence resulting from pharmacologically increased libido. Many authors recommend the use of testosterone to enhance treatment results particularly when there is a demonstrated deficiency, but they do not recommend its exclusive use or use when no deficiency exists (Kolodny et al., 1979).

Premature Ejaculation

The treatment of premature ejaculation is based on the assumption that it is possible to exert conscious control over ejaculation and that the man can learn to prolong continence even when sexually aroused, without having to control or diminish the experience of orgasm. This is in contrast to the commonly accepted view that the symptom occurs because of rapidity of the reflex and that it cannot be controlled. The main components of the treatment involve facilitating communication between the partners and increasing the ability of the man to perceive impending orgasm. Frequently, men with this problem have sought and tried a variety of means of cure. They may have been encouraged to ''think of something else'' or to use local anesthetics. When these methods do not solve the problem and, in fact, complicate it by increasing the disappointment and performance anxiety, they may seek treatment although they are often pessimistic about the possibility of cure.

Sensate focus exercises, as described earlier, may or may not be employed in the treatment of this disorder. The most frequently used treatment technique is the Semans' squeeze technique or a modification of it. The couple is instructed to engage in foreplay to the extent that the man has an erection. He is asked to focus on his erotic sensations in contrast to his previous therapeutic attempts where distraction was encouraged. He is asked to identify the sensation just prior to orgasm, before the state of ejaculatory inevitability, and to let his partner know when this occurs. The partner may then either use the squeeze technique or merely cease activity and refrain from stimulating him.

The squeeze technique involves squeezing the penis just below the glans with the thumb on one side and forefinger or second and third fingers on the opposite side (dorsal and ventral) with sufficient force to cause the erection to diminish and the sense of inevitability to decrease. This technique obviously requires communication and cooperation between the partners. In addition, the man must refrain from focusing on controlling himself, since that would defeat the purpose of the exercise.

This exercise can be repeated several times before ejaculation or intercourse is attempted. When the couple attempts coitus, it is best done in the female superior position so that it is possible for coitus to be interrupted more easily and the squeeze used. The man is asked to signal for the woman to stop thrusting or moving prior to ejaculatory inevitability, in the same way as described earlier. Some couples prefer withdrawal of the penis and use of the squeeze technique, others prefer cessation of thrusting activity. Although other intercourse positions may also be successful, it is important to remember that control is more difficult to attain in the male superior position. The couple is generally instructed to repeat these exercises periodically after they have formally terminated treatment and to use the techniques they have learned if symptoms reappear.

One problem worth emphasizing involves the active participation of the woman. This may be difficult for some couples, since sexual activity in the female may not be consistent with their values or previous adaptation. Therapy with this kind of couple may be more difficult. On the other hand, the maintenance of this attitude can also be used as a resistance to treatment.

Female Dysfunctions

Sexual Unresponsiveness ("Frigidity")

The goal of therapy is to create an undemanding, relaxed, and sensuous environment in which comfortable and mutually gratifying sexual interaction can take place, if the relationship is a good one. Thus, the sensate focus exercise is a critical component. The permission and encouragement provided by this exercise may produce dramatic effects particularly if there is no specific coital demand. It is important that treatment proceed slowly so that the woman can experience her own sexual feelings rather than perform as she feels is expected. She is encouraged to be more active in her participation.

If the exercises are too stimulating for the man, who must control his need for coital gratification, he may be brought to orgasm by means other than coitus. During this treatment program, coitus may be encouraged initially even if there is no vaginal sensation. Slow, nondemanding thrusting under the woman's control, with her in the superior position, can often be extremely effective in increasing her sensitivity. Rest periods during which time no sexual activity occurs are effective in heightening excitation and diminishing performance pressure. It is important for the woman to feel that she can maintain control of the situation.

A variety of other coital positions may also be suggested, and the couple should be encouraged to try on their own. This is often more effective than prescribing specific techniques, since they may not be comfortable or acceptable to a couple.

The resistances that frequently emerge include negative reactions to the feelings that are experienced and disbelief that there will be any positive effect of treatment. In addition, uncomfortable sensations in the most highly erogenous areas may occur either because of anxiety or the partner is too rough or direct in his stimulation. When obsessive thoughts occur, as they frequently do, it is necessary to refocus on sensual feelings.

Orgasmic Dysfunction

The basic goal of treatment for this symptom is to facilitate the patient's ability to learn how to release an overcontrolled response. This involves maximizing clitoral stimulation, while at the same time diminishing those factors that may inhibit orgasm.

Since masturbation may produce orgasm in women with this symptom, whereas coitus does not, the maximization of stimulation may initially involve teaching the woman to bring herself to orgasm through masturbation, without a partner. If she can accept this practice, she can be taught manual clitoral stimulation. At times, a vibrator is useful. Some practice in contracting her pubococcygeus muscles may also be helpful. She may also practice coital thrusting. Fantasies are encouraged, and she may be reassured that they are not "sick," regardless of the content. Treatment may then proceed to involve the partner, first in noncoital stimulation, and then progressing to coitus.

The use of the bridge technique may help to increase sexual stimulation. This technique involves manual stimulation of the clitoris while coitus is taking place. This is followed by intercourse in a position that provides maximal clitoral stimulation. The female superior position is recommended since it facilitates active thrusting and control by the woman. Clitoral stimulation may cease as the woman nears orgasm. Self-stimulation may at times also be effective.

For those women who are primarily anorgasmic, the major objective is to achieve the first orgasm. This dispels the woman's fear that she is incapable of orgasm. Treatment proceeds on the premise that the reflex has been inhibited, not destroyed, in these women. According to Kaplan (1974), approximately 8% of women are anorgasmic by any means for unknown reasons. If orgasmic inhibition has significant unconscious determinants, psychotherapy is indicated. In the context of direct sexual treatment, however, the therapist may help to foster a conscious awareness of the fear and anxiety that exists and attempt to allay them by providing support, information, and positive reinforcement. At times, a patient will be anxious about being able to transfer what is experienced in a masturbatory situation to a sexual experience with a partner. It is possible to facilitate this transfer with the cooperation and support of the partner.

Vaginismus

The successful treatment of this disorder most often utilizes behavioral techniques aimed at modifying a conditioned response. It involves progressive deconditioning of the involuntary spasm of the muscles around the vagina. Before this can be done, the patient's phobic avoidance of vaginal entry must be alleviated. Often these patients present with a history of difficulty with self-exploration or the use of tampons.

Frequently the woman can begin her self-exploration in the gynecologist's office with a gentle pelvic exam and the use of graduated-sized dilators. The partner's presence may facilitate or inhibit progress so that the therapist must make a clinical judgment about whether to involve the partner. Behavioral approaches specifically aimed at extinction of frightening fantasies may be effective in desensitization.

The objective is to reduce the patient's anxiety about penetration sufficiently to enable her to proceed. Continued encouragement and support, particularly by the partner, are of primary importance. This may be difficult if the partner is angry or feels rejected. The most important part of the treatment is to encourage the patient to stay with it. Psychotherapy in conjunction with sexual therapy may facilitate progress.

Treatment Follow-up

The fact that the new sex therapies are of relatively recent origin, coupled with the variability of the patient population, with regard to individual and couple dynamics, symptoms, and motivation make long-range projections and long-term follow-up data difficult to obtain. It is clear, however, that follow-up visits are necessary and that referral for couples or individual therapy is often indicated. The purpose may be to consolidate gains or because the therapy has uncovered other issues that have prevented successful resolution of the presenting problem.

Treatment failures occur most often when the evaluation has not been careful enough to eliminate those patients for whom this modality is inappropriate, most often because they are not sufficiently motivated or they are ambivalent about treatment. Even serious psychopathology, while making treatment difficult, does not preclude sexual therapy, especially if the partner is supportive and committed to the success of the therapy. Among the most important results is the improvement of couple communication and the quality of the relationship beyond the sexual sphere.

References

Kaplan, H. S. *The new sex therapy*. New York: Quadrangle/Brunner/Mazel, 1974.

Kaplan, H. S. *Disorders of sexual desire*. New York: Brunner/Mazel, 1979.

Kolodny, R. C., Masters, W. H., and Johnson, V. E. *Textbook of sexual medicine*. Boston: Little, Brown, 1979.

Masters, W. H., and Johnson, V. E. *Human sexual response*. Boston: Little, Brown, 1966.

Masters, W. H., and Johnson, V. E. *Human sexual inadequacy*. Boston: Little, Brown, 1970.

Nadelson, C. Treatment of sexual dysfunction. In A. Lazare (Ed.), *Outpatient psychiatry*. Baltimore, Md. Williams & Wilkins, 1979.

Sexual Concerns of Childhood

James W. Maddock

Introduction

Children enter the world as sexed beings. Prenatal processes have established the basis for a gender identity (in most cases) as well as the capacity for erotically stimulating interaction with the environment. From the moment of birth, significant persons in the infant's environment respond to the individual as a male or female. An elaborate psychosocial network forms that supports the perceived biological sex of the child. This network will provide more or less flexible choices of role-related behaviors as the child grows and struggles to develop a coherent, socially acceptable, but personally unique, sexual identity (Money and Erhardt, 1972). Numerous complexities and challenges lie along the road toward adult sexual identity. This chapter will focus primarily on erotic aspects of childhood socialization, whereas later chapters (4 and 5) will examine the pitfalls and problems of gender identity formation and sex-role socialization.

The child is born with a preprogrammed capacity for "sexual" response. Of course, sex does not have the same meaning for the infant as for the adult. Only gradually through childhood and adolescence does the developing individual learn the sexual "scripts" that are required to function effectively as an adult in his or her culture. Nevertheless, the child's sensory apparatus can experience the world in what are apparently erotic ways and can respond to this sensory stimulation with signs of physical tension increase (arousal) and discharge (orgasm). Recent studies of sexual physiology point to the possibility that a regular rhythmic ebb and flow of sexual tension may occur in the human organism from birth to death—a rhythm whose periodicity is greatest in the earlier years of life and lessens gradually, though not uniformly, through the life cycle (Gadpaille, 1975). Any reasonably observant parent of a male infant will notice frequent erections when the child is unclothed—as well as

James W. Maddock • Meta Resources, P. A., and Department of Family Social Science and School of Public Health, University of Minnesota, St. Paul, Minnesota.

the disconcerting ability, later lost, to urinate through an erect penis! Preliminary data suggest that females may experience genital vasocongestion—the analog of male erection—on a regular, periodic basis as well (Cohen and Shapiro, 1970; Abel, Murphy, Becker, & Bitar, 1979). Future research may demonstrate these phenomena conclusively and, thus, define the biological bases of sexual functioning. Against this background, it is easier to appreciate the potentially rich eroticism of infancy and childhood.

An equally important factor in determining childhood eroticism is the heavy reliance of the individual on kinesthetic experience during the early period of life. A child has learned much about his or her world before acquiring the capacity to interpret or to reproduce language. This nonverbal interaction with the environment serves as the basis for much of later personality development and adult modes of being. Thus, normal touching and body contact are the precursors of adult sexual relationships and, probably, of other forms of social interaction as well (Prescott, 1975).

Psychosexual development is a process of shaping and channeling—according to cultural norms, social values, familial expectations, and other influences—the natural erotic response potential of the human organism. The behavior of parents and other significant adults impacts upon the child's conscious and unconscious experience to help form his or her sexuality. All parents, then—as well as other important adults, such as the clinician—are inevitably "sex educators." This chapter will focus on ways in which a clinician can serve as a helpful resource for the sexual concerns and problems of children and their parents.

Parents' Sexual Concerns about Their Children

Gender Concerns

Probably the earliest sex-related problem to come to the attention of the clinician is the recognition of a physical manifestation of gender ambiguity or fear on the part of parents that such ambiguity may exist when they confront a malformation of the genitals. It is important that a clinician be sensitive to the implications of genital anomalies, even when such anomalies are clinically insignificant and easily correctable. Uncorrected genital malformations may have a significant impact upon an individual's life in childhood and/or adulthood in such a way as to strongly influence the process of gender identity formation (Chapter 6). Here, I only wish to emphasize the importance of dealing directly and thoroughly with parental concerns about genital malformation or ambiguity, since parents' conscious and unconscious attitudes toward their children's physical appearance and gender characteristics are enormously powerful in determining the outcome of those children's psychosexual development (Gadpaille, 1975). The clinician can do much to provide reassurance and accurate information that will encourage parents to be confident and comfortable rather than worried and uncertain.

Genital Health

Numerous parents bring their infants or young children to a clinician with concerns about minor genital or pelvic problems. One parent may notice the slight vaginal discharge common to newborn females. Another may be concerned about the appearance of the foreskin or glans following circumcision. Others may notice genital rashes, scabs, cuts, or abrasions and become unduly worried based upon their belief that this area of the body is extremely fragile and, therefore, subject to greater damage than other body parts. Most parents who demonstrate this concern will deny any recognition of its sexual implications. This is consistent with their tendency to desexualize their children with whom they so often have intense emotional and physical contact.

On the other hand, the clinician must remain alert to genuine inflammations, injuries, or other genital problems in those infants or young children whose parents deny their children's sexuality. Based upon unconscious taboos or their own feelings of shame and disgust, some parents may neglect appropriate genital hygiene in their children or fail to attend to diseases or injuries, some of which may be of significance. Here, the clinician and psychiatric consultant have a responsibility not only to note and treat the problem but also to encourage the parents to become more comfortable with and pay greater attention to appropriate genital hygiene for their children (such intervention may well be making an indirect contribution to the adults' *own* genital health and hygiene in this way!).

Cases

A young mother of an infant boy made three trips to the clinic in as many weeks, concerned about the appearance of the infant's foreskin and the purplish color of the coronal ridge of the penis. The medical staff took great pains to reassure her that the infant's genitals were normal. Staff consultation with a psychiatrist helped to focus on the sexual concerns of the mother. At a subsequent consultation, it was discovered that the mother had been raised in a family of all girls and had never before looked closely at a male's penis, including that of her husband.

Another mother brought to the clinic her 8-month-old daughter with severe, foul-smelling ulcerations of the inner labia, combined with unexplained chronic vaginal discharge. A careful problem history, focusing on the mother's attitudes, revealed that the mother could not tolerate touching her daughter's genitals or her feces. As a result, the girl's diapers were changed without cleaning except on those occasions when her grandmother was visiting (approximately every 2 weeks). Antibiotic therapy brought swift recovery of the daughter, and the mother was taught to carefully clean the perineum with disposable wash cloths at every diaper change. Discussion with clinic staff encouraged her to feel more comfortable with genital concerns and hygiene. Follow-up visits were scheduled for positive reinforcement of the mother and checking on results.

Toilet training is a natural occasion for attention to the genitals of children, and its practices can have a significant impact on their later sexual development. There is no single "right" way to raise children; different styles of parenting yield different results, and satisfaction with these results is relative to personal and cultural values. Toilet training practices in America seem to alternate between demanding and lenient, and there are almost as many theories of training as there are theories of child development. From the standpoint of psychosexual development, shaming should be avoided in the toilet training process (Kaufman, 1974). *Shaming* here refers to the identification of the genitals, the anus, or the body's waste products as a source of embarrassment or disgust. During the first 2 or 3 years of life, children do not have clear-cut boundaries between themselves and their worlds. They quickly identify themselves with their body products and with parts of their body that produce intense feelings—both pleasant and unpleasant. Therefore, they are likely to experience the negative reactions of adults to their excretory behavior as commentary on their still highly unstable sense of self. Rather than developing a rigid theory of toilet training, the clinician can make his/her greatest contribution by helping parents utilize techniques that promote good feelings in children about their bodies and separate the successes or failures of the children's behavior during the training process from their overall sense of value as persons.

Self-Exploration and Masturbation

Prior to the establishment of an effective language system, children's interaction with the world occurs largely through physical channels. It has been well documented by animal and human research that motion and physical touch are powerful determinants of both physical and psychological well-being. Positive, i.e., pleasurable, forms of physical contact between growing children and others in their environments make important contributions to healthy personality development (Harlow, 1974). Infant animals not touched, rocked, held, and comforted have lessened capacity for appropriate social and sexual interaction as adults. Recently, some researchers have suggested that cultural evidence links pleasurable body experiences in childhood to loving, cooperative behavior in adulthood, whereas deprivation of body pleasure in children and youth is a precursor to increased aggressiveness in adulthood (Prescott, 1975).

Outside of the family unit, the clinician is virtually unique in having social sanction to touch both children and adults in intimate places and in intimate ways. Therefore, he or she should be both an advocate and a model for the importance of touch as part of healthy child development. Just as the "laying on of hands" has particular significance for healing, so also does it have unique power in the process of effective parenting. It is virtually impossible to touch children too much—although it is certainly possible to touch children in inappropriate ways and for inappropriate reasons (Chapter 8). At every opportunity, parents should be assured that a positive climate of physical affection is an important contributor to family life.

Curiosity about the body and the urge to touch it for both exploratory and self-pleasuring reasons appear to be a relatively universal characteristic of children. Nevertheless, parents are often concerned about the self-explorations of their children. There are some parents who respond negatively even to the casual genital fingering of their infant children. Their responses may include verbal rebuke or physical punishment. Neither of these responses is appropriate. They set the stage for a generalized sense of shame in the children (and later in adults) about their bodies. Parents should be encouraged to view their children's casual self-explorations at any age as a healthy attempt to learn more about life and the nature of physical experience. Many adult women—and some adult men—have indicated that they know little or nothing about the parts of their body "down there." This promotes feelings of anxiety and guilt in relation to normal physiological processes, such as menstruation, and also in relation to sexual activity. In summary, there is no evidence that ordinary physical exploration of one's body throughout childhood leads to anything other than a greater degree of body comfort, more accurate information about anatomy and physiology, and a greater degree of self-confidence (Barbach, 1975).

Parents who are generally quite tolerant of their children's casual self-exploration will occasionally bring to the clinician concerns about what appear to be compulsive masturbation practices in children of toddler, preschool, or even elementary school age. In my experience, these concerns are more often raised about girls than about boys. Whether this reflects a greater incidence of the behavior among girls or simply greater parental disapproval of girls' sexually focused behaviors, I do not know. It might also be related to the somewhat greater frequency of minor genital or urinary tract infections among girls due to carelessness or hygienic irregularities. Some of the stories that parents tell clinicians may initially sound quite bizarre.

Cases

One mother of a 4-year-old girl reported that her daughter would not go to bed at naptime or at night without placing a rag doll between her legs and rocking rhythmically back and forth on it for 15 to 30 min before falling asleep. She had already worn out several rag dolls of a certain type in this manner, and the mother was concerned as to whether to keep replacing the dolls or to force the child to learn to fall asleep without the benefit of this apparently self-comforting activity. No objects other than this particular kind of rag doll were satisfactory to the girl, and she had screamed and carried on for several hours on those few occasions when the rag doll was not available or when her mother withheld it from her.

In another situation, the mother of a 2-year-old daughter was quite concerned that the daughter would frequently place her genitals up against a pillow, a blanket, or other object in her crib and rhythmically rock her pelvis back and forth until she became very wide-eyed, red in the face, and covered with perspiration—after which she would finally fall asleep in a seemingly exhausted condition.

These circumstances are harder to generalize than those concerning casual self-exploration. Any genuinely "compulsive" behavior can be or become a problem for children, whether or not it is sexually focused. Compulsive behaviors are frequently symptoms of unresolved tension or stress. However, the clinician interviewing the parent should be sure to listen carefully to the parents' accounts in an effort to identify whether the behavior in question is *genuinely* compulsive or simply repetitive (habitual) in nature. For some children, mild genital stimulation in connection with relaxation time or sleep is self-comforting behavior parallel to thumb sucking, hair twisting, or blanket nuzzling. It is simply a form of physical security that will be given up when it is no longer needed and/or appropriate. Parental efforts to end it prematurely will simply result in unhappiness for children, increased anxiety for both parents and children, and occasionally an overt power struggle. True, some children may be conditioned to the sensitivity of their genitals in such a way that they begin systematic masturbation at an earlier age than other children; however, this does not appear to be a problem in and of itself. Children in whom the masturbatory behavior is genuinely compulsive will often show signs of tension and stress in other areas of their lives as well. They may also continue the compulsive masturbation until, or in spite of, recognizable genital irritation. Before the behavior is labeled psychologically compulsive, however, the clinician would do well to ask a parent to bring in a child for a physical examination that might include a search for any source of genital irritation and provide the opportunity to assess the child's behavior. If a physical basis for genital irritation is found, it can be treated. If the child appears tense and stressed in ways that suggest psychological difficulties, continued assessment of the family and child is indicated. In determining the severity of the behavior as a problem, the context in which the masturbation occurs should always be taken into account. Blatantly inappropriate timing of masturbation (e.g., at mealtimes at home or overtly during school hours) is more likely to be compulsive in nature and/or symbolic of inner conflicts than is masturbation carried on privately (e.g., in bed). In the vast majority of cases, parents can be assured that even regular patterns of systematic masturbation are simply instances of natural, developmentally appropriate behavior that the child will change at some point in the future.

Problems with Sexual Values

Parents will sometimes ask the clinician to comment on issues such as the effects of family nudity on children, how to guide children away from inappropriate sexual content on television, or how to deal with differences in standards of sexual behavior between families in the same neighborhood. These concerns fall under the general heading of *family sexual values*. Therefore, simple standardized answers are not adequate. However, the clinician can supply parents with certain principles or guidelines for dealing with their growing children about these sex-related matters.

Cross-cultural evidence suggests that there is no inherent problem in exposing children to nudity, excretory functioning, or even sexual activity itself (Ford and Beach, 1951). The guidelines for such exposure are the meaning of the behavior to both the adults and children in the family, the continuity of the behavior in the family situation, and the attitudes and values of the particular culture. Standards of modesty among family members contribute to the overall sexual "atmosphere" of the home. If the physical exposure of one family member is in great contrast to that of others, his/ her beliefs will stand out and perhaps be puzzling and unsettling to children in the family. Similarly, if there is a significant change in the standards of modesty practiced by family members over time, the children involved may become anxious. Children who are exposed to parental nudity or sexual activity in a household that does not ordinarily acknowledge sexuality and the existence of sexual feelings will be affected differently than children who are used to the sight of naked family members and to some conversations about sex occurring in a casual fashion. The same is true of nearly every aspect of children's exposure to sex-related matters: *If this exposure is significantly at variance with the explicit and implicit family values, it is more likely that it will be interpreted by children as having a negative meaning.* If it is discontinuous with a child's experience of life up to that point, it is more likely to create some amount of anxiety.

The effect of television on children's behavior is currently controversial. Unfortunately, scenes depicting sex and those depicting violence are often considered synonymous by those individuals and groups who would banish "harmful" content from the television screen. Some recent evidence suggests that depictions of violent scenes on television may in fact impact negatively on children, desensitizing them to the consequences of such behavior (Eysenck and Nias, 1978). On the other hand, there is no evidence that scenes depicting natural, healthy sexual interaction—no matter how explicit—have any negative effects on children. However, the data are not all in. It is possible that such positive exposure may provide *positive* modeling. As with the issue of nudity, the problem does not appear to lie with the degree of explicitness. Rather, it is a matter of the *meaning* of the exposure to the children in relation to their family values. Much of what is depicted sexually on television can be considered to fall into negative categories—scenes that show unrealistic sexual interactions, degradation of women, and irresponsible sexual behavior. Therefore, unmonitored exposure of children to sexual activity on television or in movies constitutes a problem not because it is specifically *sexual* activity that is depicted but because the children are given no help in dealing with the value conflicts that might be raised. The clinician should certainly encourage parents to take a more responsible role in this regard.

Parents who raise questions about differing sexual values in neighborhoods should be helped to understand that it is *they* who have the responsibility and the opportunity to raise and discuss with their children differences between their own family's sexual values and those of other families, just as they would between their own sexual values and those depicted on TV or in movies. Thus, children are encouraged to recognize that value differences do indeed exist and that sometimes their own values will be challenged by the behaviors of others. Even very young children must be taught to discriminate between standards that are appropriate for one context and those that are appropriate for another.

Cases

The mother of a 4-year-old girl found the girl and a playmate using water-filled balloons between their legs as "penises." In the context of their playing house and related games, the mother decided this was acceptable behavior, so she let it continue. Later she discovered that the mother of the other girl was outraged at having the girls attempt to replicate this game in her home. This led to severe reprimands of the children, tears and unhappiness for the girl whose mother permitted the behavior, and even some tension between the two families.

The mother of a 10-year-old was extremely embarrassed upon receiving a phone call from a neighbor who took her to task for her lack of modesty and poor family standards. The irate mother reported that this woman's son had urinated in the bathroom with the door open while playing at her house with her own child. She was deeply offended by this and stated quite directly that the family who would tolerate this sort of behavior had defective moral values. Toileting behavior was openly accepted in the family of the mother who reported this incident, and the differences in these family values led to hostility between the two families and, unfortunately, to keeping the two boys from playing with each other.

These cases illustrate the intensity with which differences in families' sexual values are sometimes encountered. There is no way to immunize children against value conflicts, sexual or otherwise. Rather, parents can be helped to teach their children to discriminate between behavior appropriate in one context and that in another. Even young children can gradually be taught that certain kinds of conversation, acceptable in their own family, are not acceptable in other families. Similarly, they can be reminded that a certain kind of behavior, such as going to the toilet with the door open, will need to be altered in line with the expectations or "rules" of another family home. It should be pointed out to the children that these changes in behavior are necessary not because there is anything wrong with sex but because there are *differing standards* for dealing with sex, just as there are in other areas of life. Children have many occasions to learn discrimination between the requirements of a variety of situations. For example, at school they can talk and interact in one way in Ms. Jones' gym class and must respond and behave in an entirely different way in Mr. Smith's reading class. In summary, then, the issue becomes one of discrimination of rules and standards rather than a sexual problem *per se*.

Dealing with "Sex Play"

Most adults have memories of some kinds of sex play they engaged in as children, and not a few of these remember one or more occasions of being discovered by adults while engaging in this activity. Parents will sometimes ask clinicians about the relative health or danger of sex play or about how to handle such situations with their children if they should discover them engaging in such activity.

First of all, parents should be helped to view the sexually focused play activities of their children as natural and normal aspects of growing up. Such play is common among both boys and girls and may be focused on same-sex or opposite-sex interactions (Gagnon and Simon, 1973). Serious developmental questions should be raised about sex play only if the activities are carried on so constantly that they exclude other kinds of peer group interaction and/or if they involve interactions between children of significantly different ages (5 years or more). Otherwise, the activities can usually be seen as developmentally typical. They are usually conducted in near or total secrecy, because children have learned that overt interest in sex is not acceptable to most adults. Sexual curiosity and play activities appear to be relatively uniform throughout childhood, varying with individuals' life circumstances, availability, and the strength of parental sanctions against them. The psychoanalytic view that there is a "latency period" during which such interests and activities automatically cease is not supported by research (Broderick, 1968).

At the same time, parents need not accept any and all kinds of sex play practiced by their children. In line with their own sexual values, circumstances, and even interpersonal relationships between the children involved and/or the families, parents may rightfully choose to limit the occurrence of sex play, the type of sex play, or its location. If this is done, parents should be encouraged to impose those restrictions using terms such as *inappropriate* or *not acceptable* rather than terms like *dirty, bad,* or *shameful*. Children should not be taught that they are bad because they wish to express their sexual curiosity in this manner. Rather, they should be helped to understand that they are being limited by certain rules or restrictions placed upon them in line with social expectations. Parents should be discouraged from "spying on" or unrealistically limiting their children's experience if sex play is suspected. Similarly, if children are discovered in such behavior, the situation is best handled as rationally and unemotionally as possible. The behavior can be stopped ("David, I want you and Susan to put your clothes back on right now.") and a reasonable explanation for the limitation given to the child while acknowledging the acceptability of the motivation behind the behavior. ("David, I can understand how you and Susan are curious about each other's bodies. However, Susan's parents and your daddy and I don't believe that it is right for children to take off their clothes in front of other people outside of their own family members. And touching each other's penises and vulvas is something that we believe is only done in special situations, usually when people are adults. Therefore, I do not want you and Susan to do that kind of thing anymore. If you have any questions that you would like to ask your daddy or me about girls' bodies, we would be glad to try to answer them, and we can also find some books with pictures in them so that you can understand them better.") This kind of matter-of-fact explanation, combined with explicit recognition of sexual values and beliefs, is much to be preferred over name-calling or emotional threats.

When, like masturbation, sex play appears to be more extensive and compulsive, then further investigation is in order.

Helping Parents as Sex Educators

Frequently, parents bring to the clinician questions about their role as sex educators of their children. They wish to know how to answer specific questions that their children may ask, or they seek advice on how best to judge when children are ready for specific sex information. In these situations, the clinician has two major tasks: The first is to supply parents with accurate information about sex that they can pass on to their children; the second is to provide guidelines for the process of educating young people about sexuality.

Parents' questions about sex education for their children provides the clinician with an excellent opportunity to supply accurate sex information to the parents themselves. Relatively few parents received adequate sex information when they were children, and their questions about how to help their children may provide the perfect excuse for obtaining information that can be helpful to them personally. Nothing should be presumed; instead, a tactfully presented ''review'' of essential information can be given. The clinician must also remember that there are value aspects to many topics related to sexuality. Therefore, some statements must remain open-ended in order to accommodate the individualized value and judgments of the parents themselves. In fact, some parents may hold such highly restrictive sexual values that they refuse to acknowledge certain facts about sex. When the clinician becomes aware of this, the discussion may switch to a focus on the distinction between facts and values. In this way, the clinician can maintain his/her own sense of integrity while also respecting the values that the parent is expressing.

Case

An approach to dealing with parents is illustrated in the following sample dialogue between a clinician and a father who wishes to talk to his 12-year-old son about the subject of masturbation.

MR. J   The other day David asked me a question about what ''jerking off'' meant. I really didn't know what to say, so I told him I was busy and would talk to him later. Now I don't know what to do. I really think he's a little young to talk about that subject! But I just don't want him to hear about it from the other kids and to—you know—get involved in that sort of thing with them.

DR. A   Well, your son is 12 now, that means that masturbation could begin to be a very important subject for him. He could begin to experience ejaculation before long—that is, if he hasn't already begun. Of course, it's also possible that he's just heard other boys in his group use the term *jerking off,* and doesn't connect that with masturbation at all. What do you think?

MR. J   I don't know. But isn't 12 awfully young to be—doing that sort of thing?

DR. A   Well, actually, Mr. J., children of almost all ages play with their bodies. But most boys really don't get serious about it until after they experience their first ejaculation in connection with it. Or sometimes they hear about masturbation from other boys and just experiment with it without really knowing what's going to happen. The average age for boys in this country to first experience ejaculation is around 13; however, a good number of boys begin to experience ejaculations earlier than that, so it's not impossible that David has already matured to that point himself. Kids today mature a bit earlier than we did when we were their age. Do you remember when you had your first ejaculation, perhaps in a wet dream or something?

MR. J   Yeah, well, as a matter of fact—I guess I was just about 14 when I woke up one night after it happened. It really scared me, too, because I didn't know what to expect. At first I thought something was wrong with me.

DR. A   So you didn't really have any preparation for the experience of ejaculation. Well, perhaps that's a good reason for you to supply some information to

David ahead of time—that is, if it *is* ahead of time. Some boys talk about it with their friends, but many do not. They just hear vague slang references to it—like about jerking off. We know that virtually all males masturbate at some point in their lives, usually beginning in early adolescence, when it's the most frequent form of sexual outlet. Statistically speaking, David would be unusual if he did not at least experiment with it. I remember some myths about masturbation when I was growing up; perhaps you do also. Like the ones about making you go blind, or sterile, or get warts or pimples. We now know that masturbation doesn't cause any emotional problems either.

MR. J   Wait a minute! I think too much masturbation can cause you lots of problems, 'cause it's a sin and you're going to feel awfully guilty about it afterward.

DR. A   Well, Mr. J., it's true that masturbation can cause a lot of guilt if it violates someone's value system. So if you believe that masturbation is morally wrong, then I think you ought to let David know that when you're talking to him about it. I believe that parents should label those kind of moral values clearly, rather than trying to scare their children out of masturbating by telling them that it will cause them physical damage or make them go crazy or something. You can tell David that jerking off refers to masturbation and what masturbation is and then tell him why you believe that it's not right to do so.

MR. J   Well, actually, I don't believe it's so awful bad—as long as you don't do it too much. When I was growing up, my church told me it was a sin, but I didn't really believe that completely, and I guess I don't now either. It's just that I don't want David doing it all the time.

DR. A   I can understand your concern. Actually, it's not possible to masturbate too much, from the physical point of view. The body will quit when it gets tired. So judging whether it's excessive or not has to be based on how it fits into the rest of the boy's life. If, at any point in the next few years, David seemed to be spending most of his time in his room alone rather than in activities with friends or doing fairly well in school or being involved in a variety of other things that healthy teenagers are involved in, then there might be some concern about the role of masturbation in his life. Otherwise, I personally believe it's a healthy and normal thing to experiment with masturbation—and to do it quite a bit when one's a teenager—and even to carry it on from time to time throughout one's life.

MR. J   I guess that's true. I guess I never actually did hear about anybody going crazy or blind from doing it. If they had, I guess there'd be an awful lot more crazy, blind people around in the world than there are now, right?

DR. A   Yes, that's true. Well, it sounds to me like you can go back to talk to David about jerking off and explain to him that masturbation is a pretty natural thing for a teenager to do. You can also give him some guidelines about where and when it's appropriate—privacy, and all that. Perhaps a couple of sentences about it, and let it go at that, unless David has more questions he'd like to ask you. Just letting him know that you're willing to respond to his questions and that you're there if he needs you is a pretty important thing at his age.

The second major aspect of the parents' role as sex educators—the process of education itself—is even more important in the long run than the accuracy of sex information itself. Parents should be helped to understand that sexuality education occurs as an ongoing process in all families (Gordon, 1975). Sexual values and the modeling of sex-related behaviors pervade the entire atmosphere of the family as children develop. This is the heart of sex education—more important to the ultimate outcome of an individual's adult life than any specific piece of sex information (Kirkendall, 1970). Some parents worry that the schools will take over their responsibility as primary sex educators. This is a groundless fear. At best, schools can supply basic information on reproductive and sexual processes and serve as a forum for guided discussion of sex-related issues among children and their peers. Basic sex education is conveyed within the family through patterns of interpersonal relations, touching and physical affection, attitudes toward the role behaviors of both sexes in the family, and family members' erotically tinged feelings about themselves and each other. Thus, the clinician can remind parents of the tremendous responsibility that they inevitably have as sex educators—that it is not a question of *whether* sex education will occur, but how and when and in what circumstances. Aiding parents in achieving the greater awareness that they need in order to better take charge of the sex education of their children contributes positively to the overall task of sex education in the family.

It is also possible to give parents support and guidance with regard to the actual process of imparting information to their children. Parents can often be reassured that it is virtually impossible to "traumatize" the children by providing them with too much sex information too soon. A natural screening process—lack of understanding—will filter out any material for which the child is not experientially ready. In fact, it is important to point out that some sex information needs to be given to children several times at different ages in order for them to fully assimilate its meaning as their developmental levels change. It is also important to choose appropriate language in dealing with children's inquiries about sex. Of course, simplistic language is not one of the natural talents of many clinicians. However, appropriate language helps assure that the information will be accurately understood by the child. Parents can also be guided to refrain from excessive intrusiveness or seductiveness in interacting with their children around sex-related issues. Some parents appear to be so anxious about sex that they attempt to be overcontrolling and to intrude upon their children's legitimate privacy. This is counterproductive in that it mobilizes the children's defensiveness and leads to poorer rather than better communication. Sometimes, the clinician can aid parents in sex education by simply being an objective third party who can make suggestions.

In their acceptance of sexuality as a basic part of life experience, clinicians can serve as positive role models for parents. In fact, the overall success of interactions with parents around sex-related issues are powerfully dependent upon the clinician's own attitudes and feelings. These are expressed in his/her professional role, the ambience of the office setting, and personal comfort level when discussing sex. Through these, the clinician can facilitiate parents' understanding of the importance of touch and nonverbal interaction, serve as a clarifier of family sexual values, objectively listen to concerns, and aid in resolving sex-related conflicts within the family. The clinician can help parents recognize and deal effectively with sexual interactions in the everyday lives of their children as well as with predictable developmental "crises" and with unexpected problems. On the one hand, the clinician can help parents avoid unnecessarily exaggerating common developmental difficulties their children encounter. On the other hand, he/she can alert parents to the genuine, if sometimes hidden, traumas that can negatively affect children's development.

Thus, the clinician is a valuable resource for the sexual concerns of parents about their children. She/he can be comfortable, supportive, informative, a facilitator of problem solving, and—if the sex-related problem is severe—a more specialized source of help or a link to such a source.

Working Directly with Children's Sexual Concerns and Problems

Psychosexual Development

Basic information about childhood sexual activity patterns can provide an important reference point for the clinician working with children. Observations of children indicate that body awareness in earliest infancy includes casual exploration of body parts, apparently without any innate sense of inhibition. At least some infants seem to be capable of orgasmlike responses to either self-induced or other-induced stimulation as early as several weeks after birth. The Kinsey studies (Kinsey et al., 1948, 1953) report observations of young children, both males and females, masturbating to apparent "orgasm." The physiological responses of children to erotic stimulation appear to be general and diffuse, and they do not appear to have the sexual meaning attributed by adults nor the specific attachment to a particular erotic stimulus. Nevertheless, they seem to involve a similar pattern of tension increment and release. This response pattern has not been observed as frequently in girls as in boys. However, it may be that the response is more difficult to verify anatomically for girls, or it may be that sociosexual learning is culturally different for the sexes in this regard, as in other sex-related behaviors. Overall, research data on early childhood sexual behavior suggest that human sexuality is rooted in biogenetic factors but elaborated through highly flexible patterns of learning.

Awareness of physical differences between the sexes appears in early childhood without a full comprehension of the significance of these differences, especially their sexual significance (Gadpaille, 1975; Gagnon and Simon, 1973). Freud's theory of "penis envy" in females has not been demonstrated to be biologically innate, and many dispute its validity. More likely, the phenomenon reflects the sensitivity of female children to the male social dominance of Western culture. This is aided and abetted by some parents' insistence on treating girls' bodies as if they "lacked" something rather than emphasizing positively the possession of specific physical characteristics in girls as well as boys. Of course, this cannot be fully understood by children until the sexual as well as the excretory functions of the genitals are acknowledged by parents.

The interests of preschool children in anatomical differences and the origins of babies usually represent an exploratory, existential quest about human nature and the surrounding world rather than a highly focused sexual curiosity *per se*. The notion of coital activity in relation to reproduction is probably not fully internalized by children until around the age of 10—or even later if adults in the children's environment intentionally withhold this information (Gadpaille, 1975; Gagnon and Simon, 1973).

In recent years the concept of a "latency period," as Freud hypothesized, has become a matter of controversy in relation to sex education. Latency covers that period of time between approximately 5 or 6 years of age and the onset of puberty, during which children are thought by some to be inherently uninterested in sex and perhaps even psychologically vulnerable to trauma through inappropriate exposure to sex information. Most contemporary research evidence does not support the concept of a biologically based latency period. Rather, there appears to be a steadily increasing interest in sex among children through this period. This interest may be masked by the demands and priorities of other aspects of children's life experiences, particularly those associated with school (Broderick, 1968). During the elementary school years, then, sexual interests of children may go "underground" in response to adult prohibitions. The experience of sex educators suggests that children of latency age appear to be able to comfortably accept as much information as they are given about sex if it is conveyed in a calm, accepting, and objective way (Gordon, 1975).

Sex Education

It is surprising to some to learn that a major source of sex information for young people in the United States is sexually explicit material commonly known as *pornography*. A significant minority of individuals have been exposed to explicit sexual materials prior to adolescence. By the time they leave the teenage years, 75% of all males and females have at least encountered such materials (U.S. Commission on Obscenity and Pornography, 1970). Contrary to widespread opinion, the mere exposure of children to explicit sexual materials does *not* appear to cause psychological damage or social maladjustment in and of itself. Nevertheless, there are a small number of young people whose attention can be fixated on some aspects of pornography in such a way as to influence their sexual development in an unhealthy direction. Feminists have emphasized that the single most significant characteristic of traditional pornography is its degradation of human individuals, particularly women. Similar attitudes appear in a variety of more socially acceptable depictions of sexuality, such as in some public advertising and in certain portrayals linking sex and violence in television and movies. The most effective counter to pornography appears to be the exposure of young people to adequate sex information, positive nonsexist role models, and healthy sexual values.

Children in the United States have traditionally suffered from a "conspiracy of silence" in regard to sex education. They most often receive their sex information outside of the family setting, even though a majority of both parents and young people believe that the home should be the primary source of such information. However, surveys indicate that parents actually rank third or fourth as sources of sex education— behind peers, school or church programs, and public media as the most common sources (Gagnon, 1965). Of course, sexual attitudes and knowledge vary greatly among children of various ethnic backgrounds, socioeconomic levels, and religious orientations. Although acceptance of formal sex education programs in schools and community institutions is increasing, there is still strong opposition to such programs by a minority of adults for personal, religious, and political reasons. To date, there is little empirical evidence to support the positive outcomes of sex education programs. This results partly from lack of serious evaluation efforts and also from the difficulty in reaching agreement on desired outcomes. Most young people who participate in formal sex education programs do rate them positively (Gagnon, 1965; Carrera, 1976).

Sexual Exploration

Empirical, anthropological, and clinical data support Freud's contention that children enjoy a kind of "pan sexuality," which is shaped and channeled by environmental forces. Cross-cultural studies indicate that most societies are sexually more permissive in their childrearing practices than is the United States. In those societies that have no restrictions to the contrary, children progress from casual body exploration in infancy to systematic genital masturbation (usually without orgasm) by about the age of 8. And, if they are allowed to watch adults engage in coital activity from an early age, children will actively imitate this behavior in their own play before the age of 10 (Prescott, 1975; Ford and Beach 1951).

Casual genital exploration begins in the first year of life and becomes more systematic and goal-directed as it is increasingly given erotic meaning in the child's experience. Masturbation rates are roughly similar for males and females up to the age of 10 years, when they become more frequent for males and less frequent for females. Most boys learn about masturbation from other boys or from accidentally discovering self-induced ejaculations after they have experienced nocturnal emissions (wet dreams). Masturbation quickly becomes the major sexual outlet for males during adolescence, so that most males who will masturbate sometime during their lives (over 95%) will begin doing so before the age of 20. Research reports suggest that females are less likely to masturbate prior to adulthood, although perhaps two-thirds to three-fourths of them will do so at some time during their lives (Kinsey et al., 1948, 1953). However, it is possible that a significant number of female children or adolescents do masturbate without attaching this particular label to it and perhaps without experiencing orgasm. Masturbation is becoming an increasingly acceptable form of self-directed sexual expression for both males and females in American society, although residual elements of guilt are still present for many people.

"Sex play" in childhood is a widespread phenomenon, particularly if it is limited to looking at or casually touching the genitals of another child. The incidence of such play is slightly higher for boys than for girls up to the time of puberty. Then, the incidence of such contacts increases for males and decreases for females, probably as a result of the "protective" mentality assumed by adults for the soon-to-be reproductively vulnerable females. A small percentage of childhood sex play involves intercourse or oral–genital contact. However, the incidence varies widely according to socioeconomic class, ethnic background, and even geographic factors (Gadpaille, 1975; Ford and Beach, 1951; Kinsey et al., 1948, 1953). Children who do have a significant amount of prepubertal sexual activity are more likely to have a greater variety of sexual experiences and partners during adolescence. Sexually active preadolescents may also have more social relationship disturbances than others; however, these disturbances appear to result mostly from the violation of social expectations rather than from the specifically sexual nature of their activities (Gadpaille, 1975; Broderick, 1968). Sexual activity is frequently more problematic for children whose contacts are with adults or adolescents, a phenomenon much more common than previously thought (see Chapter 8).

More boys than girls have genital contact with members of their own sex. Kinsey reported that nearly two-thirds of all males have at least one same-sex-oriented erotic contact in their lifetimes (Kinsey et al., 1948). The incidence for females is thought to be perhaps one-half of that (Kinsey et al., 1953). However, these findings may result from the lesser visibility of female same-sex contacts due to greater social acceptability of affectional interaction. Therefore, women may be less likely to remember their early same-sex interactions as "homosexual." Erotic contacts between males are particularly prevalent around the time of puberty and in early adolescence. Rather than being a distinctly "homosexual phase" of development, this is heterosocial insecurity, and lack of available heterosexual partners. Boys of this age may even engage in group homosexual encounters (Gadpaille, 1975).

These encounters do not predispose most individuals toward a lifelong homosexual orientation. However, some individuals whose developmental backgrounds have included a particular constellation of factors (still not fully understood) that are directed toward homoerotic inclinations may at this time become aware of a feeling of "differentness" or other evidence of same-sex affectional and erotic preference. When they do occur, the same-sex contacts of girls are more likely to be private experiences with one close friend and to reflect strong affectional elements in addition to, or instead of, genital preoccupation. Developmentally speaking, a homosexual orientation cannot be said to be solidified until middle to late adolescence at the earliest, even though certain individuals are convinced of their same-sex preferences from the time of their earliest remembered sexual stirrings (Gadpaille, 1975; Broderick, 1968; Gagnon, 1965).

For some children, sex play includes experimentation with siblings. This incestuous contact is usually not problematic as long as it is not sustained and/or does not involve significant age differences (see Chapter 8). For children in rural areas, particularly males, sexual contact with animals is not uncommon. Most frequently, this activity is confined to masturbating the animal or encouraging the animal to provide erotic stimulation through oral contact. Less frequently, it may include oral–genital contact with the animal or actual intercourse. Despite the prevalence of moral and aesthetic sanctions against sexual contact with animals, this type of behavior is usually experimental and/or substitutionary in nature and is, therefore, transient. Only in a small number of instances does it fail to give way to more lasting contacts in adolescence (Kinsey et al., 1948).

The average age of first sexual intercourse is decreasing for both males and females, particularly in some segments of the population (Zuckerman, 1976). However, other than in the special instances cited earlier, heterosexual intercourse between male and female peers prior to puberty is still relatively rare in this country. Therefore, a discussion of this behavior is more appropriate in the chapter on adolescence (Chapter 5).

Responding to Children's Sexual Concerns

In their earlier years, children engage in a variety of ''sexual'' activities with little or no self-consciousness. As they grow older, children's inclination to worry about their sexual activity varies according to the content of messages about sex they have received from the adult world. Some 4- or 5-year-olds will openly engage in masturbation or in genital exploration with other children of both sexes. Some children of this age will behave similarly, but only when safely hidden from adults. Other children will demonstrate an almost phobic avoidance of any kind of intimate touching of themselves or other children, based upon their internalization of rigid adult prohibitions. None of these children are likely to talk spontaneously about sex to adults. Nevertheless, the clinician should remain sensitive to indirect evidences of difficulty that young patients may be experiencing as they sort through the myriad messages about sex that impinge upon them from their social environments.

Unfortunately, in our society, children are likely to experience increasing conflict regarding their sexual interests and activities at about the same rate that they learn how many adults disapprove of openness about sex. This deprives children of valuable resources for support and advice at the very time when they are most likely to be needed. Here, the clinician can play an important role as a somewhat removed adult who has both the authority and the permission to discuss intimate subjects. Through tactful questioning, she/he may have the opportunity to help children concerned about masturbation, sexual dreams or daydreams, or patterns of sex play with their peers. Some children express anxiety about their interest in sexual stimuli. For most of these concerns, reassurance and information are the key responses.

Body image concerns are prominent among children, particularly in the years close to puberty. Attention to the physical development of a child is important not only for reasons of health but also because body image contributes substantially to a developing individual's overall sense of self-worth (Prescott, 1975). Children who worry excessively about their height, weight, or the development of secondary sex characteristics relative to other children will sometimes experience internal stress or social maladjustment sufficient to produce significant, if temporary, psychopathology. For example, early-maturing girls and late-maturing boys are at greater risk of experiencing social maladjustment than are those children whose pubertal change patterns are more developmentally typical. Girls whose bodies develop early are more likely to be given attention by older boys and, thus, may be set apart from their same-age peers. Similarly, boys whose physical development does not keep pace with their peers' are likely to fall behind in the competition for recognition through athletics and other forms of physical prowess (Maddock, 1973). Therefore, they may find it easier to relate to younger children. Neither of these patterns is automatically a problem; however, the heightened potential for disruption deserves notice. Supportive counseling is indicated for those children whose growth patterns are noticeably atypical in timing, even if these developmental phenomena do not pose any other hazard to health.

At the same time, the clinician should watch for young patients whose physical conditions constitute genuine medical abnormalities and who can be aided by prompt and effective intervention. Developmental problems, such as endocrinologically based obesity, can significantly affect an individual's well-being by influencing comfort with social relationships, sexual responsivity, and a variety of other life experiences. In summary, no real or imagined body image concerns of young patients should be ignored by the clinician or dismissed as something that they will "outgrow." Instead, these patients should be given the benefit of sympathetic listening, support, and reassurance and, when indicated, a thorough physical evaluation (Money, 1972).

Children are most likely to be concerned with their physical characteristics around the time of puberty, when hormonal changes promote reproductive maturity. Puberty begins with the first appearance of secondary sex characteristics and concludes when full reproductive maturity (i.e., the regular production of viable sex cells) has been achieved, a span of 2 to 5 years. The average age of pubertal change has been moving steadily downward since public health records first began to be kept in the United States. The mean age of menarche in American girls is now slightly before the 12th birthday. A parallel event for boys, the first seminal emission, now occurs around the 13th birthday (Maddock, 1973). Some parents, and even some physicians, may be unprepared for these events, based upon their memories of later onset of these changes in their own lives. However, the majority of girls in our society are at least somewhat prepared for menstruation, because they have been exposed to a combination of information from mothers and older sisters, school health programs, conversations with peers, and media advertising of menstrual and feminine hygiene products. Boys are less fortunate in this regard. Many are unprepared for the occurrence of spontaneous seminal emissions, having received little sex education other than random information collected from peers. In addition, there is a widespread myth in American society that males somehow intuitively know all about sex. Thus, the clinician can be an important source of basic information for some children approaching puberty, whereas for others she/he may be more of a background resource to deal with incidental concerns as they arise. Pamphlets and booklets about sex can be supplied to young patients in the event that direct discussion is not necessary, possible, or desirable for some reason (Lief and Karlen, 1976).

The issue of sexual language is particularly important in clinical interaction with children. The clinician is cautioned to avoid the use of either belittlingly "baby talk" or highly technical language and professional jargon. Willingness to openly accept patients' sexual terminology is important, even if it includes words that the clinician does not understand or finds personally offensive. On the other hand, it is not necessary to impress children with his/her command of sexual slang, particularly if it creates personal discomfort. As long as a shared meaning with the patient is achieved, familiar and comfortable terminology is the best option. Sexual terms can have very different meanings among different ethnic groups, socioeconomic levels, or even in different neighborhoods. Therefore, patients should always be asked to define unfamiliar words so that the clinician is clear about the exact meaning of the patients' verbal descriptions.

Sexual language is itself a problem for some children. Young patients may inquire about the meaning of a particular word—either a technical term, e.g., *coitus*, or a slang phrase, e.g., *jerking off*. These children may be embarrassed to make the inquiry of their parents or to acknowledge their ignorance to their peers, and so an understanding clinician can help by offering brief, simple, and honest definitions.

The focus on sexual language can be an excellent vehicle for providing sex information to a young patient. For example, with only slight modifications, the dialogue with Mr. J. presented earlier in this chapter can be altered to suit 12-year-old David, his son.

Case

DR. A   OK, Dave. Now that you are 12 years old, some significant changes are beginning to take place in your body, and we'll want to make sure everything's developing as it should. Have you had any physical concerns or problems that you'd like to talk with me about?

DAVID   No, Doctor, I guess not. I've been fine, except for getting my leg banged up one day last fall in football.

DR. A   I guess even though minor injuries like that are fairly common, if you're involved in sports, they still cause you some concern. But I was referring to some changes taking place in your body. For example, I notice you've grown quite a bit taller this year. Also, you're beginning to develop hair under your arms and around your penis. Have you noticed any other changes in particular?

DAVID   Not really, except that my voice seems to be changing and I get teased about it sometimes.

DR. A   Yes, that voice change, your growth, and that extra hair are all signs of a growth stage we call *puberty*. As you know, they'll continue over the next couple of years. It's part of the process of maturing sexually into an adult. There will be some other changes too, one of which is the ability to ejaculate. Do you know what that means?

DAVID   Well, uh, . . . not exactly.

DR. A   Ejaculation is the body's release of fluid called *semen* through the penis. This can't begin to happen until a boy's body is producing mature sperm cells on a regular basis. When that happens, he sometimes experiences an ejaculation at night. The penis gets hard—you've probably had that happen to you—and then the semen is released in an ejaculation. It usually feels good, and sometimes it's accompanied by a dream. That's what has led to it being called a *wet dream*. Have you ever had that experience?

DAVID   No. I . . . I . . . I guess not.

DR. A   Well, it's very likely to happen to you sometime in the next year or two, and it's nothing at all to be worried about. It's a very natural process. Another way that boys can ejaculate is through masturbation. Sometimes boys call masturbation *jerking off* or *jacking off*.

DAVID   Yeah, we—the guys—talked about that. I never got to do that. The guys told me that you gotta be careful not to do it too much. . . .

DR. A   Actually, Dave, many teenage boys masturbate. And there are a lot of stories about masturbation causing problems, but most of them are not true. Masturbation doesn't cause any physical damage whatsoever, unless it's done in some unusual way. It doesn't cause any emotional problems either, unless some people do it when it's against their moral beliefs or value system. Then they might feel guilty. It's not really possible to masturbate too much, from a physical point of view. The body will simply quit when it gets tired. So judging whether masturbation is too much or not has to be based on how it fits into the rest of someone's life. If a boy seemed to be spending most of his time alone masturbating rather than in activities with his friends, doing his schoolwork, or being involved in activities that other teenagers are involved in, then I suppose there might be some concern about the role of masturbation in his life. Otherwise, I personally believe it's a relatively healthy and normal thing to experiment with masturbation. So you shouldn't believe the various stories you might hear about masturbation making you go blind, or crazy, or causing pimples or something else like that.

DAVID   My mom says I gotta watch out for pimples and not eat too much candy. Does candy really cause pimples?

Sexual language can occasionally be presented as a problem by children who have been "caught" or punished for using it. Sometimes children will actually express consternation at the unintended effects of their verbalizations. At other times, children will be very aware of the power of sexual vocabulary and will need help understanding and respecting social guidelines in order to avoid unpleasant consequences. Rarely will children demonstrate a compulsive need to use sexual language aggressively or scatologically as an expression of underlying hostility and unresolved psychic conflict. Here, the emphasis is on the anger and hostility underlying the sexual references, and these children are likely candidates for psychological treatment, perhaps involving their families as well.

The clinician may occasionally encounter children in whom fantasies, dreams, or exposure to sexual stimuli have triggered anxieties or fears, even of phobic proportions. Merely having sexual thoughts or daydreams may be disturbing to some children who have been taught that acknowledgement of sexuality is wrong. The clinician can reassure these children that such experiences are, in fact, very common. Similarly, some children are frightened by their own sexual curiosities and urges, anxious that they may be unable to control them. Here, the clinician can help distinguish between feelings and behavior, thus, encouraging the development of an appropriate sense of control. If, in fact, a particular child appears to be unable to exercise such control, then further treatment is advised. Occasionally, children will develop elaborate symptoms, such as counterphobic behavior or psychotic delusions, in an effort to resolve internal sexual conflicts. Usually these symptoms extend beyond sex into other aspects of the children's experience. These more severe disturbances may be recognized by the inclusion of bizarre behavior and/or inappropriate affect and are seldom resolved by providing calm reassurance or supplying sex information. Here, too, further treatment is warranted.

Dealing with Children's Sexual Behavior Problems

The sexual activities of children are most likely to come to the attention of the clinician on two occasions. The first is when they result in some kind of accidental injury or health problem. The second is when they are expressed in a noticeably "deviant" direction or when they are apparent symptoms of more severe emotional disturbances. On the one hand, children need reassurance that masturbation and sex play do not in and of themselves lead to physical or emotional harm, as many prevailing myths would suggest. On the other hand, it is equally important to be realistic about the potential dangers of sexual activities that subject the body or the psyche to undue amounts of stress.

Some genital injuries treated in emergency rooms or clinics result from masturbation or sex play. These include genital or pelvic cuts and abrasions, genital or pelvic rope burns or bruises, and foreign objects trapped in the urethra, vagina, or rectum. Bobby pins, fever thermometers or pencils are easily lost or lodged in the urinary tract. Similarly, the vagina and rectum can receive lipsticks, pens or pencils, candles, and other objects inserted during masturbation or in connection with childhood games such as playing "doctor."

Cases

A 5-year-old girl was brought to the clinic for investigation when her mother noticed a foul-smelling discharge and small traces of blood in her underpants. She was discovered to have a metal lipstick case lodged in her vagina. The physician learned that it was placed there approximately a week earlier in the course of playing a game of "doctor" with a neighborhood friend.

A 12-year-old boy was brought to the emergency room by his mother complaining of intense penile pain. Discoloration of the glans, abrasions at the base of the penis, and minor burns of the urinary meatus were discovered and led to a careful questioning of the boy concerning his masturbation practices. He revealed that he had been masturbating by placing a small piece of twine tightly around his penis to produce an erection while using the applicator cap from an iodine bottle to insert into the urethra. The traces of iodine remaining on the applicator led to the discoloration of the glans and to burns on the sensitive urethral tissue.

The relation of some physical injuries to sex-related activities may not always be readily apparent. Sometimes the connection is made only by careful questioning about how the injury was sustained. Rope burns on the wrists and ankles, muscle strains, dislocations, and even strangulation or suffocation have all been known to occur as side effects of masturbatory activity. Similarly, sexual games of preadolescent youth have sometimes led to unforeseen consequences, including injury and even death. In most cases, these unfortunate results are genuinely unforseen side effects of curiosity, exploration, and the desire to produce physically pleasurable feelings. In addition to treating the injury, the clinician should emphatically advise against the use of risky objects or techniques without condemning young patients for their sexual interests. This may be difficult to accomplish in the face of distraught parents, who may react with extreme anxiety and embarrassment. Usually a careful elicitation of the circumstances of the injury will provide the clinician with an opening for later warning children against repetition of the activities. while at the same time acknowledging that sexual curiosity, interest, and the wish to produce pleasurable feelings are natural and normal.

The clinician may occasionally encounter a child whose sex-related activities appear to be unusual or even pathological. When this occurs, it is important to place the sexual activity into appropriate context by noting the age and developmental level of the child as well as the environmental context in which the behavior is occurring. Children's sexual interests and activities vary greatly according to life situation. Based upon cues from the adult world, some children will be quite forthright about their sexual curiosities and interests. Other children will submerge these interests and satisfy their sexual curiosity only in the most indirect fashion. Some children may experience a sexually focused encounter with their peers very frequently while growing up. Others may refrain from any such activities, while keeping their eyes and ears open to the sexually tinged elements of the world around them. All of these children are normal but are at different points on the continuum of sexual experience. Only if there are accompanying signs of internal conflict or interpersonal difficulty should a child's relative degree of sexual experience be investigated more closely as a potential problem. *The most significant variables are the meaning of the experience to a particular child and its role in his or her total life situation.*

Cases

An 11-year-old girl was discovered to be soliciting boys in her school to have sexual intercourse with her. Upon investigation, the school psychologist discovered that this girl had been engaged in an incestuous sexual relationship with her two older brothers from the age of 8 and was inappropriately presuming sexual contact with friends to be a means of exchanging affection.

The mother of a second 11-year-old girl showed concern when her daughter reported to her quite indignantly that she was being touched and handled by 13- and 14-year-old boys in her school. Upon further investigation, however, it was learned that the girl and several of her friends had developed an elaborate teasing game directed at receiving attention from the older boys. They expected the boys to respond in kind and were quite surprised and indignant when the attentions were returned in a more explicit and sexual fashion.

It is generally inappropriate to label any of the sexual behaviors of children as "deviant" *per se*. Strictly speaking, sexual behaviors labeled *deviant*—voyeurism, exhibitionism, fetishism, pedophilia, cross-dressing, and the like—describe the sexual behavior of postpubertal adolescents or adults and may reflect unresolved developmental issues. That is, these behaviors are in and of themselves somewhat "childlike" in that they reflect the failure of certain adults to integrate developmental tasks with mature genitality. As they are sexually socialized, children are quite naturally voyeuristic and exhibitionistic: watching and being watched are ways to learn about the world (including sex) and one's potential impact upon others in the world. Similarly, children's attachment to certain objects in their lives to provide security and comfort could be said to be a precursor to fetishism if such attachment is not generalized by children as they mature. And children will often engage in a variety of cross-sex behaviors as they struggle to integrate the diverse role requirements of their respective neighborhoods, schools, peer groups, and families. Even sexual contacts with children of a significantly younger age group can signify little more than an attempt to satisfy natural curiosity without fear of censorship. In a general sense, then, many of the normal sexual behaviors of children may contain elements that, when placed in the context of a later developmental stage, may reflect psychopathology. However, at a younger age and/or in a particular life situation, these behaviors may be seen as natural steps toward the integration of adult sexuality.

Nevertheless, these behaviors can present a diagnostic dilemma. Some are symptoms of severe emotional disturbance, and some are almost certainly developmental precursors to later sexual psychopathology in adulthood. The clinician is occasionally challenged to distinguish between a normal developmental phenomenon, a temporarily disruptive sex-related incident, and a manifestation of present or future pathology. Two factors aid the clinician in meeting this challenge. The first is his/her own knowledge of developmental sexuality against which to view the behavior in question. If a young patient's behavior appears significantly out of line with developmental expectations, then the clinician would do well to make note of this and investigate further. For example, a 7-year-old girl who has had sexual intercourse, a 9-year-old boy who wishes to dress up frequently in girls' clothing, and a 13-year-old boy who habitually attempts sexual contact with preschool children are all manifesting developmentally atypical behavior that may signal emotional and/or social maladjustment.

The clinician's other resource is the ability to ascertain the *meaning of the behavior to the child* and its role in the child's current life situation. In this regard, it is often advisable to interview other family members in order to obtain a more complete picture of the context in which the behavior is occurring. For example, sex-related behavior in children may reflect a challenge to parental authority, rebellion against family values, conflicts over familial role expectations, or even generalized family disturbance. The discovery of any of these factors argues for treatment directed toward altering the family's flexibility.

Occasionally, sexual behavior of an unusual sort may be a manifestation of a severe emotional disturbance, such as a psychotic episode. Significant intrapsychic or interpersonal problems may be symbolized by conflicted sexual behavior. And it is increasingly recognized by professionals that behavioral symptoms of unexplained origin may signify that the child is or has been a victim of physical or sexual abuse (Chapter 8).

Summary

The clinician can make substantial contributions to the healthy sexual development of children, both preventatively and remedially. When sex-related injuries, difficulties, or conflicts arise, the clinician can intervene with a combination of support, a sense of perspective, helpful information, and, when necessary, appropriate medical or psychiatric treatment. On a more regular basis, the clinician can provide helpful sex education and supportive counseling as children mature through the various developmental stages in which certain sex-related concerns and conflicts are both normal and predictable.

The clinician's tools for working with children on sexual concerns and problems are: (1) the use of the special nature of the clinical situation to talk openly about intimate subjects; (2) the comfortable use of sexually explicit language; (3) a perspective on sexual normality, i.e., the range and frequency of various sexual behaviors at various ages; (4) the provision of accurate sex information in response to questions or concerns; (5) the security of patient–clinician confidentiality within the limits of moral and legal guidelines for clinical practice; (6) the potential for contact with the entire family, along with the ability to enlist parents as allies and the capacity to facilitate communication between family members; (7) the use of specialized treatment skills for sex-related problems; (8) the knowledge of resources for further specialized treatment if warranted. Finally, and most importantly, the clinician can bring a genuine concern for the total health of his/her patients and an appreciation for the role of sexuality in that total health.

References

Abel, G. G., Murphy, W. D., Becker, J. V., and Bitar, A. Women's vaginal responses during REM sleep. *Journal of Sex & Marital Therapy,* 1979, *5*(1), 5–14.

Barbach, L. G. *For yourself: The fulfillment of female sexuality.* New York: Doubleday, 1976.

Broderick, C. B. Preadolescent sexual behavior. *Medical Aspects of Human Sexuality,* 1968, *2,* 20–29.

Carrera, M. A. (Ed.). Peer group sex information and education (Special Issue). *Journal of Research and Development in Education,* 1976, *10,* 50–55.

Cohen, H. D., and Shapiro, A. Vaginal blood flow during sleep. *Psychophysiology,* 1970, *7*(2), 338.

Eysenck, H. J., and Nias, D. K. *Sex, violence and the media.* New York: St. Martin's Press, 1978.

Ford, C. S., and Beach, F. A. *Patterns of sexual behavior.* New York: Harper and Brothers, 1951.

Gadpaille, W. J. *The cycles of sex.* New York: Charles Scribner's Sons, 1975.

Gagnon, J. H. Sexuality and sexual learning in the child. *Psychiatry,* 1965, *28,* 212–228.

Gagnon, J. H., and Simon, W. *Sexual conduct: The social sources of human sexuality.* Chicago: Aldine, 1973.

Gordon, S. *Let's make sex a household word: A guide for parents and children.* New York: John Day, 1975.

Harlow, H. F. *Learning to love.* New York: Jason Aronson, 1974.

Kaufman, G. *Meaning of shame: Toward a self-affirming identity.* Paper presented at the annual meeting of the American Psychological Association, New Orleans, 1974.

Kinsey, A. C., Pomeroy, W. B., and Martin, C. E. *Sexual behavior in the human male.* Philadelphia: Saunders, 1948.

Kinsey, A. C., Pomeroy, W. B., and Martin, C. E. *Sexual behavior in the human female.* Philadelphia: Saunders, 1953.

Kirkendall, L. A. Sex education. In M. S. Calderone (Ed.), *Sexuality and man.* New York: Charles Scribner's Sons, 1970. Pp. 121–135.

Lief, H. E., and Karlen, A. (Eds.). *Sex education in medicine*. New York: Spectrum Publications, 1976.

Maddock, J. W. Sex in adolescence: Its meaning and its future. *Adolescence* 1973, *8,* 325–342.

Money, J., and Ehrhardt, A. A. *Man & woman: Boy & girl*. Baltimore, Md.: Johns Hopkins University Press, 1972.

Prescott, J. W. Body pleasures and the origins of violence. *The Futurist,* 1975, pp. 64–74.

U.S. Commission on Obscenity and Pornography. *The Report of the Commission on Obscenity and Pornography*. New York: Bantam, 1970.

Zuckerman, M. Sexual behavior of college students. In W. W. Oaks, G. A. Melchiode, and I. Ficher (Eds.), *Sex and the life cycle*. New York: Grune & Stratton, 1976.

Gender Identity and Sex-Role Stereotyping: Clinical Issues in Human Sexuality

Rona Klein

Introduction

In our complex society, the physician's understanding of human sexuality must include an awareness of the sex-role perceptions that serve to shape female and male sexual behaviors. We must realize that, as Luria and Rose (1979) note, "sexual acts are performed in a social context."

During the past two decades, our social milieu has been characterized by shifts in the roles of men and women. Numerous examples exist. Recent reports, for example, indicate that only 6% of American families now fit the traditional image of two parents with a wife at home rearing the children and the husband working (Moroney, 1978). Over the past 25 years, women have entered the paid labor force in large numbers. As of 1978, more than 50% of all women aged 20–64 were employed or actively seeking employment (Special Population Subpanel, 1978). Current studies also reflect an increasing interest on the part of young fathers in nurturing and child-care activities (Lewis and Roberts, 1979), and one author reports that 69% of college men recently surveyed expect to spend as much time as their wives in bringing up their children (Katz, 1981). For the first time, as of 1980, the U.S. Census no longer required that the male member of a household be listed as its head (Bernard, 1981).

Many such changes, however, are as yet only surface alterations, beneath which traditional sex-role stereotypes persist. Effective psychiatric and medical health care must take these developments and their consequences into consideration. For many individuals, the conflict between internalized traditional gender norms and newer

Rona Klein • Stone Center for Developmental Services and Studies, Wellesley College, Wellesley, Massachusetts.

expectations contributes to emotional, psychological, and sexual difficulties. Consider, for example, the plight of the 45-year-old husband who complained of anger and loss of sexual interest in his wife, clearly related to her recent job promotion: "I want her to work and to be good at it. But I don't understand why, if she loves me, she can't arrange her schedule to get home and have dinner on the table at six o'clock, like in any normal home."

Sex-role stereotypes are defined as shared beliefs about the differing characteristics of woman and men that we all—physicians and patients alike—have absorbed from our culture. Kagan presented a concise description of our stereotyped beliefs about masculinity and feminity:

> In sum, females are supposed to inhibit aggression and open display of sexual urges, to be passive with men, to be nurturant to others, to cultivate attractiveness and to maintain an affective, socially poised and friendly posture with others. Males are urged to be aggressive in the face of attack, independent in problem situations, sexually aggressive, in control of regressive urges, and suppressive of strong emotions, especially anxiety. (Kagan, 1964, p. 143)

These stereotypes were replicated a decade later by the work of Bem (1974, 1976, 1978), Broverman et al. (1972), and others (Bernard, 1981; Pleck and Brannon, 1978). Thus, there is currently rather wide agreement that the traits clustering around competence, independence, rationality, control, and assertion characterize the traditional male stereotype, whereas warmth, expressiveness, and relatedness predominate in the traditional female stereotype. On the whole, despite some changes in the external structures of sex-role behavior, research findings have not yet disclosed much change in underlying traditional beliefs.

A modification of this view is found in Pleck's reanalysis of accumulated sex-role data suggesting that the conventional research focus on *differences* may obscure that "male and female stereotypes in content as well as in social desirability are not so different as usually thought (Pleck, 1978). Pleck notes, for example, that the Roper Organization's 1974 Virginia Slim poll indicated that 4000 subjects considered intelligence and sensitivity to the feelings of others to be the two most important traits for *both* men and women. Feminine traits traditionally perceived as "weakness" (such as the ability to ask for help or to openly express feelings) can also be seen as strengths necessary for success as an adult in modern times (Miller, 1976). The popular press, for example, relates a growing awareness that relationship skills and concern for the morale of workers are salient to effective business and political management. Perhaps sex-role research in the 1980s will be reflective of a more flexible differentiation between the sexes.

Gender Identity, Gender Role, and Sexual Orientation

It is helpful to define the terms *gender identity* (or sexual identity), *gender role* (or sex role), and *sexual orientation*. These terms are often used in the literature in ambiguous and confusing ways. In particular, the terms *gender identity* and *sexuality* have each been used without distinction to describe both the person's internal sense of self and the preferred mode of sexual behavior. In this chapter, the term *gender identity* will be used to refer to a stable, subjective, comfortable sense of one's sex, of female-ness in females and maleness in males.

Gender role refers to everything that a person says or does to indicate the degree to which he or she is a male or a female in a particular culture. It is the public expression of gender identity. Likewise, gender identity is the private experience of gender role (Money and Ehrhardt, 1972). Gender role, as Pleck (1976) explains, includes all the psychological traits and social responsibilities that a person feels are gender appropri-ate. It is clear that the prevailing sex-role stereotypes play an important part in molding an individual's gender-role behavior.

It is important to differentiate the concepts of gender identity and gender role from those of sexual orientation. The latter refers to one's preferred adult sexual behavior as heterosexual, homosexual, or bisexual [Group for the Advancement of Psychiatry (GAP) Committee on College Students, 1975]. The traditional view of the healthy woman and man limits sexual preference to members of the opposite sex. However, current literature describes a healthy person as having a homosexual (or a bisexual) orientation without necessitating confusion in gender identity or gender role (Luria and Rose, 1979; Luria, 1980). Virtually all lesbians and male homosexuals feel that they are women and men, and, as children, they felt like girls and boys. It is likewise true that individuals can express a wide variety of gender-role behaviors without confusion in their gender identity or disturbance in sexual orientation. In fact, the evidence indicates that good psychological adjustment and intellectual performance are positively correlated with a high degree of cross-sex interests (Pleck, 1975).

In evaluating patient concerns regarding the development of gender identity, gender role, or sexual orientation, it is critical that the clinician be able to differentiate issues in one sphere of development from the others. For example, if a parent is worried that a 3-year-old son is gay because he loves playing with dolls or that a 9-year-old daughter is lesbian because she zealously plays baseball, it can be terribly important that the clinician maintain perspective and not jump to a hasty conclusion.

Although gender-identity disorders and problems in sexual orientation will not be a particular focus in this chapter, it is pertinent to note, briefly, that marked effeminate ("sissy") behavior in boys has been reported to foreshadow later homosexual, trans-sexual, or transvestite orientation (Luria & Rose, 1979; Luria, 1980; Green, 1974). Perhaps this is related to the social ostracism experienced by "sissy" boys. Young girls, however, have somewhat more latitude in acceptable sex-role behaviors (GAP Committee on College Students, 1975). For example, tomboyism is frequently part of the repertoire of the developing heterosexual female.

Changing Attitudes and Behaviors

Any discussion of sex-role stereotyping and human sexuality would be incomplete without a consideration of the "double standard" by which males are given permission to take part in premarital intercourse but females are censured for doing so. The double standard has partly been based on two misconceptions about the biology of men and women: first, that sex is biologically necessary and more enjoyable for men, and second, that women are constitutionally less interested in sex, less in need of sexual gratification, and less sexually aggressive (Gross, 1978; Schwartz and Strom, 1978). These beliefs provided a biological foundation for the late Victorian attitude that only lower-class or depraved women could engage in sex with any enjoyment (GAP Committee on College Students, 1975; Luria and Rose, 1979). Perhaps this attitude was related to the fear prevalent at the time that uncontrolled sexual activity would lead to debilitating illness in men; or it may have been related to a fear that women's enjoyment of sex would lead to a dissolution of "moral" family life. Thus, the "modest" woman, without sexual appetite, was believed to save her husband from moral depravity and from serious injury to his health. William Acton, a Victorian physician, who published what is considered to be a definitive work on Victorian sexuality, wrote

> I should say that the majority of women (happily for them) are not very much troubled with sexual feeling of any kind. What men are habitually, women are only exceptionally. It is too true, I admit, as the divorce courts show, that there are some few women who have sexual desires so strong that they surpass those of men. . . . As a general rule, a modest woman seldom desires any sexual gratification for herself. She submits to her husband, but only to please him; and, but for the desire of maternity, would far rather be relieved from his attentions. (Acton, cited in Luria and Rose, 1979, p. 104)

From these myths evolved the traditional sex-role stereotypes according to which men are to be sexually aggressive and women are to reserve their sexuality for love and marriage and to be sexually inhibited in general.

On a progressive note, Luria and Rose (1979) describe a recent decline of this double standard, at least on the American college campus. They cite several studies showing an equal incidence of premarital sex for college men and college women. Katz (1981) reports data collected from over 6000 college students, showing that by 1975, 90% thought premarital intercourse acceptable for both genders. This contrasts with pre-1950 surveys, according to which the incidence of intercourse for college women ranged from 13 to 33% and that for college men ranged from 52 to 58%. These statistics appear to reflect the emergence of new norms for sexual attitudes and behavior of females and males.

Clinical assessment of patients must incorporate an awareness of these changing norms, so that diagnostic and treatment decisions are not made on the basis of a physician's personal sex-role values. For example, when a woman makes a well-considered choice not to have children, it is important that her physician not automatically see her as "unfeminine" or "neurotic." It is likewise important that a man not be labeled abnormal just because he wishes to work part-time in order to assume more household responsibilities and to allow his wife more freedom for her own pursuits.

Early Determinants of Sex Roles

In this culture, gender distinction is a powerful organizing principle of one's cognitive and emotional orientation to others and to the world. From birth, a person's sex is a prime determinant of how he or she is treated and socialized. Parents enter labor and delivery rooms with preformed fantasies and expectations connected to the future gender of their child. The exclamation "It's a girl!" or "It's a boy!" automatically sets off a chain of dimorphic responses in language and behavior of the medical personnel, parents, and relatives. This is seen in the use of gender-specific nouns, pronouns, and even colors. Dimorphism is also reflected in nurturing; Moss (1974) reports that mothers differentially vocalize to their infants and handle them differentially according to the infants' sex. All this conveys subtle gender meanings to a baby (Money and Ehrhardt, 1972; Kleeman, 1971).

Rubin et al. (1974) have reported a study that dramatically illustrated the impact of gender labeling—that is, designating a baby "boy" or "girl." They asked primiparous parents to describe their babies during their first day. Daughters were already described as "soft, fine-featured, and little," whereas sons were seen as "hard, large-featured, and big." Interestingly, objective raters did not find a realistic basis for the parents description. Sex-role stereotypes had clearly influenced parents' perceptions.

In a parallel manner, sex-role stereotyping influences physicians' and patients' perceptions of each other. This chapter will aim at understanding the effects of these gender-related issues on patient care. Initial sections will review basic research findings and current theories in the fields of sex-role stereotyping, gender identity, gender-role development, and sex differences. The last section will more specifically discuss the influence of unconscious stereotyping on the doctor–patient relationship and on clinical interventions in human sexuality. Clinical vignettes will be used wherever possible to emphasize particular points.

Sex-Role Stereotyping in Clinical Practice: Research Findings

The past decade has witnessed the emergence of a growing body of literature exploring the role of sex bias and sex-role stereotyping in health care, particularly in psychotherapy. The reliability of the research in this field is limited by the fact that it is based almost entirely on questionnaire studies rather than on direct observations of clinical interactions. The volume of work and the extent of agreement among the studies do, however, allow for some general conclusions. Most recently, Sherman (1980) has compiled evidence from over 50 studies in the field. Based on her review of the data, she concluded: (1) that therapists' sex-role values do influence clinical interactions; (2) that sex-role discrepant behaviors are likely to be judged as more maladjusted; and (3) that there is sex-role stereotyping in standards of mental health for men and women.

A seminal study by Broverman et al. (1970) demonstrated what has come to be known as the double standard of mental health. The subjects in this study consisted of 79 practicing clinicians, ages 25–55, male and female. They were asked to rate the Stereotyped Questionnaire, an instrument consisting of 122 polarized typical masculine and feminine items, such as very aggressive/not at all aggressive, and very rough/very gentle. The subjects were divided into three groups: One group was asked to indicate on each item the pole to which a healthy adult would be closer, another group was asked to rate the items for a healthy male adult, and the third group was asked to rate the items for a healthy female adult.

For both male and female clinicians, the concept of a healthy male was synonymous with the concept of a healthy adult, sex unspecified. Mentally healthy traits, such as aggressiveness, independence, objectivity, activity, and logic, were ascribed more often to the healthy man than to the healthy woman. In contrast, the clinicians' descriptions of a healthy, mature woman was characterized by a group of socially undesirable and seemingly unhealthy traits. That is, healthy women were perceived to differ from healthy men and adults by being more submissive, more emotional, more easily influenced, less independent, less adventurous, and less competitive. The Broverman team indicated that women in our culture are in a double bind. Women who are healthy and adultlike cannot be feminine in the traditional sense; and women who are feminine cannot be competent, fully functioning adults.

Sherman (1980) reports studies by Miller (1976) and Bowman (1976) as providing corroborating evidence for the double standard. Miller administered bogus therapy protocols to 67 clinicians and found that they rated a very passive protocol as better adjusted when it was labeled *female* than when it was labeled *male*. In addition, Miller found that more therapists chose passivity as the focus of therapy when the protocol was labeled *male* than when it was labeled *female*. Bowman's results were similar in that active responses (as opposed to passive responses) were discouraged by therapists for female protocols.

The concept of a lower standard of mental health for women has important treatment ramifications. The clinician who has internalized this is more likely to see dependent, compliant, or unassertive behavior in women as appropriate rather than problematic and, therefore, more likely to be accepted than worked on. One patient recently described her own insight into this dynamic:

> Mrs. R. was a 28-year-old professional woman with a 6-year history of myasthenia gravis. Her illness had developed during the latter part of her training in a health-related field. Following thymectomy, Mrs. R's physical illness was controlled, and she was able to finish her training and obtain a good job in her field. Her return to her professional pursuits was based upon a thoughtful weighing of all the pros and cons involved.
>
> Mrs. R. was referred to therapy for treatment of depression related to her recent realization at her inability to express her own needs and feelings, particularly anger, in work relationships. She came from a traditionally oriented, large Catholic family in which "girls were born and raised to become housewives." In order to pursue her own career goal, Mrs. R. had to rebel against her family's concept of her as less competent than her brothers and less entitled to her own interests. However, Mrs. R's ability to achieve academically contributed to her sense of self-worth and encouraged her to persist in her plans.
>
> In the course of therapy, Mrs. R. learned that her lack of assertiveness and depression were connected to an underlying fear that her parents would hate her for choosing a "deviant" path. For a long time Mrs. R. had warded off her anxiety and guilt by "making sure she was extra nice and cooperative to everyone." This worked until a new person was added to the office staff whose demands could never be met.
>
> Mrs. R. also expressed concern that her internist had contributed to her

conflict by communicating in subtle ways his own disapproval of her career strivings. He could not appreciate that the sense of competence and health she derived from her job helped her to cope with her chronic illness. Despite her overall stability, Mrs. R. noted that busy periods at work were associated with the increased fatigue at the end of the day, a price she thought worth the gains in self-esteem. However, if she reported symptoms to her doctor, he would remind her that if she weren't so "stubborn" and quit her job she would not have these symptoms. He often asked her why she needed to be "so ambitious."

Mrs. R. also described that when she was accompanied by her husband, the internist related to him in a "macho manner, shooting the breeze about sports and work," subjects that she was equally interested in. "After a while, he would turn to me, his demeanor changed, and he would only be interested in my physical symptoms."

In this situation, the physician seemed to view active, independent strivings as less appropriate for his pateint than a passive acceptance of her physical problems. His inability to separate his own agenda from his patient's complicated her conflict over her own goals.

There is a general impression that sex-role stereotyping has become less pervasive in the last decade. A study by Aslin (1977) demonstrated a shift in attitude from the double standard theory. Aslin administered the same sex-role stereotype questionnaire used by the Broverman team in 1970 to female ($n = 75$) and male ($n = 55$) community mental health center (CMHC) psychotherapists and also to feminist therapists ($n = 82$). The therapists were each asked to rate one of the following four groups: mentally healthy adults, females, wives, or mothers. Female CMHC and feminist therapists were found to have consistent views of normal mental health for all four groups, suggesting that they had just one standard of mental health for everyone.

This was contrasted by the male CMHC therapists, who demonstrated a modified double standard. They perceived mentally healthy adults as more masculine than they perceived mentally healthy females, wives, or mothers. Interestingly, though, the male therapists perceived women labeled *wife* as being more similar to a healthy adult than women labeled *mother* or *female*.

Data from a study by Engelhard et al. (1976) also suggest a decline in sex-role stereotyping in therapy. However, the same study indicated a "conservative attitude toward working mothers." So perhaps not all stereotypes change equally but vary according to expectations evoked by specific labels, the term *wife* evoking more liberal expectations than the terms *mother* or *working mother*.

Given the dearth of direct observational evidence, it is very hard to be sure that sex-role stereotyping is really becoming less of an issue. Clinicians' responses on questionnaires may not be reflective of their actual behavior:

> A nod, a smile, a reinforcement may display an attitude which the therapist may not be able to appreciate intellectually or of which he may not even be aware. For example, a male therapist may indicate in a questionnaire that he values independent behavior for female clients. Nevertheless, during an actual therapy session he may smile approvingly or nod when the female client is more dependent upon him and, by

the same token, he may fail to signal his approval of her moves toward independence. Similarly, in an interactional situation, if a female client becomes assertive, he may feel that she is being aggressive and react by emitting disapproval behavior or negative reinforcement. He may be totally unaware of this tendency, and quite oblivious of this bias when asked to assess his attitudes on an "objective" questionnaire. In private, male therapists are usually willing to reveal their stereotypic attitudes toward women. But these same therapists who sincerely present themselves in public on question-naires as being very flexible and liberated may, in fact, not have flexible liberated attitudes at all when they are off guard. (Of course a similar argument applies to female therapists.) (Franks, 1979, p. 463)

Lennane and Lennane (1973) have described the role of sex-role stereotyping in producing a greater prevalence of psychosomatic diagnoses for women. They report that although scientific evidence suggests that there are clear organic etiologies for primary dysmenorrhea, nausea of pregnancy, pain in labor, and infantile colic, these problems have been persistently diagnosed as psychogenic disorders of women. Fur-thermore, women complaining of these difficulties have been perceived as "neurot-ic," "weak," and somehow responsible for their own pain and, therefore, not entitled to symptom relief. The Lennanes concluded that this was a "form of sexual preju-dice," seriously inhibiting the doctor's ability to relieve the patient's symptoms.

Patients who complain of functional, or psychosomatic symptoms present a com-plex problem to clinicians. Data regarding sex differences in psychosomatic conditions were recently reviewed by Seiden (1979) showing a general female preponderance in the incidence of almost all psychosomatic symptoms. Seiden suggests that this may reflect a "different vocabulary of distress as opposed to a differential incidence of an illness." Nevertheless, physicians react to psychosomatic symptoms as less valid, especially if they are reported by a woman patient, whose report is often anticipated to be "hysterical" or "exaggerated." This emotional reaction on the part of the physi-cian clouds his/her ability to heed the distress communicated via the symptom.

In discussing the woman patient, Notman and Nadelson (1978) note that "func-tional symptoms may be seen as manipulative, deceitful or foolish. The patient's anxiety and pain are dismissed as in her head and, therefore, not deserving of serious attention and concern." For example, a recent report given at the American Pain Society meeting indicated that even when a female is in the hospital and in pain, her discomfort is likely to be underestimated and to go untreated; pain medication was less frequently prescribed for female hospitalized patients as compared to male hospitalized patients and frequently withheld even when prescribed (American Psychiatric Associa-tion, 1981).

The following case illustrates the importance of avoiding sex-role bias in evaluat-ing physical complaints in a female patient:

Ms. D., a 26-year-old successful professional came to therapy with a variety of functional gastrointestinal symptoms associated with underlying feelings of worthlessness and work anxiety. Prior to therapy, she became very dependent on frequent contacts with her internist, and it was at his urging that she sought psychotherapy. Ms. D. was able to use therapy to understand and change her behavior and to solidify an ability to cope directly with her conflicts rather than express them somatically. Soon after establishing a termination plan with her therapist, Ms. D. developed epigastric pain and nausea, followed by a recurrence of depressive symptoms. The possibility that these emotional and physical symptoms were related to conflicts over independence and termination was actively explored in her therapy. However, by the third week it became clear to both the patient and her psychiatrist that her persisting symptoms made no sense in terms of the psychological gains Ms. D. had made. It was decided that the patient should actively pursue a medical evaluation to rule out organic illness.

Ms. D. returned to her internist, who concluded, after a negative physical examination, that her symptoms were again due to her "nerves." The internist was reluctant to do further testing at that time and encouraged Ms. D. to reconsider whether she was ready to end therapy. With the patient's permission, the therapist and internist conferred, enabling them to resolve the latter's concern that he not encourage "hysterical" or "clingy" behavior in his patient. A medical work-up was begun, in the course of which Ms. D. became jaundiced. Surgical exploration confirmed the diagnosis of carcinoma of the head of the pancreas. Two months before her death, Ms. D. told her doctors how important it had been to her positive sense of self that they had respected her psychological strength and had taken her somatic symptoms seriously.

Nadelson and Notman note the difficulties that physicians have in separating their role as patient's caretaker from their role as society's agent (Notman and Nadelson, 1978; Nadelson and Notman, 1977). A pertinent factor is that physicians are subject to the differential standard of morality in our culture that condemns its women for the same behavior it encourages for its men, especially in the sexual sphere. Awareness of this social bias is of particular importance in the treatment of the woman patient who has contracted venereal disease or who has been raped. The physician who is not alert to this may, by his or her own behavior, unwittingly contribute to the social and self-criticisms of such patients, whereas the physician sensitive to this issue will be able to respond in a more constructive manner. The following vignette is illustrative:

A beautiful, bright 33-year-old divorced woman came to therapy to understand her pattern of self-destructive heterosexual relationships. A year after her divorce she contracted herpes genitalis. After her initial outrage at her unfaithful lover abated, she was overwhelmed with feelings of guilt and shame. This affliction seemed to confirm her inner sense of defectiveness and to be just punishment for her "sin." Her gynecologist's unsympathetic and abrupt attitude served as further proof of her badness. Despite her loneliness, she avoided romantic contact with men for more than 2 years, feeling that she was doomed to "justifiable rejection." She changed gynecologists, not being able to face the old one. The new gynecologist sensitively encouraged her to discuss her feelings about her condition and gave her a chance to ask detailed questions about its prognosis. This physician's nonjudgmental and accepting intervention helped Mrs. S. to realize that she was punishing herself needlessly and that she was deserving of further help. She began psychotherapy soon afterward.

An Evolving Psychology of Sex Roles: Is Biology Destiny?

The traditional theory of sex-role development proposes that women and men differ from each other in many psychological and behavioral areas and that these differences have an extensive biological basis. It further proposes that a secure gender identity is tied to accurately learning "appropriate" sex-differentiated personality traits, interests, and behaviors that then affirm biological sex. In fact, failure to develop these sex-appropriate characteristics is believed to result in grave deficiencies in gender identity and life adjustment. These ideas are representative of what Pleck (1976) calls the "traditional psychology of sex roles," which proposes that the familiar division by sex of work and domestic responsibilities is essential to the development of healthy women and men.

The belief that biological gender is so critical has important clinical implications. This belief fosters feelings of shame and guilt when individuals diverge from stereotyped sex-appropriate scripts. Indeed, those who have chosen deviant paths have been misperceived as "ill" rather than self-directed. An equal disservice can occur if a clinician fails to understand painful intrapsychic conflict masked by conformist choices (Nadelson et al., 1978a; Lerner, 1978a). For example, a woman's decision to get pregnant may stem from strong wishes to experience motherhood as an aspect of her feminine identity, but it might also represent an avoidance of fear of failing (or succeeding) at her work.

Although the controversy about nature versus nurture is not yet resolved, recent evidence indicates that what we have traditionally held to be true about sex-role development may not be true. Several authors (Pleck, 1976; Luria and Rose, 1979) have begun to articulate a "new psychology of sex roles." They propose that individuals do not have an innate need to conform to sex-role stereotypes in order to feel secure in their sense of gender. For example, it has been noted that no one would question the masculinity of Roosevelt Grier (former defensive tackle for the Los Angeles Rams), who happens to enjoy doing needlepoint as a hobby (Luria and Rose, 1979)!

The new theory of sex-role development emphasizes a dynamic, interactive process through which biological forces are modified by social forces. Pleck (1976) points out that the important factors limiting sex-role development are more likely to be found within our social structures than within individual psychobiology. He states that

> what ultimately limits change in women's role is not women's psychological ambivalence about achievement—though women *are* socialized to have this ambivalence, and it is important—but the absence of support for this change in work and family. What ultimately limits men's ability to change is not innate male needs for dominance or for "security" in their sex role identities—though men *are* socialized to have these concerns—but the current institutionalized structure of the male work role, which is incompatible with role change. (Pleck, 1976, p. 197)

The new psychology of sex roles draws its ideas from the fields of biology, psychology, sociology, and psychoanalysis. The following sections will review some important research contributions from each field.

Biological Research

As noted by Baill and Money (1980), chromosomes do not directly determine psychosexuality, but they are the first step. Initially, each baby is equipped with primordia of both male (Wolfian) and female (Mullerian) duct systems. During the third fetal month, if an embryo is genetically male, the Y chromosome will determine the presence of H-Y antigen, which will then stimulate the fetal gonads to develop into testes. In the absence of the Y chromosome, the same fetal gonads will, in the fourth month, develop into ovaries instead of into testes.

Continued male differentiation is determined by the presence of the testicular hormones, androgen and Mullerian inhibiting substance. Androgen is required for the development of the Wolfian duct system into male internal genitalia and for the later development of male external genitalia. Mullerian inhibiting substance inhibits the development of the female duct system. The development of female internal and external genitalia is dependent only on the absence of testicular hormones. Female differentiation can be said to be "the basic blueprint" for genital differentiation (Baill and Money, 1980, p. 47). The absence of ovaries or testes (or the failure of androgen secretion) will lead to female differentiation, regardless of chromosomal sex.

Animal experiments involving rats, guinea pigs, and rhesus monkeys provide data indicating that fetal and maternal androgens have an effect not only on genital morphology but also on the developing fetal brain, mediating subsequent adult sex-linked behavior (Money and Ehrhardt, 1972; Friedman, Rickart, and Vande Wiele, 1974; Baill and Money, 1980; Luria and Rose, 1979). For example, female rhesus monkeys treated prenatally with testosterone will invariably show masculinized play and sexual behaviors (Phoenix, 1974). Obviously, similar hormonal manipulations are not ethically possible on the human level. However, clinical cases of human hermaphroditism have functioned as natural experiments for the study of prenatal hormonal contributions to human gender.

Money and Ehrhardt's (1972) studies of genetic females who were androgenized *in utero* parallel the data from animal experiments. The authors carefully observed 15 girls with adrenogenital syndrome (AGS), a condition in which an enzyme defect transmitted as a genetic recessive prevents the adrenal cortex from producing normal levels of cortisol. This enzymatic defect leads to excess production of pituitary adrenocorticotropin and adrenal androgens (androstenedione, testosterone, 11β-hydroxyandrostenedione, and possibly dehydroepiandrosterone) (Stempfel and Tomkins, 1966). The timing of the androgen release results in a female fetus with normal internal genitalia but varying degrees of masculinization of the external genitalia (such as clitoral enlargement or fusion of the labia majora). The girls included in this study were all surgically feminized early in infancy and maintained on cortisone replacement therapy to prevent postnatal developmental masculinization. They were all reared as girls.

Overall, observations indicated that the girls unquestionably developed normal female gender identities and roles. Nevertheless, Money and Ehrhardt stressed what they felt to be important differences in their subjects. When compared to normal controls, the AGS girls showed an increase in tomboyish behavior and interests: They preferred playing with boys rather than other girls, enjoyed active outdoor play rather than play with dolls, preferred slacks to dresses, showed little interest in future motherhood, and preferred careers to marriage. These results were interpreted by the Money team as indicating that the postnatal gender identity and behavior of these girls were partly determined prenatally by the effect of fetal androgens on the brain.

In retrospect, it is hard to assess whether the tomboyism found in the AGS girls was more related to prenatal androgen or to the factors in the postnatal environment. First, the girls did not *look* like normal female babies at birth and their initial appearance may have influenced parental expectations and behavior toward them. Second, the effects of maintenance cortisone treatment in childhood cannot be discounted. The behavioral characteristics of the treated girls may have resulted from as yet undetected side effects of the artificial restoration of cortisone. Furthermore, mother interviews were an important source of information in this study; but prior knowledge of their daughters' medical history may have biased maternal reporting.

Another point of caution is that Money and Ehrhardt did not consider in their discussion of the evidence the fact that the behaviors shown by androgenized girls are also frequently shown by nonandrogenized girls. For example, a 1977 study showed that tomboyism was reported more than 50% of the time by samples of female junior-high students, college undergraduates, and noncollege adult women (Hyde et al., 1977). The behavior they described is widespread and fully consistent with a normal female gender identity.

Money and Ehrhardt (1972) have studied several other clinical hermaphroditic conditions in their investigation of the determinants of gender identity. One group consisted of ten genetic males born with androgen-insensitivity syndrome (testicular feminization). These subjects were born with feminized external genitalia (but masculine internal genitalia) due to an inability of their tissues to respond to fetal testicular androgen. The syndrome involves a genetically transmitted biochemical defect that is thought to be enzymatic but has not yet been specifically identified. The proposed site of action is within any cell of the body that is usually responsive to androgen. Each of the ten subjects had been assigned and reared as a female from birth. Nine of them developed firm feminine gender identities. They rated themselves as fully content with the female role. The tenth ''girl'' was ambivalent. Thus, for 90% of the ''girls,'' postnatal environmental factors were more important in shaping gender identity than either their chromosomal makeup or the histology of their gonads.

The study of human hermaphrodites has led Money and his colleagues to conclude that prenatal factors make some contribution to gender identity (Money and Ehrhardt, 1972; Ehrhardt and Baker, 1974; Baill and Money, 1980). Nevertheless, in contrast to the lower species, human gender-identity differentiation is *not automatically* determined by prenatal biological factors.

Chromosomal and hormonal factors influence gender identity and role in subtle ways. They may perhaps contribute to the development of temperamental differences between and within the sexes or they may possibly lay down behavioral predispositions. But, in humans, these prenatal factors are strongly modified by environmental and social conditions and are not a valid basis for the prescription of social roles.

This principle is most dramatically demonstrated by a case, reported by Money and Ehrhardt (1972), in which male (XY) identical twins developed different gender identities. At 7 months of age a faulty circumcision destroyed the penile tissue of one of the twins. At 17 months, the parents began implementing a medical recommendation to reassign the injured child as a girl. The parents immediately began changing their behavior toward the penectimized child in gender dimorphic ways, giving it a girl's name and emphasizing feminine dress and hairdo. Money and Ehrhardt report several charming vignettes illustrating the mother's sex-related patterns of expectations and cues in rearing her two children. For example, the mother was stricter about sexual immodesty and genital play with her daughter than with her son. When the boy "took a leak in my flower garden . . . he was quite happy . . . I started laughing. . . ." When the girl, however, "took off her panties and threw them over the fence . . . I gave her a little swat on the rear and I told her that nice little girls didn't do that. . . ." (Money and Ehrhardt). The mother also had different attitudes regarding physical activity for her son and daughter: "of course, I've tried to teacher her not to be rough . . . she doesn't seem to be as rough as him . . . of course I discouraged that. I teach her more to be polite and quiet" (Money and Ehrhardt, 1972). By age 4½, the daughter was quite different from the son—neater, daintier, and interested in feminine activities, such as dollplay and helping her mother in the kitchen. Thus, from two genetic males (with the aid of surgery for genital congruence) socialization forces produced one male child and one female child.

Material from a second sex-reassignment case illustrates the important role of the father in reinforcing gender conforming behavior of children. The following excerpt describes the behavior of a father whose second male child was born with hypospadiac microphallus and subsequently was reassigned to be a girl:

> "It's a great feeling of fun for me to have a little girl. I have completely different feelings towards this child as a girl than as a boy." He had noticed a change in his behavior towards his daughter compared to his son: "I treat my son quite differently— wrestling around, playing ball." He said that he had done the same with the second child before sex reassignment. Now he avoided such things with the girl. He attempted to distinguish between "things you associate with fun for boys, and things for girls." (Money and Ehrhardt, 1972, p. 124)

Money and Ehrhardt propose that there is a critical point for the establishment of gender identity occurring between 18 months and 3 to 4 years. They point out that this is connected in time with the acquisition of language. Prior to 18 months of age it is possible to successfully reassign a child's sex (with appropriate surgical and hormonal aids). But they found that after 18 months, and especially after 3 to 4 years of age, sex reassignment is usually fraught with psychosexual difficulties. Individuals whose initial gender identity is ambivalent are, however, better able to adapt to late gender reassignment.

Imperato-McGinley and associates (1979) report an apparent exception to Money and Ehrhardt's formulations. The team studied male pseudohermaphrodites, all living in one of two isolated villages in the Dominican Republic, where the mutant gene for this disorder has established itself. The disorder entails a deficiency of 5-α-reductase. This enzyme normally converts testosterone in utero to dihydrotestosterone, which then virilizes the external genitalia of the XY fetus. Due to the lack of di-hydrotestosterone, the subjects studied were born with ambiguous-appearing external genitalia. At birth, many of the affected babies were thought to be girls and were reared as such. However, because synthesis of testosterone is normal, prenatal, neonatal, and pubertal exposure to testosterone proceeded normally.

At puberty, these "girls" failed to develop breasts. Instead, their voices deep-ened, testes descended into the scrotum, and they experienced growth of the phallus. However, they were sterile and did not have male placement of the urethral opening. This virilization occurred in response to normal levels of testosterone produced by the testes with the onset of puberty. According to the Imperato-McGinley team, 19 of the affected subjects had been unambiguously raised as "girls." They report the remark-able finding that after puberty 16 of these "girls" shifted to a male gender identity and male gender role, and a 17th girl shifted to a male gender identity but maintained a female role.

This natural experiment demonstrates the important contribution of androgens to the formation of a male gender identity. However, it cannot be concluded that an-drogens were solely responsible for the adolescent gender shift. The authors' statement that the gender change occurred in a "laissez-faire environment" is open to question. Their material does not rule out the operation of parental and/or societal practices that may allow for new sex-role assumption and that may, therefore, mediate the ex-pression of hormonal effects. Parents in the two villages are well aware of the existence of and familial nature of the disorder and the possibility that their daughters may later become sons. This expectation must have an important effect on how the parents relate to their children. Specific parental attitudes or practices may, thus, be instrumental in allowing the gender-identity shift to occur. Possibly, the very high status and greater privilege given to males in their culture help the adolescents to switch gender. The sheer magnitude of the biological contradictions to the original identity as girls may also be an important factor (Luria and Rose, 1979).

The authors feel that their study challenges the theory of the immutability of gender identity after 3- to 4 years of age. However, the parents' anticipation of later sex change in their daughters may lead to ambivalence in the initial female gender assignment. This initial ambivalence may lay the groundwork for future negotiation of gender change.

In summary, research evidence from the biological arena suggests that biological and sociocultural factors may all make important contributions to gender identity. The various factors are so complexly intertwined that it is not yet possible for researchers to separate the boundaries of the biological forces from the boundaries of the environmen-tal. What is clear is that prenatal, biological influences do not prevent human gender behavior from being strongly modified by social experience.

Research on the Psychology of Sex Differences

What are the actual differences and similarities between the sexes? What are the boundaries between these realities and our stereotyped beliefs? Where differences do exist, are they the result of innate forces or social stereotypes that could, therefore, be changed as society changes? The literature on the psychology of sex differences is composed of a large body of contradictory, inconsistent, and complicated studies of variable quality and validity. We cannot draw firm conclusions from this as yet rudimentary data base. We will, therefore, only be able to offer partial answers to the important questions raised.

One major limitation to accurately interpreting the evidence is that researchers tend to publish positive findings more readily than negative findings. Consequently, a few reports of sex differences become widely known and cited as representative of the whole field, whereas studies finding no sex differences go unattended. At times, even published studied are ignored. For example, Bell and Costello (1964) studied the relationship between sex and tactile sensitivity in the newborn in three separate tests. The results of the first two tests showed greater female tactile sensitivity, but these tests were characterized by low sample size and poor retest reliability. The third test, better designed and with a large sample size, found no sex differences. Despite this latter finding, Bell's work is frequently used as proof of neonatal sex differences (Birns, 1976). Moreover, there is a tendency to take the relatively few findings of early sex differences as evidence for biological determinism. Since we know that socializing forces are present from the very beginning, we cannot assume that an early occurring difference is necessarily an innate difference.

An interesting complication in sorting through the data is that studies published prior to the feminist movement of the late 1960s reported more sex differences than later studies. On the other hand, many of the earlier experiments were not aimed at studying sex differences; they used sex only as a control variable in the hopes that it would not turn out to be significantly related to the behavior under examination. Many of the early findings regarding sex differences were, therefore, incidental, rather than intentional and based on theoretical expectations. Since the late 1960s, however, researchers have been more interested in explicitly testing assumptions about sex differences.

Taken as a whole, the body of literature indicates that gender differences occur against a background of substantial similarities between the sexes. For most characteristics studied, the average differences between women and men are smaller than the range of individual differences within each sex. The distribution of gender-related characteristics can be conceptualized as two bell-shaped curves with differing means but with substantial areas of overlap. As one author comments, we would be more accurate to speak of "sex-related differences" rather than "sex differences," "meaning that an individual's score is statistically but not necessarily biologically related to the individual's sex" (Harris, 1979).

A Critique of Maccoby and Jacklin's Conclusions

Maccoby and Jacklin (1974) have published what is to date the most comprehensive review of the observational and experimental literature on sex differences. They used the "box score" method of organizing the results of 1600 studies published between 1966 and 1973. With this method, studies are categorized via various attributes and behaviors (e.g., compliance, self-esteem, and dependency). The results are then tallied as indicating either "Difference" or "None." Conclusions are drawn on the basis of the tallies.

A number of important reservations must be kept in mind about this method. The "box score" itself is a black-and-white method of tabulating the data that has a number of shortcomings. Several authors, for example, have noted the erroneous omission of studies from Maccoby and Jacklin's box score tables, as well as the inappropriate inclusion of other studies (Maccoby and Jacklin, 1974; Birns, 1976; Block, 1976; Caplan, 1979). Another concern is that the box score tally overemphasizes the null hypothesis such that results tabulated as "None" are interpreted as meaning "There is no sex difference with respect to . . ." when what is really meant is "No sex difference has been shown." (Maccoby and Jacklin, 1974, p. 5). This leads the reader to interpret the results as being strongly negative for sex differences when they are really inconclusive. Another problem is that younger age groups are disproportionately represented in the studies summarized by Maccoby and Jacklin, which may mask sex differences that require maturation or the accumulation over time of socializing influences and that may, therefore, not emerge until adolescence or beyond.

More detailed criticisms of Maccoby and Jacklin's work are available in reviews by Block (1976, 1978), Caplan (1979), and Birns (1976). These authors feel that the data substantiate more sex differences than are claimed by Maccoby and Jacklin and that socialization has a stronger role in producing these sex differences than Maccoby and Jacklin have acknowledged. For example, according to Block, evidence overlooked by Maccoby and Jacklin shows that beginning at age 2 or 3, boys are more active than girls. Boys are by then engaging in more gross motor activity, and they are more curious and exploratory, whereas girls are sitting still, attending, and being nondisruptive (Pedersen and Bell, 1970). Block also notes that numerous psychological studies indicate that girls comply with adult demands more readily than boys and that girls are more dependent in the sense that they seek more help from adults and maintain a closer proximity to home and teachers. In addition, Block's analysis of the data suggests that females do experience greater general anxiety than males.

Block (1976) and Caplan (1979) present convincing evidence that contradicts Maccoby and Jacklin's assertions that there are no differences between men and women in self-esteem and achievement orientation. Findings on self-confidence show that females underestimate their ability to perform at various tasks, in contrast to males who are optimistic in their assessments of how well they will perform, and also that females have less sense than males of being able to control their own fates (Crandall, 1969; Benton et al., 1969). Maccoby and Jacklin describe these differences as occurring only during the younger ages of 7 and 14. Girls seem to grow up believing that their achievements are due to external circumstances rather than their own skills and hard work.

Hypothesized Sex Differences

Despite these criticisms, Maccoby and Jacklin's conclusions are useful. They propose that there are sex differences in only four psychological areas. The areas are verbal ability, visual spatial skills, mathematics, and aggression. We will here summarize the evidence for these differences with an eye toward sorting out the social from the biological factors.

1. Girls appear to excel in *verbal ability*. Although somewhat inconsistent, the evidence suggests that girls acquire verbal skills earlier, presumably due to the earlier left-hemisphere maturation of females. Socialization experiences may reinforce the differences. For example, Moss noted that parents spend more time eliciting vocalizations from their infant daughters and that they in general show a "greater investment in the social behavior of their daughters than of their sons" (Moss, 1974, p. 151). Thus, it may be that girls' early neurological lead in language development predisposes them to being particularly responsive to such early-occurring social influences, which may then act to further reinforce linguistic modes of functioning.

According to Sherman's (1967) "bent twig" theory, girls early in life establish left-hemispheric, verbal modes of thought and problem solving and continue, with the influence of sex-typed experiences, to elaborate these modes (Maccoby and Jacklin, 1974). Presumably, girls' early preference for verbal modes eliminates a need for them to develop nonverbal (particularly spatial) modes of thought. Thus, although girls are practicing verbal skills and social interactions, boys are exploring the spatial aspects of their environment and are developing nonverbal modes of cognition (Harris, 1979). The accumulated effects of these differential experiences may contribute to the adolescent female's lead in verbal ability. However, as Harris notes, girls' greater reliance on verbal, left-hemispheric modes may work to their disadvantage in tasks for which these modes are not appropriate.

2. Boys excel in *visual-spatial ability*. This ability may be defined as the ability to mentally understand and manipulate two-dimensional and three-dimensional objects in space. Boys' lead in this ability begins in adolescence and increases through the high school years.

There is evidence, although not conclusive, that the sex difference in visual-spatial ability is related to a recessive X-linked gene, which is consequently expressed more frequently in males than in females. This, however, does not mean that visual-spatial ability is something that all males have entirely and that females lack completely. It means only that different proportions of each sex are likely to express the gene: 50% of men and 25% of women should show the trait phenotypically. However, as with all other human abilities, this one is genetically multidetermined, with other non-sex-linked genes playing a role as well. It is, thus, possible to have good genetic potential for spacial visualization without the X-linked gene. Indeed, the distributions of test scores for visual-spatial skills show that females and males overlap with some percentage of females doing better than the average male and some percentage of males doing worse than the average female (Harris, 1979).

Differences in cerebral specialization are also implicated in the sex difference in visual-spatial skills (Levy-Agresti and Sperry, 1968; Kimura, 1969; Galapurda et al., 1978). Early cerebral lateralization in girls seems to occur at what is a premature stage of the development of the right hemisphere (the spatial hemisphere) (Buffery and Gray, 1972). As a result, the right hemisphere in a woman is less specialized in spatial function than it is in a man, and, additionally, the right hemisphere in a woman has a greater degree of secondary cortical commitment to language (Harris, 1979, p. 171). The right hemisphere in males seems to be more efficient in its visual-spatial functioning.

Sex-typed socializing experiences, beginning in early childhood, are felt to have a salient role in the development of sex differences in spatial visualization. In fact, these differences emerge at adolescence when sex-role scripts become so important. Evidence indicates that experiences in object manipulation and visual-tactile exploration improve visual-spatial skills. Many of the cultural experiences that encourage these abilities are more available to boys. In this regard, it is important that clinicians understand the very different learning experiences provided by the kinds of toys and games typically given to boys and girls. Those for boys—cars and trucks, model planes and cars, erector sets, and balls—teach far more about form and structure than do the dolls and "domestic" toys usually given girls. This observation is supported by studies showing that training in visual-spatial skills improves functioning and wipes out the sex difference. Cross-cultural studies and studies of maternal practices indicate that opportunity to freely explore the outdoors, freedom to experiment with a variety of objects, and encouragement to be independent are all related to enhanced visual-spatial ability (Money and Ehrhardt, 1972; Harris, 1979).

The need for clinicians to understand this material is illustrated by the following case:

> A college student consulted her family physician about recurrent stomach aches, which were diagnosed as stress related. Discussions with her physician helped the student realize that a conflict between her fierce determination to become an engineer and her fear of failing in this pursuit was creating the stress. The student's parents had expressed grave doubts about any woman's ability to "make it" in a "man's profession" and, in addition, were openly concerned that she not waste the money being spent on her education. By serving as an educational resource and addressing their misconceptions about women's ability to learn engineering, the physician was able to resolve the student's and her family's anxieties.

In a similar situation, it may also be appropriate for a clinician to help a young woman sort out what extra training experiences (such as shop, drafting, and sculpture) she may need to be more prepared for training in engineering, dentistry, airplane piloting, or other fields particularly involving visual-spatial skills. Interestingly, studies show that engineering courses themselves increase spatial skills (Tobias, 1978; Harris, 1979).

3. Boys excel in *mathematics ability,* but, once again, the sex difference is delayed until age 12–13 and then increases with age beyond its first appearances. Preschool measures of quantitative ability and competence in grade school arithmetic are similar for girls and boys. Several explanations have been offered for these findings (Tobias, 1978).

One possibility is that girls' arithemetical skill reflects their greater ability to perform for their teachers in general during the grade school years but that higher levels of mathematics require more willingness to take risks and to withstand ambiguity than is characteristic of girls (Tobias, 1978; Maccoby and Jacklin, 1974). Another possibility, not yet confirmed, is that visual-spatial skills are more important in higher levels of math than in arithmetic.

Despite recent claims to the contrary, the most impressive explanations for the appearance in adolescence of the male lead in math comes from consideration of the effects of sex-role socialization (Kolata, 1980; Shafer and Gray, 1981). Tobias quotes a group of seventh graders who were asked why girls do as well as boys in math until the sixth grade but less well afterward. The girls answered: "Oh, that's easy. After sixth grade we have to do real math" (Tobias, 1978, p. 83). There is no biological evidence so far that "real math" should not be accessible to girls as it is to boys. Maccoby and Jacklin, in fact, assert that there is little evidence for sex linkage of the genetic determinants of mathematics ability. The girls' attitudes about their math ability appears to be an important variable. Evidence indicates that girls have less confidence in their ability to perform new tasks and this undoubtedly influences their attitude about math problems. Graham and Birns (1979, p. 299) report Fennema and Sherman's (1976) finding that "confidence was almost as highly related to achievement as were cognitive variables of verbal and spatial visualization."

As with visual-spatial skills, early experience with toys and games teaches boys much more about mathematical concepts than it teaches girls. Monopoly and playing store may teach girls about basic arithmetic, but these games don't give girls exposure to higher mathematics. On the other hand, boys often gain experience in applying concepts related to math and science. Boys' play involves dropping, spinning, or colliding in dramatic demonstrations of physical concepts. Boys have almost daily lessons in ratios and percentages in the computing of scores and batting averages; and the interception of footballs can give boys invaluable experience in using concepts of time, speed, and trajectory (Tobias, 1978).

Thus, girls and boys in our culture have quite different opportunities to practice mathematical concepts in situations that are meaningful to them. Another important cultural factor in the development of math skills is that children and adolescents are bombarded with cues from parents, teachers, the media, and peers that identify math and science with masculinity (Tobias, 1978). For example, packaging on erector sets, chemistry sets, and such have often shown pictures of boys alone. The textbooks used to teach mathematics further emphasize the association of math competency with boys and men by the use of examples that typically do not relate to females, or, if they do, portray them as baffled and confused. The intensified sex-role pressures of the high school years reinforce a stereotyped view of math and science as a more appropriate and more essential field of study for males than for females. The adolescent girl who doesn't want to seem different from her peers will begin avoiding displays of her mathematical ability. Hence, even girls who are talented in math and science take significantly fewer of these courses, a fact that is considered to contribute to the male lead in these areas.

It would be a mistake to underestimate the power of the message to girls that doing well in math will do them in socially! This message can interfere with their ability to learn math. Of equal concern, for those who succeed at math, it can be a source of anxiety about their femininity that lasts well beyond the high school years.

A rather successful, but depressed 40-year-old woman accountant recently provided an example of this clinical problem. In exploring the basis for her almost paralyzing fear that people will dislike her, she remembered that during her high school years her mother frequently warned her that "it is a mistake to get all A's, especially in math. You won't be popular with the boys!"

This woman had indeed been an "A" student in high school and especially gifted in math. She dealt with her fear that her mother's prophecy would come true by avoiding social interactions, and, thus, the chance of rejection. As a result, she never felt herself to be a girl or a woman but rather developed an image of herself as an unwanted, socially inept achiever.

According to Tobias (1978), the impact of the various socialization factors makes girls more vulnerable to math anxiety, which occurs when an individual is confronted for the first time with an idea or a new operation that seems totally beyond the realm of comprehension. Females who have this experience tend to assume that the problem is innate and unchangeable. They lose sight of the probability that all they need is to be patient and to give themselves extra time and help in digesting the new lesson. Instead they avoid asking the teacher questions and give up prematurely. They feel ashamed and guilty and fearful that at last everyone will find out how "stupid" they really are. Males, on the other hand, typically feel that if they are having a problem with math, it is due to a bad text or bad teaching rather than due to a nonmathematical mind. This attitude helps many males persist through bad experiences in math.

Math anxiety in women is a clinically relevant phenomenon. It can be an unrecognized cause of depression in adolescent and young adult women, particularly those who have perfectionistic academic standards. Because the wish to achieve academically often conflicts with a girl's sense of femininity, a female patient may be unable to recognize math anxiety as a legitimate cause for depression in herself.

4. Boys are found to be more *physically* and *verbally aggressive* than girls. For example, boys more than girls show modified forms of aggression such as rough-and-tumble play and aggressive fantasies as well as more direct forms of pushing and hitting (with intent to hurt). As Maccoby and Jacklin (1974) note, these differences in behavior have been observed in the school playground and wherever children are involved in free play.

Maccoby and Jacklin and other experts agree (Money and Ehrhardt, 1972; Ehrhardt and Baker, 1974) that there is a biological foundation for the sex differences found in aggression. Their reasons include: (1) Males are more aggressive than females in all human cultures for which there is data, and in subhuman primates as well. (2) Animal experiments provide strong evidence that aggressive behavior is related to levels of sex hormones, particularly testosterone, and that it can be changed by experimental manipulations of hormonal levels. For example, in one classic study, Young et al. (1964) showed that prenatal testosterone administration to female monkeys resulted in the females showing male levels of rough-and-tumble play postnatally. Experimental results indicate that prenatal and perinatal testosterone levels "set" the brain (presumably the hypothalamus) to produce sex-differentiated readiness to behave aggressively in response to relevant stimuli. Postnatally administered testosterone has also been shown to increase aggressive behavior in animals even without prenatal sensitization of the brain.

Nevertheless, hormones do not automatically determine human aggressive behavior (Ehrhardt and Baker, 1974). Maccoby and Jacklin (1974, p. 247) are careful to demonstrate that a person's aggressive behavior is strongly influenced by learning and that it is "strengthened, weakened, redirected or altered in form by her or his unique pattern of experience." The data indicate that one's testosterone level is an open system reciprocally influenced by experience. For example, an animal's testosterone will decrease when he is defeated in a fight and will increase if he wins.

Experimental observations of aggressive behavior in children show that learning plays an important role. Maccoby and Jacklin (1974) summarize pertinent experiments by Bandura, showing that sex differences in aggression may be more the result of socialization than of biological differences. In Bandura's work, children were offered a reward for performing as many of a model's aggressive responses as they could remember. Girls normally do less spontaneous copying of modeled aggression than boys do, but when a reward was offered the girls behaved similarly to the boys. Bandura concluded that girls and boys are not so different in their knowledge of aggression as they may seem to be but that girls are inhibited from expressing aggression by a fear of the negative consequences that they have been socialized to expect.

A similar conclusion was recently expressed by Caplan (1979), who noted that the experimental findings of greater aggression in boys were dependent upon the presence of an adult during the experiments. Caplan feels that evidence to date clearly indicates that girls have a stronger need to win adult approval and that it is this need that interferes with a girl's ability to express aggression in the presence of an adult. In fact, no sex differences in aggression were found in those studies where an adult was not present. Caplan stated that "Boys seem to behave more aggressively more often than girls; but when girls' concerns about adult approval are reduced, their increased freedom to express aggression seems in fact to result in an increase in the frequency of their aggressive behavior" (Caplan, 1979, p. 55).

Thus, it may be as Maccoby and Jacklin (1974) conclude that boys are, in fact, more biologically prepared to learn aggression. It, however, has become clear that the feminine woman is not by biological decree devoid of aggression. The evidence focuses our attention on a particular cultural reality: Girls are taught that truly feminine women must "learn to dismiss or suppress their anger, rather than to confront the subtleties of when and how to get mad or the rules of fair fight" (Kaplan, 1976, p. 356). Socialization restricts women in their freedom to express anger and aggression without excessive anxiety or guilt.

The research evidence points us toward the clinical prediction that our female patients will have particular difficulty with anger and aggression. Aggressive feelings threaten women more than they do men and on a variety of levels. Aggression threaten's a woman's self-concept and ego ideal. Awareness of her aggression leads a woman to feel guilty, inadequate, and to have diminished self-esteem. It also evokes intense fears of rejection from friends or loved ones. Hence, it is often very difficult for a woman to directly acknowledge or express her own aggression, which may then get channeled into less constructive outlets. It may be expressed in disguised forms, such as tears, apologies, guilt, and self-criticism and sometimes even in reaction formations, such as unsolicited favors or gifts. Aggression might also be transformed into the self-destructive symptoms or dysfunctional behaviors for which women seek professional attention (Lerner, 1978b, 1979).

Mothering is an adaptive channel for the expression of modified forms of female aggression in our culture. Women typically feel more comfortable about their aggressiveness when it exists in the form of service to others. However, for the most part, women experience taboos against their aggression to be generalized to its derivative forms as well (competition, achievement, assertion, initiation), which then become additional areas of conflict (Zilbach et al., 1979; Miller et al., 1981).

Lerner (1979) has observed that when describing a situation that should appropriately provoke anger men say "I was angry," whereas females usually say, "I was hurt." She clarifies that

> this phrase, "I was hurt," is a telling one. For when a legitimate anger cannot be acknowledged, recognized, and expressed women do, indeed, "hurt." Their hurt may take the form of headaches, fatigue, depression, or sexual disinterest. Or it may even express itself in intellectual dullness or lack of interest or capacity for creative and original work. (Lerner, 1979, p. 331)

Difficulties with aggression are so pervasive and harmful in women that it must be a priority in treating female patients to evaluate and address problems in this area (Kaplan, 1976, 1979b; Lerner, 1978b, 1979). The health professional can encourage mastery of these difficulties by acknowledging and accepting legitimate anger underlying a patient's symptoms as well as by helping patients express their anger in direct and appropriate ways. It is important, in this regard, that clinicians be open and interested rather than defensive or oblivious in response to anger directed at them by their female patients.

A common misinterpretation that clinicians make when confronted with an angry female patient stems from confusing the validity of *feelings* of anger with a problem in the *form of expression*. Since the direct expression of anger is terribly anxiety provoking and often a new experience for women, the anger may come out in a poorly controlled, incoherent, or explosive form (Lerner, 1979; Kaplan, 1976). The clinician who focuses on the form of expression of the anger without understanding the contents may conclude that the patient has more primitive emotional problems than she really does and may, therefore, write off the anger as "craziness."

The following case is a dramatic example of this kind of confusion:

> A married 38-year-old woman was referred for an emergency consultation by her internist who described her as being "problably on the verge of a nervous breakdown and perhaps suicidal." The internist received his information from the husband who described that his wife had "pushed him and made a terrible scene" at a party the night before. The husband assumed that for his wife to be so "out of control" it must mean that she was having a recurrence of the psychotic postpartum depression for which she had been treated 15 years ago. He feared that "anything might happen." As it turned out, the wife was an angry but articulate woman who for 18 years had denied her own feelings and had compliantly cooperated with her husband's desires for group sex and sadomasochistic games.

In the previous year, she had begun to reflect on her life and gained some insight into her rage at her husband and at herself. She made several efforts to explain her feelings to her husband, who had recently agreed to work with her on achieving a more mutual sexual relationship. It had been taken enormous efforts for the wife to make this request as she had always felt she "would agree to anything to keep her husband." She feared saying "no" meant losing him. When she noticed her husband embracing and kissing another woman at the party, she felt a "surge of rage" that she "deserved better treatment." She impulsively ran over and pushed her husband away from the other woman and then ran out of the house sobbing noisily.

For this patient, pushing her husband, although perhaps not the best method of assertion, expressed her sense of anger and protest. It proved to be the beginning of a phase of real personal growth rather than a regression toward insanity.

To summarize, Maccoby and Jacklin (1974) conclude that the evidence substantiates the existence of sex differences in aggression and three areas of intellectual ability, but they question other areas of presumed sex difference. They assert that the evidence disproves (1) that girls are more social and boys less so, (2) that girls are more "suggestible," (3) that girls have lower self-esteem, (4) that girls are better at rote learning and repetitive tasks, whereas boys are better at tasks requiring higher-level cognition, (5) that boys are more "analytic" in their thinking, (6) that boys are more affected by environment and girls more by heredity, (7) that girls are less motivated toward achievement, and (8) that girls are more auditory and boys are visual.

In addition, the authors review seven areas of presumed sex differences that they feel are still open to question: (1) competitiveness, (2) dominance, (3) activity level, (4) compliance, (5) nurturance, (6) tactile sensitivity, and (7) fear, timidity, and anxiety.

Self-confidence, Sex Differences, and Socialization

Hoffman (1972) suggests that sex differences in self-confidence may be secondary to the differences in early socialization experiences. Psychological studies show that girls are permitted and encouraged to be dependent upon their parents, that they receive less pressure to establish an identity separate from their mother, and that they experience less of the mother–child conflict that is so necessary to facilitate separation of self (Hoffman, 1972; Steckler and Kaplan, 1980). Boys, on the other hand, are discouraged from being dependent, pressured into giving up their childish ways, and given more opportunities to explore their environment. They learn early that they have to earn their sense of masculinity and self-esteem, whereas girls continue to depend on others for self-definition and approval (Bardwick and Douvan, 1972). Hence, boys learn to seek a "sense of effectance" through mastery and autonomous achievement. In the process, they develop important coping skills and confidence in the effectiveness of their skills.

On the other hand, girls, and women, learn from experience to seek a sense of competence through winning the help and approval of others (Hoffman, 1972). They are socialized to define achievement for women as successful affiliation rather than as mastery of their environment. This perspective challenges Maccoby and Jacklin's (1974) claim that there is no sex difference in achievement motivation. There may not be any measurable differences in the quantity of motivation, but there are important differences in the quality and direction of achievement motivation.

Given these characteristics of female and male socialization, it is not surprising that clinically we see a higher incidence of depression in women than in men (Weissman and Klerman, 1979). Women lack for autonomous sources of self-esteem, so that they are more vulnerable to loss and disappointment in interpersonal relationships. Likewise, it is not surprising that anxiety and pressure related to achievement expectations are important factors in the emotional, sexual, and physical symptoms of male patients.

From birth on, the biological and social determinants of behavior interdigitate and interact in very complex ways. Because this is so, and because the variables are so difficult to accurately define or to measure, it may be impossible at this point to definitively outline the extent to which sex differences are or are not innate. The age-old question "Which came first, the chicken or the egg?" seems applicable. Clearly, however, the evidence does prove that socialization plays an enormous role in producing and exaggerating the sex differences that do exist. This is true even for aggression and visual-spatial ability, the two areas of difference in which biology is most strongly implicated.

So, what is the clinical benefit of knowing that females and males differ in self-esteem, motivations toward achievement, aggression, etc., and that these differences are largely determined by cultural factors and learning experiences? On the practical level of service to the individual patient, such knowledge can facilitate the clinician's sensitivity to and understanding of those areas of functioning that are more likely to be a problem for one sex or the other, thereby leading to more appropriate treatment interventions. For example, a pediatrician who understands sex-role issues can more appropriately respond to parental anxieties about a female toddler's "unlady-like" forays into the world. This pediatrician can educate parents about the tendency to overprotect daughters and the ways in which this can limit a daughter's development of autonomous coping skills. On the level of more ideological goals, health professionals (in their roles as consultant, teacher, and public figure) are in a position to influence social institutions and expectations.

Currently, women and men occupy quite different political, social, and economic positions in society. Although women comprise over 40% of the labor force, they make up only a small minority of the total number of bank officials, industrial leaders, politicians, judges, scientists, and other professionals. They are instead concentrated in jobs of low prestige and low pay. Even when women have jobs or careers outside the home, they retain the primary responsibility for house and children (Special Populations Subpanel, 1978)! However, since it is socialization that largely determines these differences in social roles, societies have the option of developing parenting practices, training experiences, and other supports or structures to minimize rather than maximize sex differences that impair self-esteem and limit human potential. As put by Maccoby and Jacklin (1974, p. 374): "A society could, for example, devote its energies more toward moderating male aggression, or toward encouraging rather than discouraging male nurturance activities."

One positive outgrowth of the recent focus on sex differences has been a reassessment of traditional ideas of what constitutes a psychological strength versus a weakness. Clearly, at this point in history, women and men have different life experiences that lead them to develop different characteristics and motivations. Many of the sex differences that characterize women have been traditionally defined, by society and by women themselves, as less important. Recent psychological theory, however, recognizes that although some of these differences are problematic, some of them are very valuable (Miller, 1976). For example, women's sense of responsibility in relationships, their concern to not hurt others, and the satisfaction they derive from participating in the growth of others are all essential to the survival of our society.

The Acquisition of Sex Roles: Social-Learning Theories

What is the process by which socialization forces influence the development of the various differences between girls and boys, women and men? Several answers to this question have been proposed, falling largely within three social-learning theories: (1) direct reinforcement, also called *shaping,* (2) *modeling,* and (3) cognitive developmental. Maccoby and Jacklin (1974) conclude, on the basis of their review of the relevant literature, that all three processes are to some degree involved in the acquisition of sex-differentiated behavior.

Direct Reinforcement and Sex-Role Socialization

This process of direct reinforcement refers to the "shaping" of boys' and girls' behavior by adult use of praise or discouragement, resulting in sex-typed behavior. The term *sex-typed behavior* may be defined as "role behavior appropriate to a child's ascribed gender" (Sears et al., 1965). In regard to this process, Maccoby and Jacklin (1974, p. 339) summarize that there is "surprisingly little differentiation in parent behavior according to the sex of the child." However, despite this negative conclusion, they do report evidence that when sex-typing is narrowly defined (e.g., toy preference), parents do seem to "shape" their children differentially; they encourage sex-appropriate modes of dress, play, interests, goals, and even chores. Parents begin to exert this kind of sex-typing pressure before their children reach age 3. There is wide agreement that sex-typing, even when narrowly defined, conveys important sex-role information to the child and has broad implications for the development of adult behaviors and motivations.

Several authors, however, present evidence that Maccoby and Jacklin (1974) underestimate the magnitude of differential socialization practices (Birns, 1976; Block, 1973, 1978; Caplan, 1979). They cite a number of factors that handicapped Maccoby and Jacklin's ability to interpret the data: (1) the lack of information about the sex-typing behavior of fathers and of working-class families; (2) the small sizes of research samples; (3) the lack of information about the rearing of children over age 6; and (4) the lack of specificity of experimental hypotheses, as well as the unreliability of experimental instruments.

Block (1978), in particular, presents evidence suggesting that parents do socialize their children differentially according to sex. She presents cross-cultural data from extensive studies comparing the child-rearing practices of parents of female and male children. Her data come from a large sample (696 mothers, 548 fathers, 1227 students from six different countries) and is well balanced. It was collected from parental self-reports and from college students reporting on parental behavior.

The results describe several areas of sex-differentiated parental behavior, with striking similarity across cultures and equally striking consistency between the reports of parents and nonrelated college students. Block (1973, 1978) found that, with regard to sons, parents encourage competition and achievement, emphasize control of affect and impulse expression, and urge the assumption of personal responsibility. With respect to daughters, parents emphasize affection and physical closeness, foster introspection, and encourage "ladylike" behaviors.

One theme that emerges from the data is that parents show a much greater concern for the sex-typing of their sons (Maccoby and Jacklin, 1974; Block, 1978). They exert greater sex-typing pressure on boys to behave in sex-appropriate ways. Luria (1980) indicates that when children are as young as 20 months, parents are noted to be more upset at cross-gender activity in their sons. She quotes a study in which the authors concluded that parental attitudes underlying the toy ownership of their 20-month-old children could be characterized as "It's okay if my daughter plays with hammers and bracelets, just so long as my son doesn't play with a doll" (Luria, 1980). Pleck (1976) interprets this kind of parental reaction as related to the traditional belief that the acquisition of a healthy male gender identity is a particularly risky process, dependent on learning correct sex-role behavior. Thus, parents are more likely to interpret feminine behavior in boys as a danger signal indicative of possible homosexual tendencies, which they feel compelled to stop.

A second, very important theme is the recognition of the salient role of the father in children's development. The father "appears to be a more crucial agent in directing and channeling the sex-typing of the child, both male and female" (Block, 1973, p. 517). This realization, which is widely supported in the literature (Birns, 1976; Lamb, 1976; Rubin et al., 1974), underscores that clinicians as well as researchers must pay attention to the critical role of the father in gender-identity and sex-role differentiation.

The literature on sex-typing has also brought attention to the lessons acquired from participation in team sports, activities from which girls had been traditionally excluded. As a result of playing competitive games, boys learn much more about the process of competition, winning, losing but going on, accepting criticism without diminished self-esteem, and persisting at hard work and practice. These traits are important not only for eventual success in vocational life but for a sense of competence and security in almost any aspect of adult life (Hennig and Jardim, 1977).

The following case raises an interesting point about the role of sports in women's development:

> Jane, a 32-year-old career woman, was dissatisfied with her bureaucratic position in a large institution. During one psychotherapy session she worked on understanding how she had lost touch with the aggressively ambitious dreams of her youth. She commented that "the period in my life

when I most felt a sense of mastery and power—as if I was truly in charge of my body and my life—was when I was avidly playing baseball and other sports with the boys in the neighborhood. I was very good at it. I knew it. The boys knew it. And it made me feel very good about myself.'' She went on to describe that, ''later, when I was 13 or 14 my mother forbade me to play sports with the boys any longer. She said it was time to start acting like a young lady. . . . I didn't really know how to feel good about myself for a long time after that. It was a tremendous loss for me. I've never quite gotten back to the same sense of mastery or to feeling so free to fight to get what I want.''

Jane echoes a common theme heard from women who were successful at ''tomboy'' activities in their youth. These women typically were forced by sex-typing pressures to withdraw from activities that had been meaningful to their developing sense of self. In the process, they often lost a sense of validation of themselves and of their abilities.

Cognitive Developmental Theory

According to the cognitive developmental theory articulated by Kohlberg (1966), girls and boys first define their own gender identity (or gender label) and then actively and selectively match their behavior to their own developing constructs of ''masculinity'' and ''femininity.'' Although not yet extensively researched, this view of sex-role development offers an important perspective. It emphasizes that the child's own developing ability to absorb and organize knowledge plays a role in the acquisition of sex-typed behaviors.

Kleeman (1976) states that the ''categorization of gender (who is a girl, who is a boy), largely a cognitive function, starts around fifteen months and reaches a crescendo in the final third of the third year.'' Luria has looked at the question of what a child actually knows about gender before age 3. The data indicate that by 30 months of age a child has an imperfect but orderly and workable system for judging its own and others' gender. Children first learn to label the gender of external objects and people and then of themselves. At age 24 months, they can reliably label female and male pictures with the correct girl–boy or mommy–daddy nouns. They can also sort common objects, such as toys and tools, into girl and boy boxes, but they cannot identify the gender of their own picture, nor can they consistently use pronouns. However, by 30 to 36 months, the labeling of their own and others' gender evolves. At 36 months, when objects are experimentally labeled *for girls,* they are preferred by girl subjects, and when they are labeled *for boys,* they are preferred by boys (Luria and Rose, 1979; Luria, 1980). Thus, by 3 years of age children have solidified quite a lot of knowledge about gender and gender roles, and it becomes clearer why it is clinically so difficult to reassign children beyond age 3 to a new gender if that is seen as necessary (Money and Ehrhardt, 1972).

During the preschool years, children usually organize information about gender in terms of dichotomies and opposites. This process facilitates the learning of gender stereotypes and, as Katz (1979) notes, acts as an impediment to sex-role change in society. In the middle childhood years (6 to 12 years of age), the peer group and the media emerge as powerful influences, further reinforcing the stereotypes learned during the preschool years.

Researchers have given increasing attention to peer group formation and its role in sex-role learning during the preschool years. Preschool girls and boys already self-segregate into play groups according to sex. Moreover, girls' and boys' groups differ in that boys' groups are larger and exhibit more rough-and-tumble play (Maccoby and Jacklin, 1974; Luria, 1980). Because the peer group reinforces continuing sex-role learning via dichotomies, this early social segregation by sex probably contributes to the fact that sex differences increase over time.

In a recent study, Jacklin and Maccoby (1978) observed the social behavior of 33-month-old children who were brought together in same-sex and mixed-sex pairs in a laboratory playroom. Children were noted to show higher levels of social interaction in same-sex than mixed-sex pairs. Another striking finding was that in the mixed-sex pairs girls (who were very active when paired with girls) tended to withdraw from boys. The authors describe one piece of data that may relate to the differing behavior in girls in the presence of boys. They note that when a girl issues a prohibition, a boy partner ignores it, whereas a girl partner withdraws. When a boy issues a prohibition, a partner of either sex withdraws. It is not known why boys ignore girls' prohibitions. However,the result is that a girls' verbal efforts to protect herself are less effective with boys, and this may be what leads her to withdraw. This study suggests that by 33 months the foundations are already laid for the selection of same-sex playmates. This then further influences the course of future sex-role learning.

Modeling and Sex-Role Acquisition

Modeling refers to the process of identification with and imitation of the same-sex parent and other same-sex models. According to Maccoby and Jacklin (1974), the modeling process is involved in the acquisition of a wide range of potential behaviors. Which behaviors are then selected depends upon the child's growing understanding of what is appropriate to her, or his, sex role. Katz (1979) suggests that earlier modeling of the same-sex parents has its most profound effects on later adult behavior as parents and marital partners.

Psychoanalytic Theories and the Development of Gender Identity and Role

Psychoanalytic studies further enrich our understanding of the early origins of gender identity and sex-role differentiation. Many of the assumptions of early psycho-analytic theory have been empirically confirmed. The existence of infantile sexuality and the importance of the child's discovery of the anatomical difference between the sexes are too examples. However, other assumptions have not been validated including Freud's (1959, 1925/1961) claim that there is no femaleness before puberty and that early female sexuality is masculine in character.

Primary Feminity and Core Gender Identity

According to Freud's formula for the development of femininity, the little girl's recognition of the anatomical difference between the sexes involves a sense of castration and inferiority with consequent penis envy. The girl then renounces clitoral sexuality (masculine sexuality). She turns away from her mother, who seemingly deprived her of a penis, and toward her father who can at least supply a substitute, a baby. Thus, according to classical theory, femininity begins at the phallic stage as a "bedraggled" defense (Stoller, 1980) against castration anxiety and penis envy.

This concept of femininity was challenged soon after its publication by other early theorists such as Horney (1926–1967, 1933–1967), Jones (1927), and Zilboorg (1944). They believed that girls have an early positive sense of their sexuality. Direct observations of children by Kleeman (1971) and Galenson and Roiphe, (1976, 1980) and reconstructive data as reported by Stoller (1976, 1980) provide evidence for the existence of an early, positive, nonconflictual preoedipal sense of femininity, which Stoller has called *primary femininity*. This early stage of femininity is described by Stoller as related to a "core gender identity," which is simply a positive sense of one's biological femaleness or maleness. In the case of a girl, this exists with some of the trappings of femininity but without a conviction about role behavior. It precedes the more complex gender identity that develops later out of conflict resolution, especially oedipal (Stoller, 1976, 1980). Stoller, Kleeman, and the others point out that penis envy and the oedipus complex contribute to feminine development but are not the initiators of feminine gender identity. Cognitive functions, the availability and the quality of parental object relationships, learning conveyed through parental attitudes and behavior, separation–individuation issues, and body image all contribute significantly to the beginnings of gender identity (Stoller, 1976, 1980; Kleeman, 1971, 1976; Galenson and Roiphe, 1976, 1980).

The Role of Early Genital Awareness

Roiphe and Galenson stress the role of genital drive organization in the development of early childhood gender identity. They studied the development of 35 girls and 35 boys, noting the emergence of differential gender awareness from the first days of life, arising "not only in the course of the mother's fondling and bodily ministrations and during feeding, but also probably in connection with transmitted pressure and excitation from the adjacent anal and urinary areas, the totality of these sensuous interactions contributing to a substantially different early body image for each sex" (Galenson and Roiphe, 1980, p. 89).

In describing their observations, Roiphe and Galenson stressed the mutual influence of object relationships and progressive (anal, urinary, and genital) drive organization. They interpreted their data as indicating that, as the children move through the phases of separation and individuation, they become increasingly interested in genital derivative behaviors (including masturbation) and between 16 and 19 months of age discover the anatomic difference between the sexes. This discovery was noted to be associated with behaviors that the authors interpret as an early "castration reaction."

Roiphe and Galenson also observed that awareness of the genital difference appears to be associated in time with a divergence in the development of boys and girls. From this observation, they interpret that castration reactions induce the sex-differentiated developmental differences. Boys, they report, had less intense castration reactions characterized by a continuation of masturbation, interest in typically masculine toys and activities, such as cars and ball playing, and an increased general use of the motor apparatus, whereas girls were characterized as having decreased masturbation, evidence of temporary depressive mood, blossoming of fantasy play, and elaboration of new ego defenses. The authors state that milder reactions, those producing less dysphoria, presumably induced a shift toward the father as a new love object with a less intense but continuing attachment to the mother. Those girls who experienced a disturbance in the early mother–daughter relationship had more intense castration reactions. They exhibited the persistence of an intense, ambivalent tie to the mother instead of a turning toward the father.

Kleeman (1976) cautions that Roiphe and Galenson attribute too much power to the influence of progressive genital drive organization on the development of gender identity and of behavioral differences between girls and boys. He indicates that although genital sensation and awareness contribute to core gender identity, they are not the major organizers of behavior. Factors such as cognitive functioning and parental shaping are at least as important, if not more so.

However, familiarity with the normal development of early genital awareness can enhance the clinician's ability to respond appropriately to parental concerns and questions. The following example from the literature illustrates this aspect of normal development:

> Winnie had fluctuated in her level of manual masturbatory activity from her 19th month on. At 22 months, while bathing with two little boys, she examined her own genitalia and asked where her penis was. After her baby sister was born, when Winnie was almost 23 months old, her doll play flourished remarkably, whereas her genital play subsided. At 24 months, she persistently tried to open her father's underwear and to grab for his genitals. At 25 months, she started to masturbate again, and at 26 months, she tried to urinate while standing up in imitation of a boy. She had remained an extremely avid doll player when last seen in a follow-up, at almost 4 years of age, and her fantasy life was rich and varied. (Galenson and Roiphe, 1976, p. 50)

Contemporary psychoanalytic writings stress the important tie between gender identity and the development of object relationships. Thus, the consolidation of a secure gender identity, like a secure sense of self, requires the normal resolution of mother–infant symbiosis (the mutual sense of oneness established between mother and infant) and progressive separation–individuation. As described by Mahler (1972), this process entails a "growing away" from the sense of oneness with mother and a progressive awareness of physical and psychological separateness from the primary love objects, usually the parents. Stoller reports from his work with transsexuals that an excessively intense and prolonged sense of oneness between mother and son can produce the failure in the son "to sense himself as separate from his mother's female body" (Stoller, 1976, p. 69). On the other hand, an inadequate mother–daughter symbiosis can result in a sense of maleness in the daughter.

Chodorow (1974, 1978) focuses our attention on gender differences in the preoedipal separation–individuation process. These differences stem from the fact that, in our culture, the mother is typically the primary caretaker. Thus, a girl has the task of separating from a same-sex parent, whereas a boy must separate from an opposite-sex parent. Chodorow draws upon the contributions of earlier psychoanalytic theorists (Brunswick, 1940; Klein, 1937; Riviere, 1937; Deutsch, 1944; Horney, 1932; Chasse-quet-Smirgel, 1964; Fairbairn, 1952) in describing differences in the relationship between mothers and their daughters and mothers and their sons. Because mothers have been daughters themselves, they identify more strongly with their daughters than with their sons. This may make separation a particularly difficult issue for a woman and may lead to a feminine personality marked by less differentiated ego boundaries and by an embeddedness in relationships, often involving an unrealistic sense of "guilt and responsibility for situations that did not come about through her actions" (Chodorow, 1974, p. 59). The author states that daughters tend to develop into women who have a capacity for nurturance and intimacy but who have difficulty with issues of autonomy and self-esteem.

On the other hand, the mother of a son tends to relate to him in a way that stresses his "masculine oppositeness" to herself. Psychological and anthropological studies support the significance of this aspect of the mother–son relationship. Chodorow, based on evidence from Bibring, Slater, and Whiting, concludes that

> a mother, of a different gender from her son and deprived of adult emotional, social and physical contact with men (and often without any supportive adult contact at all), may push her son out of his preoedipal relationship to her into an oedipally toned relationship defined by its sexuality and gender distinction. Her son's maleness and oppositeness as a sexual other become important, even while his being an infant remains important as well. (Chodorow, 1978, p. 107)

This dynamic contributes to a son's differentiation.

For sons, separation–individuation involves replacing the early primary identification with a woman with a masculine gender identification. In Western society, this process is complicated by the fact that the boy may have little personal contact with his same-sex parent (Chodorow, 1974, 1978; Slater, 1961; Mitscherlich, 1963/1970). One outgrowth of these circumstances is that boys tend to gain a sense of masculinity through identification with stereotyped aspects of the father's role rather than through identification with the father as a real person who communicates feelings, values, and beliefs. Chodorow describes several factors in male development, related to the structure of families and of parenting in our culture:

> A boy, in his attempt to gain an elusive masculine identification often comes to define this masculinity largely in negative terms, as that which is not feminine or involved with women. There is an internal and external aspect to this. Internally, the boy tries to reject his mother and deny his attachment to her and the strong dependence upon her that he still feels. He also tries to deny the deep personal identification with her that has developed during his early years. He does this by repressing whatever he takes to be feminine inside himself, and, importantly, by denigrating and devaluing whatever he considers to be feminine in the outside world. (Chodorow, 1974, p. 50)

This process results in the development of a masculine personality characterized by firm, but rigid, ego boundaries, a need to deny connection to others, and a psychological need to feel superior to women. Chodorow suggests that this latter need underlies the universally found subjugation and devaluation of females (Rosaldo, 1974; Ortner, 1974). She concludes that children need fathers who participate equally in parenting. This would enable both sexes to develop an individuated sense of self and a positive, secure gender identity. Boys would develop the autonomy that comes from differentiation, but without a fear of affectional ties. Girls would have the opportunity to gain autonomy in addition to their capacity for intimacy.

Chodorow's formulation stresses that a father has an important role in his child's early development. This contrasts with Freud's work, which originally emphasized the importance of the father during the oedipal period, but not before. Recent psychological studies, however, show that children form a distinctive relationship with their fathers well before their first birthdays (Lamb, 1976). Kleeman (1971, 1976) notes that the father's availability to the child and to the mother during that time is essential for optimal separation–individuation.

As Lerner (1978b) notes, the folk saying, "A son's a son till he gets a wife; a daughter's your daughter for the rest of her life," is reflective of a daughter's greater difficulty in separating from her mother. The following vignette typifies how women experience this issue:

> An active, successful college student poignantly expressed insight into her own struggle with separation. She described that when her mother left her at the airport at the end of the last semester break she was struck by an acute realization that "this was the last time I would see my mother until the summer and it just felt devastating. I felt intense loss that she was going to be a thousand miles away. When I got back, I cried as if I had just come to school for the first time. I couldn't believe that I was a 20-year-old college junior and I could feel so much about my mother being in another city."

This concept is important in clinical work with women since female patients often manifest a particular difficulty in tolerating feelings of separateness, difference, or aloneness. These are inherent in the experience or expression of anger and may also characterize other autonomous behaviors or ambitions. Lerner notes that men may be exhilarated by the sense of "aloneness," but women may feel it dangerous, "as if it threatens a bond with a mother who would herself be left emptied out and depleted if her daughter should feel whole and complete unto herself, apart from a relational context" Lerner, 1978b, p. 9). The two cases that follow serve as examples:

> 1. Mrs. P was a 43-year-old short-term psychotherapy patient who had been married for 21 years. Although she had graduated from a college and excelled academically, an early marriage and motherhood took the place of her original career goals. For several years she had been aware of her increasing resentment of her husband's and teenage children's "adventures in the outside world." This motivated her to enroll in a postgraduate course to improve her marketability as well as her shaky self-esteem.
>
> Mrs. P arranged to spend an evening working on her term paper in the university library, away from family responsibilities and interruptions. While there she was delighted to discover that she had confidence in her ability to think and to create. She described that she felt her brain "was

working for the first time in many years." She left the library feeling exhilarated, but on the way home her thoughts drifted to "worrying how my family had managed without me and fantasizing that they would be furious with me for being so selfish." By the time she reached home, she found herself "very anxious and upset, amost panicky." She "rushed to get into the house to apologize" to her family and to "check on their love." In the process, she banged her head on a cabinet door. Her response was to collapse on the floor in uncontrollable tears. Although she maintained an intellectual awareness that her tears were way out of proportion to her mishap, she was painfully aware of an unbearable sense of being alone and helpless: "I felt like a little girl who just needed her mommy."

In the course of therapy, it became clear that Mrs. P had for many years avoided exploring her intellectual interests, because they were associated with the threat of being different from and consequently cut off from her conservative, uneducated mother.

2. Mrs. I was a 29-year-old married woman who was concerned about her inability to enjoy sexual intercourse unless she was first "pressured into letting my husband arouse me." When she felt that she was "doing it for him," either to please or appease him, she could "relax and feel good." She could not think about initiating intercourse herself without experiencing a "dreadful sense of emptiness and abandonment."

Mrs. I associated these feelings with the longings she felt as a child for her mother when her parents left for business and vacation trips without the children. Mrs. I's mother was a prim, controlled woman who was painfully uncomfortable with any display of physical affection from husband or children. For Mrs. I, her own sexual wishes and needs had come to represent disloyalty to her mother and potential loss of their relationship with each other.

Androgyny and Beyond

Our discussion of sex roles would not be complete without considering the concept of psychological androgyny. Bem is credited with introducing and operationalizing this concept in psychology. However, it is important to note that Block (1973), Spence and Helmreich (1978), and others (Pleck, 1975; Berzins and Welling, 1974; Heilbrun, 1976) have also made significant contributions to the study of androgyny.

Bem (1974, 1976, 1978) defines androgyny as the equal balance within an individual of both feminine and masculine personality characteristics, resulting in healthier, more effective functioning. She notes that for the androgynous individual it is possible "to blend these complementary modalities in a single act, being able, for example to fire an employee if the circumstances warrant it, but to do so with sensitivity for the human emotion that such an act inevitably produces" (Bem, 1978, p. 5). An individual with only those stereotyped traits considered appropriate for his/her sex, however, would be restricted in functioning in simple, everyday tasks and in more complex situations.

Most traditional theories and research instruments treat femininity and masculinity as opposite poles of a single dimension. Thus, an individual high on femininity automatically must be low on masculinity, and vice versa (Pleck, 1976). Bem's work, however, offers a different perspective. Femininity and masculinity represent "complementary domains of positive traits and behaviors" (Bem, 1978, p. 5) that can be integrated within one person. Other theorists conceptualized two fundamental domains but gave them different labels. Bem notes that according to Parsons and Bales (1955) "masculinity has been associated with an *instrumental orientation,* a cognitive focus on getting the job done, or the problem solved, whereas femininity has been associated with an *expressive orientation,* an affective concern for the welfare of others and the harmony of the group" (Bem, 1978, p. 5). Bakan (1966) uses the labels *agency* and *communion* in discussing these two domains. Agency, associated with masculinity, represents a concern for oneself as an individual and is characterized by such traits as self-assertion, self-expansion, and isolation. Communion, associated with femininity, represents concern for the relationship between oneself and others as manifested in openness, cooperation, and a sense of being at one with others. Bakan argues that unmitigated agency is destructive and that the successful integration of agency and communion (that is, androgyny) is essential for the viability of individuals and of society as a whole.

In order to establish an empirical basis for the theory of androgyny, Bem (1974) devised a new personality scale (BSRI) to distinguish the sex-typed from the androgynous individual. The data collected confirmed Bem's suggestion that femininity and masculinity are independent of each other; subjects who had high scores on femininity did not necessarily have low scores on masculinity, and vice versa. Bem reports that about one-third of these subjects could be classified as sex-typed (either feminine or masculine) and one-third as androgynous. Fewer than 10% were sex-reversed.

Bem and her colleagues designed several experiments to test their hypothesis that feminine individuals would have difficulty in situations requiring instrumentality or agency and that masculine individuals would have difficulty in situations involving expressiveness and communion but that androgynous individuals would "do well" and feel comfortable in either situation. As predicted, for both women and men, sex-typing served to restrict the behavior studied, whereas androgyny facilitated more flexible behavior. Bem concludes that the evidence regarding the androgynous male indicates that he is competent in both the expressive and instrumental domains: "he stands firm in his opinions, he cuddles kittens and bounces babies, and he has a sympathetic ear for someone in distress" (Bem, 1976, p. 58). In contrast, the sex-typed male could perform well consistently only in one sphere.

The female data are somewhat more complex. Like their male counterparts, androgynous women perform competently in both the expressive and instrumental domains and do not shun behavior just because our culture labels it as masculine. Masculine women, however, have difficulty functioning in the expressive domain and feminine women have difficulty in the instrumental domain. The feminine women, however, were not consistently high even in the expressive domain. To sum up, Bem speculates that "femininity may be what produces nurturant feelings in women, but then at least a threshold level of masculinity is required to provide the initiative and perhaps even the daring to translate those nurturant feelings into action'' (Bem, 1978, p. 19).

Several authors, including Bem, point out an implicit contradiction in the concept of androgyny (Kenworthy, 1979; Spence and Helmreich, 1980). On the one hand, androgyny indicates a conception of mental health that is free from the damaging restrictions of culturally defined sex-role stereotypes. But, on the other hand, the sex-role scales used by Bem and others to operationalize the concept of androgyny are rooted in the very sex-role stereotypes that Bem feels we must transcend.

An additional reservation regarding Bem's work is discussed by Kaplan (1979a) and Vogel (1979). They point out that it is not simply an equal balance of feminine and masculine traits (as implied by Bem's definition of androgyny) that leads to behavioral flexibility. Of essential importance are the particular configuration of traits uniquely held by each person and the degree to which feminine and masculine traits are integrated and tempered, one by the other. As Vogel notes, someone who is self-reliant, independent, and self-sufficient as well as tender, sensitive, and understanding presents a very different clinical picture than someone who is aggressive, dominant, and competitive, as well as childlike, flatterable, and loyal. Although the two configurations may be similar in terms of balance of feminine and masculine traits, it is likely that one configuration could be considerably healthier than the other.

Evidence presented by Spence and Helmreich (1980) indicates that Bem's claim that there are greater social–psychological advantages for those who are androgynous has not yet been fully tested. They show that Bem's data tap the specific personality traits of expressiveness and instrumentality, but that these traits are not fully representative of global sex-role expectations or attitudes. Thus, a woman or a man may be highly expressive without being feminine in other ways, and, similarly, an individual may be highly instrumental without being masculine in other personality domains. According to Spence and Helmreich, the personal qualities of expressiveness and instrumentality have significance for successful social interactions, some of them role related, but our understanding of these traits must be disentangled from global conceptions of masculinity, femininity, and androgyny.

A new perspective beginning to emerge in the literature is that of sex-role transcendence (Rebecca et al., 1976; Pleck, 1975). This presents a phasic view of sex-role development according to which individuals in our culture can mature beyond dichotomous sex-role stereotypes and even beyond androgyny to a stage in which choices are made for personally meaningful and adaptive behaviors without any relevance to sex-role norms. Bem herself states that ''if there is a moral to the concept of psychological androgyny, it is that *behavior* should have no gender'' (Bem, 1978, p. 19).

Clinical Issues in Sex-Role Stereotyping and Sexual Functioning

In this section we will discuss some aspects of the interplay, in clinical work, between sex-role stereotyping and sexual functioning. Human sexuality and sexual functioning are sensitive to the pressures and conflicts produced by sex-role stereotypes. Persistent myths (women are not interested in sex whereas men are) and unrealistic expectations (truly feminine women always have vaginal orgasms) contribute significantly to the spectrum of sexual complaints and symptoms presented by individuals of either sex (Nadelson and Notman, 1977). In recent years, there have been changes of sex-role norms. Women and men have new expectations for themselves and others that effect their sexual interests and behaviors. As Mathis points out,

> Sex, reproduction, and the reproductive system are almost synonymous with emotional reactions in our culture. The emotional charge invested in the genitalia makes that area peculiarly vulnerable to symptoms arising from any conflictual aspect of living. (Mathis, 1967)

The physician, having grown up in a particular culture, is likely to have responses to sexual issues presented by patients that are reflective of the physician's background. These responses are, to a large degree, determined by unconscious sex-role expectations. These, in turn, may influence clinical thinking. Thus, the physician must be prepared to cope with the treatment of individuals who may have very different concepts of sexual intercourse, marriage, parenting, pregnancy, and even the doctor–patient relationship.

As noted by Nadelson and Notman (1977), the doctor–patient relationship has traditionally been based on a parent–child model. This is particularly true when the doctor is a male and the patient female, but it occurs in other situations as well. Thus, the doctor, who has usually been male, is expected to be authoritative, informed, and helpful. This emphasizes the "childlike" position of the woman patient whose traditional role has been seen as compliant, undemanding, dependent, and naive. The physician must be aware of this transference–countertransference aspect of the doctor–patient relationship.

Successful resolution of clinical problems and patient growth is more likely to accrue from a collaborative model. An unequal relationship prevents communication and mutual respect between the patient and the physician. It may lead to regressive patient behavior and, eventually, to mistrust and antagonism (Notman and Nadelson, 1978).

Sex-role stereotyping has taught many women to handle their relationships with men by sexualization (Notman and Nadelson, 1978). Women often use this coping mechanism as a way of dealing with anxiety and insecurity and they may bring this way of responding into the doctor–patient relationship. The physician who responds to the (usually unconscious) seductiveness in the patient's style rather than attending to the underlying anxiety does his/her patient a disservice.

Male Sexuality

The response of the male patient to the authoritative "parent" physician has its own characteristic problems. Males have been socialized to experience problems, including health problems, as signs of weakness. Men tend to avoid the direct expression of wishes and needs for help and comfort. Thus, it can be very difficult for men, who fear being perceived as "unmanly" to seek medical attention. But even when they do consult a clinician, it can still be very difficult for them to openly convey their fears, anxieties, or concerns. The physician who understand this sex-role issue can be more supportive and skillful in giving male patients opportunities to articulate their needs.

This aspect of the physician's relationship with the male patient becomes crucial in considering the assessment and treatment of sexual problems. Central to the notion of the male sex-role identity is the notion of the male as sexually aggressive, powerful, and fully in control. Hence, the male patient will often experience sexual or reproductive difficulties as a threat to his masculine identity, producing feelings of shame, guilt, and loss of self-esteem. One man who developed impotence related to diabetes wrote the following about his own sense of lost manhood:

> My own erective dysfunction started at a time when, by all logic and reasoning, it shouldn't have. I was shifting gears in my attitudes toward myself . . . everything was looking up. But over this scene was the big shadow—my sexual spirit was willing, but the flesh was occasionally weak.
>
> I didn't know why then, but my reflex action was that nobody must know. If the secret homosexual is in a closet, I was locked in a large, barren room. The women I went to bed with were given stories of fatigue, nervousness, crises on the job, or just too much gin.
>
> Then came the guilt. My sex role was supposed to be that of initiator, enticer, schemer, promise-maker—and I was failing to deliver. The penalty for nondelivery is guilt. (July, 1974, p. 36)

Sensitive and thoroughgoing management of male sexual dysfunction, independent of etiology, requires the clinician to address psychological and emotional meanings for the patient, who is likely to feel that his sexual identity has been threatened.

Other problems related to gender-role stereotyping occur in the context of the infertility workup. Current reports in the literature describe the depression, anxiety, guilt and anger, self-doubt, and loss of libido experienced by couples who consult physicians for infertility problems or who undergo artificial insemination (Mazor, 1978, 1980; David and Avidan, 1976). The inability to produce a baby is a threat to the sexual identity of each partner, independent of which one has the medical problem. However, the husband is often unable to recognize or to express his feelings and needs for support during the infertility workup, and it is often assumed that he needs less support. In fact, the structure of the infertility workup often does not include the husband until it is far along, typically assuming first that it is the "wife's fault." The male physician treating the infertile couple may also identify with the husband and experience unconscious anxiety, leading the physician to avoid open discussion of the husband's feelings.

Having a semen specimen counted, having to produce it on demand, or having to make love on a schedule determined by the physician are all clearly stressful. These experiences are contrary to the stereotyped notion of the male who is always "on top" or "in charge" of his sexual relationships. Walker has been cited as reporting that during the infertility workup, in more than 50% of the cases, transient ejaculatory disturbances and impotence occur (Mazor, 1980). This occurrence is not surprising given the stresses involved. As one man expressed it,

> At first I thought I was doing something wrong, that there was something about sex I didn't know. I felt like a scared teenager, and a couple of times I couldn't keep an erection. Then we started with the doctors and the temperature charts, and it was like having programmed sex. You have to have it on such-and-such a day whether you feel like it or not. It was a long time before we could ever think about having sex for pleasure. (Mazor, 1980, p. 43)

The supportive and understanding clinician who addresses these issues with his patients can help to prevent or ameliorate sexual and emotional alienation within the infertile couple.

Another important issue in clinical work with men is the tendency to focus on issues related to achievement concerns and to overlook problems with closeness and intimacy as an important area for therapeutic work. The following case example underscores this issue:

> Mr. W was a 45-year-old scientist who began weekly individual psychotherapy complaining of depression with insomnia, fatigue, and diminished libido. He reported that he had been depressed for about 8 months, knowing how long it had been because he knew that the onset of his symptoms occurred shortly after his middle child left home for college.
>
> At first Mr. W persistently related his depression to lack of fulfillment in his career. However, after several months of exploring the issues, it became clear to both himself and his therapist that he had actually achieved what he had hoped to achieve in his career. The "sense of something missing or lacking in his life" that he spoke of had to do really with the emptiness in his marital relationship, coupled with his growing awareness that his children were one by one leaving the home before he "had the time" to get to know them.

Social scientists suggest that traditional male sex-role socialization focuses on training men to become successful, competitive, aggressive, "good providers," but it does not encourage them to develop interpersonal and emotional skills (Pleck and Sawyer, 1974; Pleck and Brannon, 1978; Bernard, 1981). London discusses the effects of this masculine sex-typing on male sexual behavior. He states that to "be a man" in the American sense is to be emotionally sterile and, thereby, sexually inadequate:

> Machismo and aggressiveness are in direct contradiction to sensitivity and intimacy. "Taking a woman" is supposed to fulfill this masculine urge. Perhaps this explains why 90% of all men ejaculate within the first two minutes of intercourse! It's not surprising that frigidity is extremely common. Sex as a means of communication is sorely lacking. (London, 1974, p. 42)

Gross (1978) points out that one of the most limiting features of the male sex role is that the male is required to appear as the sexual expert and to hide ignorance and even uncertainty. As a result, sexual information is often acquired by men accidentally and relatively late in life.

Male sexual behavior has been characterized by the same goal orientation that has characterized the male sex role in general, and male sexuality has been measured by the number of women a man could "make it" or "score" with. In more recent years, the focus has shifted to a concern with being a technically proficient lover who is interested in knowing what his partner needs and wants so that he can provide her with multiple orgasmic pleasure. Gross (1978) explains that this apparent shift toward more considerate lovemaking actually represents a new variation on the old theme of goal orientation. Only now the goal has shifted from the number of conquests to the number of orgasms produced. Thus, concern that the female partner reach orgasm each time becomes evidence of the man's sexual adequacy and can lead to problems in sexual performance. Further, it can evoke tension and anxiety in the man's sexual partner. The couple may then attempt solutions that unwittingly compound their sexual difficulties. The alert clinician can ameliorate such a situation by encouraging open discussion and by clarifying basic information. Fisch reports an excerpt from a case that captures this kind of problem:

> "I can't reach orgasm and my husband tries to help by holding back his own orgasm; during intercourse he keeps checking with me as to how I'm doing but this makes it worse. After he has climaxed, he always asks me how it went, and I'm afraid to tell him that I couldn't have an orgasm." (Fisch, 1981, p. 69)

Female Sexuality

Although some aspects of the traditional female sex role contribute positively to sexual expressiveness, other aspects, such as the expectations that women be passive and sexually disinterested, do not. Optimum sexual satisfaction for a woman and her partner involves a degree of self-assertion and initiative not prescribed by the traditional female script.

Some women reject the traditional stereotypes and may use counterdependent mechanisms and deny sexuality, achieving a self-concept as competent and strong (Nadelson et al., 1978b). This dynamic may be partially motivated by a wish to deny identification with a mother who is perceived as weak and ineffectual, but it is also partially accounted for by cultural factors. A college student who, equating femininity with heterosexuality, explained her fear of "committing" herself to a heterosexual life-style. She explained that to do so would mean "accepting a feminine identity as it exists in our culture—dependent, weak, acquiescent, dependent, emotional, dependent, unconfident and unintelligent."

The following case presents a young woman's attempt to apply a counterdependent solution to her problem with feminine identification:

> B.L. was a 25-year-old junior medical student who had always performed well academically. She was seen in short-term psychotherapy after she became acutely depressed during her clerkship on the high-pressured active medical service of a local hospital. She worked long and hard, asking for no help and interacting minimally with her colleagues. She was generally seen as distant, aloof, and asexual. When one of the interns asked her what she did with her free time, and suggested that they might spend some of it together, she told him to "bug off." Initially she was angry, feeling that he had been attempting to "put her down," and that he was not taking her seriously as a colleague. As she thought more about the incident she found herself in tears, recognizing her loneliness and emptiness. She began to consider that her life up until that point had avoided close relationships and intimacy with men. The recognition of some of

her passive, dependent and sexual feelings frightened her. She was fearful that she would be overwhelmed by them and be rendered helpless if she did not maintain her strong and distant position.

She had come from a family where her father had been a successful, enterprising business man who accepted her as the "boy" when her sister was born. She was identified with him and determined to please him and gain his respect. Her mother, a self-deprecating woman, had always been the object of her scorn. She felt distant from her and unable to relate. The therapy brought her some recognition of the ambivalence and her desire for closeness and identification with the parts of her mother which were warm and caring. She began to be able to integrate some aspects of both her parents. (Nadelson et al., 1978b, p. 208)

Recently, changes in sexual behavior have fostered a shift away from another sex-role script that views female sexuality as existing only in the context of love and a committed relationship and that censures women for participating in other sexual activities such as premarital intercourse. Although behavior may have changed, the double standard still has covert but profound effects on how women feel about themselves.

M, an attractive woman of average weight, consulted her internist about her increasingly desperate struggle to control compulsive eating. She had for 5 or 6 months been almost constantly preoccupied with thoughts about weight and dieting, associated with painful feelings of guilt and ineffectiveness. The internist explained that M was not medically overweight but that she would benefit from understanding her painful feelings about food. M accepted a referral for psychotherapy.

In reviewing her history, M discovered that she had experienced several episodes of inability to control her eating. They all seemed to occur at times when she was involved in a sexually active relationship. At the present time, M is involved with a young man whom she loves. But she does not yet feel ready to make a long-term commitment.

M described an episode that occurred after a telephone conversation with her mother in which they discussed M's relationship with her boyfriend. M's mother conveyed disapproval of her daughter's "giving it away" without a marriage commitment. After the conversation, M found herself finishing off a box of crackers. She felt disgusted with herself for "binging," and "teary," but her thoughts led to an important insight—that her disgust was really about her sexuality. Despite the fact that her now divorced parents were each living with partners to whom they were not married, they had instilled in her a belief that "good girls make love only to their husbands."

In her next therapy session, M stated that "I know intellectually that values have changed and that I'm supposed to feel liberal and free. But underneath, they wind up making you feel bad and dirty just the same. It's the same old double standard all over again!"

M came to recognize that she used her compulsive eating to punish herself for violating her parents', and particularly her mother's, expectations of her. When she feels stuffed she experiences painful feelings of shame about her body. She wants "to hide herself." At these times it is impossible for her to feel sensual or to enjoy lovemaking no matter how much she may love the person she is with.

M had been reared to value "acting like a lady." Her internalized image of the appropriate female sex role incorporated the ethos of the traditional double standard. When her behavior deviated from this stereotype, unconscious anxiety and guilt led to symptom development.

The case of M raised another important clinical issue—the role of weight, dieting, and self-control in the lives of women. Female sexuality in our culture is more closely tied to standards of physical attractiveness than is true for male sexuality (Schwartz and Strom, 1978; Wooley and Wooley, 1980). For the man, standards are based on achievement, status, etc. (Luria and Rose, 1979). There is little doubt in our society that the acceptable female body is the slender one. It was recently shown that most women not only value smallness, they also overestimate their own size (Halmi et al., 1977). These cultural values contribute to the emotional intensity that surrounds weight control. Wooley and Wooley (1980, p. 145) hypothesize that, for many women, the ability to control eating and weight becomes a metaphor for the ability to be in control of one's life, "with the result that successes are experienced with a pleasure disproportionate to the tangible social or physical benefits of reduced body weight, while failure is experienced as profoundly demoralizing."

Another effect of sex-role stereotyping occurs when the clinician who values a traditional view of female sexuality ignores sexual complaints from women patients that would be acknowledged from male patients. For example, Mrs. R, the patient with myasthenia gravis who was discussed previously, tried several times to discuss her sexual dissatisfaction with her doctor (muscle fatigue at the end of the day gravely diminished her ability to make love at night).

> The internist dismissed her concerns and advised Mrs. R to accept her limitations. She began to think that she was wrong to be so unhappy about the lack of sexual activity in her marriage. However, when given the opportunity to discuss the details of her sexual functioning with her psychotherapist, Mrs. R realized that having sex in the morning instead of at night might drastically improve her situation. This simple solution resulted in increased sexual satisfaction and intimacy for both Mrs. R and her husband.

Mrs. R. is typical of female patients who often need to have their interest in sexuality or concerns about their sexual functioning validated. This concept may be of particular importance in clinical work with the partners of those who have sexual dysfunctions related to chronic illness.

Thus, sex-role stereotyping has a number of important effects on the sexual functioning of men and women. Recognition and understanding of these effects facilitates effective clinical intervention in human sexuality.

Conclusion

Gender identity and sex-role distinctions begin their development very early in life and very much under the influence of interpersonal and cultural forces. These forces have the power to strongly modify biological determinants. Evidence indicates that most sex differences are the result of gender stereotypes and sex-differentiated patterns of child-rearing. Clinicians who have grown up in this culture have internalized the same sex-role values and stereotypes that effect their patients. These values have significant effects on therapeutic thinking.

Rigid sex-role stereotypes have been shown to limit human potentials for interpersonal and individual growth and happiness. Current knowledge about sex-role socialization provides a point of entry for conceptualizing broader sex-role definitions that can include less restrictive views of female and male sexuality. Some changes have already begun. As Block summarizes: "In our review, the socialization changes now feasible within our civilization can permit self- and sex-role definitions that can transcend the stark and limiting conceptions of masculinity and feminity imposed in the past" (Block, 1978, p. 85).

References

Aslin, A. L. Feminist and community mental health center psychotherapists' expectations of mental health for women. *Sex roles, 1977, 3,* 537–544.

Baill, C., and Money, J. Physiological aspects of female sexual development. In M. Kirkpatrick (Ed.), *Women's sexual development explorations of inner space.* New York: Plenum Press, 1980. Pp. 61–62.

Bakan, D. *The duality of human existence.* Chicago: Rand McNally, 1966.

Bardwick, J. and Douvan, E. Ambivalence: The socialization of women. In J. Bardwick (Ed.), *Readings on the psychology of women.* New York: Harper & Row, 1972. Pp. 52–57.

Bell, R. O., and Costello, N. S. Three tests for sex differences in tactile sensitivity in the newborn. *Biologia Neonatorium,* 1964, *7,* 335–347.

Bem, S. The measurement of psychological androgyny. *Journal of Consulting and Clinical Psychology,* 1974, *42,* 155–162.

Bem, S. M. Probing the promise of androgyny. In A. G. Kaplan and J. P. Bean (Eds.), *Beyond sex-role stereotypes: Readings toward a psychology of androgyny.* Boston: Little, Brown, 1976. Pp. 47–62.

Bem, S. Beyond androgyny: Some presumptuous prescriptions for a liberated sexual identity. In J. A. Sherman and F. L. Denmark (Eds.), *The psychology of women: Future directions in research.* New York: Psychological Dimensions, Inc., 1978. Pp. 3–23.

Benton, A. A., Gelber, E. R., Kelley, H. H., and Liebling, B. A. Reactions to various degrees of deceit in a mixed-motive relationship. *Journal of Personality and Social Psychology,* 1969, *12,* 170–180.

Bernard, J. The good provider role. *American Psychologist,* 1981, *36,* 1–12.

Berzins, J. I., and Welling, M. A. *The PRF-ANDRO scale: A measure of psychological androgyny derived from the personality research form.* Unpublished manuscript, 1974. (Available from J. I. Berzins, Department of Psychology, University of Kentucky, Lexington, Ky. 40506.)

Birns, B. The emergence and socialization of sex differences in the earliest years. *Merrill-Palmer Quarterly,* 1976, *22,* 229–254.

Block, J. H. Conceptions of sex role: Some cross-cultural and longitudinal perspectives. *American Psychologist,* 1973, *28,* 512–526.

Block, J. H. Issues, problems, and pitfalls in assessing sex differences: A critical review of the psychology of sex differences. *Merrill-Palmer Quarterly,* 1976, *22,* 283–308.

Block, J. H. Sex differentiation. In J. A. Sherman and F. L. Denmark (Eds.), *The psychology of women: Future directions in research.* New York: Psychological Dimensions, Inc., 1978. Pp. 31–85.

Bowman, P. R. The relationship between attitudes toward women and the treatment of activity and passivity. (Doctoral dissertation, Boston University School of Education, 1976). *Dissertation Abstracts International,* 1976, *36,* 5779B (University Microfilms No. 76-11, 644)

Broverman, I. K., Broverman, D. M., Clarkson, F. E., Rosenkrantz, P., and Vogel, S. R. Sex-role stereotypes and clinical judgements of mental health. *Journal of Consulting Psychology,* 1970, *34,* 1–7.

Broverman, I. K., Vogel, S. R., and Broverman, D. Sex-role stereotypes: A current appraisal. *Journal of Social Issues*, 1972, *28*, 59–78.

Brunswick, R. M. The preoedipal phase of the libido development. *Psychoanalytic Quarterly*, 1940, *9*, 293–319.

Buffery, A. W. H., and Gray, J. A. Sex differences in the development of spatial and linguistic skills. In C. Ounsted and D. C. Taylor (Eds.), *Gender differences: Their ontogeny and significance*. Baltimore, Md.: Williams & Wilkins, 1972.

Caplan, P. J. Beyond the box score: A boundary condition for sex differences in aggression and achievement striving. *Progress in Experimental Personality Research*, 1979, *9*, 41–85.

Chassequet-Smirgel, J. Feminine guilt and the oedipus complex. In J. Chassequet-Smirgel (Ed.), *Female sexuality*. Ann Arbor: Univ. of Michigan Press, 1970. Pp. 94–134. (Originally published, 1964.)

Chodorow, N. Family structure and feminine personality. In M. Z. Rosaldo and L. Lamphere (Eds.), *Women, culture and society*. Stanford, Calif.: Stanford Univ. Press, 1974. Pp. 43–68.

Chodorow, N. *The reproduction of mothering*. Berkeley: Univ. of California Press, 1978.

Crandall, V. C. Sex differences in expectancy of intellectual and academic reinforcement. In C. P. Smith (Ed.), *Achievement related motives in children*. New York: Russell Sage Foundation, 1969.

David, A., and Avidan, D. Artificial insemination donor: Clinical and psychological aspects. *Fertility and Sterility*, 1976, *27*, 528–532.

Deutsch, H. *The psychology of women*. New York: Grune & Stratton, 1944.

Ehrhardt, A. A., and Baker, S. W. Fetal androgens, human central nervous system differentiation, and behavior sex differences. In R. C. Friedman, R. M. Richart, and R. L. Vande Wiele (Eds.), *Sex differences in behavior*. New York: John Wiley, 1974. Pp. 33–52.

Englehard, P. A., Jones, K. O., and Stiggins, R. J. Trends in counselor attitude about women's roles. *Journal of Counseling Psychology*, 1976, *23*, 365–372.

Fairbairn, W. R. D. *An object-relations theory of the personality*. New York: Basic Books, 1952.

Fennema, E., and Sherman, J. *Sex-related differences in mathematics learning: Myths, realities and related factors*. Paper presented to the American Association for the Advancement of Science, Boston, 1976.

Fisch, R. Preventing minor sexual difficulties from becoming sexual problems. *Medical Aspects of Human Sexuality*, 1981, *15*, 61–77.

Franks, V. Gender and psychotherapy. In E. S. Gomberg and V. Franks (Eds.), *Gender and disordered behavior*. New York: Brunner/Mazel, 1979. Pp. 453–485.

Friedman, R. C., Richart, R. M., Vande Wiele, R. L. (Eds.). *Sex differences in Behavior*. New York: Wiley, 1974.

Freud, S. *Three essays on the theory of sexuality* (Standard ed.). London: Hogarth Press, 1959. Vol. 7, pp. 125–243. (Originally published, 1905.)

Freud, S. *Some psychical consequences of the anatomical distinction between the sexes* (Standard ed.). London: Hogarth Press, 1961. Vol. 19, pp. 241–258. (Originally published, 1925.)

Galapurda, A. M., Le May, M., Kemper, T. L., and Geschwind, N. Right-left asymmetries in the brain. *Science*, 1978, *199*, 852–856.

Galenson, E., and Roiphe, H. Some suggested revisions concerning early female development. *Journal of the American Psychoanalytic Association*, 1976, *24*, 29–55.

Galenson, E., and Roiphe, H. Some suggested revisions concerning early female development. In M. Kirkpatrick (Ed.), *Women's sexual development*. New York/London: Plenum Press, 1980. Pp. 83–106.

Graham, M. F., and Birns, B. Where are the women geniuses? Up the down escalator. In C. B. Kopp (Ed.), *Becoming female*. New York: Plenum Press, 1979. Pp. 291–312.

Green, R. The behaviorally feminine male child: Pretranssexual? pretransvestic? prehomosexual? pre-heterosexual? In R. C. Friedman, R. M. Richart, and R. L. Vande Wiele (Eds.), *Sex differences in behavior*. New York: Wiley, 1974. Pp. 301–314.

Gross, A. E. The male role and heterosexual behavior. In J. H. Pleck and R. Brannon (Eds.), Male roles and the male experience. *Journal of Social Issues*, 1978, *34*, 87–107.

Group for the Advancement of Psychiatry Committee on the College Student. *The educated woman prospects and problems*. New York: Charles Scribner's Sons, 1975.

Halmi, K. A., Goldberg, S. C., and Cunningham, S. Perceptual distortion of body image in adolescent girls: Distortion of body image in adolescence. *Psychology and Medicine*, 1977, *7*, 253–257.

Harris, L. J. Sex-related differences in spatial ability: A developmental psychological view. In C. B. Kopp (Ed.), *Becoming female*. New York/London: Plenum Press, 1979. Pp. 133–182.

Heilbrun, A. B., Jr. Measurement of masculine and feminine sex role identities as independent dimensions. *Journal of Consulting and Clinical Psychology*, 1976, *44*, 183–190.

Hennig, M., and Jardim, A. *The managerial woman*. Garden City, N. Y.: Anchor Press/Doubleday, 1977.

Hoffman, L. W. Early childhood experiences and women's achievement motives. *Journal of Social Issues*, 1972, *28*, 129–155.

Horney, K. The dread of women. *International Journal of Psycho-Analysis*, 1932, *13*, 348–360.

Horney, K. The flight from womanhood: The masculinity complex in women as viewed by men and women. In H. Kelman (Ed.), *Feminine psychology*. New York: Norton, 1967. Pp. 54–70. (Originally published, 1926).

Horney, K. The denial of the vagina: A contribution to the problem of the genital anxieties specific to women. In H. Kelman (Ed.), *Feminine psychology*. New York: Norton, 1967. Pp. 147–161. (Originally published, 1933.)

Hyde, S., Rosenberg, B. G., and Berman, J. A. Tomboyism. *Psychology of Women Quarterly*, 1977, *2*, 73–75.

Imperato-McGinley, J., Peterson, R. E., Gautier, T., and Sturla, E. Androgens and the evolution of male-gender identity among male pseudohermaphrodites with a-reductase deficiency. *New England Journal of Medicine*, 1979, *300*, 1233–1237.

Jacklin, C. N., and Maccoby, E. E. Social behavior at thirty-three months in same-sex and mixed-sex dyads. *Child Development*, 1978, *49*, 557–569.

Jones, E. The early development of female sexuality. *International Journal of Psycho-Analysis*, 1927, *8*, 459–472.

Julty, S. A case of "sexual dysfunction." In J. H. Pleck and J. Sawyer (Eds.), *Men and masculinity*. Englewood Cliffs, N. J.: Prentice-Hall, 1974. Pp. 35–40.

Kagan, J. Acquisition and significance of sex-typing and sex-role identity. In M. L. Hoffman and L. W. Hoffman (Eds.), *Review of child development research*. New York: Russell Sage Foundation, 1964. Vol. 1, p. 143.

Kaplan, A. G. Androgyny as a model of mental health for women: From theory to therapy. In A. G. Kaplan and J. P. Bean (Eds.), *Beyond sex-role stereotypes: Readings toward a psychology of androgyny*. Boston: Little, Brown, 1976. Pp. 352–362.

Kaplan, A. G. Clarifying the concept of androgyny: Implications for therapy. *Psychology of Women Quarterly*, 1979, *3*, 223–230. (a)

Kaplan, A. G. Toward an analysis of sex-role related issues in the therapeutic relationship. *Psychiatry*, 1979, *42*, 112–120. (b)

Katz, P. A. The development of female identity. In C. B. Kopp (Ed.), *Becoming female*. New York/London: Plenum Press, 1979.

Katz, J. Changed sexual behavior and new definitions of gender roles. In J. R. Brown and J. D. Sawyer (Eds.), *Sex and the college campus*. San Francisco: Jossey–Bass, 1981, in press.

Kenworthy, J. A. Androgyny in psychotherapy: But will it sell in Peoria? *Psychology of Women Quarterly*, 1979, *3*, 231–240.

Kimura, D. Spatial localization in left and right visual fields. *Canadian Journal of Psychology*, 1969, *23*, 445–458.

Kleeman, J. A. The establishment of core gender identity in normal girls. II. How meanings are conveyed between parent and child in the first three years. *Archives of Sexual Behavior*, 1971, *1*, 117–129.

Kleeman, J. A. Freud's views on early female sexuality in the light of direct child observation. *Journal of the American Psychoanalytic Association*, 1976, *24*, 3–27.

Klein, M. Love, guilt, and reparation. In M. Klein and J. Riviere (Eds.), *Love, hate, and reparation*. New York: Norton, 1964. (Originally published, 1937.)

Kohlberg, L. A. A cognitive-developmental analysis of children's sex-role concepts and attitudes. In E. E. Maccoby (Ed.), *The development of sex differences*. Stanford, Calif.: Stanford Univ. Press, 1966.

Kolata, G. B. Math and sex: Are girls born with less ability? *Science*, 1980, *210*, 1234–1235.

Lamb, M. E. *The role of the father in child development*. New York: Wiley, 1976.

Lennane, K., and Lennane, R. Alleged psychogenic disorders in women—A possible mainfestation of sexual prejudice. *The New England Journal of Medicine*, 1973, *288*, 288–292.

Lerner, H. Adaptive and pathogenic aspects of sex-role stereotypes: Implications of parenting and psychotherapy. *American Journal of Psychiatry,* 1978, *135,* 48–52. (a)

Lerner, H. *Internal prohibitions against female anger.* Paper presented at annual meeting, American Psychiatric Association, Atlanta, Ga., 1978. (b)

Lerner, H. Taboos against female anger. *Cosmopolitan,* 1979, *187,* 331–333.

Levi-Agresti, J., and Sperry, R. W. Differential perceptual capacities in major and minor hemispheres. *Proceedings of the National Academy of Science,* 1968, p. 61.

Lewis, R. A., and Roberts, C. L. Postparental fathers in distress. *Psychiatric Opinion,* 1979, *16,* 27–30.

London, I. Frigidity, sensitivity and sexual roles. In J. H. Pleck and J. Sawyer (Eds.), *Men and masculinity.* Englewood Cliffs, N.J.: Prentice–Hall, 1974. Pp. 41–43.

Luria, Z. Psychosocial determinants of gender identity, role, and orientation. In H. Katchedourian (Ed.), *Human sexuality a comparative and development perspective.* Berkeley: Univ. of California Press, 1980.

Luria, Z., and Rose, M. D. *Psychology of human sexuality.* New York: Wiley, 1979.

Maccoby, E. M., and Jacklin, C. N. *The psychology of sex differences.* Stanford, Calif.: Stanford Univ. Press, 1974.

Mathis, J. Psychiatry and the obstetrician-gynecologist. *Medical Clinics of North America,* 1967, *51,* 1375–1380.

Mazor, M. D. The problem of infertility. In M. T. Notman and C. C. Nadelson (Eds.), *The woman patient.* New York/London: Plenum Press, 1978. Pp. 137–160.

Mazor, M. D. Psychosexual problems of the infertile couple. *Medical Aspects of Human Sexuality,* 1980, *14,* 32–49.

Miller, J. B. *Toward a new psychology of women.* Boston: Beacon Press, 1976.

Miller, J. B., Nadelson, C. C., Notman, M. T., and Zilbach, J. Aggression in women: A reexamination. In S. Kelbanow (Ed.), *Changing concepts in psychoanalysis.* New York: Gardner Press, 1981.

Mitscherlich, A. *A society without the father: a contribution to social psychology.* New York: Schocken Books, 1970. (Originally published, 1963.)

Money, J. and Ehrhardt, A. *Man & woman, boy & girl,* Baltimore, Md.: Johns Hopkins Univ. Press, 1972.

Moroney, R. Note from the editor. *Urban and Social Review,* 1978, *II.*

Moss, H. A. Early sex differences and mother-infant interactions. In R. C. Friedman, R. M. Richart, and R. L. Vande Wiele (Eds.), *Sex differences in behavior.* New York: Wiley, 1974. Pp. 149–164.

Nadelson, C. C., and Notman, M. T. Emotional aspects of the symptoms, functions and disorders of women. In G. Usdin (Ed.), *Psychiatric medicine.* New York: Brunner/Mazel, 1977. Pp. 334–400.

Nadelson, C. C., and Notman, M. T. Women as patients and experimental subjects. In *Encyclopedia of bioethics.* Washington, D.C.: MacMillan, 1978. Pp. 1704–1713.

Nadelson, C. C., Notman, M. T., and Bennett, M. Success or failure: Psychotherapeutic considerations for women in conflict. *American Journal of Psychiatry,* 1978, *135,* 1092–1096. (a)

Nadelson, C. C., Notman, M. T., and Bennett, M. Achievement conflict in women psychotherapeutic considerations. *Psychotherapy and Psychosomatics,* 1978, *29,* 203–213. (b)

Notman, M. T., and Nadelson, C. C. (Eds.) *Sexual and reproductive aspects of women's health care.* New York: Plenum Press, 1978.

Ortner, S. B. Is female to male as nature is to culture? In M. Z. Rosaldo and L. Lamphere (Eds.), *Woman, culture and society.* Stanford, Calif.: Stanford Univ. Press, 1974.

Parsons, P. and Bales, R. F. *Family, socialization and interaction process.* Glencoe, Ill.: Free Press, 1955.

Pederson, F. A., and Bell, R. Q. Sex differences in preschool children without histories of complications of pregnancy and delivery. *Developmental Psychology,* 1970, *3,* 10–15.

Phoenix, C. H. Prenatal testosterone in the nonhuman primate and its consequences for behavior. In R. C. Friedman, R. M. Richart, and R. L. Vande Wiele (Eds.), *Sex differences in behavior.* New York: Wiley, 1974. Pp. 19–32.

Pleck, J. H., and Sawyer, J. (Eds.) *Men and masculinity.* Englewood Cliffs, N.J.: Prentice–Hall, 1974.

Pleck, J. H. Masculinity—feminity: Current and alternative paradigms. *Sex Roles,* 1975, *1,* 161–178.

Pleck, J. H. The psychology of sex roles: Traditional and new views. In L. A. Cater and A. F. Scott (Eds.), *Women and men: Changing roles, relationships, and perceptions.* New York: Aspen Institute for Humanistic Studies, 1976, Pp. 181–198.

Pleck, J. H. Males' traditional attitudes toward women: Conceptual issues in research. In J. A. Sherman and

F. L. Denmark (Eds.), *The psychology of women: Future directions in research*. New York: Psychological dimensions, 1978. Pp. 619–644.

Pleck, J. H., and Brannon, R. (Eds.) Male roles and the male experience. *Journal of Social Issues*, 1978, *34*.

American Psychiatric Association. Women in pain said frequently ignored. *Psychiatric News*, Febraury 20, 1981, pp. 1, 26–27.

Rebecca, M., Hefner, R., and Oleshansky, B. A model of sex-role transcendence. In A. G. Kaplan and J. P. Bean (Eds.), *Beyond sex-role stereotypes readings toward a psychology of androgyny*. Boston: Little, Brown, 1976. Pp. 89–97.

Riviere, J. Hate, greed, and aggression. In M. Klein and J. Riviere (Eds.), *Love, hate, and reparation*. New York: Norton, 1964. (Originally published, 1937.)

Rosaldo, M. Z. Woman, culture, and society: A theoretical overview. In M. Z. Rosaldo and L. Lamphere (Eds.), *Woman, culture and society*. Stanford, Calif.: Stanford Univ. Press, 1974.

Rubin, J. Z., Provenzano, F. J., and Luria, Z. The eye of the beholder: Parents views on sex of newborns. *American Journal of Orthopsychiatry*, 1974, *44*, 512–519.

Schwartz, P., and Strom, D. Female sexuality. In J. A. Sherman and F. L. Denmark (Eds.), *The psychology of women: Future directions in research*. New York: Psychological Dimensions, 1978. Pp. 151–175.

Sears, R. B., Rau, L., and Alpert, R. *Identification and child rearing*. Stanford, Calif.: Stanford Univ. Press, 1965.

Seiden, A. M. Gender differences in psychophysiological illness. In E. S. Gomberg and V. Franks (Eds.), *Gender and disordered behavior*. New York: Brunner/Mazel, 1979. Pp. 453–485.

Shafer, A. T., and Gray, M. W. Sex and mathematics. *Science*, 1981, *211*, 1.

Sherman, J. A. Problem of sex differences in space perception and aspects of intellectual functioning. *Psychological Review*, 1967, *74*, 290–299.

Sherman, J. A. Therapist attitudes and sex-role stereotyping. In A. M. Brodsky and R. T. Hare-Mustin (Eds.), *Women and psychotherapy*. New York: Guilford Press, 1980. Pp. 35–66.

Slater, P. E. Toward a dualistic theory of identification. *Merrill-Palmer Quarterly of Behavior and Development*, 1961, *7*, 113–126.

Special Populations Subpanel. *Report on Mental Health of Women*. Submitted to the President's Commission on Mental Health, February 15, 1978.

Spence, J. T., and Helmreich, R. *The psychological dimensions of masculinity and feminity*. Austin: Univ. of Texas Press, 1978.

Spence, J. T., and Helmreich, R. L. Masculine instrumentality and feminine expressiveness: Their relationships with sex role attitudes and behaviors. *Psychology of Women Quarterly*, 1980, *5*, 147–163.

Steckler, G., and Kaplan, S. The development of the self: A psychoanalytic perspective. *The Psychoanalytic Study of the Child*, 1980, *35*, 85–105.

Stempfel, R. S., and Tomkins, G. M. Congenital virilizing adrenocortical hyperplasia (the adrenogenital syndrome). In J. B. Stanbury, J. B. Wyngarden, and D. S. Frederickson (Eds.), *The metabolic basis of inherited disease*. New York: McGraw–Hill, 1966. Pp. 635–664.

Stoller, R. J. Primary femininity. *Journal of the American Psychoanalytic Association*, 1976, *24*, 59–78.

Stoller, R. J. Femininity. In M. Kirkpatrick (Ed.), *Women's sexual development*. New York/London: Plenum Press, 1980. Pp. 127–146.

Tobias, S. *Overcoming math anxiety*. Boston: Houghton Mifflin, 1978.

Vogel, S. R. Discussant's comments symposium: Applications of androgyny to the theory and practice of psychotherapy. *Psychology of Women Quarterly*, 1979, *3*, 255–258.

Weissman, M. M., and Klerman, G. L. Sex differences and the epidemiology of depression. In E. S. Gomberg and V. Franks (Eds.), *Gender and disordered behavior*. New York: Brunner/Mazel, 1979. Pp. 381–425.

Wooley, S. C., and Wooley, O. W. Eating disorders: Obesity and anorexia. In A. M. Brodsky and R. T. Hare-Mustin (Eds.), *Women and psychotherapy*. New York: The Guilford Press, 1980. Pp. 135–158.

Young, W. C., Goy, R. W., and Phoenix, C. H. Hormones and sexual behavior. *Science*, 1964, *143*, 212–218.

Zilbach, J., Notman, M. T., Nadelson, C. C., and Miller, J. B. *Reconsideration of aggression and self-esteem in women*. Paper presented at the International Psychoanalytic Association, August 4, 1979.

Zilboorg, G. Masculine and feminine: Some biological and cultural aspects, *Psychiatry*, 1944, *7*, 257–296.

5

Adolescent Sexuality and Pregnancy

Carol C. Nadelson

Introduction

The implications of sexual activity in teenagers have become an important concern in our society. Although there is some disagreement on the incidence of coitus among teenagers, there is substantial evidence of an increase in the past three decades. In 1948 and 1953, when Kinsey published his data, he reported that 3% of females and 40% of males under age 15 and 20% of the females and 71% of the males between 16 and 20 were sexually active (Kinsey et al., 1948, 1953). A study by Kantner and Zelnick (1972), however, reported that 13.8% of 15-year-old females and 46.1% of 19-year-old females had had intercourse. Seventy-five percent of this group did not use contraceptives regularly, and 26% had become pregnant (Kantner and Zelnick, 1972). Sorenson (1973) reported somewhat higher figures with 19% of females and 38% of males having had intercourse by age 15. The impact of this sexual activity is clearly seen in the high incidence of pregnancy and in its repercussions for the adolescent.

Sorenson has reported that sexual activity is not conflict free. He found that adolescent girls more often report negative emotions afterward, i.e., guilt, regret, discomfort, worry, and disappointment, and they often wished they had waited. These negative feelings, however, tended to diminish with subsequent experiences. Interestingly, girls under 15 reported fewer negative effects than older girls. This can perhaps be attributed to the use of denial and rationalization in this age group, coupled with a tendency to take less responsibility for actions. Boys, on the other hand, reported emotions like excitement, pleasure, satisfaction, and power, with no age differential (Sorenson, 1973).

From the abundant literature on the emotional status and life history of sexually active teenagers and their families, it is evident that the majority of these youngsters are neither very disturbed nor promiscuous. What is most consistently reported is their

Carol C. Nadelson • Department of Psychiatry, Tufts-New England Medical Center, Boston, Massachusetts.

lack of contraceptive use and their poor understanding of sexuality (Nadelson et al., 1980; Furstenberg et al., 1969; Osofsky, 1968; Goldsmith et al., 1972).

Although studies of teenagers often reveal familiarity with the technical details of contraception, it is clear that a significant number of those who are sexually active do not use contraceptives, and a large number of those who initiate contraception discontinue it because of pressure from friends, boyfriends, or family or because they fear possible harmful effects (Addelson, 1973; Thiebaux, 1972; Line and Shafkin, 1971; Pregnancy Counseling Services, 1972). It has also become apparent that lack of information and access to contraception alone are not enough to account for the nonuse of contraceptives (Nadelson et al., 1980; Kane et al., 1972). Among the other factors involved in contraceptive nonuse are guilt about sexual activity and fear of being discovered. Psychological and adolescent developmental issues, such as conflict about separation, impulsivity, and lack of future orientation, are also important. Likewise myths about the dangers of contraceptive use and conscious or unconscious motivation to become pregnant are factors (Nadelson, 1975).

For some adolescents, nonuse of contraceptives is a way of "controlling" their sexual activity when they are fearful of being "too" sexual. It may also be a means of punishing themselves for their sexuality. For others, effective contraception may be relatively unavailable, since a medical examination involves initiative toward medical intervention and acknowledgment of sexuality. Uncertainty about what is considered appropriate sexual behavior is also a problem for adolescents. Parents are often uncertain or insecure themselves and do not provide clear guidelines. Practices and standards have changed, and the conventions supported by parents may not seem consonant with the mores of young people confronted with current peer standards (Notman, 1975; Nadelson, 1979).

Many parents, although punitive and restrictive about sexuality, present a confusing picture, because they seem overinvolved. For example, they may focus excessively on the girl's sexual behavior with questions, prohibitions, and rigid attention to the occurrence of menstrual cycles. Thus, sexual activity may be seen as consistent with the family communication, that she is "bad" or sexual.

For the young adolescent, since denial is a prominent defense mechanism, acknowledgment of the consequences of unprotected sexual intercourse may not occur. The use of contraception implies acknowledgment and responsibility for sexuality, and it may be inconsistent with the developmental stage of many adolescents (Nadelson, 1975).

It is also important to distinguish between failure to use contraception and unconscious motivation for pregnancy, since for many they are very different issues. The adolescent does not necessarily conceptualize a clear connection between sexual activity, pregnancy, and motherhood. The statement then that nonuse of contraceptives indicates that there is a positive motivation for pregnancy is simplistic.

Adolescent Pregnancy

Despite the decline in the total birth rate in the United States, there has been a dramatic increase in adolescent pregnancy during the past decade (Jaffe and Dreyfoos,

1976; Sugar, 1979). According to recent estimates, one out of ten American women becomes pregnant during her high school years, and two-fifths of 15- to 19-year-olds risk unintended pregnancy (Jaffe and Dreyfoos, 1976; National Institute of Child Health and Development, 1974). Two-thirds of all pregnancies and one-half of all births to adolescents are unplanned (Goldsmith et al., 1972).

Teenage pregnancy is a concern because of the major psychological, social, and economic sequelae of early childbearing. Premature birth, perinatal loss, and complications of labor and delivery are more frequent in the young adolescent, and they appear to be related to poor prenatal care (Mecklenberg, 1973). In addition, the younger pregnant adolescent is less likely to develop and realize life plans and goals, and the recidivism rate is alarmingly high (Mecklenberg, 1973; Sarrel, 1967). Pregnancy has been cited by one-half to two-thirds of female dropouts as the principal reason for leaving school (Nadelson, 1975; Mecklenberg, 1973; Sarrel, 1967; Coombs and Cooley, 1968). Furthermore, if an adolescent marries because she is pregnant, there is a greater probability of eventual marital dissolution (McAnarney, 1978; Lowrie, 1965).

The child born from an unintended pregnancy may have difficulty because of maternal ambivalence or rejection, which has long been acknowledged as a major contributing element in the development of psychopathology and physical illness. Furthermore, recent studies suggest that there is a higher incidence of developmental problems and child abuse than occurs with older mothers (Sugar, 1979; Lynch and Roberts, 1977). Much of this undoubtedly relates to the psychological issues that were factors in the occurrence of the pregnancy and the lack of stable support systems and resources in the family and community.

Intrapsychic Considerations

Early in adolescence, sexual fantasies and feelings are handled by direct expression in action, by symptom formation, or by repression, withdrawal, or denial. At times, the coping mechanisms employed by an adolescent is inconsistent, unpredictable, and ambivalent. The development of a stable self-image, a sexual identity, and a self-concept as separate from parents does not proceed in a fixed and orderly sequence. Thus, it is not surprising that the adolescent girl does not necessarily integrate the events and implications of menarche with a perception of herself as a physiological woman capable of procreation. The consequences of sexual activity may be perceived in vastly different ways, and often there is little focus on, or understanding of, the repercussions of sexual acts. The adolescent may feel empty or isolated, and she may see a baby as a means of receiving the care she lacks or of replacing a loss in her life. The urge to mother may be an expression of the need to be mothered and a failure to resolve early conflicts around closeness and separation (Schaffer and Pine, 1975). If the adolescent feels guilty about her sexual activity, she may see her pregnancy as a just punishment. Pregnancy may be perceived by the adolescent who is unsure of her sexual identity as an affirmation of her femininity and womanhood. It can also seem to be a vehicle for achieving independence from parents and asserting adulthood, or it may provide a sense of security and status. At times the family may communicate, overtly or covertly, that a pregnancy is desirable. Often this occurs after the last child has been born to the parents, or when there are family stresses or disruptions (Schaffer and Pine, 1975).

Schaffer and Pine (1975) discussed pregnancy as an expression of and solution to the conflict between the wish to be mothered and the urge to be mothering. Bernard (1944) described the interplay of social and familial forces with the girl's internal strivings for independence and sexual maturation. She also pointed to the significance of disorganization and deprivation in the families of the young pregnant adolescents she studied.

Deutsch emphasized unconscious motivation and mentioned flight from incestuous fantasies by means of intimacy with the first man encountered, passivity, identification with a pregnant mother or sister, revenge toward the family, and depression (Deutsch, 1945). She pointed out that no specific dynamic constellation is present for all pregnant adolescents. She also stated that the "ego is too weak to escape the dangers and temptations of the outside world or to achieve more favorable conditions under which to satisfy the urge for motherhood." Friedman (1972) commented on defective ego functioning in pregnant adolescents she saw as evidenced by "massive repression and denial of interest and knowledge of their own sexual lives." She postulated that similar unconscious dynamics exist in other women but "integrated ego function resists their expression in such disruptive form as an illegitimate pregnancy."

Although attempts have been made to study personality characteristics in pregnant and nonpregnant adolescents in order to better understand the dynamics, the diversity of motivations, stresses, and situations makes it unlikely that this is a particularly fruitful pursuit. There are, however, a few studies that provide useful insights.

One interesting report points to differences in sex-role attitudes. Among sexually active adolescents, high contraceptive users (the nonpregnant group) saw themselves as more rational, assertive, and oriented toward self-fulfillment than did those who were pregnant (Crovitz and Hayes, 1979). This suggests that those girls who assume a passive-dependent, more traditionally feminine position may also lack assertiveness with regard to sexual interactions and contraceptive use.

Although it is clear that for some adolescents pregnancy is neither disruptive nor inconsistent with the expectations and mores of their culture, the problems that do occur in our society suggest that interventions and programs for the care of these youngsters and their children are important. Even those with positive motivation toward pregnancy and the ability to mother, may require support (Fisher and Scharf, 1980).

The Dilemma of Pregnancy

When an adolescent becomes pregnant, there is often no "good" alternative. She can continue the pregnancy and care for a child or face the pain of separation and loss; or she can have an abortion and attempt to work through the conflict inherent in that choice. For the adolescent, this conflict is of particular developmental significance. It may represent the first time in her life she must make a decision with such serious implications. Even passive acceptance of pregnancy represents a decision to continue it (Nadelson, 1974). The consequences cannot be avoided or permanently denied.

Pregnancy may constitute a developmental step in the life cycle. However, it is often difficult for the adolescent to move from the position of being a "daughter" to seeing herself as the adult member of a combined mother–child unit (Nadelson, 1975). This conflict is important. It can either become a significant maturational experience in which the adolescent assumes control and direction for her life-long decision, or it can increase her feeling of failure, inadequacy, and inability to cope. An adolescent who has not recognized or worked through maturational issues or the conflicts that relate to the occurrence of the pregnancy is more at risk of becoming pregnant again (Addelson, 1973; Pregnancy Counseling Services, 1972).

Recent data indicate that a high percentage of adolescents, even those who choose to continue their pregnancies, do see abortion as a possible solution, despite their own personal choice, and few see marriage as a solution. This study also reported that a substantial number of those continuing their pregnancies stated that adoption should be considered. Few of these girls, however, actually relinquish their babies for adoption (Nadelson et al., 1980).

Decision Making

For the pregnant adolescent, the first encounter with medical care may be in the context of the decision-making process surrounding a pregnancy. This is often complicated by the delay in acknowledging or dealing with pregnancy, which is so frequent. This results in the need for an immediate decision about termination or continuation of the pregnancy, without sufficient time to work through this decision. Denial, fear, and ignorance are important reasons for the delay in the recognition of the pregnancy.

In this situation, there are two primary goals: (1) short-term intervention including decision making about the pregnancy and (2) facilitation of the psychological integration of the experience of pregnancy. This includes some understanding of motivation and circumstances.

Although pregnancy in a teenager may be considered a crisis, it is not in itself either an indication of psychopathology or a reason for recommending psychotherapy. In fact, the conditions of urgency and heightened emotionality inherent in the situation may preclude the development of the kind of therapeutic situation that is optimal (Nadelson and Notman, 1977).

Paradoxically, the objective pressure for a rapid decision about whether to terminate a pregnancy or carry it to term may serve a defensive function. In the atmosphere of urgency, the pregnant adolescent may be drawn toward activity and at the same time deny the implications of the pregnancy and the need for resolution. Conversely, the teenager may avoid active participation in the decision, because she views herself as helpless, unable to effect changes, or powerless (Osofsky, 1968).

The adolescent who is making a decision about having an abortion or continuing a pregnancy needs an ally who can help her understand her motivations, explore her ambivalence, consider her alternatives, and help her work through those family problems related to the pregnancy.

The capacity to take responsibility and to consider long-term consequences are often not part of the adolescent's ego resources at the time that a pregnancy occurs. The person who works with a pregnant adolescent is in a sensitive position. He or she must maintain objectivity and neutrality and, at the same time, avoid communicating his or her own values. He or she must offer support, concern, care, and respect for the adolescent, while also encouraging exploration of painful issues (Nadelson, 1975). In addition, suggestions for future prevention can often best be made in the context of the experience with an unwanted pregnancy, when motivation for future prevention may be higher (Nadelson, 1974).

At times, the counselor or therapist may feel strongly about the girl's choice. Thus, it may be particularly difficult to be supportive of her autonomy and objective about the realities facing her. On the other hand, it is important that the counselor or therapist not be drawn into a totally laissez-faire attitude of "anything she decides is fine." The counselor or therapist must serve as an auxilliary ego to the girl to provide the perspective she lacks and also be available to the family to help them regain their perspective. In their distress and disappointment, they may threaten abandonment, or they may precipitate rejection by the putative father, thus intensifying the girl's sense of worthlessness.

An assessment of motivation and ambivalence, as well as other aspects of ego functioning, including stress tolerance, object relations, and impulse control, are also important in the initial contact. Expectations and planning must be adapted to the developmental level and the maturity of the particular girl.

Working with a more troubled pregnant teenager may be particularly difficult, since she may be unwilling or unable to give up comforting and supportive fantasies, and she may be too terrified to face her own emptiness and inadequate resources. Repetition of the pregnancy is likely to occur if the basic issues are unresolved. An important goal of intervention involves working toward the integration of the experience, so it is not repeated, self-destructively. A distinction must be made between the girl who is seen in counseling or therapy as a consequence of the crisis of the unwanted pregnancy and those girls for whom the pregnancy is a signal of disturbance and who may be referred for psychotherapy with long-term goals.

Family Influences

Family influences, cultural and class differences, and social circumstances play a large role in determining what is acceptable and possible. Social patterns strongly influence the family reaction to a teenage pregnancy (Notman and Zilbach, 1974). Although some families are accepting, most respond with intense distress. The result then may be a family crisis where the members are anxious, fearful, angry, and guilty, and the presenting picture is confusion. Their attempts to cope with these feelings often result in a tendency to blame the girl or, more often, the boy (Nadelson, 1974; Nadelson and Notman, 1977).

Since the adolescent is often attempting to separate from her family at this time, she may attempt to polarize behavior and ideas in order to differentiate herself. She may choose a solution primarily because she feels her family wants the opposite, instead of considering the alternatives that exist for her as carefully and as objectively as possible. The family may be guilty and react by displacing their feelings onto their daughter and the punative father. At times their anger may cause them to seek to punish their daughter and "teach her a lesson" by insisting that she continue a pregnancy that she doesn't want or that she have an abortion against her wishes. Since the adolescent will likely continue to live with her family, it is difficult to help her to make a decision without their participation. This is sometimes resisted by the girl who sees the immediate problem of confronting her parents and may feel that she is unable to deal with her guilt, fear, and anxiety about their reactions (Nadelson, 1974).

The Putative Father

The putative father is usually another adolescent. If the relationship is casual, the girl may not tell him about the pregnancy. She (and her family) then assumes the major burden of the decision making and planning. If he knows about the pregnancy and remains involved, he most likely is frightened and guilty. At times, he may be attentive and concerned, at other times he may be rejecting. Family reactions and institutional arrangements may punitively exclude the boyfriend, often as a way of projecting guilt onto the person who is "really" guilty. This isolates the girl and removes from her a potential support and the person who actually does share the responsibility.

Generally, the boyfriend is more difficult to enlist in a therapeutic program than the girl; he is either too anxious and fearful and has been rejected by her either as part of her denial or in response to her guilt, or he attempts to deny responsibility himself. In those girls whose motivation for the pregnancy involves regressive wishes, with a strong identification with the baby, or the wish to become closer to her mother as an important factor, the father of the baby may indeed become consciously incidental, as far as the girl is concerned.

It may be developmentally important for the putative father to be included and involved, when possible. He may need help in dealing with the reality of the pregnancy and its implications. The tendency to conduct sex education programs and counseling for girls or to focus on the girl's responsibility often belies our own ambivalence and fosters the possibility for withdrawal and noninvolvement. The ability to avoid taking responsibility for actions can be fostered by excluding the boy. The putative father may be the vehicle for initiating important communication in both families (Nadelson and Notman, 1977).

What the Future Holds

There is an increasing tendency for those young mothers who do not have abortions to want to keep their babies (Sugar, 1979; Nadelson and Notman, 1977). A girl, thus, places herself in the position of combining her own maturational processes with the care of a baby whose needs she is not fully prepared to separate from her own.

Motivations for keeping the baby may arise from feelings of emptiness and depriva-tion. The baby may be seen as a possession or as a gift to the mother in order to enable her to receive the caring she feels she lacks. Pressure for adoption, which ignores these needs, may result in repetition of the pregnancy.

For the girl who continues her pregnancy, realistic planning is important. The young adolescent who is passive and regressed may turn the responsibility for the baby over to someone else, e.g., parents or an institution. Denial of the real implications of having a baby and sensitivity to social criticism make exploration of these issues difficult, since they are often avoided. Later, when the baby is older, alternative choices are closed, since attachments have developed and the repercussions for both mother and child can be more serious and difficult.

Conclusion

Although in a teenage pregnancy there is no ''good'' alternative, in the sense of achieving uncomplicated resolution, or the possibility of erasing the reality, there are sometimes developmental gains from this difficult experience. With the help of coun-seling and/or therapy, the crisis can be resolved with understanding. A confrontation with the issues and the involvement of family and others who are helpful and suppor-tive can introduce new possibilities for the adolescent and her family. The result may foster growth and maturation.

Adolescents live in a changing society where values are being questioned, sexual mores are changing, traditions are weakening, and social performance pressure is high. Although undoubtedly helpful, providing information or making contraceptives more available will not alone diminish the rate of teenage pregnancy. The issues are more complex and involve developmental and situational determinants as well as lack of information or resources. Becoming pregnant during adolescence may be related to unresolved familial issues and difficulty in making the transition to adulthood. Moti-vations for the nonuse of contraceptives as well as the messages communicated by an unwanted pregnancy are diverse. Clearly there is no single resolution for an unwanted pregnancy that is appropriate for all young women. The handling of this stressful period for the unmarried adolescent is critical, since its lifelong implications are instrumental in the young woman's development.

Educational programs should begin early and must be geared toward understand-ing the complexity of the determinants of adolescent pregnancy rather than merely providing information. Adolescents can use problem-solving techniques with each other in order to probe the important consequences of sexual activity. They must be able to learn to make informed decisions and to talk *with* each other and *with* adults.

In addition, programs must be developed that provide peer and professional supports and concrete guidance and advice during pregnancy, as well as for young mothers. These resources must be available beyond the immediate postpartum period, since ongoing developmental issues for both mother and child will evolve. Further, the important role of the father must be recognized and his involvement should be fostered whenever possible (Fisher and Scharf, 1980).

References

Addelson, F. Induced abortion: Source of guilt or growth? *American Journal of Orthopsychiatry* 1973, *43*, 5.

Bernard, V. M. Psychodynamics of unmarried motherhood in early adolescence. *Nervous Child,* 1944, *4*, 26–45.

Coombs, J., and Cooley, W. Dropouts: In high school and after school. *American Educational Research Journal,* 1968, *5*, 343.

Crovitz, E., and Hayes, L. A comparison of pregnant adolescents and non-pregnant sexually active peers. *Journal of American Medical Women Association,* 1979, *34*(4), 179–181.

Deutsch, H. *Psychology of women.* New York: Grune & Stratton, 1945. Vol. II.

Fisher, S., and Scharf, K. Teenage pregnancy: An anthropological, sociological and psychological over- view. *Annals of the American Society for Adolescent Psychiatry,* 1980, *8*, 393–403.

Friedman, C. Unwed motherhood: A continuing problem. *American Journal of Psychiatry,* 1972, *128*, 85–89.

Furstenberg, F., Gondis, L., and Markowitz, M. Birth control knowledge and attitudes among unmarried pregnant adolescents: A preliminary report. *Journal of Marriage and Family,* 1969, *31*, 34–42.

Goldsmith, S., Gabrielson, W., Gabrielson, I., Matthews, V., and Potts, L. Teenagers, sex and contracep- tion. *Family Planning Perspectives,* 1972, *4*(1), 32–38.

Jaffe, F., and Dreyfoos, J. Fertility control services for adolescents: Access and utilization. *Family Planning Perspective,* 1976, *8*(4), 167.

Kane, F. J., Lochenbruch, P. A., Lipton, M. A., and Baram, D. *Motivational factors in abortion patients.* Presentation at the American Psychiatric Association Meeting, Dallas, Tex., May, 1972.

Kantner, J. F., and Zelnick, M. Sexual experience of young unmarried women in the United States. *Family Planning Perspectives,* 1972, *4*(4), 9–18.

Kinsey, A. C., Pomeroy, W. B., and Martin, C. E. *Sexual behavior in the human male.* Philadelphia: Saunders, 1948.

Kinsey, A. C., Pomeroy, W. B., Martin, C. E., and Gebhard, P. H. *Sexual behavior in the human female.* Philadelphia: Saunders, 1953.

Line, R., and Shafkin, E. Pregnancy and therapeutic abortion: A critical issue in adolescence. *American Journal of Orthopsychiatry,* 1971, March *41.*

Lowrie, S. Early marriage: Premarital pregnancy and associated factors. *Journal of Marriage and the Family,* 1965, *27,* 49.

Lynch, M. A., and Roberts, J. Predicting child abuse: Signs of bonding failure in the maternity hospital. *British Medical Journal,* 1977, pp. 624–626.

McAnarney, E. R. Adolescent pregnancy—A national priority. *American Journal of Disabled Children,* 1978, *132,* 125–126.

Mecklenberg, F. Pregnancy: An adolescent crisis. *Minnesota Medicine* 1973, *56*(2), 101–104.

Nadelson, C. Abortion counseling: Focus on adolescent pregnancy. *Pediatrics,* 1974, *54,* 6.

Nadelson, C. The pregnant teenager: Problems of choice in a developmental framework. *Psychiatric Opin- ion,* 1975, *12*(2), 6–12.

Nadelson, C. Pregnancy in adolescence. In J. Noshpitz (Ed.), *Basic handbook of child psychiatry.* New York: Basic Books, 1979. Vol. IV, pp. 354–359.

Nadelson, C., and Notman, Treatment of the pregnant teenager and the putative father. In J. Masserman (Ed.), *Current psychiatric therapies.* New York: Grune & Stratton, 1977. Vol. 17, pp. 81–88.

Nadelson, C., Notman, M., and Gillon, J. Sexual knowledge and attitudes of adolescents: Relationship to contraceptive use. *Obstetrics and Gynecology,* 1980, *55,* 340–345.

National Institute of Child Health and Human Development. Center for Population Research, RFP No. NICHD-BS-75-7, Washington, D.C., 1974.

Notman, M. Teenage pregnancy: The non-use of contraception. *Psychiatric Opinion,* 1975, *12*(2), 23–27.

Notman, M., and Zilbach, J. *Family factors in the non-use of contraception in adolescents.* Presentation at the Fifth International Congress on Psychosomatics in Obstetrics–Gynecology, Tel Aviv, Israel, Octo- ber 1974.

Osofsky, H. J. *The pregnant teenager.* Springfield, Ill.: Charles C Thomas, 1968.

Pregnancy Counseling Services. *1972 Statistics.* Boston, Mass.: Author, 1972.

Sarrel, P. The university hospital and the teenage unwed mother. *American Journal of Public Health,* 1967, *57*(8), 1308–1313.

Schaffer, C., and Pine, F. Pregnancy, abortion and the developmental tasks of adolescence. *J. Child Psychiatry,* 1975, *14,* 511–536.

Sorenson, R. C. *Adolescent sexuality in contemporary america.* New York: World Publishing Co., 1973.

Sugar, M. Developmental issues in adolescent motherhood. In M. Sugar (Ed.), *Female adolescent development.* New York: Brunner/Mazel Inc., 1979. Pp. 330–343.

Thiebaux, J. H. Self-prescribed contraceptive education by the unwilling pregnant. *American Journal of Public Health,* May 1972, *62.*

Sexual Counseling in Student Health

Oliver Bjorksten

Student counseling is of particular interest to many counsellors because we feel close to students chronologically and often in fantasy. At times, we eagerly enter and romanticize the events in students' lives, without tempering our view with a realistic perspective on the particular developmental issues for the student. As students enter adulthood, they are often conflicted. They experience ambivalence regarding identity, autonomy, relationships, and their future life goals. They have reached the point in their lives where they are struggling to separate from primary relationships and to leave home in order to find their own directions and establish their own life-style. They are often unaccustomed to the degree of personal freedom they experience, nor have they had the experience of making decisions for which they must assume final responsibility. The fact that there are no longer authority figures on whom to depend may increase insecurity, although it often brings a welcome relief.

Students also experience what Tofler (1970) has called "over choice." They are bombarded by theories, ideas, and potentials with regard to their own choices, but they have little experiential base on which to make a choice. There is a paradox inherent in the need to make a choice: one cannot know if the right choice is made until it is tried out in practice, but in order to practice one must be trained. Thus, students often feel unsure of their choices and have no way of assessing the wisdom of them. Further, they must cope with unpredictability, which engenders anxiety regarding their inability to control their life circumstances. They may also be insecure about the adequacy of their coping mechanisms, especially since those mechanisms that were tolerated in their families are not always acceptable in the world at large. They may not have the opportunity to explain themselves when they have missed a deadline or performed poorly, and they may find that effort alone may not be enough to guarantee success. They are faced with the impersonality of a system that knows no excuses. They must deal with competitive feelings and with jealousies. They are being judged! These

Oliver Bjorksten • Department of Psychiatry, Medical University of South Carolina, Charleston, South Carolina.

issues may be reflected in the kinds of concerns that become focused in interpersonal relationships and often their sexuality is the means for their expression of anxiety.

This review may suggest several potential areas of conflict that students may experience. These general problems have been studied and discussed (Reifler & Liptzin, 1969; Segal, 1966; Walters, 1970; Weiss et al., 1965; Braaten and Darling, 1961; Buckle, 1972; Comstock and Slome, 1973; Deutsch and Ellenberg, 1973; Edwards and Zimet, 1976; Farnsworth, 1957; Fox and Reifler, 1967; Frary, 1968; King, 1968; Monks and Heath, 1954; Raskin, 1970; Schuckit et al., 1973; Winer et al., 1974). This should not imply that all students have problems requiring counseling, as most adolescents do not require it (Oldham, 1978). Sexual problems are only one kind of problem students have, albeit an important one (Evrard, 1974; Melton, 1967; Baldwin and Wilson, 1974). As attitudes and cultural values change, some problems are "automatically" resolved whereas others are created (Bauman and Wilson, 1974a, 1974b, 1976), so our discussion must be viewed as only a cross section of student sexual problems.

Sexual Problems of Students

There are six main categories of sexual problems that students experience.

1. Educational problems. These represent the lack of sexual information or experience necessary for a person to have a satisfactory sexual adjustment. These problems may be due to inadequate education in school but usually represent the failure of parents and other authority figures to sufficiently discuss sexual matters with their children. Closely related to educational problems are inhibitions due to the feeling of lack of permission to engage in sexual behaviors. This is slightly different than problems due to morality or religious restriction, since these latter people experience normal urges and impulses, but accompanied by considerable anxiety and guilt due to the feeling that they are breaking important rules.
2. Relationship problems are one of the most common categories of sexual difficulties. Problems can arise in the context of marriage or students living together and people who are dating. Our discussion will not be limited to heterosexual relationships but to homosexual ones as well.
3. Specific sexual dysfunctions, including premature ejaculation, seminal seepage, impotency, and ejaculatory incompetence in men, as well as orgasmic dysfunction, vaginismus, dyspareunia, etc., in women.
4. Object-choice difficulties in students, as well as sexual identity problems.
5. Psychiatric problems with sexual ramifications. Important in this category are depression, state and trait anxiety, and schizophrenia.
6. Sexual problems related to pharmacological agents.

Each of these specific problem areas will be covered in greater detail after a brief discussion of the general assessment of students, treatment planning, and implementation of therapy services.

Assessment

Aside from examining the patient's chief complaint and history of the present problem, there are a number of other issues that the physician should touch upon in the course of assessing students (Bjorksten, 1978; Keats and Bjorksten, 1978). Not all of these issues need to be explored in great depth, but at least should be appreciated for whatever contribution they make to the student's general life difficulties.

1. Developmental-stage issues. (These issues have already been discussed.) The physician must determine what kind of student and individual he is dealing with in order to be alert to age- and stage-specific problems.
2. The context and demand characteristics of the student's life situation. Important to assess are the demands from school and family, as well as the support system within the family, school, and friendship circle.
3. Student's goals.
4. Learning history with respect to coping strategies, family norms, and psychological issues.
5. Individual capacities, including overall intelligence, preparation for the course of study, and personality characteristics. All of these individual capacities are very important in determining how difficult a course of study will be for the student. This directly relates to the amount of stress the student will experience.
7. The presence or absence of individual psychopathology.
8. Peer relationships.
9. Amount and number of recent life changes. This may often reflect the overall level of life stress.
10. Sexual knowledge, experience, and functioning (Keats and Bjorksten, 1978).

Only when one has an overall picture of the student's stresses and support system can one begin to understand the potential sources for sexual difficulty. In our experience, sexual problems remain an enigma only when the physician has not inquired deeply enough into the student's background.

Treatment Planning

The main principle in treatment planning should be parsimony. Students are, by definition, developing, and as counselors it is incumbent upon us to help catalyze change and development, not to restructure personality. Psychotherapy and/or counseling itself implies that there is something wrong with the student, and often this message is more powerful than any specific help that one can render. Thus, counseling should be kept short whenever possible and should focus on removing blocks to development.

The largest single cause of treatment failure is the difficulty that a person has going from one service-rendering agency to another. Students tend not to keep appointments when referred unless there is some prior contact with that person or unless the referring physician facilitiates the referral by calling the consultant on the phone in the presence of the student and/or having the student speak to the consultant in person. The student health counselor can act as a central clearinghouse for students so that if, for some reason, they decide not to continue with the consultant, they can return for another referral.

It is easy to assume that bright, knowledgeable young people have virtually the same assets and experience as an adult, but this is often not so. Students are ignorant in some areas, whereas highly knowledgeable in others. It is important to assess the broad spectrum of a student's knowledge regarding sexuality rather than assuming that he is knowledgeable in most areas. The overall approach to the treatment of sexual difficulty involves four steps: (1) education; (2) permission giving; (3) specific advice; and (4) therapy. These steps have been fully elaborated elsewhere (Annon, 1975a, 1975b, Kaplan, 1974) and will not be repeated here.

Implementation of Services

Most colleges and universities make some provision for the delivery of health care to their students, and although students utilize these health services, many are apprehensive about consulting them for mental health problems. Their fears usually revolve around confidentiality. These concerns are especially prevalent in professional schools. For that reason, it is vital that student health services, especially mental health services, strive for genuine confidentiality with colleagues even in one's own department. In the student health psychiatry section at the Medical University of South Carolina, we will not release information about students to administrators unless the student has been informed *before* an evaluation has been conducted that this information would be shared. Aside from designated mental health consultants that the student health service refers to, students also obtain counseling from other faculty members, from the administrative offices of the deans, through some physicians who are not part of the school system, and from friends. It is extremely difficult to assess how many students obtain services officially and how many obtain them unofficially. Studies conducted at the Medical University of South Carolina Department of Psychiatry suggest that fully 50% of the students who are seen by psychiatric faculty found their way into therapy by unofficial routes. One of the most important implications of this finding is that it is very important for psychiatric faculty members to be responsive to the educational needs of their colleagues, especially around sexual problems, because it is possible that the internist or family physician colleague may be treating several students for sexual and/or psychiatric difficulties. One way of meeting these educational needs of nonpsychiatric colleagues is by interdepartmental teaching by conferences, consults, and Grand Rounds.

Another excellent method of providing sex counseling services is by utilizing peers. The Human Sexuality Information and Counseling Service at the University of North Carolina was founded at a time when the health education resources at the University were inadequate to provide sufficient services in the areas of sex information and education, crisis intervention counseling, and intermediary referrals. Table 1 shows the utilization of this service by students and reflects their concerns. One

TABLE 1 Student Utilization Patterns Since Inception of the Service[a]

Service categories	Spring 1972				Fall 1972				Spring 1973			
	M	F	Total	%	M	F	Total	%	M	F	Total	%
Contraceptive information/ referral	57	123	180	21.1	117	193	310	31.4	84	151	235	26.5
Pregnancy information/re- ferral	48	69	117	13.7	61	90	151	15.3	50	87	137	15.4
General information on human sexuality	70	64	134	15.7	49	61	110	11.2	40	50	90	10.1
Abortion information/re- ferral	63	68	131	15.4	33	50	83	8.4	55	36	91	10.3
Venereal disease/infections	48	23	71	8.3	63	30	93	9.4	66	28	94	10.6
Marital/relationship problems	23	25	48	5.6	32	26	58	5.9	38	16	54	6.1
Books requests/research information	30	29	59	6.9	11	29	40	4.1	25	22	47	5.3
Reproductive physiology/ sexual technique	31	18	49	5.8	26	19	45	4.6	26	23	49	5.5
Sexual inadequacies	2	12	14	1.7	26	12	38	3.9	27	7	34	3.8
Homosexuality	32	2	34	4.0	21	7	28	2.8	25	3	28	3.2
Speakers/discussion leaders	5	10	15	1.8	1	9	10	1.0	7	15	22	2.5
Prank/crank calls	0	0	0	0	12	1	13	1.3	3	0	3	0.3
Legal information	0	0	0	0	5	2	7	0.7	1	3	4	0.4
Totals	409	443	852	100	457	529	986	100	447	441	888	100
Student contacts/semester week	25.6	27.7	53.3		28.6	33.1	61.7		27.9	27.6	55.5	

[a]From Baldwin and Wilson (1974, p. 404).

important advantage that peer counseling programs have over official programs is that they may deliver service to students who would otherwise be reluctant to present themselves at official counseling services (Wilson, 1974a, 1974b).

Management of Specific Sexual Problems in Students

Educational Deficits

There are three major forms of educational deficits: lack of information, misinformation, and lack of experience. Frequently all three of these deficiencies coexit within the same individual. Students who lack information may seek counseling for a variety of reasons but most often to verify the sexual information they have heard. Information may be sought about contraceptive devices and venereal disease but also about sexual functioning. Students are often concerned about whether they are sexually "normal" and have questions regarding the frequency of intercourse, patterns of coitus, and so forth. Educational deficits are often closely related to sexual inhibitions caused by conflicting feelings about sexual behavior, since the inhibited person tends to avoid thinking about sex and, thus, doesn't learn as much as he might. A difficult problem in dealing with students is to differentiate the inhibited, anxiety-prone student who avoids sexual contact from the student who is experiencing a genuine morality conflict regarding his sexual behavior. Students who are inhibited often blame moral and religious teachings for their reluctance to engage in even the most rudimentary sexual behaviors. One approach to this most difficult differential diagnosis is to consult the family and minister in order to learn what acceptable behaviors are. If nothing else, it is often beneficial for the student to hear his parents and/or religious authority figures clearly state their limitations with respect to sexual and moral issues. Frequently, parents do not realize that injunctions against sexual behavior that were given to their children at age 13 or 14 still remain inappropriately in force when they are in their twenties.

Ms. X is a single, 26-year-old, third-year medical student who presented herself for treatment of extreme social inhibition, anxiety, and fear of heterosexual relationships. She was struggling with the decision of whether or not to embark on a life-style that would include celibacy but, before doing so, wanted to examine her motivations; was her wish to do so based on moral considerations or simply fear of men?

Initially she presented herself as having strong moral feelings that sex should not be a part of her life but also recognized her fear of men. During her early adolescence, she was seduced by an older boy, and, unbeknownst to her, his friend watched them have intercourse. When she discovered this later, she was mortified and became furious. She felt such extreme shame that she withdrew from social relationships, especially potentially sexual ones. Her suspiciousness of men generalized and at presentation she had virtually no heterosexual relationships except with one man who had equally severe inhibitions and with whom she felt safe. Her masturbatory behavior was normal.

The patient exhibited no signs of ego problems and manifested an obsessive–compulsive personality style. During the first few months of individual therapy, she felt extremely reluctant to speak freely with the therapist but would anxiously wring her hands and flush with embarrassment unless she could discuss intellectual topics. As she became more comfortable with the therapist, she could express her thoughts with appropriately attached affect, and she was encouraged to begin making some contact with other people, especially men. As she gradually became able to do this, she found that her efforts were rewarded and social relationships began to occur. At this point, she noticed that some of her "moral" beliefs didn't seem to have the same intensity, although they were still present.

Soon she was confronted with sexuality since some of the men she dated were interested in having a sexual relationship with her. She decided to allow one of her relationships to become sexual, and with great pride she reported to the therapist that she had had intercourse. Intercourse was not altogether unpleasant for her, although she did report being very tense and not being able to let herself go and have orgasm. As the sexual relationship continued, she soon became excited and able to have orgasms. Her greatest problem occurred only during the initiation of foreplay when she would feel very anxious.

At this point in therapy, she experienced a major adjustment of her moral belief system. She changed her attitude about sexual behavior and no longer felt it to be immoral or something she should exclude from her life. At no point in the therapy was her moral system of beliefs either questioned or attacked by the therapist. The changes that occurred were due entirely to the change in anxiety about sexual activity. It became clear to her that much of her "moral" belief system was in the service of her fear of sexuality.

Educational mislearning or sexual myths are closely related to ignorance and often are more difficult for the physician to discover, since most patients do not complain of having sexual misinformation. The best way to assess the possibility of mislearning is to question patients routinely about at least a few of their sexual behaviors to see not only what they know but also their degree of comfort in talking about sex. An uncomfortable student who is extremely inhibited about even mentioning the topic of sex will, very possibly, be not only inexperienced but also ignorant or misinformed as well. It is vital that the physician be clear about his own moral and legal limitations regarding sexual behavior so that he can state them from the outset. This is especially important when dealing with students who are in the process of learning what works well for them sexually and what doesn't. Much of this learning occurs by trial and error so that ambiguous messages from the physician are frequently taken as negative judgments about the student's behavior.

College and graduate school days are usually times when students begin to gain experience in relating to sexual partners. Students usually need support and advice on what to do, how to do it, and when to do it. They need specifics rather than vague generalities and are often more interested in specific sexual information. The physician must be prepared to quickly and easily provide this specific information to students because attempts to dodge specifics are seen as escape attempts and the physician may lose credibility.

Mrs. X is a 25-year-old, third-year dental student who has been married to her 30-year-old, self-employed businessman husband for 1 year. The X's have known each other for 4 years and decided to marry even though they were aware of conflicts about marital roles: He has more conventional attitudes about marriage than she does and resents her school work since he wants her home most of the time. Raised as an only child, Mrs. X is used to a great deal of personal freedom and resents the feeling of constriction that her marriage places on her.

The couple presented themselves for treatment of different levels of sexual desire (he desired sexual activity more often than she did), marital-role problems, and arguments mainly due to a power struggle. Both members of the couple are highly intelligent and psychologically minded, and neither has major neurotic or psychotic illness.

Marital therapy was started, and it was quickly discovered that Mr. X was feeling demoralized about the relationship since he felt that his wife would not change and neither could he unless he could see improvement in some aspect of their relationship. It was decided to begin focusing on the sexual difficulties, since that was the single most important problem according to the patients and seemed to offer some chance of rapid solution. The therapist agreed to this with the idea that if the sexual problems could be alleviated, it might combat the couple's pessimism.

The couple's sex problem was that Mrs. X didn't feel like having sex unless she was "in the mood" for it, but she was never in the mood. When the couple did have sex on occasion, it took a long time for Mrs. X to get sexually aroused, but otherwise both members of the couple functioned normally. Mrs. X was able to identify a strong sexual "script," which consisted of the belief that foreplay had to proceed in a very prescribed pattern. If her husband deviated from that script in any way, she became disappointed and angry, which inhibited her sexual feelings. Further, she felt a great deal of pressure, from herself, to hurry and become aroused. This script was learned during her adolescent years and also had the additional aspect that she felt that sexual thoughts and fantasies were inappropriate for women. Thus, she could not use her own internal associations to help provide sexual stimulation.

Treatment was aimed at her paucity of sexual fantasies and her sexual script. She was given permission to have fantasies and also reading material to help her develop them. Her response was rapid as she quickly began to fantasize, which led to increased responsiveness. The couple was also told to completely dispense with foreplay and begin sexual activity with guided clitoral stimulation in which she would start sex by guiding her husband's hand on her clitoris. Again the response was excellent. She found that bypassing foreplay (the conflicted part of the sexual activity) relieved her of performance anxiety, and she could become excited. At this point, Mr. X objected since he enjoyed foreplay a great deal, and the couple began to engage in foreplay *backward*. That is, they would begin sex play with clitoral stimulation until both were excited and then stop it and engage in their more usual foreplay activities and eventually have intercourse. The outcome has been that the sexual desire discrepency problem is resolved, and the couple feels optimistic about working on their other marital problems. Mr. X feels much less reluctant to engage in therapy and actively participates in working on the power and marital-role issues.

Although one of the tasks of young adulthood is to gain some sexual and interpersonal experience, most young people are somewhat apprehensive about sexual experimenting but nonetheless face their fears and begin relating with partners sexually. With each success comes an increase in self-confidence and an increased willingness to try new behaviors and new depths of intimacy. Unfortunately, some students cannot overcome their fears of sexuality and intimacy, and instead, avoid them. The consequences of this avoidance behavior are decreased self-confidence and increased fear that the next time they try to engage in intimate behavior they will be less experienced and, therefore, more prone to failure. If this persists, a person can actually regress in social ability so that she/he does need to fear that rejection and failure is possible.

The patient is a 22-year-old, single, second-year medical student who presents himself with the main complaint of depression and the inability to form heterosexual relationships. Further, he complains of sexual identity difficulties in that he feels as though he has strong homosexual impulses although he has never had any homosexual activity. The patient came from a home in which his mother was described as extremely domineering and specifically engaged in a pattern of behavior with her son that involved coaxing him to insult her or hurt her feelings so that she would feel justified in hostile behavior toward him. This led the patient to feel extremely fearful of women, which in turn retarded his ability to relate to them. Largely as a consequence of his inhibitions around women and lack of experience with them, he began to question his own sexual adjustment and concluded that he, in fact, must be homosexual in orientation, although he did not feel particularly attracted toward members of the same sex.

Mr. X's closest relationships were with males, especially homosexual males, who on numerous occasions tried to engage him in sexual activity, which he refused. Whenever this would happen, he would become extremely anxious and quite depressed. Therapy was directed toward his inhibitions around women and as he became more comfortable with them, he found his social relationships improving considerably. Within a few months, he found himself in a warm relationship with a woman, which quickly became sexual. Shortly thereafter, most of his concerns about sexual identity diminished, and after 7 months in this relationship, he had no question at all about his sexual orientation. His interpersonal anxiety diminished in general, and he has not been plagued with depression.

There are many forms that this avoidance of sexual and intimate behavior may take. A few of them are mentioned below.

1. Excessive interest in other things such as studies, sports, etc.

2. Adherence to religious "dictates" that prevent intimate contact with other people. There is virtually no religion that prevents intimate contact with other people, although some religions discourage specific sexual behaviors before marriage. Students who claim that their religions prevent them from dating fail to mention that those same religions provide many situations for young people to get together intimately and encourage responsible intimate behavior. They encourage courtship and marriage and usually only make some minor restrictions on the *form* of social contact rather than social contact itself.

3. Confusion of goals. Some students use dating only as a means for finding a future mate instead of as a method of learning how to relate to and enjoy other people. The result is that these people sometimes form prematurely close relationships, only to be frustrated if this occurs repeatedly. They often either avoid dating altogether because of its lack of reward or they cling to an early relationship and exclude others.

4. Perfectionism. Closely related to the "looking for a mate" syndrome is the perfectionist idea that there is only one "right" person to date or marry. As a consequence, these people find something wrong with virtually all of their dates and eventually use that as an excuse to avoid intimate contact. Both the diffusion of goals and perfectionistic approaches are usually thin rationalizations by which to avoid intimate contact.

5. Family restrictions. Some students pretend that their family is so restrictive as to prevent them from having intimate relationships with other people. Other students pretend that they are responsible for their families' well-being, especially emotional well-being, and, therefore, avoid intimate contact with peers out of "concern" for their parents' feelings. This is usually expressed as "If my mother knew I was sleeping with him, she'd be terribly upset."

6. Substance abuse. Substance abuse can be an excellent way to avoid intimacy. Not only can the anesthesia produced by some substances prevent intimacy, but it can also seriously interfere with sexual performance. Finally, there is the possibility that the intimate behaviors that do occur during drug intoxication may represent "state-dependent learnings" so that when students are not intoxicated, they may view their feelings as not being as significant or intense as they were while abusing substances.

7. Eating disorders. Obesity and anorexia are often thought to be ways by which young people, especially women, avoid intimate contact with others by way of making their bodies seem less sexually appealing.

8. Most of these forms of avoidance, if excessive, can be seen as pathological. In addition, however, schizophrenia and clinical depression are other causes for the avoidance of intimate social contact. The cognitive triad of depression (negative assessment of self, future, and world) can lead to such a pessimistic perspective of relationships that those individuals don't make even the most rudimentary attempt at intimate behaviors. Depression during young adulthood can severely affect a person's social skills and can lead to permanent deficits.

Principles of Management for Educational Deficiencies

1. Public education. Although physicians may regard their primary focus as being on individual patients, it is incumbent on them to share expertise with the public and with the student body in general. This can often do more good in preventing problems than secondary preventive measures in the office. Public presentations are often excellent practice for students and residents, and most physicians can request speakers from their nearest medical school or medical society to help them in educating local organizations and student groups. Television, radio, newspapers, especially school newspapers, and presentations to private organizations within and outside schools are all methods that the physician can use to help in treating educational deficits. Audiovisual materials, which can provide excellent information on sexual topics, are also available from a number of sources (see Appendix) (Bjorksten, 1976).

2. Include sexual questions as part of the medical history. The psychiatrist, especially in his or her role as consultant and educator, should encourage his or her colleagues to ask specific sexual questions as part of the medical history. Needless to say, these questions should also routinely be included in the psychiatric workup. If the patient is embarrassed, this must be respected but never colluded with. For further discussion of the sexual history, please see Chapter 1.

3. In summary, sexual ignorance may be due to a lack of information, misinformation, or lack of experience. The best form of treatment is education to remedy these deficits, and it is extremely important to recognize common forms of avoidance of sexual contact so that these specific problems can be addressed.

Relationship Problems

A. *Marriage.* The key concepts of the *married student syndrome* can best be summarized as anxiety, anger, and absence. This syndrome appears to occur in couples in which either the husband or the wife is a student and the nonstudent takes the supportive role. The student is usually very anxious about academic performance and feels a considerable amount of pressure to succeed for his new family. In order to justify not working, the student must do well in school. Aside from this pressure, the student is usually quite dependent on the partner and can become quite anxious when signs of disillusionment or dissatisfaction appear in the spouse. This anxiety may promote a defensive self-preoccupation, which the partner may feel is his/her fault.

If the spouse supports the family, she/he often experiences *role expansion* in contrast to the student's *role contraction*. Role expansion refers to the spouse's taking over almost all of the household duties including the job of financial support so that the student can devote him/herself entirely to studies. The problem with role expansion is that it is usually based on the assumption that there will be an adequate, if not abundant, reward later. Unfortunately, role expansion can only last for a limited period of time before the partner wishes some degree of acknowledgment. It is usually at this point that the partner makes some covert or possibly overt demand on the student, who is felt to be taking the partner for granted. These demands often lead the student to feel angry at the partner and withhold the very acknowledgment that would quickly settle the situation. The marital partner usually feels abused, left out intellectually and socially, somewhat inadequate and unattractive, and usually very needy and somewhat hurt by the degree of preoccupation of the student as well as the student's absences.

Finally, the student is usually gone, if not physically, then at least psychologically. Most professional schools require an inordinate amount of class time, followed by huge amounts of studying, which are not only anxiety producing but also extremely tiring. The married student syndrome is summarized in Fig. 1. It is very common and

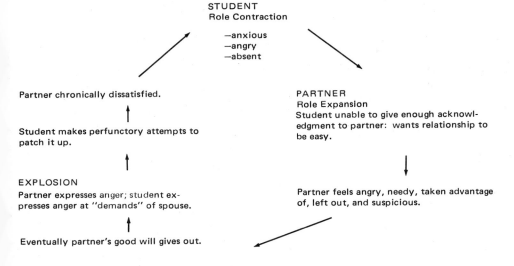

Figure 1 Married student syndrome.

often comes to the attention of professionals when the needy and hurt feelings escalate to the point of severe marital distress, most commonly manifested by arguments. Both partners feel overextended; the student wants to avoid turmoil as much as possible and usually makes some perfunctory attempts to assuage the partner, who in turn wants the student to express some genuine sense of caring. This sometimes takes the form of requesting that the student choose the partner over the schoolwork. It should be clear that in this context, intimate warm sexual relationships do not flourish. The most common complaints that students present with are decreased frequency of sexual contact and difficulties in reaching orgasm.

Marriages between two students appear to have better balance and, thus, seem to be spared the married student syndrome as described earlier. Since both students are experiencing more or less the same pressures, which can themselves create difficulty in the relationship, there is not the same feeling of unfairness and educational disparity that occurs in the married student syndrome. Problems in the two-professional marriage often revolve around the inability of partners to give adequate support to each other, lack of time, and professional competition.

Principles of Management for Married Students

1. The most important single factor in the treatment of difficulties in married students is early detection. The longer a pathological pattern continues, the more it tends to produce secondary complications of anger, acrimony, and demoralization, which often makes the prognosis for the relationship poor.

2. Increase the marital partner's support system. It is vital that the marital partner get acknowledgment and support for the effort that is being put forth to maintain the student. This can be done sometimes by contact with peers, but often established organizations that could potentially provide this kind of support fail to do so and, instead, become superficial socially oriented get-togethers.

3. The student may need to learn to manage his/her study time as much as possible so that adequate time can be budgeted for the family. This cannot only be done during the course of study but also can be done by planning some easy semesters with the express purpose of creating some extra time for the marital partner.

4. One can encourage the marital partner to increase involvement in the student's life. This may be done by asking the partner to go to the student's classes and see what they are like and even help with homework assignments.

5. Encourage role expansion by the student. Students tend to waste inordinate amounts of time worrying about academic performance. Often this wasted time comes out of the time that potentially could be devoted to the family and takes the form of sitting around and doing very little under the guise of "thinking about schoolwork." I would encourage students to take on more chores around the house, which still permit them to worry while they are contributing to the overall welfare of marital endeavor.

6. Individual psychotherapy and marital therapy. Although the earlier suggestions may appear quite simplistic, they can be highly effective for many student couples in which there is not major psychopathology or marital pathology. It is best to treat minor marital adjustment problems in a straightforward, relatively simple fashion first, and

only upon failure of these simple measures resort to in-depth therapy or long-term marital therapy. It is beyond our scope to deal with the principles of individual or marital therapy, but suffice it to say that students who have major self-esteem problems leading to depression or excessive competition probably need to be treated by individual psychotherapy. Further, patients who exhibit excessive degress of self-absorption, which are characteristic of many neuroses, also require indepth therapy. If difficulties with the experience and expression of intimacy, competition, dependency, impulse control, and symbiotic family relationships are manifest, long-term psychotherapy is usually required.

7. Finally, it is important to deal with the fantasy of "it will be better after graduation." It usually is not. People who are motivated enough to go through a strenuous professional graduate program tend to continue living in that fashion even after graduation. Things generally do not get better in the marriage, and it is important for the marital partner to become aware of that as early as possible. Either that becomes an accepted mode of the relationship or the couple will not do well later on. For example, a married freshman medical student's partner may think that after 4 years the worst is over. That's far from the truth because there usually is an internship year and at least 3 residency years, all of which require as much time away from the family as medical school did. After the residency program, there usually are the early years of establishing a practice and/or an academic position, either of which is also highly stressful and requires a considerable amount of time away from home. So, instead of a 4-year stint, the partner really has to look forward to 8 or even 10 years after college before the student reaches some semblance of equanimity and can contribute to the marital relationship. The point of this is that it is vital for both marital partners to learn ways of enjoying the present marital relationship during the student period rather than believing in the marital fantasy that rewards will be forthcoming later on.

If marital therapy is successful, then usually sexual difficulties that are based on relationship difficulties improve as well. However, it is important to emphasize that not all sexual difficulties will improve when a relationship does.

B. *Students living together*. Students living together are remarkably similar to married students but appear to have fewer difficulties with expectations of the relationship, since each partner tends to be equally involved with his/her own pursuits. One partner usually is not supporting the other, expectations of the other's role behavior are usually lower, and duties around the household are usually shared a bit more equally. The problems that couples do complain of resemble those of nonstudents in companionate marriages. There are usually fewer fights about finances, children, and role behaviors and more about affection, jealousy, and the limits of the relationship. Relationship distress usually leads to a change in the nature of the relationship and so seldom escalates to the point at which the couple desires sex counseling, although they may occasionally present themselves for couples' therapy. Sexual problems in students living together are (1) the usual sexual dysfunctions and (2) inexperience/ignorance. It is often assumed that couples living together are very sexually sophisticated. This is not always the case. It takes a certain amount of time and experience for that sophistication to develop, and, in the process, some people have difficulties. They often need information not only about contraception and venereal disease but about sexuality. If the problem is a basic educational one, it can be treated by the methods outlined earlier. If, on the other hand, guilt and inhibition are problems, then issues as well as other psychopathological problems must be considered.

C. *Dating*. Motivations for dating include simply having fun, looking for a marital partner, social pressure, loneliness, and the possibility of a sexual encounter. If two people differ in their reasons for dating, conflict will very naturally arise, which, if poorly handled, can lead to frustration and anger. Often people who date do not know each other very well. The dating situation, by definition, is designed to facilitate getting acquainted. However, since the expectation is that dating will be fun, there is demand on each person to try to have fun with someone whose preferences they don't know. The issue of whether or not a sexual encounter will occur, and if so, when and how, is often on both people's minds. On the one hand, a male may feel that it is part of his masculine role to initiate some sexual behavior in order to make his date feel attractive. On the other hand, a woman may feel that being too forward sexually might turn off her date and so might tend to inhibit herself more than she otherwise would. Thus, in the various combinations of demand characteristics, motivations, and personality factors, there is enormous potential for conflict.

Sexual problems in people who are dating are often caused by:

1. Conflicting motivations. If one person is interested in finding a marital partner but the other is interested in having a sexual relationship, there is enormous potential for feelings of rejection, hurt, sadness, and, of course, sexual dysfunction. The dysfunction might take virtually any form, including lack of desire or any of the dysfunctions mediated by anxiety.

2. Peer pressure. Some people feel an enormous pressure from their peer group to engage in sexual behavior, even though they are not particularly inclined to do so themselves. The resulting conflict can lead to half-hearted attempts at sex or lack of responsiveness once in the sexual situation.

3. Ambiguity as to when and how to initiate sexual behavior. Initiating sex has traditionally been the male's role, and it has usually been the female's role to communicate whether that initiation is welcome and if so, when. The situation is inherently ambiguous, and this can cause a considerable amount of anxiety in both partners with the potential for a consequent dysfunction.

4. Fear of failure and/or ridicule is an important inhibitor of sexual behavior in relationships. Men often are afraid that they will not perform adequately or that they are physically inadequate in some fashion for their partners. Women occasionally fear that they will look funny when they are sexually responsive and also fear being used by a somewhat heartless male. All of these will have a deleterious effect on sexual functioning.

5. Drugs. In an effort to alleviate some of the anxiety surrounding the sexual situation, some people use various pharmacological agents. These agents may have deleterious effects on sexual functioning as described in Chapter 15.

6. There can be a number of sexual "games," that is vicious interactive cycles, that people experience in the dating situation. These are self-perpetuating interactions that often have a double bind quality to them and may be caused by a large number of

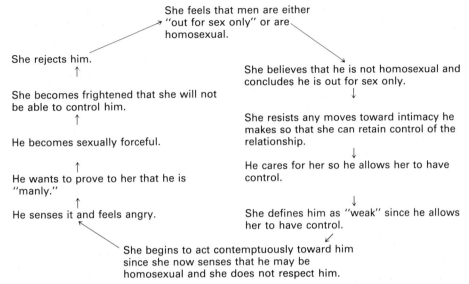

Figure 2 Polarized thinking: "Men are sexually uncontrollable or homosexual."

beliefs, expectations, communication difficulties, and so on. The most important feature of them is that complimentary assumptions and coping styles between partners allow these unpleasant interactions to continue unless something is done about them. These interactive cycles can be broken at any step and so treatment occasionally requires in-depth therapy and at other times fairly superficial marital counseling. It can be seen from inspection of Fig. 2 that treatment could be aimed at several steps in the cycle, including the woman's beliefs about sexuality, the man's need to prove himself manly, the woman's need to control the relationship, and the man's passivity. Specific intervention at any of these steps would stop this particular self-perpetuating interaction and should have important consequences to the relationship as a whole.

Specific Sexual Dysfunctions

Sexual dysfunctions have already been covered in Chapter 2 and will not be discussed in detail here. All of the usual sexual problems that have been described occur in students. Sex therapy is generally the same, the only issue being who the partner will be and whether the partner can or should come in if the students are not married. This frequently becomes a moot point, since students who present themselves in my office are generally married or living together. There is a potentially significant complication to the application of sex therapy to couples who are unmarried. Sex therapy will often artifically strengthen the relationship between two people because of the symbolic connection between it and marriage. Each are emotional "public" endeavors in which the relationship, or at least parts of it, are focused on.

Identity and Object-Choice Problems

Most physicians make a heterosexual assumption about their patients and orient all questions and comments in that direction. Although this may be a statistically reasonable presumption, it may not be on an individual basis. Thus, it is important for physicians to leave room for patients with homosexual feelings to express themselves and present their unique concerns and problems.

Students who present themselves with a specific sexual-identity problem or the complaint that they do not like their homosexual feelings must be questioned closely in order to distinguish a simple fear of the opposite sex from a genuine sexual attraction for members of the same sex. It is also important to distinguish pseudohomosexual concerns from homosexual ones. Pseudohomosexuality (Ovesey, 1969) is a condition in which homosexual thoughts and feelings result from sex-role failure either in the spheres of occupation, sex, or personality traits. As a consequence of sex-role failure, a person feels less masculine or feminine and concludes that they must in fact be homosexual even though they do not feel a genuine sense of sexual attraction as manifested by physiological arousal for members of the same sex. This condition is very different from genuine homosexuality in which individuals feel a sense of sexual attraction including physiological arousal for members of the same sex. Both of these situations are very different from patients who are simply afraid of members of the opposite sex and tend to manifest social avoidance in many forms, including sexual ones. The approach to these patients includes education, support desensitization, and/or psychotherapy. Pseudohomosexual patients generally require a considerable amount of support and possibly psychotherapy, whereas patients complaining of homosexuality generally must learn to adapt to their own sexual preference and the negative attitudes in society, unless they choose to attempt to change their sexual orientation. Generally, psychotherapy has not been of great benefit to homosexuals who wish to change their sexual orientation.

Pharmacological Agents Causing Sexual Problems

The drugs of abuse of particular concern are amphetaminelike substances and soporifics. Most students in our experience have not abused narcotic agents but use amphetaminelike substances to stay awake for examinations and soporifics for recreation. Medications that are particularly troublesome are the antihypertensives and anitcholinergic substances as well as substances with anticholinergic side effects, such as antidepressants and major tranquilizers.

Psychiatric Problems with Sexual Complications

The psychiatric conditions that cause most sexual problems in students are depression, anxiety, and schizophrenia. Depression, whether it be unipolar or bipolar, may be severe enough to decrease a person's sexual interest and drive and also may lead to significant relationship problems. Frequently, couples presenting themselves for marital difficulties or sexual problems have one or both partners who are clinically depressed. It is important to distinguish between marital difficulty in which depression is primary and causes the marital problem or one in which the depression is secondary as a result of the marital or sexual difficulty. Needless to say, the treatments for these conditions would be quite different. It is beyond the scope of this chapter to discuss the psychiatric treatment for depression. The usual treatment would be either psychotherapy alone or in a combination with antidepressants. With a bipolar illness, lithium carbonate would probably be the treatment of choice.

There are some forms of situational depression that are particularly common among students.

1. Poor academic performance can often lead to demoralization, which further reduces academic performance. Frequently, the students who are doing very poorly in school are dissatisfied with their course of study and may need to reconsider their career choice.
2. Social disconnection that occurs when students move to new institutions can often be a source of depression, anxiety, and loneliness. Often this condition improves as they develop a new social network.
3. The uncontrollability of the academic environment is occasionally such that the individual cannot cope and begins to feel depressed. If therapeutic efforts directed toward improving coping skills fail, then it may be best for these students to leave the academic enviroment rather than struggling against an impossible adaptive task.

Anxiety Syndromes

A distinction is usually made between situation-specific anxiety and nonspecific anxiety states. Spielberger (Zuckerman and Spielberger, 1976) refers to these as "state anxiety" and "trait anxiety," respectively. Situation-specific anxiety is commonly found in test situations, career decisions, and often in relationship to sexual issues. Nonspecific anxiety, on the other hand, is often related to the general unpredictability of the environment (Seligman, 1975) and psychodynamic factors that are usually unconscious.

The net result of either state or trait anxiety is that an individual experiences a state of hyperarousal and excessive preoccupation with himself. He tends to pay inadequate attention to a broad range of environmental stimuli that becomes important in the sexual situation, since the ability to openly experience environmental stimuli helps determine the ability of an individual to respond sexually. Moreover, the sympathetic arousal that accompanies these anxiety states is often incompatible with the early stages of sexual arousal, which are mediated by the parasympathetic system.

These conditions are managed by a variety of techniques including desensitization for state-anxiety symptoms and long-term outpatient psychotherapy for nonspecific anxiety states. Minor tranquilizers can be a temporary adjunct to the management of these conditions but by no means should be seen as the primary therapeutic modality. In the student population, who have to contentrate effectively on the homework material and class presentations, the use of *minor* tranquilizers is at best questionable except for the management of panic states.

Depression and anxiety often occur simultaneously and must be distinguished from the signs of schizophrenia. Both state and trait anxiety feel different, subjectively, than the experience of apprehensiveness and restlessness or schizophrenia. When schizophrenia has definitely been ruled out but both depression and anxiety are present, I would usually consider both to be related to a depressive syndrome and begin by treating that. Often tricyclic antidepressants will alleviate both the anxiety and depression in these people.

It is beyond the scope of this chapter to cover the signs and symptoms of schizophrenia, but suffice it to say that this condition is a common one that most student health physicians are extremely reluctant to diagnose. Without question, one should be reluctant to make too definitive a diagnosis of schizophrenia until one has gathered sufficient evidence to warrant it. However, it is not in the best interests of the patient to pretend that the condition is not present until a major emotional upheaval takes place. If one has adequate grounds to make the diagnosis presumptively, one can begin the appropriate treatment with major tranquilizers, usually starting in low doses, and observe the clinical response of those agents. Most commonly, the schizophrenic has severe difficulties in relating to other people and the sexual difficulties that arise are usually secondary to relationship problems rather than an integral part of the disease.

Summary

Sexual problems seen in students are fundamentally the same as problems seen in any other population, except students differ from others in their life circumstances. These circumstances include leaving home for the first time, being sheltered from the "real world" by their school situation, the demand characteristic of the school situation itself, and the vicissitudes of the stage of adult development that they are in. Marital relationships in students are extremely difficult, but the sexual problems found in those marriages are not unique to students.

Principles of management are fundamentally the same for student sexual problems as for any others, except that because the academic institution can be involved, there may be greater potential for primary prevention as well as secondary prevention of sexual difficulties.

Appendix: Sources for Audiovisual Materials about Sex Education and Sex Therapy

1. Focus International, 505 West End Avenue, New York   10024
2. Multi-Media Resource Center, 1525 Franklin Street, San Francisco   CA   94109
3. Sex Information & Education Council of the U.S., 84 Fifth Avenue, Suite 407, New York   10011
4. EDCOA Productions, 12555 East 37th Avenue, Denver   CO   80239
5. Planned Parenthood/World Population, 810 Seventh Avenue, New York   10019

References

Annon, J. S. *The behavioral treatment of sexual problems,* Vol. 1, *Brief therapy.* Honolulu, Hawaii: Enabling Systems, Inc., 1975. (a)

Annon, J. S. *The behavioral treatment of sexual problems,* Vol. 2, *Intensive therapy.* Honolulu, Hawaii: Enabling Systems, Inc., 1975. (b)

Baldwin, B. A., and Wilson, R. R. "A campus peer counseling program in human sexuality." *Journal of the American College Health Association,* 1974, *22*(5), 399–404.

Bauman, K. E., and Wilson, R. R. Contraceptive practices of white unmarried university students: The significance of four years at one university. *American Journal of Obstetrics and Gynecology,* 1974, *118,* 190–194. (a)

Bauman, K. E., and Wilson, R. R. Sexual behavior of unmarried university students in 1968 and 1972. *The Journal of Sex Research,* 1974, *10,* 327–333. (b)

Bauman, K. E., and Wilson, R. R. Premarital sexual attitudes of unmarried university students: 1968 vs. 1972. *Archives of Sexual Behavior,* 1976, *9,* 29–37.

Bjorksten, O. J. W. Sexually graphic material in the treatment of sexual disorders. In J. K. Meyer (Ed.), *Clinical management of sexual disorders.* Baltimore, Md.: Williams & Wilkins, 1976. Chap. 8.

Bjorksten, O. J. W. Basic principles of counseling for the physician. In R. C. Buckle (Ed.), *Adolescent Obstetrics and Gynecology,* 1978, pp. 557–565.

Bjorksten, O. J. W. In A. K. K. Kreutner and D. R. Hollingsworth (Eds.), *Circles: A guide to self-perpetuating interactions.* Chicago: Yearbook Medical Publ., in press.

Braaten, L. J., and Darling, C. Mental health services in college: Some statistical analyses. *Student Medicine,* 1961, *10,* 235–253.

Buckle, R. C. University students: Psychological problems and their management. *The Medical Journal of Australia,* 1972, *1,* 455–459.

Comstock, L. K., and Slome, C. A health survey of students: I. Prevalence of perceived problems. *Journal of the American College Health Association,* 1973, *22,* 150–159.

Deutsch, A., and Ellenberg, J. Transience vs. continuance of disturbances in college freshmen. *Archives of General Psychiatry,* 1973, *28,* 412–417.

Edwards, M. T., and Zimet, C. N. Problems and concerns among medical students—1975. *Journal of Medical Education,* 1976, *51,* 619–625.

Evrard, J. R. Sexually transmitted diseases on the college campus. *Journal of the American College Health Association,* 1974, *22,* 427–430.

Fransworth, D. L. *Mental health in college and university.* Cambridge, Mass.: Harvard Univ. Press, 1957.

Fox, J. T., Jr., and Reifler, C. B. Student health psychiatry at the University of North Carolina, 1956–1964. *North Carolina Medical Journal,* 1967, *28,* 129–137.

Frary, R. A. School health services: Kindergarten through college. *Journal of School Health,* 1968, *38,* 207–212.

Kaplan, H. S. *The new sex therapy: Active treatment of sexual dysfunction.* New York: Brunner/Mazel Inc., 1974.

Keats, C. M., and Bjorksten, O. J. W. Adolescent sexuality. In R. C. Buckle (Ed.), *Adolescent Obstetrics and Gynecology,* 1978, pp. 3–23.

King, S. H. Characteristics of students seeking psychiatric help during college. *Journal of the American College Health Association,* 1968, *17,* 150–156.

Melton, A. W., Jr. The sexual problems of college students. *Journal of the American College Health Association,* 1967, *15,* 10–14.

Monks, J. P., and Heath, C. W. A classification of academic, social and personal problems for use in a college student health department. *Student Medicine,* 1954, *2,* 44–62.

Oldham, D. G. Adolescent turmoil: A myth revisited. *Medical Digest,* 1978, pp. 23–32.

Ovesey, L. *Homosexuality and pseudo-homosexuality.* New York: Jason Aronson, Inc., 1969.

Raskin, M. Psychiatric crises of medical students and the implications for subsequent adjustment. *Journal of Medical Education,* 1970, *47,* 210–215.

Reifer, C. B., and Liptzin, M. B. Epidemiological studies of college mental health. *Archives of General Psychiatry* 1969, *20,* 528–540.

Schuckit, M. A., Halikas, J. A., Schuckit, J. H., McClure, J., and Rimmer, J. Four year prospective study on college campus: II. Personal and familial psychiatric problems. *Diseases of the Nervous System,* 1973, *34,* 320–324.

Segal, B. E. Epidemiology of emotional disturbance among college undergraduates: A review and analysis. *Journal of Nervous and Mental Diseases,* 1966, *143,* 348–362.

Seligman, M. E. P. *Helplessness: On depression, development and death.* San Francisco: Freeman, 1975.

Toffler, A. *Future shock.* New York: Random House, 1970.

Walters, O. S. Prevalence of diagnosed emotional disorders in university students.. *Journal of the American College Health Association,* 1970, *18,* 204–209.

Weiss, R. J., Segal, B. E., and Sokol, R. Epidemiology of emotional disturbance in a men's college. *Journal of Nervous and Mental Diseases,* 1965, *141,* 240–249.

Wilson, R. The sexual revolution vs the quiet revolution. In G. Connolly (Ed.), *Population activist's handbook.* Population Institute, New York: Macmillan, 1974. Chap. 13. (a)

Wilson, R. Targets For change. In G. Connolly (Ed.), *Population activist's handbook,* Population Institute. New York: Macmillan, 1974. Chap. 14. (b)

Winer, J. E., Dorus, W., and Moretti, R. J. Sex and college year differences in students' presenting psychiatric complaints. *Archives of General Psychiatry,* 1974, *30,* 478–483.

Zuckerman, M., and Spielberger, C. (Eds.) *Emotions and anxiety: New Concepts, methods and applications.* Hillsdale, N.J.: Erlbaum, 1976.

7

Gender-Identity Problems

Alayne Yates

Introduction

Parents are frequently concerned about gender identity and gender role. Questions about the adequacy of a boy's penis, a girl's preference for playing baseball, adolescent homosexual experimentation, and cross-dressing in preschool or latency years are frequent. In no other area are parents more worried and confused about what is "normal." Physicians are in the position to render an essential service by allowing parents to express their fears and by providing accurate information and assessment. Since education in these areas is often lacking, the physician will often seek consultation.

When a 7-year-old boy prefers to play "house" rather than baseball, he seems "odd" in terms of how we expect little boys to behave. This is but one example of identity dissonance: any discrepancy between a person's behavior, activities, or convictions and that which the culture defines as expectable behavior for a person of that age and gender. Identity dissonance in children and adolescents, as in adults, ranges from a preponderance of interests toward those of the other sex to transsexualism in which the individual is absolutely convinced that he or she is imprisoned in the wrong-sexed body. In differentiating various forms of identity dissonance, one must consider the following possibilities.

Cases

1. Nonmaladaptive variation from the traditional male/female stereotype. Several generations ago, girls only wore dresses to school, and boys always kept their hair close cropped; girls wished to become mothers and teachers, whereas boys would be pilots, engineers, or physicians. Now, even the girl who studies to become a police

---

Alayne Yates • Department of Psychiatry, University of Arizona Health Sciences Center, Tucson, Arizona.

officer, or the boy who would be a nurse, is no longer seen as maladjusted; in fact, girls with "masculine" interests are reported to become happier, more productive adults than those who maintain the more traditional stance (Jones et al., 1978; Schiff and Koopman, 1978; Bem, 1975; Chesler, 1972). Those clinicians who respond to parents' concerns who are older, or who were reared in "traditional" homes, must be aware of their biases as this has a potential impact on the advice they offer to parents.

> Nancy's mother had taken large doses of progesterone during pregnancy to avoid a threatened abortion. Nancy was born with an enlarged clitoris. A sex chromatin stain was ordered and a specialist was summoned to aid in sex assignment. At 6 months of age, Nancy's parents complained to the family physician that Nancy acted "more like a boy than a girl." She didn't like to cuddle but preferred to pull over wastebaskets and pester the family cat. In spite of this, the parents were pleased with Nancy, and there were signs of a positive attachment. They appeared relieved when it was suggested that there was considerable variation in temperament, interest, and activity among both boys and girls. The consultant also commented that girls who are active and assertive adapt more easily to current cultural expectations, and she discussed the significance of the earlier chromatin stain and noted Nancy's normal genitalia and potential for bearing children.

2. Homosexual expression in the course of normal development. It is common and nonpathological for children and adolescents to experiment with members of the same sex. Heterosexual adolescents who are involved in homosexual liaisons remain confident in their identity as male or female and continue to enjoy erotic fantasies about the other sex. It is also common and nonpathological for young children to enjoy erotic games, such as "mommy and daddy" or "doctor," with playmates of either sex.

> Beverly's parents sought consultation after they found their 12-year-old daughter, Beverly, and a friend who was staying overnight masturbating each other. At 2:00 in the morning, the father walked into the family room where the two were supposed to be sleeping in order to turn off the television, and he discovered what the girls were doing. Neither girl had a boyfriend and both were members of an all-girls club for backpacking and camping. Both girls had had "crushes" on older boys and male teachers. Both attended school socials but were seldom asked to dance as they were taller than any of the boys in their class. The psychiatrist reassured Beverly's parents that her erotic enthusiasm was normal and that she was not likely to be a homosexual. He pointed out the strength of the sex drive in early adolescence and the paucity of heterosexual experiences allowable.

3. Gender-identity conflict: The patient has covert or overt anxiety and/or depression about gender identity. The attitudes and behaviors expressed can lead to social rejection by peers and may suggest a later homosexual preference.

> Bart was born with hypospadias in which his ureter opened at the penoscrotal junction. This was corrected through several operative pro-

cedures, which began when Bart was 2 years old. In nursery school, at age 5, he was reprimanded for repetitively trying to pull down little girls' panties. He preferred playing with girls and would stay in the bathroom to see them urinate whenever possible. At home he avoided his father and brothers, preferring the company of his mother. Eventually, he was seen in the mental health clinic, where, in the second month of therapy, he wished to see the genitals of his female therapist. Shortly thereafter, Bart was reassigned to a male therapist, because the clinic staff felt that Bart would profit by a same-sex role model. This therapist explained, at some length, the difference between boys and girls. Through working with the therapist, the family became less involved and protective of Bart, and his father began to take a special interest in his activities. Over time, Bart became less anxious and started to play with boys as well as girls.

Ten-year-old Harold was brought by his mother to the family physician because of obstinacy, angry outbursts, and sullen withdrawal. His mother suspected a physical problem, as Harold had been a happy, outgoing child 2 years before. When the physician spoke directly to Harold, he appeared sad and silent. Physical examination and all laboratory tests were negative. On each of three follow-up visits, the physician tried to get close to Harold, with little success. Finally, on the fourth visit, Harold asked if the tests had shown that he was more like a girl than a boy. Then, in a flat voice, he described how his stepfather had been forcing rectal intercourse for the past 2 years. Harold did not think that mother knew anything about this as it only occurred when she was at work. Harold did not know why his stepfather had selected him instead of his brothers; he wondered if he were not more like a girl. After a family conference, the physician reported the case to the legal authorities. Harold was removed from the home and began therapy. The stepfather persistently denied the allegations and refused to be involved in family therapy. Although allegations of incest are often difficult to prove, it would perhaps have been a different solution for Harold if his stepfather had left the home, with his return contingent upon successful involvement in family therapy. This would have communicated to Harold that his stepfather was responsible for initiating inappropriate sexual activities as well as applying pressure on the parent to engage in treatment. In Harold's case, the District Attorney elected not to prosecute and the stepfather remained at home with Harold's two younger brothers.

4. Homosexuality: The patient has pronounced conscious or unconscious erotic interest in and fantasies about individuals of the same sex. This is sometimes accompanied by behavior, such as cross-dressing, or mannerisms intended to mimic the opposite sex or attract members of the same sex. When preferences and fantasies vacillate, the individual is termed *bisexual*.

Clyde, age 16, was brought by his irate parents to the family physician after Clyde was arrested in a gay bar dressed in female attire. Ever since this incident, more than 2 weeks before, Clyde's parents had confined him to his room. Father lectured and mother cried. Clyde didn't see why they were so upset and claimed that the whole thing had been a lark. He denied ever being in that bar before, although a cache of women's clothing and high-heeled shoes had been discovered under his dresser. Both parents wanted to know if Clyde was homosexual. On physical examination, Clyde appeared as a normal, but slightly effeminate, adolescent. When alone with his physician, Clyde confided that he had been a weekend prostitute for almost a year. It was somewhat dangerous, but exciting and lucrative. He had not cross-dressed in childhood but had always felt more attracted to males than females. Although he occasionally fantasized about girls, he had never participated in heterosexual intercourse. He assumed both the male and the female role with his parents and was proud of his ability to "put people on" by dressing as a woman. He was very active sexually and expressed no desire to change his orientation, although he was concerned about his parent's distress. Family therapy was recommended. In the sessions that followed, Clyde's parents began to understand Clyde's homosexuality. They expressed grief over the loss of their "normal" son and guilt over ways in which they might have contributed to his homosexuality. Eventually they accepted Clyde's decision to remain a homosexual, and Clyde agreed that he should find a less risky way to make liaisons.

5. Transvestitism: The patient, invariably a male, is erotically stimulated through cross-dressing, as he identifies with the alluring or erotic woman that he pretends to be. He may also employ women's clothing (commonly underwear or a nightgown) as a fetish, holding or rubbing the garments while he masturbates. Transvestites who use clothing in this fashion are most likely to do so in adolescence; when maturity is attained, fetishism decreases while cross-dressing increases. The continuum of transvestitism ranges from the man who is happily married and who sometimes likes to wear a nightgown while having intercourse to the man who obtains enormous satisfaction living and dressing as a woman. The latter demonstrates a greater degree of gender dissonance. The transvestite does value his penis and does derive enjoyment from it. The symptom of cross-dressing may be marked even in the preschool years.

> Robin was a 4-year-old boy who was reluctantly brought to our clinic by his mother after his paternal grandmother insisted that there was something wrong. Robin appeared as a large-eyed, anxious little boy who, on questioning, stated clearly the wish to be a girl. This was because boys were "bad" and girls were "nice." He enjoyed putting on his mother's clothes and assuming her role when playing "house" with other children. Robin played exclusively with girls and had acquired a number of expressions used by adult women. In family evaluation, it soon became apparent that his father viewed Robin as "queer" and had sided with his own mother in requesting the evaluation. There was little closeness or communication between the parents, and the mother's major emotional investment lay with Robin, her only child. She had longed for a girl prior to his birth. She saw no problem in Robin's "cute" behavior and described him in entirely favorable terms as artistic, sensitive, and kind. On the other hand, she presented men as irresponsible, self-centered, and undependable. Family therapy was recommended; however, the father was not prepared to participate because of work responsibilities. The mother soon stopped coming after several "forgotten" sessions and refused to discuss the matter further with the therapist.

6. Transsexualism: The patient is convinced that he or she was assigned the "wrong" body and is actually of the opposite sex. The genitals are devalued, and the adolescent or adult may wish to live as a person of the opposite sex. This may include taking hormones and having sexual reassignment surgery.*

> Eighteen-year-old Bud called for an appointment without his parent's knowledge. He appeared as a depressed, well-built young man with no unusual mannerisms. He gazed directly at the examiner as he spoke. A year before, he had read an article that described hormonal and surgical treatment for transsexuals. At that time, he had felt "neuter," since he did not masturbate, seldom dated, and preferred not to think about marriage. As a child, he had enjoyed playing girls' games, but he had never cross-dressed. In the months after Bud read about transsexualism, he became more and more convinced that he was truly a woman in a man's body. For a while he pilfered his mother's hormone pills and secretly enjoyed the bodily changes. When the supply of hormones was exhausted, he had become more and more depressed. Bud's physician asked for a consultation with a psychiatrist, who saw him at monthly intervals for 3 months for further assessment. Bud appeared essentially unchanged in his mood and desire. The consultant then suggested that Bud discuss his predicament with his family. He saw Bud and the family together, and although he was not able to obtain their support, they agreed not to object if his final decision was gender reassignment. Bud was referred to a center for the evaluation of gender disturbance.

Surgical reassignment is controversial following a recent long-term follow-up of 15 transsexuals who were reassigned and 35 who were not. There were no differences in marital, job, or educational adjustment between the two groups (Meyer and Reter, 1979).

7. Gender-identity dissonance: Certain cases of gender identity dissonance are more apparent than real, and great care must be taken in evaluation. Family assessment is essential since parents often project their sexual anxieties on their children.

> Robert was the first-born infant of a well-to-do professional couple. He had been incompletely circumcised at birth and, therefore, the procedure was repeated when he was 3 months old. When his parents first examined Robert's penis shortly after the operation, they summoned the surgeon and accused him of taking more than was warranted. In actuality, Robert's penis was obscured by a large fold of edematous adipose tissue. Later, Robert's father described his own penis as small and commented that if Robert's was small, he must have inherited that deficiency. Would Robert be less aggressive and more artistic than other boys, also? Follow-up at age 4 confirmed none of these fears.

> Fourteen-year-old Richard was brought to his pediatrician by his mother who wondered if some drug could not be given that would stimulate

*Further information is available in the works of Stoller (1976), Green (1974), and Meyer et al. (1978).

growth in Richard's penis. Physical examination revealed an overweight, prepubertal boy with moderate gynecomastia and normal penis and testes. During the examination, mother commented that she might have to buy Richard a bra. The physician diplomatically arranged for mother to leave the room during the rest of the examination. He spoke to Richard of his concerns about the breast tissue and reassured the youth that the swelling was a sign of "getting ready for adolescence." It would most likely be gone within a year without any specific treatment. Later he spoke to both mother and son about general principles of diet and exercise. He stressed Richard's development as perfectly normal. The consultant suggested that they consider family therapy to include Richard's father.

In yet other families, the apparent dissonance is related to the child's feelings of anger, hopelessness, or fear.

Eight-year-old Lisa had been raised by her father after her mother abandoned the family when Lisa was 3 years old. Lisa and her father were very close, and she seemed well adjusted until her father remarried. Then Lisa began to demand all of father's attention whenever possible. She insisted that he play baseball, climb trees, and take her horseback riding. Her father complied because he knew that the adjustment to having a stepmother might be difficult. After several months, the marital relationship had deteriorated to the point where the couple requested marriage counseling. Both parents described Lisa as a tomboy, who had no friends of either sex. During the initial assessment, Lisa sat huddled against her father. The stepmother was dressed in high heels, with an elaborate hairdo, whereas Lisa wore close-cropped hair, jeans, and a tattered shirt. Couples' therapy was initiated and without any direct intervention, Lisa became less dependent, less controlling, and less "masculine" as the months progressed. Lisa continued to wear jeans and to prefer playing baseball although she now enjoyed shopping expeditions with her stepmother. In therapy, both parents had come to understand that not all little girls delight in wearing dresses.

In any evaluation of gender-identity dissonance, there are two components to be assessed. The first of these is sex-role dissonance or the extent to which the patient adopts the attributes and interests of the other sex; the second is the extent to which the individual is erotically aroused by members of the same sex. If the individual's fantasies and erotic responses are dissonant with the anatomical gender, the sense of maleness or femaleness is affected and the patient may question his or her gender identity or, in the case of the transsexual, may be convinced that he or she is imprisoned in the wrong-sexed body. Although sex role and gender identity are certainly related, a modification in one does not necessarily connote an alteration in the other. For instance, weight lifting and professional sports are not in the least incompatable with male homosexuality; nor are homemaking or esthetic interests inconsistent with lesbianism. Most homosexuals of either sex behave as do heterosexuals and the underlying identification may or may not be ambiguous. In assessing gender disconsonance, both the behavior and the identification must be considered.

Variation in Sex Role (Interests and Attitudes)

On the basis of clinical experience, it would seem possible to construct a continuum of sex-role change: from that which is most consonant with the cultural definition of maleness or femaleness to that which is the least consonant.

1. *Consonance:* All of the child's interests and attitudes are consistent with the cultural stereotype. None of the individuals in this category question their maleness or femaleness and all will select partners of the opposite sex. Such an individual has often been raised in a working-class, stereotypically traditional family in which male and female roles are sharply demarcated. A boy in such a family may have been punished by both parents for behaving like a "sissy." Such rigid role modeling can be maladaptive (Lerner, 1978; Heilbrum, 1976) and associated with poor adjustment (Bem, 1975) and lower self-esteem (Schiff and Koopman, 1978; Spence and Helmreich, 1978), especially if the individual attempts to move into another social class or group. The girl whose sex role is strongly consonant may suffer more than her counterpart, as flexibility and adjustment are linked to masculinity (Bem, 1975), and feminity may be associated with emotional disorders in both men and women (Jones et al., 1978; Chesler, 1972). "Masculine" girls tend to be less anxious and more egalitarian in their sex-role attitudes. They date more often and are more likely to be accorded both academic and extracurricular honors (Heilbrum, 1976). The increased drive toward achievement may explain why these androgynous women also have been reported to score higher on intelligence tests than those who conform (Kagan and Freeman, 1963; Ehrhardt and Money, 1967). Any polarization of role would seem less propitious than an integration of those qualities that we perceive as masculine or feminine.

2. *Mild to moderate disconsonance:* Individuals in this category blend some interests and attitudes of the other sex. For instance, a boy may enjoy artistic activities or listening to classical music while playing almost exclusively with other boys. A girl may refuse to wear dresses and be a member of the debating team while she reads *Teen* magazine and idolizes pop heroes. This mingling of attitudes and interests connotes better self-esteem, greater openness, and flexibility. Such individuals adapt with ease to varying situations and role requirements. Most prefer heterosexuality, but some may be bisexual or homosexual. An example is the young woman who had been heterosexual prior to her involvement in the women's movement but who subsequently chose another woman "for political reasons."

3. *Marked disconsonance:* These individuals adopt mannerisms, attitudes, and interests predominantly of the other sex stereotype. They are perceived as different by most observers and may suffer social ostracism. Examples would include the adolescent boy who competes for female parts in the school plays or the grade-school girl who rejects other girls as "silly" and only participates in rough-and-tumble play with boys. Although such behavior may cause concern about later transsexualism, homosexuality, or transvestitism, this does not necessarily occur. Many of these individuals go on to make heterosexual choices. Some youngsters express both components within themselves and may become bisexual. Many girls in this group change at puberty, losing their blatant boyishness to adopt feminine interests and attitudes. The predomi-

nantly feminine male is less likely to change at puberty, perhaps due to the greater rejection by other males and family factors, to be discussed later.

4. *Exaggerated disconsonance:* Individuals in this group reject the culturally prescribed stereotype to adopt an extravagant stance. For example, an adolescent girl might always stand with legs apart and arms akimbo, swear like a truck driver, and be aggressively seductive toward other girls. One such girl wore jockey shorts instead of underpants and had her forearms tattooed. A grade-school boy in this category might strut in front of company wearing his mother's wigs, jewelry, and dresses or actively arrange games in which he plays a mother or female fashion model. He might wave his hands, "swish" about the classroom, speak in a falsetto voice, and be unusually loquacious, attention getting, or dramatic. He could express a violent dislike for competitive sports and describe other boys as crude, dirty, insensitive, or stupid. By adolescence, this caricature may have become so preposterous that the classroom is disrupted and the teacher antagonized. Individuals in this category are well aware of their divergence from the norm. Erotic fantasies revolve about members of the same sex and those who are sexually active are homosexual, although a few have experimented with other alternatives.

As the youngster's attitudes and interests become characteristic of the other sex, they bespeak personal, family, and cultural strain. Although homosexuality is relatively well accepted in certain subgroups, the culture at large still discriminates against the homosexual. When a boy appears effeminate, he is often rejected by his father and other males unless they also show "feminine" characteristics. Anxiety and depression are common concommitants of this psychosocial strain (Green et al., 1972).

The second, unrelated variable to be assessed is the degree to which the patient assumes a gender identity that differs from his or her biological sex.

Gender Identity

1. *Consonance:* The individual in this category feels assuredly a member of his or her assigned sex. Erotic fantasies are conventionally directed and the erotic response is evoked by the other sex. Even when a youngster has never had a conscious homosexual thought, there is likely to be an unconscious homosexual component, which is denied or repressed. In a heterosexually confident individual, this is easily accomplished and/ or the homosexual urges are relatively weak. There is little internal conflict, and protests of masculinity (the macho) or femininity (the clinging vine) are unnecessary. In a boy, such confidence allows flexibility in sex-role definition and the inclusion of "feminine" traits, such as sensitivity and artistry.

2. *Mild to moderate disconsonance:* The individual in this category entertains some question as to his or her masculinity or femininity. This may evoke considerable anxiety with efforts to counter or deny the perceived deviation. Boys who are slightly built, delicate in feature, clumsy, or late in entering puberty often worry about their masculinity. Girls who are hirsute, whose breats are small, or who are late in beginning menstruation entertain similar doubts. When youngsters compare their bodies and

abilities with those of the peer group, even minor differences can cause concern. A boy or girl may panic and assume that he is homosexual after an overt erotic response to a member of the same sex. This commonly occurs during wrestling contests, while sleeping with a chum in the same bed, or when fondling or being fondled by a parent. As our culture restricts children's physical contact across the sexes, the youngster may not recall a similar response to heterosexual body contact.

3. *Marked disconsonance:* An individual in this category not only perceives many opposite-sex characteristics of his or her own but feels of mixed or neutral gender. Such a person seeks stimulation through contact with the same sex or through activities, such as cross-dressing, which connote membership in the other sex. At the same time, he or she continues to value and "own" the genitals and anticipates with pleasure some of the privileges accorded to his own sex. An adolescent boy might dress in "drag" in order to attract another male, and yet be proud of, and enjoy using his penis in the activities that follow. In his idle moments, he might fancy becoming a woman, but he would not really wish to rid himself of his penis and would prefer to remain as a male who could attract and make love to other males. They may have no history of feminine behavior and don't appear feminine in the least but derive major gratification through erotic fantasies about, or sexual congress with, the same sex. Although most individuals in this category are homosexual, some are bisexual.

4. *Complete disconsonance.* Individuals in this category are true transsexuals. They receive little erotic gratification from their genitals and persistently seek gender reassignment through surgery. The conviction of being a man contained in a woman's body (or vice versa) is fixed and persistent, although this belief may not have crystalized until adolescence. Overall sexual activity, including masturbation, is often half-hearted or sporadic. A certain proportion of transsexuals insist that they have no erotic drive at all (Stoller, 1976). Although a male transsexual may have intercourse with another male, he will refuse to make love to one who recognizes, values, or stimulates his penis. The true transsexual wishes to alter the genitals in order to live as the other sex rather than in order to attract or cohabit with members of the same sex. All of the male transsexuals in Green's sample (Green et al., 1972) reported a compelling preference for girls' games, clothing, and activities in childhood. Others (Newman, 1970; Weitz, 1977) have made similar observations.

Transsexuality cannot be definitely diagnosed in the child, as the gender identity remains malleable at least until puberty and the response to treatment may be excellent. Unfortunately, parents are less likely to recognize or seek help for gender-identity problems per se than for the more obvious changes in role-modeling behavior. Parents of an effeminate son often equate his behavior with homosexuality and request an evaluation, whereas the parents of a true transsexual may not be alarmed even when he requests sex reassignment, because he doesn't act "swish." Thus, the more serious problems are less likely to be identified early. However, identification is possible if there is a high index of suspicion and if a sexual history is routinely included, as one would with an adult.

An older male adolescent transvestite or effeminate homosexual may claim to be a woman contained in a male body and request surgical correction. In these cases, the request is precipitated by a personal crisis, and the conviction of femaleness is neither fixed nor persistent over time (Newman and Stoller, 1974; Kirkpatrick and Friedmann, 1976). The boy may have read all about transvestitism so that he presents a convincing history. However, on closer questioning it is evident that he has been erotically active and has enjoyed his penis. In a transvestite, the crisis that precedes the request may have been his family's discovery of his cross-dressing or an inopportune arrest for lewd conduct or disturbing the peace; in an effeminate homosexual, it may have been rejection by a lover or an episode of impotence. If such individuals are mistakenly referred for reallocation surgery, great damage can result; both Benjamin (1966) and Bieber (1972) emphasize the potential for suicide.

The term *homosexual* simply connotes a preference for erotic activity with the same sex. As we have already noted, this preference does not necessarily affect sex roles; male homosexuals can be aggressively athletic and females can be unassertive and nurturant. In addition, the term *homosexual* does not necessarily connote doubt about gender identity. Transient homosexual adaptations occur in boarding schools, prisons, and in early adolescence in individuals who have never doubted their gender identity and who develop an exclusively heterosexual adaptation later on. Some homosexuals do entertain doubts about their masculinity or feminity, but they continue to value the genitals and rarely seek a sex change operation; they do not feel betrayed by nature and cruelly imprisoned in a body of the wrong sex.

In most cases of gender dissonance, social, cultural, and family influences seem the most significant. Certainly the recognition of and responses to the child as boy or girl in the earliest years is crucial, and a change in gender assignment made after the third year of life can be disastrous. However, there are also biological forces at work, and in some cases this may be of overriding importance. For instance, Money and Dalery (1976) have studied girls born with the adrenogenital syndrome, who had been exposed *in utero* to increased androgenic hormones. These girls grew to become tomboys who preferred playing boys' games and who adopted masculine dress and functional rather than "pretty" clothes and hair styles. Although this study is open to criticism, because it was poorly controlled and because variables, such as parental attitudes, were not thoroughly studied, other descriptions by Ehrhardt and Money (1967) and Goodman (1976) also implicate early exposure to virilizing agents in girls who have "masculine" interests and/or are aggressive, hirsute, and hypersexual. Males also may be affected by early exposure to estrogen. Yalom and associates (1973) have shown that boys exposed prenatally to an estrogen–progesterone compound are less assertive and less skillful in sports. Males afflicted with the testicular feminizing syndrome (androgen insensitivity syndrome), in which a chromosomally male individual's cells are insensitive to circulating androgens, develop not only a feminine appearance but act like females in all respects (Money et al., 1968). They may present for evaluation because of delayed menarche. Stoller (1968) presents seven cases in which a child was mistakenly raised in a fashion consistent with the appearance of the external genitalia. These children developed a pattern of interests characteristic of the other sex, and, from an early age, the child was convinced that he or she actually belonged to the other sex. At puberty, it became evident that the child had been correct all along, and entities such as Sertoli Cell Only syndrome, hermaphroditism, Klinefelter's syndrome, and testicular failure of unknown etiology were discovered. Perhaps the most compelling evidence to date is a recent report by Imperato-McGinley and associates (1979) who studied 18 male pseudohermaphrodites in the Dominican Republic, who were raised as girls. These chromosomal males suffered from a hereditary deficiency of the enzyme 5-α-reductase and were born with female-appearing genitalia. They remained testosterone responsive, so that during puberty the ''girls'' developed a deep voice and enlarged genitals. They experienced erections and ejaculation but were incapable of insemination because of the location of the urethral orifice. Seventeen out of the eighteen subjects began to realize that they were different from the other girls in the village when they were between 7 and 12 years of age. Over several years, they adopted a male gender identity. Although this study may be criticized because cultural factors were not clearly delineated and because the inhabitants were aware of others in the village who had changed from female to male (in fact they were called *machihembra*—first woman then man), it does strongly suggest that androgen can override the sex of rearing to promote a male gender identity. Gender identity, then, may not be as ''fixed'' in childhood as we have assumed.

There is also considerable variation within groups of boys and girls without gender-identity problems, so that biological forces may be commonly present to interact with social, cultural, and familial factors. Psychoanalytic literature has often presented ''characteristic'' family dynamics said to cause or contribute to homosexuality. Prototypes include the overprotective, seductive mother and the distant, uninvolved father (Bieber, 1972; Socarides, 1968). These theories are biased in that they emanate from studies of homosexual patients. A recent report from the Institute for Research (Bell and Weinberg, 1978) is more descriptive of the nonpatient homosexual population. However, it is quite conceivable that the lack of an appropriate role model or an overly close relationship with the same-sex parent could influence a child whose biological ''givens'' do not weigh heavily toward his/her anatomical sex. The concept of the biological given is extremely important since parents are often anxious, guilty, and overly dutiful when the youngster appears to have a gender-identity deviation. Parents can cooperate far better if they do not continue to assume the entire responsibility for the child's state. It is important to communicate that the child may be innately influenced toward other sex characteristics in order to enlist the parent's support in helping the youngster to better define his/her identity. The parent must also be made aware that the child does not choose to be different because he or she is obstinate, evil, or perverse. Children and adolescents who feel or appear more like the other sex suffer ridicule and rejection in school, if not at home. Parents can aid the child in maintaining self-esteem by remaining objective and empathetic. The parents also need to know that effeminate behavior is not equivalent to homosexuality. Many effeminate youngsters, with or without treatment, proceed toward an exclusively heterosexual adaptation.

The emergence of psychosexual gender identity occurs in several stages. First, the infant is declared male or female by the physician and then the parents. The infant is ''told'' of his gender identity in countless ways: for instance, parents behave differently in the amount and kind of touching and the amount of verbalization they accord the infant depending on the perceived sex (Lewis, 1972). Innate temperamental differences in the infant may interact to prejudice the parental response. In the second half of the first year, male infants are already more autonomous with respect to their mothers, spending less time in visual and physical contact. By age 3, boys play more aggressively, explore, and manipulate toys more. Girls are more sedentary, persistent, attentive, and imitative. By the end of the second year, children seem already to have identified themselves as male or female and can distinguish other children as the same or other sex (Lewis, 1975; Moss, 1974; Will et al., 1976; Birns, 1976). The conviction of maleness or femaleness, the "core" of gender identity (Stoller, 1968), exists from age 2 or 3. Role-modeling behavior, the selection of interests and activities characteristic of one sex, begins in toddlerhood and is fairly consistent by the time the child enters school, although there are class and sex differences (Rabban, 1950). Gender identity and role modeling are separate but related processes: for instance, a girl who feels intrinsically female is more likely to select "feminine goals" and interests if she is "expected" to make these choices.

Evaluation

When the gender-identity evaluation of a child is solicited, it is almost always requested by a mother who is concerned about effeminate behavior in her son. Gender-identity disconsonance is indeed more frequent in the male, as virtually all transvestites are men and perhaps only one female wishes to become male for every three to six males who request a sex change (Green, 1974). The predominance of male patients is also related to the greater cultural acceptance of masculine behavior in females. Increased assertiveness in the female is supported by feminists, and boyishness in girls can be seen as a normal developmental stage or a continued reasonable adaptation by parents, peers, and the physician. Not so the effeminate boy who is deemed a "sissy" or "mother's boy" by his father and needled as a "faggot" or "queer" by his age-mates. Once rejected by his peers, he may perpetuate the problem through a retreat to the tender ministrations of a solicitous mother.

The parent's presenting complaint is often vague: The boy doesn't look right, act right, or even smell right. A girl won't learn how to cook or a boy isn't good at baseball. In the course of a routine physical examination, mother may ask if the penis is "all right" or if it is safe for a girl that age to be riding motorcycles. The mother may complain that her son cannot get along without her or that he should join the boy scouts in order to make friends. It may be that the boy prefers to play with dolls, avoids sports, hates his male teacher, and for years has been strutting about the house dressed in mother's jewels, lace, and high heels. The mother may have made the appointment only because the father, teacher, or her neighbor insisted that something was strange. If questions are not asked directly in response to mother's "casual" comments, she may return home to report that the "doctor didn't think there was anything wrong." Occasionally the parent views the child as "queer," and the evaluation reveals nothing out of the range of normal. In that case, the parents' own sexual identification or the marital relationship might be examined. The mother may single out a few more feminine qualities in her son to rationalize her anger at her husband who is distant and emotionally uninvolved, or the father may complain about a daughter's masculinity when he really wonders if his wife is having an affair with a woman.

A detailed history from the parents should include the existence of any genital abnormality, such as cryptorchidism, traumatic experiences, such as circumcision or urethral dilatation during childhood, early sexual misuse or abuse, early usage of suppositories or other rectal manipulations, homosexual exploitation by an older individual, and discipline by frequent spankings of the bare buttocks. One must also inquire about hormones taken by the mother during pregnancy, the physical habitus and gender-identity consonance of relatives of the same sex, early ambiguity of the child's genitals, and, if the patient is postpubescent, the time of appearance of secondary sexual characteristics. Family factors that may be relevant include overt or covert conflicts between the parents, the patient's status as mother's ''special'' or only child, mother's devaluation of males as crude or stupid, father's absence or lack of involvement, father's brutality, drunkenness, or devaluation of mother and child, and mother's encouragement or bland acceptance of her son's cross-dressing and feminine mannerisms. Physical examination might include assessment of general habits, secondary sexual characteristics, size of penis, location of meatus, presence of testes within the scrotum, size and consistency of testes, presence of uterus and adnexa (examined rectally in the young girl), and distribution of pubic and body hair. Short stature, web neck, broadened chest, and cubitus vulgus are suggestive of Turner's syndrome.

Through a kind, nonjudgmental approach, one can assess the boy's underlying conviction of maleness or femaleness. How flexible is the child's view of sex-role behavior? Must boys only play competitive sports and never enjoy poetry? Must girls always choose home economics class and never woodshop? How would it be if mother worked and father cared for the children? It is helpful to ask the child if he would prefer to become a female when he grows up, if he would like to marry and bear children were this possible, and with whom he would like to live as an adult. What are his favorite activities and does he play with boys or girls? If he plays with girls, would he like to have more boys as friends? His perception of his father, and the closeness of that relationship, is extremely important. This can be determined by asking questions, such as ''What are the three things that your father likes to do in his spare time?'' ''What things has your father taught you?'' ''What has your father done just with you?'' and ''If you could choose just one thing to do with your father, what would that be?'' The relationship with mother may be similarly assessed. The boy's perception of his parents' relationship can be appraised by asking, ''What do your mother and father do together just for fun?'' or ''Could your father get along without your mother?'' (and vice versa). How the parents argue, who makes the rules in the house, and which parent is in charge of discipline help to determine the child's perception of the balance of power. A conversation about dreams, favorite TV programs, books, and life goals may reveal underlying fantasies. Role-modeling behavior is easy to assess either by taking a history of the child's preferences or by observing the child at play. The basic gender identity is suggested by projective tests, drawings, and favorite themes in stories or TV programs and by eliciting the child's fantasies. When a boy is asked to draw ''a person,'' and his first portrait is of a girl, this suggests a disconsonant gender identity (Green, 1974; Jolles, 1952; Skilbeck et al., 1975). He may be asked to draw a picture of his ''whole family doing something'' on one sheet of paper (KFD or Kinetic Family Drawing). The boy who identifies with mother may depict himself closest to her or engaged in the same sort of activity. He may omit the father figure entirely from the drawing, place him in a separate room watching television, or depict him taking out the garbage (Birns, 1976). These, of course, are cues to be taken only with other supporting evidence.

It is important to exercise great caution in interpreting unusual behavior to parents. Poorly informed, rigid, or anxious parents are prone to overreact and may assume "the worst," i.e., that their child is homosexual. This can precipitate rejection by at least one parent and lower the child's already precarious self-esteem. Both parents may believe that homosexuality is untreatable and refuse further intervention. Such a reaction demands patience and perseverance on the part of the consultant as he/she explores the parents' perception of homosexuality. If gender disconsonance does seem to exist, it is better to present the evidence as suggestive while emphasizing the need for family involvement and shared responsibility in therapy. An optimistic approach is warranted when the family is open and the boy prepubescent. In some cases, there is no abnormality whatsoever in the child, but the parents can only accept a son who rides motorcycles, fights, and plays football. Such families may develop tolerance while in therapy. Other families resist any concept that differs from their own and will negate even the kindest suggestions. Occasionally they will permit the child to enter therapy, hoping that he will achieve masculinity through the male therapists, but the prognosis is poor without the parents' and child's full cooperation.

Therapy

When the patient is an adolescent and there is evidence of overt homosexuality, transvestitism, or transsexualism, immediate intervention may best be slanted toward exploring the parents' and the youth's understanding of, and feelings about, the gender disconsonance. If the adolescent expresses internal discomfort with his identity and the desire to change, long-term therapy may be warranted. If the patient is a transsexual, he or she may benefit by information about available programs or referral to a treatment center.

Newman (1976) has reported on his experience in treating extremely feminine prepubescent boys. Although the treatment was lengthy, the results were highly gratifying and sometimes dramatic. He stresses early intervention as gender disturbances seem to crystalize in adolescence. He recommends individual therapy and work with the mother, who may covertly encourage her son's femininity, and the father, who is commonly emotionally unavailable or turned off by the child's behavior. An attempt is made to provide the child with an involved, adequate male role model, ideally the father, and to enhance the boy's individuation through work with his mother. In most cases, the parents' relationship with each other will eventually demand a major share of the therapist's attention. This approach can reverse the role-modeling behavior and even the apparent gender identification in the effeminate prepubescent boy. Effective intervention with the masculine girl has not been clearly outlined, although it would presumably follow the same guidelines. Davenport and Harrison (1977) do report a case of gender-identity reversal in an early adolescent transsexual girl.

Common Errors in Management

Perhaps the commonest error on the part of clinicians is to disregard seemingly irrelevant questions and statements made by parents in the course of the routine examination. When parents press the issue in spite of their own anxiety and embarrassment, the physician may feel that they are exaggerating or that the complaints are "silly." He/she may mislead the parents by omitting a thorough evaluation and then dismissing the problem as something that the child will outgrow without consultation. If the clinician is convinced that a problem exists, he or she may experience anxiety or anger at the "deviant" child because of his/her own unresolved feelings about homosexuality. As a result, he/she may refer too quickly, state that he/she doesn't handle "emotional" problems, or assume that nothing can be done anyway. This nihilistic approach is particularly unfortunate in the case of the prepubescent, cross-dressing youngster, as treatment must be instituted before puberty to be effective.

Another common error in management is to discount the importance of the family in initiating and maintaining the child's symptomatology. In families who present for evaluation because of outside pressure, resistance is usually extremely high. Unless there is rapid assessment and energetic follow-up, they are likely to sink back into complacency. A significant omission occurs when the father is omitted from the evaluation process. The father may appear disinterested or unavailable as he has already assumed that his son is a "queer" and that nothing can be done about it. Unless the father participates in family therapy, it may be difficult or impossible for the son to identify with father or to individuate from mother. Also, the mother's investment in the boy's feminine stance may be ignored. Unless the mother is fully involved in treatment and has made a therapeutic alliance, she may continue to allow her son to cross-dress and even supply him with wigs and high heels "as long as he does it in his own room." The mother's easy rationalizations hide her sadness and anger at the prospect of losing her special child. Her loss may only become tenable if she can derive greater satisfaction from her marriage, a job, or community activities. Thus, the only reasonable approach must include the family.

In deciding whether or not he or she should treat the gender-incongruent patient, the psychiatrist must assess his or her own level of comfort. If anxiety, distaste, or boredom are experienced, referral is most likely indicated. Professionals need to give themselves permission not to treat patients to whom they react with discomfort by recognizing their own very "human" limitations. In that case, however, the psychiatrist does have the responsibility for either resolving that ambivalence or making a considered referral. Unfortunately, patients such as homosexuals are more often rebuffed than referred. Masters and Johnson (1979), in their recent study of dysfunctional homosexuals, found that 23 out of 26 had been turned away, often repeatedly, by health care professionals when they requested treatment.

Other considerations include the psychiatrist's level of expertise in dealing with sexual issues and the amount of time he or she has available for what may well be a lengthy and complex problem. Certainly most psychiatrists could counsel the postpubertal transvestite or the homosexual who wishes to moderate certain kinds of behavior to avoid dangerous or upsetting consequences. The psychiatrist could also treat most cases related to parental rigidity or homophobia by providing parents with information, perspective, and a chance to ventilate. Occasionally a parent's perception of the child is not only unrealistic but bizarre, in which case the parent, not the child, warrants psychiatric evaluation and treatment. Most psychiatrists may also wish to treat the mildly or moderately effeminate preadolescent youngster when the parents are open and amenable to intervention. Therapy is then geared toward supplying adequate male role models, decreasing the boy's dependence on his mother, and enhancing the parental relationship. The homosexual who wishes to become bisexual or heterosexual, the impotent homosexual, and the true transsexual are best treated by extensive intervention.

Summary

With adequate time, patience, sensitivity, and knowledge, the phychiatrist can evaluate and treat most cases of gender-identity dissonance. He or she can assess the accuracy of parental perceptions and provide parents with a broad and valid perspective.

References

Bell, A. P., and Weinberg, M. S. *Homosexualities: A study of diversity among men and women*. New York: Simon & Schuster, 1978.

Bem, S. L., Sex role adaptability: One consequence of psychological androgeny. *Journal of Personality and Social Psychology, 1975, 31,* 634–643.

Benjamin, H. *The transsexual phenomenon*. New York: Julian Press, 1966.

Bieber, I. Homosexual dynamics in psychiatric crisis. *American Journal of Psychiatry,* 1972, *128,* 1268–1272.

Bieber, I., Dain, H. J., Dince, P. R., Drellich, M. G., Grand, H. G., Gundlach, R. H., Kremer, M. W., Rifkin, A. H., Wilbur, C. B., and Bieber, T. B. *Homosexuality; A psychoanalytic study*. New York: Basic Books, 1962.

Birns, B. The emergence and socialization of sex differences in the earliest years. *Merrill-Palmer Quarterly of Behavior and Development,* 1976, *22,* 229–254.

Burns, R. C., and Kaufman, S. H. *Actions, styles and symbols in kinetic family drawings (K-F-D); An interpretive manual*. New York: Brunner/Mazel, 1972.

Chesler, P. *Women and madness*. New York: Doubleday, 1972.

Davenport, C. W., and Harrison, S. I. Gender identity change in a female adolescent transsexual. *Archives of Sexual Behavior,* 1977, *6,* 327–340.

Ehrhardt, A. A., and Money, J. Progestin induced hermaphroditism: I.Q. and psychosexual identity in a study of ten girls. *Journal of Sexual Research,* 1967, *3,* 83–100.

Goodman, J. D. The behavior of hypersexual delinquent girls. *American Journal of Psychiatry,* 1976, *133,* 662–668.

Green, R. *Sexual identity conflict in children and adults*. New York: Basic Books, 1974.

Green, R., Newman, L. E., and Stoller, R. J. Treatment of boyhood transsexualism. *Archives of General Psychiatry,* 1972, *26,* 213–217.

Heilbrum, A. B. *The derivation of negative sex stereotypes from the adjective checklist*. Unpublished paper, 1976. Available from Johns Hopkins University.

Imperato-McGinley, J., Peterson, R. E., Gautier, T., and Sturla, E. Androgens and the evolution of male-gender identity among male pseuhermophrodites with 5α-reductase deficiency. *New England Journal of Medicine,* 1979, *300,* 1233–1237.

Jolles, I. A study of the validity of some hypotheses for the qualitative interpretation of the H-T-P for children of elementary school age: Sexual identification. *Journal of Clinical Psychology,* 1952, *8,* 1113–118.

Jones, W. H., Chernovetz, M. E., and Hansson, R. O. The enigma of androgny: Differential implications for males and females? *Journal of Consulting and Clinical Psychology,* 1978, *46,* 298–313.

Kagan, J., and Freeman, M. Relation of childhood intelligence, maternal behaviors and social class to behavior during adolescence. *Child Development,* 1963, *34,* 899–911.

Kirkpatrick, M., and Friedmann, C. T. H. Treatment of requests for sex-change surgery with psychotherapy. *American Journal of Psychiatry,* 1976, *133,* 1194–1196.

Lerner, H. E. Adaptive and pathogenic aspects of sex-role stereotypes: Implications for parenting and psychotherapy. *American Journal of Psychiatry,* 1978, *135,* 48–52.

Lewis, M. Parents and children: Sex role development. *School Review,* 1972, *80,* 229–240.

Lewis, M. Early sex differences in the human: Studies of socioemotional development. *Archives of Sexual Behavior,* 1975, *4,* 329–335.

Masters, W. H., and Johnson, V. E. *Homosexuality in perspective.* Boston: Little, Brown, 1979.

Meyer, J. K., and Reter, D. J. Sex reassignment; Follow-up. *Archives of General Psychiatry,* 1979, *36,* 1010–1015.

Meyer, W. J., III, Keenan, B. S., de Lacerda, L., Park, I. J., Jones, H. E., and Migeon, C. J. Familial male pseudohermaphroditism with normal leydig cell function at puberty. *Journal of Clinical Endocrinology and Metabolism,* 1978, *46*(4), 593–603.

Money, J., and Dalery, J. Iatrogonic homosexuality. *Journal Homosexuality,* 1976, *1,* 4–12.

Money, J., Ehrhardt, A. A., and Masica, D. N. Fetal feminization induced by androgen insensitivity in the testicular feminizing syndrome: Effect on marriage and maternalism. *Johns Hopkins Medical Journal,* 1968, *123,* 105–114.

Moss, H. A. Early sex differences and mother-infant interaction. R. C. Friedman, R. M. Richart, and R. L. Vande Weile (Eds.) *Sex differences in behavior.* New York: Wiley, 1974.

Newman, L. E. Transsexualism in adolescence: Problems in evaluation and treatment. *Archives of General Psychiatry,* 1970, *23,* 112–121.

Newman, L. E. Treatment for the parents of feminine boys. *American Journal of Psychiatry,* 1976, *133,* 683–687.

Newman, L. E., and Stoller, R. J. Nontranssexual men who seek sex reassignment. *American Journal of Psychiatry,* 1974, *131,* 437–441.

Rabban, M. Sex-role identification in young children in two diverse social groups. *Genetic Psychology Monograph,* 1950, *42,* 82–158.

Schiff, E., and Koopman, E. J. The relationship of women's sex-role identity to self-esteem and ego development. *Journal of Psychology,* 1978, *98,* 299–305.

Skilbeck, W. M., Bates, J. E., and Bentler, P. M. Human figure drawings of gender-problem and school-problem boys. *Journal of Abnormal Child Psychology,* 1975, *3,* 191–199.

Socarides, C. W. *The overt homosexual.* New York: Grune & Stratton, 1968.

Spence, J. T., and Helmreich, R. L. *Masculinity and feminity: Their psychological dimensions, correlates and antecedents.* Austin: Univ. of Texas Press, 1978.

Stoller, R. J. *Sex and gender,* Vol. II, *The transsexual experiment.* New York: Jason Aronson, 1976.

Weitz, S. *Sex roles: Biological, psychological and social foundations.* New York: Oxford Univ. Press, 1977.

Will, J. A., Self, P. A., and Datan, N. Maternal behavior and perceived sex of infant. *American Journal of Orthopsychiatry,* 1976, *46,* 135–139.

Yalom, I. D., Green, R., and Fisk, N. Prenatal exposure to female hormones: Effect of psychosexual development in boys. *Archives of General Psychiatry,* 1973, *28,* 554–561.

Incest and Other Sexual Contacts between Adults and Children

Noel R. Larson and James W. Maddock

A sizable minority of children—perhaps 25–30% of girls and 15–20% of boys—have inappropriate sexual contact with an adult prior to adolescence (Kinsey et al., 1953; Rossman, 1976). "Inappropriate" here refers to an explicit, genitally focused contact whose major purpose is erotic gratification of the adult regardless of the child's feelings. These contacts are exploitive of children, because they largely ignore the feelings of the child in favor of adult gratification and because they reflect (overtly or covertly) the dynamics of coercion (i.e., "big" overpowering "little"). This contrasts with the natural, sexually tinged touching, which is a normal part of growing up—being bathed by a parent, being examined by a physician, being discovered during masturbation or sex play, even the hugging, kissing, and stroking that are part of the sensual and erotic fabric of everyday family life.

In determining the extent of trauma or damage—if any—to a child as a result of sexual contact with an adult, four factors should be considered:

1. *The status relationship of the child and the adult.* This can usually be determined rather easily and is often part of the story that the child or parent reports.
2. *The duration of the contact (single incident vs. repetition).* Good rapport and effective interviewing skills will usually elicit this kind of information; however, the children will occasionally minimize the extent of the content for fear of being blamed for its occurrence. On rare occasions, they may also exaggerate for a variety of reasons, including the fear that they will not otherwise be believed.

Noel R. Larson • Meta Resources, Psychotherapy and Training Institute, St. Paul, Minnesota. **James W. Maddock** • *Department of Family Social Science, University of Minnesota, and Meta Resources, St. Paul, Minnesota.*

3. *The nature of the contact, particularly with regard to elements of force and coercion (both physical and psychological).* Obtaining an accurate description of sexual contact from the child will require effort, patience, and sensitivity. Beyond the details of the child's conscious experience, some cautious interpretations of the incident(s) will probably have to be made.

4. *The meaning of the experience to the child.* This factor is the key to appropriate intervention, and yet it is the most difficult to assess. It requires observation of the child's behavior as well as interpretation of the child's expressed thoughts and feelings. Since the meaning of the experience may very well change for the child over time, careful follow-up is necessary.

Based upon these factors, we will discuss four common types of sexual contact between a child and an adult, with particular emphasis upon the most complex of these—incest (Flammang, 1975; Schultz, 1975; Lester, 1975; Walters, 1975).

Violent Sexual Assault of a Child by a Stranger

Parents understandably fear the possibility that a child will be attacked, raped, and even murdered by a stranger. These incidents, through relatively rare, are emotionally charged and dramatic. They are further sensationalized by coverage in the news media and popular press. However, beyond some basic precautions that can lessen the child's chances of being chosen as an object of sexual attack, parents are relatively helpless to prevent such an incident from occurring. Most such "sex crimes" are perpetrated by highly disturbed individuals who have a well-thought-out and methodically rehearsed strategy (Gebhard et al., 1965; Stoller, 1975). When such an incident occurs, the child is usually a victim of forcible rape and should be treated as such (see Chapter 10).

Parents may also require emergency intervention measures to help them deal with their mixed feelings of terror, rage, and grief. Such an incident is genuinely an acute family crisis. When one of their children is forcibly assaulted by a stranger, many parents also feel violated, as if they themselves had been assaulted. This feeling of having been victimized can render them of little value in supporting the child. Therefore, additional support and treatment resources for the child, as well as the family, may be necessary. Some adults, when severely traumatized, tend to become emotionally numb and appear to function in a relatively rational and coherent fashion. This form of coping can be effective for carrying on the everyday routines of life despite the trauma; however, such individuals should be watched carefully for later signs of erosion of this superficial calm. At some point, most adults will need to confront their feelings of grief, anger, and even guilt for the incident.

Some parents will react to the trauma immediately, becoming emotionally agitated and moderately or severely dysfunctional. Some will express angry, even murderous feelings about the attacker. Others will rage at each other, or even the child. Feelings of guilt and remorse are common. It is particularly important to give considerable attention to working with parents, because the child's trauma can be greatly reduced if the parents are able to be sensitive and nurturing to the child.

Violent sexual assault of a child should be considered a crisis of significant proportions to the entire family. Special resources for crisis intervention and ongoing counseling or psychotherapy are often necessary. The family's regular physician can aid in several ways: to provide emotional support; to advise on medical and/or legal options; to facilitate communication between family members; to facilitate communication between family members and the medical and legal professionals who are commonly involved in such cases; to refer the family to a community resource for counseling or psychotherapy, such as a family service agency or mental health center.

Incidental, Nonviolent Sexual Contact with a Stranger

Most sexual contacts of children with strangers are incidental and nonviolent, although varying degrees of seduction and/or subtle coercion may be involved. The exact incidence of such contacts is unknown, although it is thought that they occur more often than most parents realize. Even the children themselves may be unaware of the specifically *sexual* nature of these contacts. A voyeur with an interest in young children may disguise this interest by pretending to have a legitimate reason for being in a washroom, bathhouse, or dressing area. Some voyeurs will watch children through windows of their own homes and, if seen, will make up excuses for their presence that seem satisfactory to the child. Younger children may react to contact with a masturbating exhibitionist by noting only that he was "peeing" or "doing something funny with his penis." Even instances in which actual physical contact takes place between the adult and the child may be satisfactorily "explained" by the adult so that the contact is dismissed from the child's conscious mind with little or no notice. Therefore, evidence of such contact may not show up at all, or it may show up in indirect ways at a later point in time. Unexpected sex-related questions or comments, unusual fears or anxieties, or a variety of generalized psychological symptoms *may* be reactions of a child to an incidental sexual contact with an adult.

Although not as traumatic as violent sexual assault, a child's coincidental contact with an exhibitionist, voyeur, or fondler can become a family crisis, particularly if the parents are prone to expect a significant developmental impact on the child. If a child directly reports that such an incident has occurred, parents should be encouraged to begin by obtaining further information from the child in a direct, but thoughtful and reassuring, fashion. Frequently, children feel ambivalent about such an incident. They may feel anxious and distressed but also curious and somewhat aroused. They may also feel guilty about behavior on their part that they believe caused the incident to occur. Some children do indeed have a role in instigating certain kinds of sexual contacts with adults, even though they do not recognize the full consequences of their teasing and/or seductive behavior. Some children of prepubertal or early adolescent age may even consciously instigate sexual contact with an older adolescent or adult as a result of what they perceive as a "prank" or peer group challenge. For a minority of children, seeking sexual contact with an adult will be a manifestation of a complex emotional disturbance or of an early antisocial character disorder. Nevertheless, the child should not be labeled ''responsible'' for the contact, since an adult whom a child consciously or unconsciously seeks to seduce has a choice. In addition, adults are charged with the maturity to guide children or to correct the inappropriate choices of the child.

Few children will voluntarily come to a physician or psychiatrist's office complaining of sexual molestation by a strange adult. Most often, they will come at the insistence of a parent, either because a sexual incident has recently taken place or because the parent is at a loss to explain certain physical or psychological symptoms in the child. Though they seldom occur in this type of incident, physical symptoms (e.g., evidence of gonorrhea) should be investigated and treated appropriately. If a specific incident is reported, the clinician should arrange to interview the child and the parent alone as well as together, in order to learn the details of the incident. Most likely, the focus of the interview will be on ascertaining the meaning of the incident and aiding the child and the parent in taking steps to avoid its recurrence. Unless there is clear-cut evidence to the contrary, the child's word should be taken at face value, since credibility is an important issue for those who have been victimized. If there is a strong reason to doubt the child's account of the incident, it is wise to refer the family to an appropriate investigatory agency and/or counseling resource.

Parents need to express their feelings about the reported incident in a supportive, reassuring context where they can obtain a sense of perspective. This may also be a good opportunity for the clinician to bring parents and child together in order to facilitate communication about the incident, and to develop mutual strategies for future prevention. Finally, parents should be alerted to watch for indirect effects of the incident at a later point in time. These may be sleep disturbances, or regression with symptoms, such as bedwetting, overdependent behavior discrepant with the child's developmental stage, changes in school behavior, severe acting out, or withdrawal.

If, instead of a specific incident, vague complaints, such as genital pains with no physiological cause, overly emphatic needs for modesty, or overreactions to previously unnoticed adult nudity are reported, parents may seek consultation. The consultant should be aware of the possibility of earlier sexual trauma of some kind, even when minor events are reported. If an incident is finally revealed by the child, it should be investigated. Parents, in this context, should not convey negative feelings to the child despite their own anxieties and anger. Parents' inappropriate reactions to a sex-related incident may further discourage the child from revealing such incidents or from talking freely and openly about other sex-related concerns and experiences. This communicates that it is wrong to talk about sex openly, even at times when this silence is to their own disadvantage.

Incidental or Occasional Contact with Someone Known to the Child

Experts estimate that the greatest frequency of sexual contact occurs between a child and an adult who is known to that child, either an acquaintance or a relative (Finkelhor, 1979; Gagnon, 1965). This includes neighbors, babysitters, older siblings, and friends, relatives, and others with whom the child has had at least intermittent contact. A child's sexual contact with an acquaintance is often repetitive and may include sexual intercourse or oral–genital contact. The interpersonal dynamics of the contact are likely to be more complex in this situation. The meaning of the sexual behavior to the child, both in short-term and long-term perspectives, is less predictable. The child is more apt to have a role, even unwittingly, in the interaction. Sometimes the child's cooperation is elicited through enticements or rewards (e.g., money, candy). Other times, the child feels a subtle but powerful sense of coercion due to the authority of the adult (e.g., a neighbor with whom the child has a great deal of contact). As a result, the child is likely to feel ambivalent about reporting the incident and to report it in such a way that the roles of the participants are confused and/or distorted.

Parents also have greater ambivalence in handling this type of sexual molestation. They may have considerable anxiety about how to confront someone they know. Or they may be conflicted about whom to believe, particularly if the adult in question denies that any such incidents took place. All of these complexities and ambiguities increase greatly when the duration of the sexual contact between adult and child has been lengthy prior to discovery. Another question is whether more than one child in the family has been affected.

All in all, then, the discovery of this type of sexual contact between a child and an adult is complex and probably will require extensive intervention. The family's regular physician is most likely to encounter this type of sexual molestation when it has been brought to light following a specific incident, or when parents have noticed some change in their child's physical status or behavior that they are at a loss to explain.

An individual interview with the child should be undertaken if the parents approve and the child seems willing. This interview should include the following components: (1) privacy; (2) careful listening; (3) reassurance that it is okay to talk and ask questions and that blame is not being attributed for the incident; (4) "what," "where," and "how" questions rather than "why" questions since the latter can sound accusatory; (5) attention to the *meaning* of the contacts to the child; (6) ascertaining how much one child has told others about the sexual contact, including the parents; (7) reassurance that steps are being taken to protect the child from further molestation; (8) preparation for a physical examination by explaining its purpose and the procedures; (9) open-ended questions, depending upon the child's level of comprehension and general emotional state, are most helpful. The clinician should also be explicit with the child about the sexual content (e.g., "And where did he touch you with his penis?") while at the same time gearing language to the child's own vocabulary (e.g., "thing," "wienee," or "dick" for penis).

If a special examination has not previously been done on an emergency basis, a complete physical should be done with emphasis on symptoms, such as vaginal discharge in girls or urethral discharge in boys (possible gonorrhea); oral lesions of an unexplained nature (gonorrhea transmitted through oral sex); rectal pain or discharge (from anal insertions or anal gonorrhea); and genital lacerations, bruises, or abrasions. Findings from the physical examination and laboratory tests should be carefully documented, since there is a potential need for medical evidence if later court procedures are instituted.

It is also important to plan to talk with the parents privately about their views of the molestation. In an atmosphere of calm reassurance and support, important information can be exchanged by all parties. Parents should be:

1. Reassured that children are not usually violently attacked or physically hurt during a sexual contact with an adult. At the same time, they need information on medical findings and treatment possibilities, if appropriate.

2. Advised to believe their child's report of the sexual contact and cautioned against blaming the child or expressing their anger or anxiety directly to the child.

3. Given an opportunity to express their own personal feelings, and helped to respond rationally and thoughtfully to the situation.

4. Encouraged to respect their child's privacy and to maintain an open and positive atmosphere of communication with the child.

5. Advised to continue to take a positive approach to sexuality and sex-related matters in the home. The discovery of an incident of inappropriate sexual contact on the child's part should not lead the parents to unduly restrict the child or to shut out all sexual stimuli from the child's life in an effort to keep the incident from recurring.

6. Alerted to possible indirect evidence of upset in the child that may be a result of the sexual contacts or of the bringing of these contacts out into the open. Common postmolestation problems, as noted earlier, include sleep disturbances, bedwetting, generalized fears, regressive dependent behaviors, or general manifestations of anxiety such as stomach aches, crying spells, or loss of appetite.

7. Advised and aided in putting an immediate stop to the sexual contact or the threat of contact between the child and the adult in question. Appropriate authorities might also be contacted, such as the children's protective services agency (welfare department), police, or the local county attorney's office. All states have a mandatory reporting law that requires that the physician supply information to the appropriate authorities or face possible misdemeanor charges, or even a civil suit, for failure to protect the child.

Since, as noted earlier, parents tend to suffer some of the same victimlike responses as do their children, they will require support and, at times, more specialized therapy. Interviews or counseling sessions undertaken with all family members present should be done in an atmosphere of reassurance, support, and facilitative communication rather than with an aura of investigation. The clinician's goal is to facilitate a return to the state of equilibrium in the family while taking steps to assure that inappropriate sexual contacts do not recur.

Sexual Contact within the Family—Incest

Although incest—sexual contact between a child and a close relative—was previously estimated an infrequent activity (such as one to nine cases per million in the general population) (Weinberg, 1955), current estimates are running as high as one or two cases of adult/child incest out of ten, i.e., 10–20% (Halleck, 1962; Lukianowitz, 1972; Malmquist et al., 1966; Finkelhor, 1979; Tormes, 1968; Gagnon, 1965). At best, this estimate is highly speculative and projects the belief of experts in the field that the reported incidence of incest (7000 cases in the United States in 1976) is merely the tip of the iceberg (Rosenfeld et al., 1976). It is speculated by some health professionals that sexual abuse is a more common childhood problem than broken homes or tonsillitis.

It is difficult to elicit exact incidence figures for incest, because it frequently goes on undetected by most health professionals unless they specifically ask the patient whether or not such an activity has occurred or is currently occurring. Most physicians consider it "invasive," if not "dangerous," to ask children if their parents or other adults have been sexual with them. Many who do so, do so in a form that children may be unable to understand. For example, asking a 7- or 8-year-old if an adult has ever "masturbated" or "fondled" their genitals, had "sexual intercourse" with them, or "seduced" them is unlikely to produce an accurate response, because the child is unfamiliar with the words and their meaning.

The literature seems divided about the overall impact of incest on the child, with some authors viewing incest as most frequently nontraumatic for the child, and other authors always predicting a traumatic psychological impact on the child, persisting into adulthood (Meiselman, 1978; Justice & Justice, 1979). Although few generalizations can be made about the overall effects of incest on children, the authors believe that the following variables are important in assessing the potential impact.

1. *The discrepancy in ages between children or between child and adult.* Generally speaking, the greater the distance in ages between the parties involved, the greater the potential for trauma to the child. For example, one could generally expect little or no traumatic impact on children involved in sibling incest if their ages are 6 and 7, or 15 and 17. However, if the children involved are 4 and 12, or 9 and 19, the potential for trauma substantially increases. Similarly, one could expect less psychological trauma when incest occurs between a 17-year-old and her 22-year-old uncle than when sexual contact is between a 12- or 13-year-old and her 22-year-old uncle or 25-year-old steparent. The important variable behind this principle is, again, "big" doing something to "little," with "little" unable to cognitively and emotionally respond with an age-appropriate choice.

2. *The amount of force or threat used to coerce the sexual activity.* Actual physical violence or physical force are used infrequently to coerce sexual contact between children and their parents or parent-substitutes. In instances where force or violence are used, the major vehicle for trauma is the intense fear of physical harm or even death rather than the sexual contact itself. Similarly, in situations where violence is threatened, the child is potentially more traumatized from the fear and associated loss of trust in the nurturing adult than from the sexual contact.

3. *The duration of the contact.* The longer the time frame in which incest occurs, the greater the potential for trauma. For example, sibling incest occurring for a 1- or even 2-year period pre- or midpuberty could perhaps be considered to be developmentally normal childhood curiosity. However, if the sexual relationship were to persist throughout adolescence, the potential for a negative impact from the experience increases dramatically. One of the most important sources for trauma from prolonged sibling incest is the shame and resulting negative self-concept from having experienced a life with the family so discrepant from what society at large condones. Children who

are sexually socialized by family members frequently grow up feeling inadequate, morally defective, and sexually perverse, because their life experience was so different from what they perceive as normal and because they blame themselves for this discrepancy.

4. *The degree of social isolation.* Children who experience prolonged sexual contact with each other or with a parent or parent figure over a prolonged period of time, frequently do not experience normal social development outside the home. If a 16-year-old adolescent girl, for example, has been having sexual contact with her father since she was 12 years old, her father could be expected to discourage and even forbid her dating as long as she lived at home because such contact would be experienced by him as "competition" or an "affair" outside of his relationship with his daughter. Because the desire and emotional need for peer contact is so strong during adolescence, children who experience severe social isolation in order to be maintained as sexual partners for their parents often run away from home and/or request foster placement.

5. *The ability of the other parent to nurture.* The family dynamics in most incest families preclude a nurturing parent. If a parent is available to meet some of the child's needs, the child most likely will be more able to emotionally handle the other parent or parent figure's inappropriate sexual behavior. Premature adulthood, the loss of nurturing parent figures, and the responsibility for meeting parents' sexual needs hamper the normal development of children in incestuous families. The presence of an adult, even a grandparent who can respond to the child's needs for protection, structure, nurturing, and support can potentially minimize the trauma the child experiences from the loss of appropriate parenting. (It is interesting to note that incest victims frequently express rage at their mothers for not protecting them from the experience while at the same time feeling that the only nurturing they received in the family was from their fathers, through sexual contact.)

6. *The meaning of the experience to the child.* The meaning of sex to children is different at different ages and tends to move from a simple meaning of pleasurable physical sensations to a much more complex set of meanings as puberty approaches. Generally, nonviolent, seductively coercive sexual contact with a 5- or 6-year-old will be less traumatic than for an 11- or 12-year-old child, who has begun to associate power, self-concept, love, and probably fear with sexuality.

7. *Direct or indirect sexual contact.* Children who receive "indirect" sexual contact, such as having their genitals looked at or being exposed to an adult's genitals, will probably be less traumatized than children who are actually sexually touched or forced to touch. It seems easier for children to minimize the importance of contacts that are not physically intrusive or painful.

Thus, a number of factors must be considered when assessing the degree of trauma actually or potentially associated with incest. The greater the frequency of the negative factors just listed, and the greater the severity, the more likely the existence of trauma. For example, the 12-year-old socially isolated child who is being forcibly raped by her 35-year-old father has an emotionally immature mother who operates out of the framework of experiencing her daughter as "competition" for her lover (father), and has been sexually abused by her father for 3 years will probably experience considerable psychological damage. Conversely, the 6-year-old who is sexually fondled "lovingly" on one or two occasions by her alcoholic father prior to his chemical dependency treatment, or the adolescent sisters who mutually fondle each other to orgasm frequently for a year or so while developing positive age-appropriate sexual and social contact with peers of both sexes are less likely to experience psychological damage.

Incest Family Patterns

Until 1970, only one book and several dozen clinical research articles were written about the phenomenon of incest (Meiselman, 1978; Justice and Justice, 1979; Kroth, 1979; Armstrong, 1978; Burgess et al., 1978; Walters, 1975). There is general agreement among leaders in the field that incest is a symptom of family problems rather than the result of the psychopathology of an individual family member. Incest offenders seem to defy consistent categorizations by traditional psychiatric diagnoses, as do their spouses. Abuse can best be described as a "family affair" and is the result of a complex system of interaction between spouses, parent and child, child and environment, parent and environment, and parent and society (Justice and Justice, 1979).

It seems possible to hypothesize that incest families and their members have problems with boundaries in four specific areas:

1. Overly rigid boundaries between the family and the outside world; societal boundaries
2. Inappropriate boundaries within the extended family system, characterized by overflexibility of boundaries between generations: intergenerational boundaries
3. Symbiotic relationships (Bowen, 1978) characterized by boundary diffusion between family members: interpersonal boundaries
4. Diffuse internal personal boundaries, characterized by poor reality testing and distortions: intrapsychic boundaries

By conceptualizing that the incest families exhibit disturbed boundaries in their intrapsychic, interpersonal, intergenerational, and societal interaction patterns, the authors can explain a range of behaviors that occur with some frequency among the population of incest families.

1. Social isolation and/or subculture membership (rigid societal boundaries), e.g., rural isolated families who are suspicious of all outsiders
2. Erotic contact between generations, whether nuclear or extended family (inappropriate intergenerational boundaries), e.g., children sleeping in the same bed with grandparents—some erotic behaviors
3. Sex-role exchange between mother and daughter (interpersonal boundary diffusion), e.g., teenaged daughter who assumes maternal role with other children and is assigned role of homemaker
4. Genital interaction between mother and daughter (interpersonal bound-

ary diffusion), e.g., inappropriate sexual curiosity of mother with her child to include sexual touching

5. Abandonment theme: "If you leave, I lose part of me" (interpersonal boundary diffusion), expressed by all or some members of family

6. Extreme dependency and low self-esteem of family members

7. Maternal collusion in regard to an awareness of and covert acceptance of sexual activities of spouse and children; usually fear that the family will disintegrate if the mother acknowledges the behavior (interpersonal boundary diffusion): "My survival depends upon your survival"

8. Incest as a stabilizer of the family system: Mother: "If you (husband) leave, I won't survive"; daughter: "If Dad leaves, I won't survive, nor will Mom" (interpersonal boundary diffusion); any change in the family system will be perceived as a threat to the survival of the family

9. Strong family cohesiveness (rigid societal boundaries, diffuse interpersonal boundaries), e.g., the family perceives itself as enmeshed without separate identities that form a bulwark against outsiders

10. Chaotic family patterns where no sense of privacy or separation of family members is acknowledged (diffuse interpersonal and intrapsychic boundaries) (Kantor and Lehr, 1975)

11. Compulsiveness of the incestuous behavior pattern: "I (father) must complete myself and fill my deficit" (diffuse interpersonal and intrapsychic boundaries), e.g., incestuous behaviors compensate the father for feelings of sexual inadequacy when compared to other men and/or allow specific forbidden behavior (anal intercourse, oral sex)

12. Denial and rationalization as major defense pattern of parents: "Taking care of me (parents) is taking care of you (children)" (diffuse interpersonal boundaries), e.g., sexual behavior is rationalized as initiation into adult sexuality

13. Seductive child: "It's my (child) job to take care of us" (inappropriate intergenerational boundaries); "Taking care of you (parents) is assuring my survival" (diffuse interpersonal boundaries), e.g., the converse of the above concept clearly places the child in a position to rationalize their compliance

When one considers the concept of either overly rigid or porous boundaries as central to understanding incestuous family dynamics, it is quite possible to develop a treatment model based on this theoretical assumption. The tasks of the clinician/therapist then become:

1. To increase the flexibility of the overly rigid boundary between society and the family

2. To restructure role relationships that are consistent with parental and child roles and are age-appropriate to the developmental stage of the family

3. To enable family members to individuate and become separate people who express themselves individually as opposed to the amorphous "we" of an enmeshed family

4. To provide a structure for consistent reality testing

A treatment model with these tasks will primarily be family-focused with intervention strategies consistent with the given theoretical assumptions.

Although it is clear that incest is a family problem with each family member having a stake in maintaining both the behavior and the "secret", in no circumstances is the child *responsible* for the sexual abuse, even if the child is responsive emotionally or physically (including being orgasmic). Children will accept "love" in whatever form it presents itself from their parents and, in fact, will even initiate "incestuous loving" once they have been taught the process, in a misguided attempt to meet their needs for love and nurturing.

Common Clinical Indications

Incest or childhood sexual abuse rarely presents to the clinician in straightforward terms, such as "I'm an incest victim and I need help," or "My daddy is touching my genitals and I don't like it." Most frequently, a symptom or cluster of symptoms that seem unrelated to incest are presented. It is important for the clinician to have a degree of suspicion when certain signs or symptoms appear so that she/he can pursue an appropriate series of questions.

Psychological Recognition Signs in Children and Adolescents

1. *Adolescent prostitution.* Adolescent prostitution replicates the incest family system in that in both instances the child is expected to use or "give up" her body primarily for the benefit of others. (A recent Minneapolis study of 80 adolescent prostitutes found that 33% had experienced incest, half of which incidents had occurred before the age of 10 (Enablers, Inc., 1978; James, 1977).

2. *Child/adolescent suicide threats or attempts.* Child incest victims who attempt suicide believe that their families would be better off, i.e., free of the major problem (themselves) if they were dead. In this way the "shame" of the family remains a secret.

3. *Unusual accumulation of money, candy, and clothes.* Candy in large amounts is a frequent "bribe" used by abusing adults as a means of ensuring secrecy outside the family; similarly, money and clothes are frequent bribes given to adolescents in an attempt to ensure their silence about the incestuous activities at home (Armstrong, 1978).

4. *Moderate to severe depression or anxiety.* Depression or anxiety, with no situational correlate, such as a move to a new house, a divorce, or death in the family, is a common symptom among incest victims, especially if the onset is sudden and/or dramatic (Armstrong, 1978; Berliner, 1977; Maisch, 1972).

5. *Dramatic change in the child's behavior.* A sudden change in a child's behavior, either in the direction of acting out and becoming unruly, or pulling in and becoming introverted and sullen, uncommunicative, etc., frequently marks the onset of incestuous behavior (Muldoon, 1979; Berliner, 1977).

6. *Sudden weight gain or loss.* Adolescent incest victims frequently experience eating disorders, including both compulsive overeating and compulsive undereating, in

an unconscious attempt to make themselves unattractive to the abusing or potentially abusing parent (Kroth, 1979).

7. *Alcoholism of one or both parents*. Although there is little consensus about which started first, the alcoholism or the incest, there is consensus in the field that alcoholism of the incest perpetrator and/or spouse is *extremely* frequent among incestuous families (Muldoon, 1979; Anderson and Shafer, 1979; Nakoshima and Zakus, 1977; Rada, 1976; Virkkunen, 1974).

8. *Habitual use of alcohol/drugs by the victim*. Adolescent victims of incest frequently abuse chemicals in an attempt to "modify" or "anesthesize" their reality, since the open expression of feelings is not allowed in their families (Benward and Densen-Gerber, 1975; Maisch, 1972).

9. *Running away from home*. Running away from home is perhaps the most common symptom among adolescent female victims, but it is also seen in children as young as 8 or 9 (Giarretto, 1976; James, 1977).

10. *Unexpected sexual utterances*. A sexual language system or vocabulary inappropriate to the child's age or developmental stage sometimes indicates a parent asking a child to perform certain sexual behaviors and labeling those for the child (Herjanic, 1978; Branch and Paxton, 1965).

11. *Parent reports molestation by a "stranger."* Sometimes parents are able to bring their child to the doctor for help with incest or incest-associated physical problems even though they are unable to report that they or their spouses were responsible for the problem (Herjanic, 1978).

Physical/Medical Recognition Signs in Children and Adolescents

1. *Unexplained abdominal pain*. Psychosomatic abdominal pain, usually with a sudden onset, frequently signals anxiety or stress associated with sexual abuse (Larson, 1980).

2. *Body mutilation*. Children who purposely inflict physical injury, such as cutting, burning, inhaling toxic fumes, or carving initials on their bodies, are often acting on their extreme self-hate and shame associated with being incest victims (Larson, 1980).

3. *Adolescent pregnancy*. Adolescents pregnant with a family member's baby (father, brother, grandfather, uncle, mother's boyfriend) will rarely report the actual identity of the father. Frequently they will present vague stories about a peer who no longer lives in town or who went off to the army, and they do not know his name, etc. (James, 1977).

4. *Venereal disease*. Oral and/or anal VD is more common among young incest victims (1 to 10 years), and genital VD more common among adolescent victims (Herjanic, 1978; Branch and Paxton, 1965).

5. *Vaginal discharge in girls, urethral discharge in boys*. Bacterial infections associated with oral and/or anal contact with adults show up frequently with young victims (Herjanic, 1978).

6. *Pain on defecation*. Pain on defecation is a common symptom among young male incest victims but also might be seen among young female victims as well. The

pain might be physiologically based, due to trauma or gonorrhea, or it could be psychologically based (Herjanic, 1978).

7. *Urinary tract infection, especially in young girls.* "Honeymoon cystitis" is frequently seen in young female incest victims (Larson, 1980).

8. *Parental obsession with discharge of child.* Parents who are obsessed about a discharge or blood on their child's underpants, with no physiological evidence to support such concerns, are showing their concern for the child without being able to expose the cause for their concern. They may not even know consciously why they are bringing the child in for a checkup (Larson, 1980).

9. *Gagging response.* Incest victims, especially very young ones, frequently display gagging behavior with no apparent physiological cause when they "remember," either consciously or unconsciously, oral sexual abuse (Herjanic, 1978).

10. *Parental obsession with child's bowel patterns.* A common method for maternal incest victimization is the frequent use of enemas (one to three times per week) on one of several of their children without a medical reason for the enema. This behavior may or may not be associated with sexual fantasies on the part of the mother (Larson 1980).

Psychological Recognition Signals in Adults

1. *Hospitalization for depression.* Multiple hospitalizations for depression, often with an adolescent onset, is perhaps the most common adult psychological recognition sign (Lukianowicz, 1972; Meiselman, 1978; Rosenfeld, 1979).

2. *Frightening fantasies or dreams.* The most common recurring fantasy or dream among adult victims appears to be about themselves as a child, usually in bed, with a dark, ominous creature coming toward them, usually of unknown identity (Larson, 1980).

3. *Lack of clear memory of childhood.* The childhood incest victim frequently protects him/herself by repressing certain parts of childhood memories or sometimes massive periods in the child's life ranging from 5 to 15 years.

4. *Compulsive sexual behavior.* Young women who are prostitutes or who feel compelled to have sexual contact with every potential partner, or middle-aged women who choose married partners with whom to have sex, are often simply compulsively reenacting their experience of their early incestuous activities.

5. *Chemical dependency.* The use of chemicals and drugs to abusive proportions is a common symptom among adults who were victims of incest as children, as an attempt to "anesthetize" psychic pain associated with their sexual abuse.

6. *Sexual dysfunction.* The most common sexual dysfunction associated with early incest history is sex aversion (sometimes of phobic proportions, and symptoms may reflect areas of the body violated as a child), vaginismus, and dyspareunia (Scharff, 1978). (Anorgasmia is also frequently present; however, its high incidence in the general female population may simply mask other causes (Meiselman, 1978; Scharff, 1978; Boekelheide, 1978b).

7. *Defective body image.* Shame might be genital or breast focused or could be

more generalized, including virtually the entire body. Women with this symptom often elect multiple cosmetic surgeries, including breast augmentation or reduction, stomach or intestinal bypass surgery (for weight control), facial surgery, etc. (Larson, 1980).

8. *Sadomasochistic sexual fantasies or behavior*. Although many women utilize episodic sadomasochistic fantasies during sexual activity, victims of incest frequently report that such fantasies or actual sadomasochistic behavior are *necessary* in order for them to become sexually aroused (Larson, 1980).

9. *Sexual attraction issues*. Victims may manifest an aversion rather than an attraction to members of the opposite sex, based on fear and anger. This is not usually an expression of positive attraction to members of the same sex; rather it is confusion about their lack of attraction to the opposite sex (Meiselman, 1979; Muldoon, 1979).

10. *Suicide attempt(s)*. Adults who were childhood incest victims may attempt suicide as a result of feelings of guilt and shame. They may think that their families would be better off without them, since they see themselves as the source of problem in their families (Meiselman, 1979).

Physical/Medical Recognition Signs in Adults

1. *Persistent pain in the lower abdomen*. Victims often describe persistent abdominal pain with no physiological cause, usually with adolescent onset. The pain subsides with successful psychological treatment, which includes focusing on the early abusive experiences (Larson, 1980).

2. *Body mutilation*. The most common forms of body mutilation among adult victims appear to be razor cuts (not necessarily suicidal wrist slits), cigarette burns, facial gouging (compulsive digging into the skin), and sometimes breast and genital mutilation (Larson, 1980).

3. *Eating disturbances*. Both compulsive overeating and undereating are frequently associated with early incest victimization. A third eating disturbance, bulimia (compulsive eating followed by spontaneous or induced vomiting), is also being identified among adults who were victims as children (Meiselman, 1978).

4. *Severe emotional reaction to medical pelvic examination*. The frightened powerless feelings of being sexually exploited by an adult, i.e., a person in power, is often replicated for incest victims during a medical pelvic examination. Victims sometimes experience vaginismus, or more commonly, an extreme fear reaction to being examined, coupled with intense feelings of shame and humiliation (Larson, 1980).

5. *Pain in the genitals*. The pain experienced by some victims in their genitals is psychogenic and usually occurs immediately prior to sexual contact, even if the partner is the victim's spouse or lover (Meiselman, 1978).

Certainly none of these symptoms or symptom clusters confirms the presence of incest or incest history; they are merely cues which suggest that questions concerning sexual abuse and/or incest are indicated during history taking. Although discomfort is frequently associated with asking direct questions of children about sexual contacts with adults, it is important to do so in order to protect the child from further abuse. Likewise, adults should be asked if they had been abused as children in order to institute appropriate treatment.

Methods of Intervention

Methods of Intervention with Children

Incest families are characterized by three general defense patterns: denial, rationalization, and projection. These mechanisms have generally enabled the families to live with behavior that is highly discrepant with the majority of society's mores, therefore, they tend to be rigid and resistant to intervention. The most important single intervention the clinician can make is to report confirmed or suspected incest or family sexual abuse to the local child protective services agency (usually the welfare department), regional mental health center, or police department. Every state requires that such a report be made for the protection of the child, and failure to report could result in a criminal charge against the clinician. In cases of severe threat to the child, where physical abuse and/or the survival of the child is in question, the child should be hospitalized until the protective services division of the local child welfare agency should be called in.

It is, therefore, important that the clinician *not* accept the parents' denial of incest or sexual abuse as evidence that the child is deluding him/herself, lying, fantasizing, or projecting oedipal wishes (Spencer, 1978) Children *rarely* openly report the presence of sexual behavior that *does* exist and certainly are even more reluctant to report sexual behavior that *does not* exist between themselves and their own parents. In fact, the child in an incest family, where the behavior occurs as part of the family denial pattern, tends to minimize incest behavior rather than exaggerate it (Anderson and Shafer,1979; Machotica et al., 1967).

If incest is confirmed, it is important that the clinician try to enlist the support of the concerned parent who brought in the child, in an attempt to protect the child from his/her other parent. If the support of the concerned parent (usually the mother) is not enlisted early, she may become frightened that her husband/boyfriend will abuse or abandon her and may subsequently join the perpetrator in denying the abuse. However, if she is actively emotionally supported by the clinician until help is available from the child protective services agency, she will be more likely to maintain her support of the child.

The presence of alcoholism or other chemical abuse on the part of the perpetrator or spouse enhances denial and complicates treatment considerably (Hindman, 1977; Maisch, 1965). It is common for chemically dependent parents to use alcohol as an excuse for the behavior and "bargain" with the clinician *not* to report the incident if the parents stop drinking or go through chemical dependency treatment. This response pattern, although typical, should not be taken seriously. Treatment for chemical dependency does not ensure that the incestuous behavior will cease (Rada, 1976).

In situations where an adolescent is presenting him/herself as an incest victim and is sharing the "secret of incest" for the first time, it is important to ask if the child wishes to go home, knowing that an investigation will occur. If the child feels the need for protection, even temporarily, this should be provided, with hospitalization or foster care placement. Exposing the family secret can indeed be traumatic for an adolescent and his/her family, and fears of reprisal at home for "getting the family into trouble" are not necessarily ungrounded. Often the child has been told by the perpetrator *never* to tell anyone and threatened with physical harm if she/he does so. Additionally, the child may have told the nonperpetrating parent about the abuse and been chastised for causing the behavior or creating problems for the family. It is not unusual for children to be told that they were "asking for it" by running around the house in their flimsy nightclothes, not locking the bathroom door, or sitting on daddy's lap (Nakashima, 1977).

Most incest families require long-term treatment in programs or settings that are designed to effectively intervene in the family's network of rigid defense patterns (Giarretto, 1976; Sholevar, 1975). Many treatment centers throughout the country are reporting success with family treatment models focused on restructuring the family's inappropriate generational boundaries around sexual- and role-related behaviors. Prison as a form of "treatment" is being used more and more selectively, mainly with perpetrators who are multiple offenders, physically violent, likely to disappear, or are resistant to family, marital, individual, and/or group therapy. Treatment centers are reporting that many families are able to restructure themselves and that the presence of incest no longer need mean automatic prison or divorce and permanent disruption of family relationships (Meiselmann, 1978; Giarretto 1976).

Methods of Intervention with Adults Who Were Victims as Children

As the shroud of silence surrounding incest lifts, more and more adults with histories of childhood sexual abuse are exposing their tightly held, painful secrets to physicians who sensitively ask the appropriate questions during history taking. Sometimes the adults experience seemingly little or no major negative long-term effects of their early abuse. Others may be experiencing symptoms of various sorts, including depression, sexual dysfunction, lack of sexual interest, chemical dependency, abusing their own children, and weight problems, and might not link their symptoms to their earlier abuse experiences. Generally, if an adult has experienced childhood sexual abuse and has not had therapy, it is indicated. Denial of the need for treatment can be appropriate, *or* it could be another instance of the use of denial to maintain the family secret.

Even though the adult patient has had counseling or therapy earlier, further work may be indicated in a new adult life stage. Further, since incest or family sexual abuse is relatively new as a legitimate arena for scientific investigation and practice specialization, many therapists are not familiar with the problems and with the new models for treatment which are emerging. The most promising form of therapy appears to be same-sex group treatment with other victims of incest (Tsai and Wagner, 1978). The group mode can provide an effective support system for their extreme dependency while at the same time helping them expand their network outside of the group.

One of the major rationales for referring adult patients with a history of incest to counseling or therapy is one of prevention. Children from sexually abusive families marry abusers, or they abuse their own children, regardless of the gender of the child. It is not uncommon for three generations of family members to be actively involved in sexual abuse, including uncles, aunts, and cousins as well as grandparents, parents, and children. Referring the adults for treatment is an attempt to prevent further abuse of the vulnerable next generation of children (Meiselman, 1978; Justice and Justice, 1979; Walters, 1975).

Case Examples

George and Margaret are a middle-class couple. She is in her early thirties and he is in his mid-thirties. They have two girls (ages 13 and 16). The girls are Asian and were adopted when they were 9 and 12. They were referred after the oldest girl revealed a long incest history to her high school counselor. She disclosed the incest because it was beginning to occur between her adoptive father and younger sister. She stated that she wanted to protect her sister.

A psychosexual history of George revealed that he was an extremely isolated adolescent, emotionally rejected by his parents at an early age. He described himself as socially shy and naive, with few friends and no dates with girls while in high school. At 17, he enlisted in the military service and was sent to Asia. While there, he received the majority of his adolescent sexual socialization with Asian prostitutes, who were young adolescents. When he returned to the United States, he married a 15-year-old girl and was subsequently divorced. He remarried, this time to a 16-year-old girl, and this marriage also ended in divorce after a couple of years. His third marriage was to an 18-year-old, his current wife.

Margaret's history revealed years of early sexual abuse, first by an uncle when she was prepubescent, and later by older adolescents in her neighborhood. She reported being molested several times in movie theaters when she was quite young. She was sexually active with her dates during adolescence, frequently having intercourse because she did not think she could say "no." When she married George she was unaware of his previous marriages to a 15- and 16-year-old, but she did not think of it as unusual at the time. Margaret was unaware of her husband's sexual experiences in Asia until this history was revealed during the course of treatment.

George began fondling the oldest girl shortly after her arrival from Asia. Within a year he was actively engaging in sexual intercourse with her several times a week. During this period he continued his pattern of sexual intercourse with his wife four or five times a week. When the youngest Asian girl reached puberty, George began spending time with her in the family room watching late movies, the same pattern he had established with the older girl. Recognizing this, the older girl became alarmed and decided to report the incest.

After initially denying that incest had occurred, George did eventually admit that he had been engaging in sexual activity with his daughters but only to help them feel loved and more accepted in their adoptive family. His rationalization was developed in response to the mother's hostility toward the girls, which resulted in continual conflict between her and them. Margaret denied that she had any knowledge of her husband's sexual activity with their daughters and maintained this denial throughout treatment. The father chose to voluntarily terminate his parental rights rather than participate in treatment. The mother eventually made the same choice, following months of ambivalence about her desire to continue her marriage versus her desire to continue to parent the girls. Throughout the legal process she vacillated between being extremely angry with the girls for having an "affair" with her husband and being angry with her husband for choosing the girls as sexual partners and "cheating" on her. She was eventually hospitalized after several suicide threats and was diagnosed as severely depressed.

Alice is a 43-year-old divorced mother of three boys, ages 12, 13, and 17. She was referred following a psychiatric hospitalization precipitated by a suicide attempt. During Alice's two previous hospitalizations for depression she had talked with the hospital staff about her vague memories of a man engaging her in sexual activity when she was 5 or 6. Both times she was told that she was projecting her feelings of *wanting* to have been loved sexually by her father who had abandoned her at birth. During her last hospitalization, the staff recognized the cluster of symptoms suggestive of an incest history, and she was referred for treatment.

Alice, a fraternal twin, was placed in a foster home shortly after birth following the death of her mother (from postdelivery complications). At the age of 3, Alice and her twin brother were placed in a permanent foster home with a couple in their early fifties. Alice described her foster father as verbally and physically abusive, frequently drunk and angry. She described her foster mother as manipulative and rejecting, both when she was a child and currently as well. The couple had no other children.

Initially during treatment, Alice remembered little about her childhood. As treatment progressed (weekly group treatment with other incest victims), her memory gradually revealed a long history of childhood sexual abuse. When Alice was 6, her foster father began asking her to take naps with him, especially after he had been drinking. Alice would join him, fall asleep, and wake up to find her father touching her genitals. Although Alice could remember having disliked this, she was frightened of being beaten if she did not comply with his wishes. Subsequently Alice would lock herself in her room whenever her foster father had been drinking. Alice has no memory of her mother's whereabouts during the incest episodes.

At the age of 8, Alice commenced a pattern of running away from home that persisted until, at the age of 14, she was placed in a correctional facility for adolescent incorrigibles. Alice has no memory of anyone from the welfare department or juvenile correctional agency asking her if there was anything occurring at home that prompted her runaway pattern.

At the age of 14 Alice was released from the correctional facility and sent to live with her sister and brother-in-law. Shortly thereafter, Alice became pregnant out-of-wedlock by her brother-in-law who was 35. At 17, Alice married an alcoholic. Following a divorce after 12 years of marriage, Alice found herself compelled to engage in sexual intercourse with any man who appeared interested; she enjoyed the sex but would experience extreme anger and feelings of shame after each episode, only to compulsively repeat the sexual contact again and again. Even the violent sexual patterns of some of her partners were not deterrents from her compulsive sexual behavior.

During the course of treatment, Alice experienced relief from a number of her incest-related symptoms; her depression lifted and she was able to function without antidepressant medications; her abdominal pain, which began when she was 10, disappeared; she recovered much of her memory of early childhood, which had been dim and filled with gaps in information, especially during the time her foster father was sexually abusing her; she stopped her pattern of compulsive sexual contact with men; and she was able to learn how to develop satisfying relationships with both women and men. Additionally, with the help of family therapy, she was able to take a much firmer stance at home with her children, who were victimizing her as well.

Terrance and Vera are a couple in their mid-forties. They have five children, ranging in age from 13 to 25. Three of the children, including the youngest (the only child currently living at home), are girls. Jenny, the third oldest child in the family, was referred following a psychiatric hospitalization precipitated by a suicide attempt. Jenny reported an early history of learning and behavior problems in school, coupled with extreme withdrawal and depression. The onset of her school and social problems coincided with the onset of her sexual abuse by her father, which began when she was 8. When Jenny was 13, she lost 60 pounds. Anorexia nervosa was suspected, although it was not diagnosed as such at that time. Jenny was hospitalized when she was 19 and again when she was 21, diagnosed as severely depressed. It was noted at that time that she was scarred on many parts of her body from self-inflicted razor blade cuts and cigarette burns.

Shortly after commencing outpatient treatment in an incest victims group, Jenny discovered when talking with her sisters about her own treatment that both of them had also experienced sexual contact with their father. Since the youngest (aged 13) was still actively sexually involved with her father, a report was filed with the local child protective services division of the welfare department, and the entire family was referred for treatment.

Although Jenny was a behavior problem throughout her grade school and high school years, she was never questioned about the possibility of incest by the psychologists and psychiatrist who worked with her. Her postpubertal eating disturbance, which went undiagnosed, persisted into adulthood.

During the course of treatment, Jenny began dating men who were not verbally or physically abusive toward her (unlike the men she had dated previously). She stopped mutilating her body, her depression lifted, and she secured a new, challenging job. Her younger sister, who also was becoming a school behavior problem, quickly changed her disruptive pattern shortly after she began treatment. Although the parents eventually decided to divorce, the prognosis for each of the family members appears to be good.

Common Errors in Management

Overreaction

Many adults, including physicians, experience feelings of extreme anger or horror when confronted with sexual abuse, especially if a very young child is involved. They naturally may want to protect a 4-year-old child with vaginal trauma from forced intercourse or a 6-year-old boy with anal gonorrhea. It is helpful to remember that incest in a family is the result of a "system of interaction between spouses, parent and child, child and enviroment, parent and enviroment, parent and society (Meiseleman, 1978). Every family member is involved in the problem. Although the adults in the system certainly bear responsibility for the inappropriate sexual behavior, every family member is experiencing emotional pain. Despite the strong feelings one might have about the behavior, it is important to maintain a professionally tolerant attitude toward incest families, dealing firmly but sensitively with *each* family member in order to avoid further shaming the family members or increasing the trauma for the child.

Interviewing the Child while the Parent Is Present

Because of the fear of malpractice or libel suit, clinicians sometimes hesitate to interview children without their parents. In identifying and confirming sexual abuse, however, choosing a private location away from parents may greatly facilitate obtaining accurate information about the sexual contact. Children in incestuous families are assigned the task of taking care of the needs of their parents, for example, their sexual needs, and often other emotional needs as well. During an interview at which his/her parents are present, a child may look to them for cues about how to respond to questions, giving only those answers that appear to meet with their approval. Although it may be necessary to check with parents about the meaning of sexual terms, it is imperative that the child be interviewed alone at some point to ensure obtaining information as accurately as possible.

Not Recognizing Boys as Victims of Family Sexual Abuse

Although the majority of reported incest victims are female, an increasing number of abused males are appearing clinically and in the literature. Young men in treatment for a variety of problems are reporting intrafamily sexual exploitation by a variety of adults, adolescent male and female babysitters, relatives who "taught" them how to have intercourse, fathers who stimulated their sons' penises regularly "to help them grow," and mothers who invited their adolescent sons to join them in bed when fathers were absent from home. These reports emphasize the importance of recognizing the possibility of incestuous histories in males, even though the occurrence in females is more common.

Failing to Surmount Family Defensiveness

A common concern of physicians investigating incest is distinguishing an actual occurrence from a fantasy, projection, or actual lie told by a child or by a nonperpetrating parent. The defense patterns of incest families often make it difficult to ascertain facts and details until well along in psychotherapeutic treatment. Family members are understandably frightened when their secret is exposed, and the entire family may feel threatened by intrusion from the outside world.

When the possibility of incest is raised by any family member and sufficient evidence is found to at least suspect that abuse might be present, then it is best to refer the family for investigation and appropriate treatment. Given current social taboos, there is relatively little likelihood of false report, although this is not impossible. More likely, however, helping persons tend to err in the direction of missing the signs or failing to report an actual occurrence.

Referring to an Inappropriate Resource

Unfortunately, every counselor or therapist is not equipped to deal with incest. It is important that the consultant know the available resources in the community if he/she is not going to be the therapist.

Forgetting to Help the Parents

Particularly with young children, the clinician should recall the general principle that the most powerful factor affecting the child who has experienced adult sexual abuse is probably the reaction of the parents. This is also true of incest. The clinician can contribute to minimizing the ultimate trauma to the child by continuing to act positively, supportively, and reassuringly with the parents, even in the face of some hostility.

Depending upon Admonition to Stop Incest

Although most clinicians have considerable authority with their patients, it cannot be assumed that simply telling a parent to stop having incestuous contact with a child will be sufficient to control the activity. Research and clinical knowledge to date suggest that incest is a compulsive behavior pattern that is not fully under the conscious control of the perpetrator. Although a warning might serve to suppress the behavior for a time, chances are great that the abuse will recur and may continue undetected for another indefinite period. Therefore, the abuse should be reported to the appropriate agency as soon as possible so that a program of treatment can be instituted, and the abuse halted permanently.

Summary

Incest is usually more emotionally traumatic than physically harmful, thereby requiring psychological assessment and extended therapeutic treatment. The risk is very great that, left untreated, incest will be passed on to another generation of children. Therefore, the clinician's responsibility for facilitating treatment of family sexual abuse is ethical and social as well as medical.

References

Anderson, L. M., and Shafer, G. The character-disordered family: A community treatment model for family sexual abuse. *American Journal of Orthopsychiatry,* 1979, *49*(3), 436–445.

Armstrong, L. *Kiss daddy goodnight: A speak-out on incest.* New York: Hawthorn Books, Inc., 1978.

Bagley, C. Incest behavior and incest taboo. *Social Problems* 1969, *16,* 505–519.

Benward, J., and Densen-Gerber, J. Incest as a causative factor in antisocial behavior: An exploratory study. *Contemporary Drug Problems,* 1975, *4*(3), 323–340.

Berliner, L. Child sexual abuse: What happens next? *Victimology* 1977, *2*(2), 327–331.

Boekelheide, P. D. Incest and the family physician. *Journal of Family Practice,* 1978, *6*(1), 87–90. (a)

Boekelheide, P. D. Sexual adjustment in college women who experience incestuous relationships. *Journal of American College Health Association,* 1978, *26*(6), 327–330. (b)

Bowen, M. *Family therapy in clinical practice: The collected papers of Murray Bowen.* New York: Jason Aronson, 1978.

Branch, G., and Paxton, R. A study of gonococcal infections among infants and children. *Public Health Reports,* 1965, *80,* 347–352.

Burgess, A. W., Groth, A. N., and Holstrom, L. D. *Sexual assault of children and adolescents.* Lexington, Mass.: Lexington Books, 1978.

Dixon, K. N., Arnold, L. E., and Calestrok, K. Father-son incest: Underreported psychiatric problem? *American Journal of Psychiatry,* 1978, *135*(7), 835–838.

Eist, H. I., and Mandel, A. U. Family treatment of ongoing incest behavior. *Family Process,* 1968, *7,* 216–232.

Enablers, Inc. *Juvenile prostitution in Minnesota: The report of a research project.* Minneapolis, Minn.: Author, 1978.

Finkelhor, D. Psychological, cultural and family factors in incest and family sexual abuse. *Journal of Marital and Family Therapy,* 1978, *4*(4), 41–49.

Finkelhor, D. A survey of sexual abuse in the population at large. In D. Finkelhor (Ed.), *Sexually victimized children.* New York: Free Press, 1979.

Flammang, C. J. Interviewing victims of sex offenders. In L. G. Schultz (Ed.), *Rape victimology.* Springfield, Ill.: Charles C Thomas, 1975.

Gagnon, J. Female child victims of sex offenses. *Social Problems,* 1965, *13*(2), 176–192.

Gebhard, P. H., and Gagnon, J. *Sex offenders: An analysis of types.* New York: Harper & Row, 1965.

Gebhard, P. H., Gagnon, J. H., Pomeroy, W. B., and Christenson, C. V. *Sex offenders: An analysis of types.* New York: Harper, 1965.

Giarretto, H. Humanistic treatment of father-daughter incest. In R. E. Helfer and C. H. Kempe (Eds.), *Child abuse and neglect: The family and the community.* Cambridge, Mass.: Ballinger, 1976.

Goodwin, J., and Gross, M. Pseudo-seizures and incest. *American Journal of Psychiatry,* 1971, *36*(9), 1231.

Halleck, S. L. The physician's role in management of victims of sex offenders. *Journal of the American Medical Association,* 1962, *180*(4), 273–278.

Herjanic, B. Medical aspects of sexual abuse of children. *Medical Aspects of Human Sexuality,* 1978, *12*(2), 139–140.

Hindman, M. Child abuse and neglect: The alcohol connection. *Alcohol Health Research World,* 1977, *1,* 2–7.

James, K. Incest—The teenager's perspective. *Psychotherapy: Theory, Research and Practice,* 1977, *14*(2), 146–155.

James, J., and Meyerding, J. Early sexual experience as a factor in prostitution. *Archives of Sexual Behavior,* 1978, *7*(1), 31–42.

Justice, B., and Justice, K. *The broken taboo: Sex in the family.* New York: Human Sciences Press, 1979.

Kantor, D., and Lehr, W. *Inside the family: toward a theory of family process.* San Francisco: Jossey-Bass, 1975.

Kinsey, A. C., Pomeroy, W. B., and Martin, C. E. *Sexual behavior in the human female.* Philadelphia: Saunders, 1953.

Kroth, J. A. *Child sexual abuse: Analysis of a family therapy approach.* Springfield, Ill.: Charles C Thomas, 1979.

Larson, N. R. *An analysis of the effectiveness of a state-sponsored program designed to teach intervention skills in the treatment of family sexual abuse*. Ph.D. Dissertation, University of Minnesota, 1980.

Lester, D. Unusual sexual behavior: The standard deviations. Springfield, Ill.: Charles C Thomas, 1975.

Lukianowicz, N. Incest: I. Paternal incest. *British Journal of Psychiatry*, March 1972, *120*, 301–313.

Machotka, P., Pittman, F. S., and Flemenhoft, K. *Incest and family affair*. *Family Process*, 1967, *6*(1), 98–116.

Maisch, H. *Incest*. New York: Stein & Day, 1972.

Malmquist, C. P., Kiresuk, T. J., and Spano, R. M. Personality characteristics of women with repeated illegitimacies: Descriptive aspects. *American Journal of Orthopsychiatry*, 1966, April *36*, 476–484.

Meiselman, K. C. *Incest: A psychological study of causes and effects with treatment recommendations*. San Francisco: Jossey–Bass, 1978.

Muldoon, L. (Ed.). *Confronting the silent crime*, Coordinated by P. Specktor, S. Sayles, and S. L. Burt. St. Paul, Minn.: Program for Victims of Sexual Assault, 1979.

Molnar, G., and Cameron, P. Incest syndromes: Observations in a general hospital psychiatric unit. *Canadian Psychiatric Association Journal*, 1975, *20*(5), 373–377.

Nakashima, I. I., and Zakus, G. E. Incest: Clinical experience. *Pediatrics*, 1977, *60*(5), 696–701.

Rada, R. T. Alcoholism and the child molester. *Annals of the New York Academy of Science*, 1976, *273*, 492–496.

Rosenfeld, A. A. Incidence of history of incest among 18 female psychiatric patients. *American Journal of Psychiatry*, 1979, *136*(6), 791–795.

Rosenfeld, A. A., Krieger, M. J., Nadelson, C., and Backman, J. The sexual misuse of children: A brief survey. *Psychiatric Opinion*, 1976, *13*(2), 6–12.

Rossman, P. *Sexual experience between men and boys: Exploring the pederast underground*. New York: Association Press, 1976.

Scharff, D. E. Childhood origins of sexual difficulty. *Medical Aspects Human Sexualty*, 1978, *12*(2), 61–70.

Schultz, L. G. The child as a sex victim. L. G. Schultz (Ed.), *Rape victimology*. Springfield, Ill.: Charles C Thomas, 1975.

Sholevar, G. P. A family therapist looks at the problem of incest. *The Bulletin of the American Academy of Psychiatry and the Law*, 1975, *3*, 25–31.

Spencer, J. Father-daughter incest: A clinical view from the corrections field. *Child Welfare*, 1978, *57*(9), 581–590.

Stoller, R. J. *Perversion: The erotic form of hatred*. New York: Pantheon Books, 1975.

Summit, R., and Kryso, J. Sexual abuse of children: A clinical spectrum. *American Journal of Orthopsychiatry*, 1978, *48*(2), 237–251.

Tormes, Y. M. *Child victims of incest*. Denver American Humane Association, Children's Division, 1968.

Tsai, M., and Wagner, N. N. Therapy groups for women sexually molested as children. *Archives of Sexual Behavior*, 1978, *7*(5), 417–527.

Virkkunen, M. Incest offenses and alcoholism. *Medical Science Law*, 1974, *14*(2), 124–128.

Walters, D. R. *Physical and sexual abuse of children: Causes and treatment*. Bloomington: Indiana Univ. Press, 1975.

Weinberg, S. K. *Incest behavior*. New York: Citadel, 1955.

9

Premarital Counseling

John W. Grover

Introduction

Few couples take advantage of premarital counseling, whether it is medical, religious, or social in origin. There is very little opportunity in our society to prepare us for marriage, sexual and reproductive function, and parenting. Sex education or "education for family living" is viewed suspiciously by school boards. Home economics classes rarely teach anything but the bare facts of living in a family, slighting or ignoring interpersonal communication, sexuality, decision making, and parenting. Churches generally have little practical input into the basis of living together for most couples, tending rather to enhance guilt than to educate about behavior. The besieged nuclear family is unable to provide its children with an adequate education for sexuality and marriage because of ignorance, hesitancy, embarrassment, lack of perception of need, and barriers to communication.

Thus, many couples enter relationships with much misapprehension and anxi__, about their sexuality and with inappropriate expectations for their sexual function after marriage. The long-term results of inadequate preparation for marriage can include sexual dysfunction, reproductive difficulty, marital discord, and divorce.

With an awareness that inadequate preparation of couples for sexuality and marriage exists in our society, this chapter will look at some of the opportunities for premarital counseling open to physicians, including those in primary care and mental health professions. It is important for the physician–counselor to be nonjudgmental, thorough, informed, and able to provide information on sexual matters objectively. By affirmation of their healthy and appropriate sexuality, couples may alter their expectations for sexual function in marriage and may learn to share and communicate more freely with each other about their needs and experiences (Grover, 1981).

The couple's level of sexual knowledge and experience needs to be assessed, as

John W. Grover • Department of Obstetrics and Gynecology, Lutheran General Hospital, Park Ridge, Illinois.

well as their expectations for function. They often need to be educated or informed about sexual function; their needs for birth control also must be considered. The uniqueness of the physician–counselor, as contrasted with other resource persons, lies in the opportunity to use the physical examination of the patient as well as the client–physician relationship in the counseling process.

Since couples come to the physician with divergent experiences and needs, the chapter is subdivided with this in mind. A detailed description of the counseling approach to a sexually inexperienced couple will be followed by counseling approaches to experienced couples, couples where the woman is pregnant or has a history of abortion, older couples, remarriages, and relationships where one member is disabled by a physical or medical condition. The interviewing and counseling skills of medical and mental health professionals are utilized extensively. Although each physician is likely to develop a pattern of history taking and counseling that is unique and appropriate, guidelines for sexual history taking and counseling exist in current literature (Green, 1979; Group for the Advancement of Psychiatry, 1974).

In all of our premarital counseling, we accept and espouse the universality of our human and sexual natures and believe that it is reasonable and appropriate to promote healthy and positive feelings about sexuality for couples who are preparing themselves for marriage.

Counseling of the Sexually Inexperienced Couple

In what appears to be an age of great sexual freedom, we still often encounter a sexually inexperienced couple who is planning marriage. This may be because of their youth, due to their inhibitions and inexperience or to their religious or moral views. A few couples of all ages have not been successful at attempted coitus and may already have a sense of failure, which leads to increased anxiety and uncertainty about their future together.

Ideally, the couple should be interviewed together at the first visit. Enough time must be allowed to establish rapport and gain their confidence. An agenda should be agreed upon for this and subsequent visits. After determining that they wish counseling as well as medical examination, a complete medical history is taken, modified by their responses and expectations. Most details of pertinent medical information can be elicited with both partners present, while they may be examined separately as seems appropriate. With each party privately, their previous sexual experiences (which may not have been revealed heretofore) and their own expectations for their relationship can be discussed. When the couple does not specifically request premarital counseling, through the process of interview and examination, the physician is reassuring and may give them information and feedback. Although many may be reluctant to discuss sexual matters, most people are gratified to be told that they are anatomically and functionally normal. The physician's openness and objectivity sets a tone that makes the couple more receptive to future encounters. The appropriateness of ongoing counseling or referral should be established and discussed, especially if a traumatic or sexually dysfunctional history is revealed by either partner.

When an inexperienced couple desires more information, the dual interview proceeds in more depth, after it is established that the couple is comfortable with the process. Additional information that is used to help assess their present level of function is gained by asking how they feel about the prospect of becoming fully sexually functional. The physician should inquire if they like physical contact, whether they find caressing sexually arousing, and what an awareness of sexual feelings means to them. Do perceived sexual feelings also cause them to feel anxious or guilty? Have they petted heavily or experienced orgasm? Have they had external genital or oral–genital contact? What were their feelings about these experiences? Their responses to this line of questioning helps the physician or counselor to form a framework around which to construct and pattern their counseling program.

Pertinent questions should be asked of the couple about their families' attitudes about sexuality. It will also be helpful for their counselor to learn their perceptions of the sexual attitudes and activities of their peers, and how they react to them. By learning about this broader milieu in which the couple lives, it is possible to construct a more individualized and appropriate counseling program for them.

After the background health and behavioral information has been obtained, their physical examinations are usually performed separately. This offers the opportunity for the physician to talk privately about any experiences or questions that they could not share in the other's presence. Some concerns may appear to be simple, such as expressing guilt over wet dreams or masturbation and sexual fantasies. There may be more complicated revelations of prior sexual experiences, pregnancies, or venereal disease. Or there may be no new information; what is important is to provide an opportunity for each of them to share in a privileged relationship information that is pertinent to the growth and development of their marriage. The timing of the opportunity for sharing of private information may vary from one patient to another, depending on the comfort levels that develop in the interview.

A thorough general physical examination is performed to rule out physical problems and includes measuring weight and blood pressure, examining the heart, lungs, abdomen, and extremities, and providing for routine blood and urine tests. The general examination helps the patient to develop confidence in the physician, adds additional medical information, and prepares the patient for the more anxiety-producing genital examination.

The genital examination of the female partner begins with the visualization and palpation of the external vulvar and perineal structures. The patient can be given the option of observing with a mirror. A warmed speculum is gently inserted into the vagina and adjusted to visualize the cervix. A pap smear is taken. The speculum is removed, and the patient prepared for the bimanual examination, which completes the process. Her emotional responses to examination are carefully observed, and she is informed about every new step in the exam. When a woman is normal by examination, it is meaningful to reassure her that this is so and that she will be capable of sexual function. This helps to clarify her total health status and eliminates many misapprehensions she may have about herself. This is an example of the effective use of positive feedback from the physician to the patient, during what might otherwise be a frightening or negative experience.

The genital examination of the male should be equally detailed and includes careful inspection of the penis, scrotum, and testicles, examining for hernia and vari-cocoele, and a careful rectal and prostatic examination. It is important to note whether circumcision was performed. As with the female, he should have an opportunity to talk privately about possible unrevealed experiences, anxieties, or other concerns. He, too, should be reassured about his normal capabilities for sexual function (Green, 1979).

With sexually inexperienced couples, it is unlikely that one partner would ask to observe the examination of the other. However, this need not be discouraged, since both the experience and the discussion of the partner's examination may lead to a more productive counseling interaction. Both partners may benefit from an opportunity to learn more about each other and may correct misapprehensions they have about their anatomy. However, no shared examination should be performed without mutual agreement.

Birth control issues are appropriately raised and discussed at the first visit, where-as the actual institution of a birth control program depends upon the evolution of their sexual interaction and their stated needs.

Following the individual physical examination, it is important to have a joint conference during which additional questions are answered and plans made for further counseling, if indicated, or desired. Some couples may choose to arrange for additional counseling and discussion, whereas others may wish to defer until they have more experience on which to base their questions. Usually, it is appropriate to recommend suitable reading materials for their study (Bird, 1976; Kelly, 1980; Masters and John-son, 1974).

Occasionally, genital abnormalities are detected during the physical examination that may impede or even prevent intercourse. In my experience, 1 or 2% of young women examined premaritally have an inelastic, rigid, or fenestrated hymen, which prevents intromission or would make it painful. They can be treated successfully by careful instruction in vaginal dilatation, using their own fingers or simple dilators. In rare patients, a previously undetected gonadal dysgenesis with an absent or rudimen-tary vagina will be encountered. She will, of course, need more extensive diagnosis, therapy, and surgical treatment. Problems that may be discovered in young males include athletic trauma to the penis or testicles, undescended testes, previously undiag-nosed hypospadias, inguinal hernia, and prostatitis. Although these anomalies occur only infrequently, when they are detected, appropriate plans must be made for referral and treatment. When male or female anomalies occur, the emotional needs of the couple must not be neglected, as they will need psychological support during an unexpectedly difficult time in their lives (Kolodny et al., 1979).

Case 1

A 25-year-old medical student and his 24-year-old fiancée, a social worker, presented for premarital counseling and birth control advice. They stated that their orthodox religious background, their personal feelings, and their busy work and study schedules precluded sexual intercourse before the wedding. In addition to examination and birth control information, they both expressed a desire to discuss their sexual function objectively. The joint interview revealed no preexisting health problems. They had known each other for 2 years and felt strongly drawn to each other physically and emotionally. They were familiar with sexual arousal and had petted to orgasm in recent months. They were firm in their decision not to progress any further sexually until marriage. Neither had attempted sexual relations with other partners. The family background of each was unremarkable. Both parents were described as loving and supportive, as well as religious.

Further discussion with the young woman revealed that she was accustomed to using tampons during menses and was comfortable with her body. Her general physical examination was normal. She wished to watch the progress of her pelvic examination with a mirror and was interested in viewing her cervix, which she had not seen before. Her vagina admitted two examining fingers snugly, and her uterus and ovaries were normal. Rectal examination completed the normal pelvic examination. Her attitude was one of general interest, with little anxiety, and she responded well to information and feedback.

The examination of the young man was unremarkable, and he, too, had no further experiences or anxieties to share. He was familiar with masturbation, had occasionally experienced erotic dreams, and apparently had no overt guilt or anxiety related to his sexuality.

In their joint conference, it was clear that their decision not to have intercourse appeared to be a conscious choice related to their personal and religious beliefs and was not because of guilt, anxiety, or ignorance. We subsequently discussed aspects of sexual behavior in detail. Included were descriptions of heterosexual function and response, variations and differences between the sexes, fluctuations in sexual needs or drives, and birth control methods. We discussed particularly their expectations for their first intercourse after marriage. In addition to more technical details, they were encouraged not to expect "perfection" on their initial attempt and were advised that satisfactory coitus is a complex physical and emotional process that becomes more satisfying with experience and practice. The couple felt positively reinforced, both from the knowledge of their potential for normal function and from my support of their decisions about their own sexual behavior.

In later years, after completion of his medical training in another city, the couple returned to the area and came to me for obstetrical care. They had positive memories of their original counseling and felt that it had initiated for them a meaningful pattern of expression and communication in sexual and other areas of their life.

Counseling of the Sexually Experienced Couple

The general counseling format, which has been described in detail in the previous section and case report, remains the same. However, specific attention should be directed to their previous sexual experiences and their feelings about them. Useful questions for their private interviews include whether they had experienced sexual intercourse with other partners. How satisfactory was coitus for them? Have they any negative experiences about which they have questions? What are their expectations for sexual function after marriage? What are their plans for children? Their answers will indicate the structure needed as their counseling progresses and can be integrated into their mutual discussions.

In spite of what may appear to be appropriate sexual experience, one or both partners may reveal that a serious sexual dysfunction exists. Premature ejaculation in the male and orgasmic dysfunction in the female partner are the dysfunctions most frequently encountered. These generally are considered to be psychological in origin and may be related to the often covert and hurried nature of premarital intercourse. In this situation anxiety levels are high, time for foreplay is shortchanged, and attention to many physical and emotional aspects of satisfying coitus is lacking. In counseling such a couple, it is important to reassure them that generally after marriage, when they have more time, and less guilt and anxiety, satisfactory sexual function can develop. If for any reason it does not, they are encouraged to return for follow-up counseling or for referral. Other more or less common sexual dysfunctions that may be encountered are dyspareunia, vaginismus, secondary impotence, and sexual disinterest. When these problems persist, referral for ongoing counseling or therapy is indicated.

There are other past experiences that may have important implications for the couple's relationship. For instance, the sexually active female partner may have a history of pregnancy, with the birth of a child that was adopted or a pregnancy that was aborted. In many instances, the partner has not yet been informed of the pregnancy and its outcome. The woman may need an opportunity to explore her feelings about these events, and make a decision about whether or not to inform her future marital partner. She will need support, no matter which choice she makes. In addition to her anxiety about communicating her pregnancy history, she is very likely to have concerns about the effects of her prior pregnancy experiences on her potential for future childbearing.

Just as a prior pregnancy may be part of the woman's history, so, too, the man may reveal that he was responsible for a pregnancy with another partner. He also needs the opportunity to work out his feelings and will have to decide what to tell or whether he will tell his partner. Generally, his reproductive capacity is not threatened, since he has "proven" himself fertile. His emotional conflicts, however, may make him feel anxious and depressed. These issues acquire special meaning when the prior pregnancy and adoption or abortion involve the couple that has come for examination and counseling. In many cases, referral for sexual or psychiatric therapy may be necessary, and the physician needs to be aware of appropriate consultants and therapists (Grover, 1981). If either partner has had a sexually transmitted disease, their concerns and our counseling approach will be similar, with attention to their feelings and potential effects on fertility.

Case 2

A 19-year-old female presented for medical examination and birth-control advice prior to her marriage. She was in good general health, and her physical examination was normal. Her 20-year-old fiancé was unable to join her for the first visit; both of them were students, and he was preoccupied with classes. They recently had become sexually active, and they were concerned about preventing pregnancy. Careful and supportive interviewing revealed that they practiced withdrawal or coitus interruptus, lacking access to other means of birth control. She felt that although she enjoyed the intimacy of coitus, she was frustrated, anxious, and unhappy with her failure to experience orgasm.

After discussion, she chose to use birth control pills to prevent pregnancy, and a suitable program was provided. After a general review of sexuality and sexual behavior, she was encouraged to return with her fiancé for additional counseling. In their joint interview, both were relieved to be able to express their anxieties about potential pregnancy and were happy to have chosen a more effective birth control program. Although he declined further examination for himself, the young man did express concern over his failure to bring his partner satisfactorily to climax. Together, they were able to understand her potential for sexual response more effectively and learned more about the importance of foreplay and the relatively slow arousal patterns of the inexperienced female. They were also able to understand more clearly the detrimental effects of hurried intercourse, with withdrawal at male climax, on their mutual satisfaction. They did not ask for any further counseling at this time. Six months later, after marriage, she returned for a routine follow-up visit and reported that, though improved, their sexual relations were still only minimally satisfactory and that her husband continued to have difficulty in discussing their sexual needs. They were referred for family therapy, at their request.

Counseling of Couples Who Are Already Pregnant

When a couple presents for premarital counseling knowing that pregnancy is already underway, there usually has been little time or opportunity for them to talk with each other about their sexual relationship or their future plans. Often, they have delayed seeking medical care until they are sure that the woman is really pregnant. Some couples feel compelled to marry because of the pregnancy, and they may need to discuss this decision objectively. Other pregnant couples might need to discuss their feelings about a previous abortion or their decision to marry rather than to have the present pregnancy terminated.

Since both marriage and pregnancy in these circumstances are likely to be new ideas, they may also have inappropriate expectations for sexual function. For example, the man may not perceive how pregnancy and the urgency of planning for marriage may diminish his partner's sex drive and responsiveness. She in turn may not understand that he avoids intercourse because he is afraid of harming the fetus or that he remains ambivalent about making a marriage commitment because of his own uncertainties about the future.

The aim of counseling, after establishing the duration and status of the pregnancy, is to help plan for obstetrical care and to guide and support them through the physical and emotional changes associated with premarital pregnancy. If pregnancy termination is chosen, they will need support as that process takes place. Whether or not marriage is the appropriate decision may remain uncertain until it actually takes place.

Case 3

A 28-year-old resident in surgery and his fiancée, a 24-year-old medical assistant, were seen because of pregnancy, which they had already decided to terminate. They had been engaged for 6 months and planned to marry upon his completion of training. They had known each other for 2 years and believed that they had a good relationship. Neither of them had been involved with other partners during this time, and the pregnancy was the first for either of them. Elective abortion appeared to be a rational solution to their dilemma of dealing with a premarital pregnancy during a difficult training period for him. However, when each was seen individually, more reluctance was expressed about terminating the pregnancy than had been communicated to each other. After confirmation of the pregnancy, a sensitive and supportive joint interview ensued in which they shared their feelings. They decided to discontinue their plans for abortion and scheduled an earlier marriage. They became more comfortable in planning for the pregnancy and were relieved when they changed their decision about abortion. As their sexual adjustment appeared to be satisfactory, specific sex counseling was not indicated; they were more in need of objective help with communication and decision making about the pregnancy and the timing of their wedding.

Counseling of Midlife Couples Planning Marriage

"Midlife" couples (35 or older) represent a special challenge to the medical counselor for several reasons. Physical problems are found more often, and sexual behavior patterns and expectations are sometimes more restricted and rigid. Reproduction carries increased risks and may cause more conflicts, especially if energies for parenting are diminished (Daniels and Weingarten, 1979).

Couples in their late thirties or early forties planning marriage for the first time may or may not have had previous sexual experience. Those who are inexperienced can be difficult to counsel, since they are likely to have remained celibate to this point in their lives because of moral convictions, strong sexual inhibitions, significant personal conflicts, or for all of these reasons. They may have "self-selected" each other because of their diminished sexual interest. They are likely to need reassurance that lower sex drives are an acceptable variation in the normal spectrum of human sexual behavior and that they need not be compelled to compete with others whose drives may be higher. Those with sexual experience may also be difficult to counsel because their sexual encounters may have given them inappropriate expectations for their own marital sexual function. Although likely to be less sexually inhibited than those in the inexperienced group, they may be "set in their ways" and less amenable to personal growth and change than younger people. They, too, will need reinforcement of the view that satisfactory sexual activity is a part of the spectrum of human behaviors open to them and that even though they are starting late, it is appropriate for them to include it as one of the goals in their new relationship.

A careful physical examination of both parties is vital in order to detect chronic conditions, such as hypertension, diabetes, and heart disease, or other health factors important to their marital and sexual relationship. Sexual counseling of midlife couples is similar to that already described, with special attention to their emotional needs. Should there be a physical disorder, they will need appropriate counseling about the condition and its impact on their marriage, their sexuality, and their potential for childbearing.

Both sexually inexperienced and experienced couples will need information about childbearing in this older age group. Fertility is diminished as a complication of intercurrent diseases, diminished coital frequency, and gonadal dysfunction. Spontaneous abortion may occur in 25% or more of cases of pregnancy in women over 40 because of increased chromosomal abnormalities and defective placentation. Fetal abnormalities, including Down's syndrome more than double (from 2 to 5%) and complications of pregnancy, such as preeclampsia, fetal growth retardation, and vaginal bleeding, increase (Daniels and Weingarten, 1979). Although classified as "high-risk" for pregnancy management, the older couple can be reassured that most of their potential problems are not limiting. If they are willing to accept the known risks, it is reasonable for them to attempt to have a baby. When pregnancy occurs, prenatal genetic diagnosis may detect some abnormalities, especially Down's syndrome and neural tube defects. These two anomalies constitute about half of all abnormal fetuses in this age group, and prenatal genetic diagnosis with the choice of abortion for affected fetuses should be provided.

Sophisticated perinatal care can help the high-risk older mother to successfully negotiate a complicated pregnancy. Couples with these potential problems should be referred to a perinatal center for obstetrical care. In spite of the known drawbacks and potential problems, more and more couples are opting to marry late and to defer their childbearing until after the age of 35.

Some of these couples will need counseling because one or the other has a medical problem whose treatment prevents or alters their sexual function. When such is the case, as with the medical therapy of hypertension, counseling must be highly individualized and supportive. There must be careful consideration of whatever sexual function they can enjoy. Referral is often necessary, in order to provide for ongoing sexual counseling and psychotherapy (Kolodny et al., 1979).

Case 4

A 42-year-old female librarian presented just prior to marriage with known uterine fibroids and several months of amenorrhea. She had no symptoms of pregnancy, and she questioned her potential fertility. She was looking forward with pleasure to marriage with a 48-year-old divorced accountant, who had two grown children. She indicated that they hoped they would be able to have a child. Her general health was good, and she was in excellent physical condition on examination. To her surprise, pelvic examination and laboratory tests revealed that she was 3 months pregnant. Prenatal genetic counseling was discussed. Although an ultrasound examination confirmed the presence and duration of the preganncy, it also showed that the uterine fibroids had enlarged from hormonal stimulation. In fact, the fibroids obstructed the pathway of planned fluid aspiration (amniocentesis) and increased the procedure's risks to the fetus. Together, the couple decided against further efforts at prenatal genetic diagnosis. Their marriage took place as planned, and their healthy and normal daughter was born 6 months later, after surprisingly few perinatal complications. Counseling for decision making for this couple involved providing them with appropriate information during the course of the pregnancy and offering support while they decided upon which course they would take.

Counseling of Couples Planning Remarriage

Couples planning remarriage after divorce or the death of a spouse may have special needs relating to their age, experiences, feelings, and expectations that inevitably have been influenced by their previous relationship. If the first marriage was unhappy and ended in divorce, their sexual functioning may also have been unhappy and their expectations influenced. If the first marriage was happy, but death ended the relationship, the new partnership can suffer by comparison. In both instances, individual counseling or therapy may be necessary in order to help them deal with these past issues and to project more realistic expectations on the new relationship. The primary physician, however, can accomplish a great deal by being interested and supportive and taking time to listen to their concerns.

Case 5

A middle-aged couple (ages 50 and 48) was referred by a minister for examination and counseling prior to a second marriage for each. They both had grown children who were away from home. The woman's first husband had been accidentally killed several years before. She described their life together as good, with a fulfilling sexual component. The man's first marriage, on the other hand, was reported as extremely unsatisfying. He described his former wife as passive, unaffectionate, and completely disinterested in sex. The marriage had ended recently in a bitter divorce. The present couple had known each other socially for several years but had not become emotionally involved until after his divorce. His health was good, but she had recently been told by another physician that she "needed a hysterectomy" because of uterine fibroids, a benign muscle change in the uterus. They were puzzled about their present sexual difficulties, which included premature ejaculation on his part and orgasmic dysfunction on hers. Both problems had worsened since she was advised to have surgery.

In her interview, she confessed that the prospect of hysterectomy was of deep concern. It made her wonder if she was becoming unfeminine and unattractive. She found herself less interested in intercourse, although she was happy about her plans for remarriage. Her general physical examination was normal, but the pelvic examination revealed that she had a slightly enlarged uterus, consistent with her prior diagnosis of fibroids. However, since they caused her no clinical problems and were asymptomatic, she was advised that hysterectomy was not indicated. In fact, as she could expect menopause during the next few years, with consequent shrinking of the uterus and the fibroids, she might not require surgery. She was greatly relieved by this advice and felt more comfortable about her sexuality.

His interview revealed that he had been intensely unhappy for many years in his first marriage, particularly because of his wife's sexual unresponsiveness. Though long contemplating it, he chose to delay the divorce until after their children were grown and away from home. Because of his wife's lack of interest, his sexual pattern was to seek coitus with her only when he felt sexually driven, and then to do it as quickly as possible. This fostered a pattern of rapid or premature ejaculation and devalued the sexual relationship. At other times, months would pass without coital sexual activity, during which masturbation was his only sexual outlet. In the later years of the marriage, he had occasional extramarital sexual contacts, but within that casual context he also experienced premature ejaculation. Following the divorce, he had a "flaming affair" for several months that reassured him that he was still desirable and helped him to feel more competent sexually. In the present relationship, he was unhappy to note that he continued to experience premature ejaculation and stated that it had become more frequent as their plans for marriage evolved.

In a joint interview they were able to communicate more openly about their concerns, and they realized that, although important, their previous experiences were not limiting. Her anxiety over possible major surgery and loss of attractiveness was lessened, and his concerns about again being committed to marriage were eased. A follow-up visit several months after their marriage verified that their sexual relationship was much improved, and they felt they had made the right choices, because of better communication with each other.

Counseling of Handicapped Couples Planning Marriage

Sexual function in couples where one member is handicapped recently emerged into our clinical awareness as an important issue as we have learned more about the possibilities for sexual function in the handicapped (Green, 1979; Grover, 1981; Kolodny et al., 1979). An important initial aspect of counseling is to be sure that the couple's expectations for sexual function are defined and that all the levels of function possible for them are fully and objectively explored. The variety of ways that human beings can express themselves sexually gives us an ample basis for educating and counseling couples who are unable to experience coitus. Indeed, some couples may be helped just by learning that cuddling, touching, stroking, and loving conversation may be satisfying to the handicapped person. The unhandicapped partner may need to learn to be content with noncoital sexual gratification, such as oral–genital stimulation or self-pleasuring assisted by the partner, as well as nongenital touching and holding. The unhandicapped partner may need support while learning that nonorgasmic function for the handicapped partner is acceptable sexual behavior.

Whatever the disability, the nonhandicapped partner must clearly understand the sexual and reproductive implications of living with a handicapped spouse. They must openly and honestly communicate their commitment to the marriage, as the spouse may be concerned about being the recipient of pity or sympathy, rather than love. If pregnancy is possible, and is considered, both counseling and obstetrical care will need to be highly individualized, depending on the nature of the handicap.

Case 6

A 38-year-old male carpenter and his 28-year-old second wife of 2 years were referred for fertility evaluation. It was her first marriage. Between marriages, he was discovered to have cancer of the penis, with therapy resulting in penile amputation. He retained the capacity for orgasm and ejaculation from perineal stimulation but clearly was no longer capable of vaginal intromission. In spite of his disability, they worked out a pattern for their satisfactory sexual interaction that involved mutual caressing and cunnilingus. However, in addition to emphasizing his inability to perform coitus, oral sexual activity caused him to feel significant anxiety and guilt. They hoped that artificial insemination using his sperm would allow them to have a baby. Her general health and examination was normal, and no gynecologic conditions were found that precluded pregnancy. Aside from his absent penis, he appeared to be free of disease and was eager to try for pregnancy. Unfortunately, multiple semen analyses revealed that he was azospermic, and urological consultation indicated that he very likely had always been sterile. When they learned that artificial insemination with his semen would be futile, they were emotionally crushed. Both individual and joint interviews reinforced their strong commitment to each other in the face of their multiple serious problems. They were referred as a couple for long-term psychotherapy.

Summary

Premarital counseling by physicians who are comfortable with issues that relate to sexual behavior and reproduction is both urgently needed and generally not available. The opportunity to counsel and educate couples about the broader aspects of human sexual behavior and to initiate therapy for specific problems within the context of primary care is exceptional. Preparation for premarital and sexual counseling is an important component of medical education, especially for primary care physicians.

The keys to effective premarital and sexual counseling are to establish rapport with the couple and to obtain a careful mutual and individual medical and sexual history and to carry out a thorough general and specific (genital) physical examination. With the information and perspective thus obtained, the physician will be able to structure a counseling program that will help the couple with the continuing process of their sexual growth and development.

In order to provide appropriate counseling, the physician needs to allocate the time needed and must be nonjudgmental, objective, informative, and supportive as well as a "permission giver." The physician needs to know when to refer the couple for additional counseling or therapy and should be aware of a network of resource people who are sensitive, supportive, and alert to the complexities of couples therapy.

As is true in many areas of medicine, the results of premarital sexual counseling may not be clearly evident or evaluated scientifically. The art of medical practice lies in effecting our desires and capabilities for caring for other people, knowing that what we do benefits them as human beings, who, like ourselves, share in the common voyage through life, and who are happy when our intervention is beneficial.

References

Bird, J. L. *Sexual loving—The experience of love*. New York: Doubleday, 1976.

Daniels, P., and Weingarten, K. A new look at the medical risks in late childbearing. *Women and Health,* 1979, *4,* 5–36.

Green, R. *Human sexuality, a health practitioner's text* (2nd ed.). Baltimore, Md.: Williams & Wilkins, 1979.

Group for the Advancement of Psychiatry. *Assessment of sexual function*. New York: Jason Aronson, 1974.

Grover, J. W. Human sexuality—Management for the primary physician. *Primary Care,* 1981, *8,* 55–76.

Kelly, G. F. *Sexuality: The human perspective*. New York: Barron's Educational Series, 1980.

Kolodny, R. C., Masters, W. H., and Johnson, V. E. *Textbook of sexual medicine*. Boston: Little, Brown, 1979.

Masters, W. H., and Johnson, V. E. *The pleasure bond*. Boston: Little, Brown, 1974.

Caring for Victims of Rape

Daniel C. Silverman and Roberta J. Apfel

Introduction

Rape is the most rapidly increasing violent crime in the United States (Federal Bureau of Investigation, 1978). As incidents of rape and requests for treatment of its aftereffects continue to grow in number (McCombie, Bassuk, Savitz, & Pell, 1976), more health care providers find themselves confronted with the responsibility of responding to the medical and psychologic needs of rape victims. Providing care to the rape victim is especially challenging because this traumatic experience profoundly affects the individual and evokes strong feelings in the caretaker as well (Silverman, 1977). Myths and misconceptions (Brownmiller, 1975) about rape are common and often influence the attitudes, expectations, and behavior of not only the victims but the important people in their lives including their friends, families, and medical caregivers.

The clinician's beliefs about sexuality, life-styles other than his/her own, and rape as a crime can affect the quality of communication, empathy, and care offered to the victim. A necessary prerequisite to providing competent medical treatment to victims of rape is a personal exploration of those values, identifications, and ideas that might interfere with the delivery of nonjudgmental, respectful care. The clinician should be familiar with the sociologic and psychologic aspects of rape, understand its common physical and emotional sequellae (Burgess and Holmstrom, 1974, 1976; Kilpatrick, Vernon, & Resnick, 1979), and be able to respond appropriately to the special needs of rape victims. In addition, he/she must be willing to be disabused of the misconceptions and personal biases that so often surround this emotionally charged topic.

Myths and Misconceptions about Rape

Perhaps the most common and potentially harmful misconception that surrounds rape is that it is in essence a sexual crime (Table 1). Rape, in fact, represents an act of

---

Daniel C. Silverman and Roberta J. Apfel • Department of Psychiatry, Beth Israel Hospital, and Harvard Medical School, Boston, Massachusetts.

TABLE 1   Rape Mythology[a]

Misconception	Fact
All rape victims are sexy young women.	Rapes have been reported for male and female victims ranging in age from 18 months to 85 years.
Anyone who is raped asked for it by being careless or walking alone late at night.	33% of rapes occurred after forced entry into the victim's *own home*; 50% occurred *inside* a residence.
Flirting with strangers invites rape.	48% of victims knew their assailant prior to being raped.
Rape is a crime of spontaneous lust.	90% of group rapes and 58% of single rapes were *planned* in advance.
Rape is committed by sexually frustrated, antisocial misfits.	In Amir's study, 60% of rapists were married men with active sex lives.
Rape is most often a crime of blacks against white victims.	93% of rapes were perpetrated by men against women of the *same race*; 4% were white men attacking black women; 3% of rapes were carried out by black men against white women.

[a]From *Rape: a crime of violence*, Rape Crisis Intervention Project, Beth Israel Hospital, Boston. Adapted from Amir (1971).

extreme violence, not an erotic event. It has been described as a deviant act of aggression, where sex is used as a weapon (Groth and Burgess, 1977). Rape victims are frequently subjected to the sadistic use of physical force, threatened with death or mutilation by knife or gun, made to cooperate in humiliating or perverse sexual activity, and often sustain serious external and internal injuries. Victims, in describing their feelings about the experience, seldom discuss it in sexual terms. Rather they experience themselves as having been exposed to a "brutal," "terrifying" situation in which their greatest concern is fear for their lives. Other prevalent misconceptions about rape include the notions that "all rape victims are sexy young women," "women who are raped ask for it by being flirtatious with strangers or careless about walking alone at night," "rape is a spontaneous act of uncontrollable sexual passion" and "rape is a racially motivated crime most often involving black men against white women."

Evidence from sociologic studies of rape (Amir, 1971; Chappell, 1971; Rabkin, 1979; Schultz, 1975) provide data to challenge these ideas. Not all victims are young women; a review of cases of patients seen in a general hospital reveal male and female victims with ages ranging from 18 months to 85 years. The belief that rape is the predictable result of "carelessness" or "flirtatiousness with strangers," is refuted by statistics indicating that in almost one-half of reported cases, the rapists were previously known to their victims. Even the exercise of considerable caution offers no absolute protection from rape victimization since it has been reported that 50% of all rapes occur inside a residence; in 33% of the instances the rapist forcibly enters the victims's home (Amir, 1971). As to the belief that rape is most commonly interracial (Brownmiller, 1975) and, in particular, that black men assault white women, evidence indicates this is the case in only 3 to 4% of reported cases. White males attack black women with a frequency equal to blacks against white victims.

Some myths seem to grow out of a need to view rape as a sudden, uncontrollable and aberrant act carried out by antisocial individuals. Again, the facts fail to support explanations that would make it easier to minimize the prevalence and unpredictability of rape's occurrence. Approximately 90% of group rapes (those involving more than one attacker) and 58% of single rapes are planned in advance of the crime. Sixty percent of rapists are married men with active sex lives, not typical of the expected profile of the "common criminal" or "sexually deprived psychopath" (Amir, 1971).

It would seem that the strong feelings of fear, helplessness, and anger this violent crime evokes make it necessary for society to mystify and mythologize rape so it will seem alien to our everyday existence, less of a continuing threat to our safety, and something that is perpetuated and experienced only by people very different from ourselves.

The Caregiver's Response: Common Errors in Interventions with Victims of Rape

The Male Caregiver and the Female Victim

At present, it is most likely that the victim of rape requiring acute medical care will be a woman. More often than not, the first or only caregiver available to the patient is a man. Clinical experience indicates there may be difficulties when a male practitioner is called upon to assist a female rape victim (Silverman, 1977). The male clinician called to see the female rape victim may experience a number of understandable concerns. He may wonder if the patient would prefer to be seen and examined by a woman, whether or not the rape victim requests it. He may imagine that the patient will feel guarded with a man and see him as symbolizing the masculine brutality from which she suffered. At the other extreme, in response to such concerns, he may deny that the patient could have any feelings at all about seeing a man. In the case in which a female victim insists upon seeing a female caregiver, if possible, her request should be honored. If it is not possible, the presence of another woman during the examination may be reassuring. Seeing that a man can be respectful, concerned, and worthy of trust may help the woman begin to reestablish a sense of safety and comfort with other men in her life.

The special concerns the male clinician may bring to the situation can, however, lead to attempts to "rescue" the victim from the pain she has suffered by being overly solicitous or changing his customary way of relating to patients. The wish to convince the woman she need not fear "all men" may lead to attempts to make the interaction an "emotionally corrective" experience that proves some men can be gentle, caring, and compassionate. Changes in the tone of one's voice, amount of reassurance offered, use of terms of endearment (e.g., "honey," "dear"), obvious avoidance or overuse of physical contact (varying from increased distance to handholding or hugging) may serve to offer the patient communications difficult for her to trust or feel comfortable with because of their exaggerated quality.

Perhaps the most common error of management made by the male practitioner is the tendency to focus more attention on the sexual aspects of the victim's rape experience than upon her emotional response to this life-threatening experience. Such a tendency is often a result of misunderstanding about rape and the woman's subjective experience of it. As indicated earlier, victims feel they have been exposed to a terrifying life-and-death experience, not a sexual event. Premature or primary emphasis on the details of the sexual assault can lead the victim to experience the caregiver as lacking in understanding or as generally unempathic.

Certain patterns of communication may indicate that the clinician's own feelings are interfering with the care being provided. Practitioners who find themselves consistently questioning the victim's credibility ("Jilted women often make false accusations of rape" is one rationalization) or degree of responsibility for the rape ("Did she somehow cause this to happen?") may be protecting themselves against uncomfortable feelings of helplessness and vulnerability stimulated by identification with the patient's genuine plight. At times the male clinician may find himself strongly allied with the victim's boyfriend, husband, father, or brother, feeling angry with the "woman as an extension of her man" for "allowing" herself to be raped. Seeing the woman as "property" (Brownmiller, 1975) and the rape as an attack upon "her man" is not an unusual response, perhaps because the sense of indignation is easier to cope with than sharing the victim's distressing feelings of an inability to control her own life and safeguard herself from harm. Caregivers too strongly identified with the men in the victim's life may express it by being paternalistic or overly protective of the woman in an attempt to reduce feelings of guilt and responsibility for what has happened to this "poor, defenseless girl." The danger here is that of reinforcing the woman's understandable sense of vulnerability and powerlessness during the time of her acute crisis. This can produce in the victim even greater feelings of being overwhelmed, inadequate, and unable to cope.

Another cause of unintentionally distancing communications on the part of men working with victims may be born of attempts to deny that he has any troubling feelings at all about rape. Trying to show that one is "liberal and liberated" concerning sexuality, rape, and women's issues, in general, may lead to patronizing, facile, or pressured efforts to prove one's "politics are in the right place." It is far better to make an honest effort to understand the center of the patient's concerns and suffering than to convince her of one's "raised consiciousness."

The Female Caregiver and the Rape Victim

The management errors previously described are not necessarily specific to the male caregiver. Female clinicians may be just as prone to the difficult feelings aroused by rape and their potentially problematic effect on the interaction with the patient. One particular pattern, which seems to be relatively common among female physicians, nurses, and mental health workers new to rape crisis intervention, is sometimes referred to as the "smoking gun phenomenon." This response centers around a persistent need to find some detail, fact, or "clue" that rationally explains why the woman was raped (Sutherland and Scherl, 1970). "She wasn't cautious enough," "if she only had window locks," "she should have suspected that the guy had a potential for violence," "if only her car hadn't broken down," and "she's the masochistic type anyway" are examples of rationalizations that may be used to explain why a particular woman was raped. The reason for such thinking may be apparent. There is often a strong need for the woman professional confronting the frightening brutality of rape victimization for the first time to maintain her belief that "this will never happen to me as long as I don't make the same mistake she did." The unfortunate truth is that rape often occurs where no carelessness, unconscious self-destructive tendency or fateful error of judgment existed. Most often, rape represents a situation in which the victim is subjected to forces that would be beyond any individual's ability to resist. To accept this harsh truth is of course to admit one's own potential vulnerability in an unpredictable world. It is a disturbing self-admission to make, and the hesitancy to do so seems very understandable.

The woman professional's wish to maintain a sense of invincibility can lead her to search for the "smoking gun" in a somewhat "prosecutorial" style during history taking. A tendency to repeat questions, point out minor inconsistencies in the victim's story, hypothesize the presence of unconscious motives, or criticize certain decisions and behavior can leave the patient feeling guilty, ashamed, or unreasonably responsible for an event over which she had little or no real control. Victims are often prone to self-recrimination and painful rumination about what they could have done differently. It is critical that caretakers help them put such unrealistic self-expectations into perspective rather than heightening them. It is often useful to remind the victim she coped well enough to escape a life-threatening situation intact and that this is an achievement the practitioner can admire.

The Victim's Response to Rape and Its Effects upon the Relationship with the Caregiver

The Acute Phase

A wide variety of affective responses may be manifested in the acute period following rape victimization, ranging from shock and numbness to anxiety, uncontrollable crying, and panic states with loss of emotional composure. Feelings of a deep sense of helplessness associated with guilt and self-criticism seem almost universal among victims (Burgess and Holmstrom, 1973; McCombie, 1976; Hilberman, 1976). The intense affects stimulated by the exposure to a life-threatening situation mobilize the individual's psychological defenses in an attempt to protect the ego from feeling overwhelmed by the sense of vulnerability and loss of control over one's life that are inherent in the experience of rape assault. The adaptiveness of the defenses and coping behaviors mobilized by the individual are ultimately a function of her developmental history, personality structure, and the emotional support available at the time of the crisis (Notman and Nadelson, 1976; Hilberman, 1976). In the most acute stages of responding to the psychological disequilibrium caused by the rape, victims are likely to regress to less adaptive forms of behavior and may rely upon more primitive defense mechanisms. Denial of the painful feelings of helplessness and inadequacy may make it difficult for the woman to establish a trusting relationship with the clinician in the immediate post-traumatic period. Victims may be somewhat guarded in answering questions and hesitant about entering into a "working alliance" with the caregiver regardless of how well intentioned the practitioner may be. The need to maintain a heightened vigilence and "safe" distance should be anticipated by those treating the woman. Caregivers may experience her as "withholding information" or "not making it easy to help." The victim may express her denial of the seriousness of the trauma she has experienced by refusing to accept follow-up appointments for medical and psychological aftercare.

Another common and remarkable early defensive response of victims is reflected often in an absence of observeable anger. Victims may find it impossible to express directly the outrage they feel toward their assailant. Fear of reprisal ("He knows where I live—he might come back again!"), difficulty in expressing aggressive feelings resulting from earlier social conditioning, or the denial of murderous fantasies may all contribute to the difficulty in expressing the resentments openly. The anger may be dealt with by displacement onto friends, family, police, or helping professionals. Ironically, those people who have been most caring and so seem "safest" may become objects of the victim's frustrations. The aggression may be indirect as well as redirected. It can be expressed through passivity or uncooperativeness, a sense of entitlement to special treatment, or devaluation of attempts to be helpful. The clinician trying hard to be of assistance may experience these hostile communications as confusing, discouraging, or a personal rejection. As in the case of the victim's use of distancing maneuvers, if the clinician is prepared in advance for the victim's reactions to repressed anger and understands their basis, he/she will be better able to respond in a nondefensive, accepting manner.

Other defense mechanisms used by victims to cope with conflicted feelings of rage and vengeance may include turning anger against the self or identification with the aggressor. These victims may feel they were responsible for or deserving of their misfortune, blame themselves excessively and generally feel undeserving of the professional's concern or attempts to be of help. Such patients often refuse all attempts to assist them and persistent efforts on the part of the practitioner may be needed to allow them to accept necessary medical and psychologic treatment.

Other patients seem to undergo major dissociative experiences in response to the traumatic episode. They seem "perfectly composed" or "completely calm" in describing their experience and may discuss it in a matter-of-fact or apparently indifferent fashion. The patient who appears almost "too good to be true" probably isn't. She may be mobilizing a pervasive but brittle dissociative defense against the emergence of difficult feelings that can break down under continued stress at a later time. Such patients should not be discharged without continuing care plans. It is wise to encourage all victims to return for a post-rape checkup because the range of initial presentations is so broad and delayed reactions to stress are so common.

Finally, because feelings of shame and humiliation are frequently associated with rape victimization and may be related to the sexual aspects of the crime, the physical part of the examination should be approached carefully and with special consideration of the woman's needs. Victims often feel themselves to be "soiled," "repulsive," or "disgusting" and may be worried about evoking similar feelings in their caregivers when examined. Fears concerning loss of control, inability to protect one's personal space, or painful penetration may arise during the physical examinations, especially the pelvic exam. It may be helpful to integrate the following suggestions into the physical examination of the rape victim:

1. Avoid examining the patient immediately. The history should not be obtained while doing the physical. It is best to indicate to the victim a clear distinction between the interview and physical parts of the medical intervention. It helps to let the woman know in advance that as much time as is necessary will be taken to listen to and answer questions before the examination begins. The physician will be seen as more empathic if he or she takes time, paces things slowly, and does not appear to be pressured by a particular agenda. In the busy emergency ward where time is often at a premium and caregivers often attend to several patients simultaneously, it may help to have an identified person (e.g., rape crisis counselor) remain with the victim throughout her stay. This can offer the victim a reassuring sense of continuity of attention that may offset the effect of the unavoidable interruptions of the fast-paced, task-oriented emergency ward setting. The history should be taken with the woman and clinician sitting on the same level rather than with the victim lying on a stretcher or an examining table. This can help the victim maintain a sense of equality and active participation in the process, while lessening feelings of passivity and dependency.

2. It is helpful to offer the victim the opportunity to have a supportive friend or medical assistant remain in the room throughout the physical examination. The rape victim should be given the chance to decide who will be present. There may be some people she would prefer to exclude (for example, parents or partner) because of immediate feelings of embarrassment or her concern about their responses. Such wishes should be respected whenever possible.

3. All aspects of the examination should be described before beginning. The more difficult parts and the degree of discomfort that can be expected should be described in advance. It is better not to underemphasize the possible discomfort but to state the facts accurately indicating that every attempt will be made to be as gentle and quick as possible.

4. The clinician should be prepared to stop the examination at any point to reassure the woman, answer questions, or to acknowledge that her concerns are reasonable and will be respected. (See section on the medical needs of the patient.) It helps to anticipate that this examination will take longer than those done under more usual circumstances. The victim may also need to pause periodically to compose herself emotionally.

5. When a rape victim seems markedly anxious about the examination because of its closeness in time to the rape and reassurance seems insufficient to contain anxiety, the administration of small amounts of an anxietolytic agent (e.g., 5–10 mg po Diazepam, or if the patient seems panicked, 25–50 mg po chlorpromazine) may be

helpful. Intramuscular injections should be kept to a minimum as the patient is likely to require them for venereal disease prophylaxis following the examination.

Familiarity with characteristic ways of coping with anxiety can help guide the clinician's treatment of the rape victim. Typically, each person will respond as she would following other traumatic events. The rape trauma syndrome (Burgess and Homstrom, 1974) is similar to post-traumatic stress-related syndromes described for victims of war, natural disasters, and accidents. The initial acute or "shock" phase described earlier is followed by a second post-traumatic readjustment phase and a third reintegration phase.

Beyond the shock common to other natural disasters, rape victims have experienced a life-threatening violation of their bodies and assault on their sexuality. Furthermore, the social misunderstanding of rape and the victim's own socialization can lead to an inordinate sense of guilt and self-criticism. The usual ability to cope in a disaster that derives from internal ego strengths and external supports can break down in the acute phase of rape trauma. The disaster is personal and attacks the very essence of one's sense of competence. The environment is ambivalent in supporting the victim and individuals of importance as well as strangers (including physicians and other health providers) can amplify rather than minimize the victim's sense of loss, guilt, and blame.

Post-traumatic Readjustment Phase

Days to weeks after the acute phase, many rape victims *appear* to return to their usual level of functioning. This stage has been termed a *pseudoadjustment,* because an outward appearance of composure may belie continuing but masked feelings of vulnerability. The victim may resume work or school activities, social and sexual relationships and, to the casual observer, seem recovered from the traumatic shock of the rape. However, on talking with the rape victim at this time, one may learn of the persistance of nightmares, anxiety states, flashbacks, phobic behavior, physical symptoms, or intrusive thoughts related to the original event. Patients may acknowledge such experiences only after the clinician has indicated his/her familiarity with these types of reaction patterns. The rape victim often feels distressed by such persistant reminders of the rape. Learning that these kinds of experiences are not abnormal may be reassuring, and open discussion of them can frequently bring some relief of symptoms. Occasionally rape victims will deny that they still experience feelings, thoughts, or dreams about the rape and may become angry at the interviewer for rekindling painful memories. Offering "permission" to have such thoughts (e.g., "after rape, many women do continue to dream about it . . . you may find that you do too") may allow the victim to share her inner fears, thus reducing the sense of isolation she may be experiencing in her attempts to readjust. It is important not to confront the denial of the victim as it may be a fragile but necessary defense against feeling overwhelmed. Offering support and a continuing availability may make it possible for the victim to discuss her concerns and doubts more openly at a later time.

During this phase there may be an increase in feelings of helplessness and dependency. The clinician may see victims who have abandoned a previously independent life-style to move back home with family or close friends. The self-reproach and loss of self-esteem that can follow rape continues in less obvious forms during this phase and may be expressed more clearly in behavior within the context of the health care setting by canceling appointments, failing to comply with recommended treatments, or frequently questioning the right to help and concern. It is important to reassure the victim of the necessity for as well as her right to medical care, psychological counseling, and the genuine concern of family, friends, and helping professionals.

Reintegration Phase

Months to years after a rape, patients may present with symptoms related to the original traumatic experience, e.g., depression, anxiety, sexual problems, phobic behaviors, or vague somatic complaints (Burgess and Holmstrom, 1979). The clinician who has followed the victim through the acute and post-traumatic readjustment phase should be alert to the emergence of rape-related problems long after the patient has resumed normal functioning. A common pattern is presentation with a ''new'' problem that is linked to the past rape only in the course of history taking or treatment. In the simplest situation, clarifying the connection of symptom and rape and validating the patient's experience is sufficient, e.g., saying "It is not uncommon to experience flashbacks of the rape during subsequent relationships and this may cause you to feel uncomfortable about current sexual activities,'' may be enough to allow the woman to begin to separate specific behaviors in the present from the traumatic aspects of the rape.

In more complex presentations, symptoms brought on by an event or situation that reminds the victim of the rape experience may signal the reemergence of unresolved past feelings. One patient, a 45-year-old woman, presented to her doctor with complaints of severe vaginal pain on intercourse. A complete medical workup failed to indicate a physical explanation for the problem. Further gentle attempts by the physician to understand what might be troubling the patient led to the history that a niece had been recently raped. This stimulated previously unexpressed feelings about the patient's own rape 1½ years earlier, an event about which she felt so much shame that she had not only refrained from obtaining medical care but had kept it a secret from her husband as well. Incomplete grieving over the loss and pain of rape or the persistence of physical and psychological symptoms related to an earlier rape experience despite clarification by the physician may indicate a need for counseling referral.

The reemergence of memories of and feelings about rape experience may also occur regularly in less dramatic ways. Anniversaries of the event may be difficult and the victim may transiently display some of the same constellation of symptoms experienced at the time of the original trauma. New situations or stimuli (e.g., movies, articles about rape) that recall the extreme sense of vulnerability, defenselessness, and fear experienced in relation to the rape are likely to evoke conscious associations to the traumatic event for an indefinite period of time. The victim will be reassured to learn that such patterns of response are to be expected and may be helped by prospective suggestion that these reactions are a possibility.

Treatment Interventions in Rape

Meeting the Psychological Needs of the Victim

In attending to the emotional needs of the rape victim, the following goals should guide the clinician's actions:

1. To lend emotional support and contain the extent of psychological trauma
2. To validate the victim's experience and reinforce adaptive coping behaviors
3. To assess the patient for evidence of gross psychological stress
4. To make a workable plan, specific to the individual patient, for necessary medical and psychological follow-up care

If the initial interaction with the clinician is one where treatment is humane and respectful, compassionate, but not patronizing or infantilizing, the extent of the trauma can begin to be circumscribed. A caregiver who treats the victim as an adult under extreme stress rather than a helpless child for whom everything must be done will be stimulating the reemergence of adaptive behavior on the part of the woman.

Support offered in the form of validation of the victim's experience is crucial. The clinician can help the patient identify clearly the feelings being experienced, e.g., numbness, shock, disbelief, anxiety, helplessness, or humiliation, and explain that these reactions are not unusual or "abnormal" but instead appropriate to the extraordinary life-threatening circumstances to which she has been exposed. Victims are often concerned that caregivers as authority figures will be critical of their behavior, question their responsibility for what has happened, or will feel revolted by the circumstances of the rape experience. Comments such as "you showed good judgment in not resisting an armed attacker," "you showed quick thinking in dealing with the rapist," "you were wise to seek medical attention immediately," or "staying calm in the face of this takes great courage" can mean much to a distressed victim who is feeling powerless, vulnerable, and self-critical. By discussing real and practical concerns with the woman, the caregiver can help her mobilize adaptive behaviors. In the period immediately following rape, discussing plans with the victim for temporary lodgings, which persons to contact for support, how to arrange legal counsel, or methods of caring for physical injuries suffered can convey the idea that the practitioner sees her as a competent adult able to cope effectively.

Follow-up planning for medical treatment or psychological counseling is an extremely important and sensitive matter. The clinician should be careful to offer the victim considerable latitude in arranging future contracts. Initially a phone call may seem less invasive and offer the woman more control and needed distance. Because rape victims frequently change their phone numbers, move, or temporarily leave home to stay with friends or family following rape, it is helpful for the clinician to obtain all numbers where the woman can be reached as well as the names of people who will know her whereabouts. A call at a prearranged time from the caregiver may help the woman to accept his/her interest and concern as genuine, allowing for an in-person return visit later. The call will indicate both the caregiver's reliability and availability as well as providing an opportunity to ask follow-up questions. In all future contacts the clinician should inquire about the woman's emotional and physical states, social relationships, and sexual functioning. Significant persistent difficulties in these areas may be an indication for referral for crisis counseling of psychiatric treatment.

Some victims will desire no more than occasional phone contact. This wish should be respected with gentle reminders that if the situation or the victim's needs change, the clinician is available and willing to help.

Interventions with the Victim's Partners and Family

Rape precipitates a life crisis not only for the victim but for the partners, family, and friends of the individuals as well (Silverman, 1978). Changes in relations with important others are inevitable following rape. Disruption in the normal functioning of friendship, couple, or family relationships can occur as a direct response to the psychological disequilibrium experienced by the victim. Clinical experience has shown that involving the members of the patient's support groups in medical and counseling interventions can be instrumental in helping them provide the victim with a safe setting in which to recover.

Ironically, it may be difficult at first for those closest to the victim to respond in a compassionate and supportive way. Loved ones may unknowingly be influenced by the same partial truths and prejudices about rape victimization shared by the public at large. Husbands may question their wife's degree of "responsibility for what has happened," harbor unrealistic ideas that somehow the "experience was enjoyable," or express resentment over the loss of "exclusive rights" to the sexuality of "their women." Parents sometimes fear that the victim will "never be the same," or find themselves uncomfortable at the prospect of having to acknowledge that their child is a mature sexual being. Lovers may struggle with urges to abandon the victim now that she has become "damaged merchandise" or "tainted." Clearly, such feelings, when experienced by partners or family members, make it difficult for them to respond to the victim in an unambivalent way. If these feelings are expressed openly or acted upon, they run the risk of reinforcing the victim's own sense of devaluation and make the psychological "revictimization" of the person a real possibility. The clinician must also be alert to his/her own negative reactions toward family members or partners for holding such "uninformed" or "chauvinistic" attitudes. Being critical of them for having such views can increase their sense of being attacked or humiliated, feelings that may already be present because of strong identifications with the victim. If the clinician is quick to judge, it may make the useful expression of difficult feelings less likely. The most helpful approach tends to be one in which people are gently encouraged to share misapprehensions and their associated feelings. Seeing the husband, boyfriend, or family members in private may offer them a safe and confidential way to discuss such concerns while protecting the absent victim.

It is useful to identify the injury that those close to the victim feel and to acknowledge that they share in the individual's trauma or loss. Partners and family can be helped to see that although rape is a terribly traumatic experience that causes reactions much like acute grief (Lindemann, 1944), the victim can regain the capacity to function effectively. Although one never "forgets" painful or traumatic experiences, such memories will decrease in intensity with time and need not make it impossible to enjoy life again after an adequate opportunity to grieve the loss or hardship sustained.

It is most important for the clinician to remember that the anger, resentments, and frustration directed toward the victim by those who should be ready sources of support result from shared feelings of guilt, devaluation, fearfulness, and embarrassment. Partners and family members must be given the chance to mobilize and explore these uncomfortable feelings in an atmosphere of uncritical acceptance.

Certain responses are typical of family members and partners in the acute stages of rape crisis. Prior awareness of these patterns can facilitate the choice of clinical intervention to be made by the clinician. During the immediate post-traumatic period, parents, partners, and siblings often experience feelings of shock, numbness, vulnerability, outrage, or physical distress that mirror the responses of the victim. Pressured attempts to help the victim through direct action often come from such feelings of shared distress.

Family members or partners may try to mobilize the support of the victim's friends, physicians, co-workers, clergy, or teachers. The victim may find these efforts intrusive. Initially, she may feel the need to deny what has happened or to share her experience with only a few carefully chosen people. The need for privacy, confidentiality, or simply to not discuss the matter should be respected by both family and clinician alike. The caregiver may want to offer the family or partner a chance to talk about the frustration of being unable to magically relieve the victim's suffering. Not infrequently, victims refuse medical and counseling follow-up because of a strong need to avoid feelings of vulnerability. In such cases, it may be extremely useful to hold meetings with family members to help them understand the reasons for the victim's refusal of professional help and to discuss ideas for assisting the patient in less formal ways.

Those individuals who see themselves in the role of the victim's "protector" may have recurring thoughts about taking revenge on behalf of the injured person. Such ideas may serve to protect the individual from awareness of his own feelings of helplessness and vulnerability. Unfortunately, if vengeful fantasies are expressed too concretely (e.g., buying a gun and going to "look" for the rapist), they may burden the victim with the added responsibility of having to calm or restrain the protecting person. The clinician should be prepared to point out that such behavior can cause added stress for the victim.

Another common and recognizable way in which families and partners respond is the tendency to be patronizing or overly protective of the victim. Parents may demand that the victim "come home where we can watch you" or "at least move to a safer neighborhood." They may insinuate themselves into the victim's daily routines, insisting upon chauffering her to and from jobs, school, or shopping. Such actions may be the result of guilty feelings about having failed to protect the victim from being raped. Although the motivation for such expression of concern is sincere, they run the risk of increasing the victim's sense of defenselessness as well as suggesting that important people see her as unable to cope and in need of constant supervision. This can make it difficult for the victim to use more adaptive coping strategies, ones that might not foster as much regression or loss of self-esteem and independence. The clinician can support the family's wish to be caretaking and available while pointing out the disadvantages of overprotectiveness.

Distraction is another strategy used by families and partners. In this case, the victim is kept continually involved in activities, such as vacations, shopping trips, or social gatherings, in an effort to prevent the person from "dwelling too much on what's happened." The wish to "undo the rape" leads to the theory that "if you don't think about it, it will go away." In other families, rather than becoming overly involved or controlling, an attempt is made to keep the rape a secret from the others in order to "protect" them. This is the result of fantasies that "mother would never be able to handle it," "Dad would be so upset it would kill him," or "the children will be harmed because they are much too young to understand." Born of a parent's discomfort with her own or a child's sexuality, fear of blame for carelessness, hidden alliances, or chronic interpersonal problems, family secrets generally fail to accomplish what they are designed to do. Most often, people in the family will know what has occurred on some level of consciousness, but the "conspiracy of silence" will make open sharing and support impossible.

Hiding the truth, as in keeping a rape a secret or trying to distract one from it through frenzied activity comes from the family or victim's belief that unrestricted discussion of the rape will only serve to keep the painful trauma alive in a destructive way, or worse, will victimize and overwhelm other "innocent" people. The unfortunate result of such thinking is to deny the victim the chance to mourn personal loss, deprive her of necessary support, and confirm the victim's worse fears by implying that what has happened is too awful to discuss openly.

Interventions with members of the victim's support system should be designed to facilitate the following:

1. The open expression of their own emotional responses to the shared crisis
2. Greater understanding of what the crime of rape represents
3. Constructive efforts to help the victim regain effective control of her life
4. Preparation of the family for the expectable emotional and physical aftereffects of rape
5. Modeling for the family and partners of the victim, the concept of emotional "containment"

The last point involves displaying how to create a safe environment in which the victim can ventilate troubling thoughts, feelings, and fantasies without fear of the confrontation or condemnation that comes from a shared sense of vulnerability. Families can learn that there is no "perfect" thing to say to do that will make everything all right. Disappointment over such a realization can be shared while the family is encouraged to continue being sensitive, caring, and emotionally available.

Indications for Referral

Victims, partners, and family members seen in the primary medical setting may need referral for psychiatric evaluation or treatment. Although it is possible for primary caregivers to become experienced in offering rape crisis counseling, time constraints, unavailability of supervision, personal preference, or severe psychological reactions in the victim may make referral appropriate.

The following kinds of situations may be ones in which the clinician will wish to triage patients, partners, and family for specialized interventions:

1. Situations where formal rape crisis intervention counseling programs exist, staffed by trained and experienced counsellors; they may offer the victim and the family immediate entrance into a support system specifically designed to meet their needs.

2. In instances where the victim wishes to seek legal recourse against the assailant and will need expert advice and assistance concerning police and court procedures.

3. Situations where the rape precipitates a profound decompensation in the thinking, affect, or behavior of the victim or members of the family, necessitating evaluation and treatment. This may be more likely in cases where significant psychiatric problems have existed prior to the rape (e.g., past history of depression with suicidal thinking or behavior, psychosis, severe personality disturbance). It may be appropriate to suggest referral prophylactically in cases where serious psychiatric illness (e.g., schizophrenia, manic-depressive illness, or borderline personality) predates the rape, even when acute decompensation is not apparent.

4. Situations where the rape exacerbates preexisting problems in sexual functioning, marital harmony, or family relationships. Rape may uncover longstanding interpersonal problems. A traumatic event can stimulate a self-awareness of problems that leads individuals to undertake psychotherapeutic treatment (e.g., individual, couple, or family therapy, sexual dysfunction counseling). The clinician's concern and help in arranging a referral may be a way of offering the victim or family members permission to get intensive professional assistance for serious, chronic emotional difficulties.

5. Severe psychological or physical symptoms persisting more than a month after the rape, i.e., inability to resume usual activities, unwillingness to discuss the rape with anyone, withdrawal from friends, persistant, severe anxiety or phobic behaviors, marked anorexia, weight loss, constant self-reproach, or suicidal ideation.

6. Severe symptoms that occur in the later phases of readjustment that persist despite clinical interventions, e.g., migrating physical complaints with minimal organic basis, psychosomatic reactions, apathy, or chronic feelings of depression with or without suicidal thinking. This may represent crystallization of a maladaptive state following the crisis and will require further intervention for a constructive outcome.

Conclusion

Rape is an increasingly prevalent, violent crime that can profoundly affect the lives of the patients and families seen in medical and psychiatric practice. The caregiver may be called upon to treat the acute emotional and physical sequelae of rape, support and counsel victims, partners, and families in their attempts to recover from its effects, and help patients cope with the dysfunctions and symptoms that may arise later in the course of readjustment following rape trauma. Clinicians who share old myths and labor under misconceptions about rape may reinforce feelings of guilt, shame, and helplessness in victims and so impede recovery from this trauma in a fashion that promotes psychological growth and restoration of self-esteem. Provision of sensitive and informed care can do much to prevent an acute crisis from becoming the basis of permanently maladaptive patterns of emotional, sexual, and physical functioning in rape victims.

Appendix: Treatment Interventions in Rape

Meeting the Medical Needs of Rape Victims

The medical needs of the rape victim are most significant in the acute phase. Subsequently, however, clinicians should be alert to rape as a factor in the etiology of somatic disorders and complaints of sexual dysfunction. The examination of rape victims involves an interface between the medical and legal professions. Detailed and carefully documented information is needed to aid in police investigation and to provide corroborating evidence in court as well as for the health needs of the victim. The medical record will be subpoenaed if the case is brought to trial. There are five goals to the examination:

1. Diagnosis and treatment of trauma
2. Collection of medical evidence
3. Venereal disease protection
4. Pregnancy prophylaxis
5. Emotional support

Since the medical record is a legal document, it must be complete, detailed, legible, and without conclusions or judgments. The clinician should not attempt to determine whether a "real" rape occurred; his/her primary responsibility is to meet the health needs of the victim and to observe, describe, collect, and record findings. A standardized protocol, such as the one below, will aid in this process. It should be written with full awareness that it may be read in court and frequently carries more weight than the victim's verbal testimony. The clinician's observations of signs of penetration and/or force, his/her record of the victim's account of the incident, and the integrity of the laboratory results are critical elements in the court case.

All individuals reporting a rape or attempted rape should be urged to have a medical examination. Those clinicians counseling victims of rape *must* be aware of the details of the medical exam if he or she is to be helpful to the medical staff or the patient. The following guidelines were developed by the Beth Israel Hospital Rape Crisis Intervention Program and are adapted from American College of Obstetrics and Gynecology (ACOG) Technical Bulletin, Number 14, (1970).

History and Review of Symptoms

1. *History of the assault incident.* It is necessary to take a detailed history of the circumstances of the assault in the victim's own words. A rape counselor, emergency

room nurse, or medical assistant should be present to give emotional support and to act as witness. The report should contain the following:

    a. A history of the time, place, and circumstances of the assault, including descriptions of any threats, weapons, physical contact, violence, and resistance and a description of the assailant or assailants

    b. A description of sexual contact attempted or completed, including whether the patient sustained oral, rectal, or vaginal penetration and ejaculation; if instruments were used; whether other sexual or degrading acts (e.g., urinated upon) were committed; the presence of condoms or tampons

    c. A description of the victim's general condition at the time of the assault (e.g., presence of alcohol, drugs)

    d. A history of the victim's behavior immediately after the assault, including whether the patient washed, douched, changed clothes, etc.

  2. *General medical history*

    a. Obtain a history of allergies, medications, major medical disorders, migraine, hypertension, seizures, coagulation defects, stroke, etc.

    b. Obtain a gynecological history, including menstrual history, last menstrual period, contraceptives, and infections

    c. Obtain a statement concerning physical complaints

  3. *Description of emotional state.* Note the victim's subjective report of her current feelings in her words and briefly indicate your own observations (e.g., shaking, nervous laughing, crying).

The Physical Examination

  1. *If the victim is wearing clothing from the time of the assault, note its condition* and record any rips, blood or semen stains, mud, soil, or foreign fibers.

  2. *Examine the entire body and external genitalia for signs of trauma* and record the location and condition. Use a figure drawing to illustrate the location of bruises, lacerations, bleeding, fractures, etc. Use the history of the assault to guide the examination of specific areas for findings that corroborate the history as given.

    a. Clothing, particularly undergarments, should be collected and stored in clean paper bags, separately labeled with the victim's name, date and time of the emergency ward or office visit, and the name of the examining physician. These should be stored until retrieval by police.

    b. The victim is to be instructed to preserve the clothing herself should the items be at home or should she refuse to permit the hospital to collect them.

  3. *Examine the entire body and external genitalia for evidence of seminal fluid, foreign pubic hair, and foreign matter,* such as mud, soil, splinters, fibers, etc.

    a. If necessary and appropriate, comb the pubic hair for hairs transferred from the assailant to the victim. These should be placed in a clean vial or envelope, sealed, and carefully labeled. Take approximately 10 pubic hairs from the patient for comparison, place them in a separate container, and label carefully.

    b. If any foreign matter is located, collect and label it as above including the source (e.g., sand found in the vagina).

    c. Fingernail scrapings are to be taken for traces of blood or flesh if the victim scratched the assailant. Scrape under each nail, place specimens in a clean vial or envelope and label (''hand,'' ''finger''). Scrapings from each nail should be kept separately.

  4. *Examine the internal genitalia for signs of trauma.* The pelvic examination is to be done with a *nonlubricated, water-moistened speculum.*

    a. If appropriate, examination of the urethra, rectum, and pharyngeal cavity are to be performed. Carefully record any evidence of trauma.

    b. A bimanual examination of the vagina is to be done only *after all laboratory specimens have been collected.*

The Laboratory Specimens

The laboratory specimens must be obtained by the examining clinician in the presence of a witness (emergency room nurse, medical assistant, or rape counselor). The specimens must be carefully labeled, using a diamond pencil to mark slides. *They should not be put in a routine collection box* but rather stored in a locked box until personally handed to the pathologist or laboratory technician. The following specimens are to be taken:

1. *Wet mount for motile sperm.* Specimens should be taken from the vagina, cervix, and vulva. A coverslip is placed on the slide to keep it moist. The slide is to be examined immediately and the results recorded. If this is not possible, swabs should be placed in separate tubes with a saline solution.

2. *Vaginal aspiration for acid phosphatase.* This is a qualitative test to establish semen presence in cases where the male is aspermatic. The fluid may be aspirated by using a disposable syringe. The vaginal pool and any other likely areas should be aspirated. All aspirated fluid should be stored in a labeled screw-top jar and frozen if the test cannot be done immediately. Diagnostic tablets can be of use in indicating immediately if there is the presence of semen. These tablets should be available in the emergency room or doctor's office. Items of clothing or dried areas of semen on the skin may be tested by touching those areas with moistened filter paper for 15 sec. The paper is then tested for acid phosphatase. (The acid phosphatase test is potentially effective up to 6 months after contact.)

3. *Cervical culture and sensitivity for gonorrhea* taken on an appropriate medium, such as Thayer-Martin, should be done. If appropriate, cultures of the rectum and pharynx should be done.

4. *A baseline serological test for syphilis: Hinton or VDRL.*

5. *PAP smear of vaginal pool.*

Treatment of Victim

1. *Treat all injuries.*

2. *Prophylactic treatment for the prevention of venereal disease* is to be given:

    a. Procaine penicillin, 4.8×10^6 units i.m., plus 1 g of oral Benemid. The Benemid is given simultaneously with Procaine penicillin.

    b. Penicillin is adequate for incubating syphilis. Serology tests for syphilis are to be drawn prior to treatment and repeated in 4 to 6 weeks if there is an allergic reaction to penicillin. If they are nonreactive, then the above dose is adequate. If the tests are reactive, then institute full treatment for syphilis. (Gonorrhea and syphilis coexist less than 1% of the time.)

3. *Postcoital contraception.* It is critical to obtain a detailed menstrual history from the woman in order to advise her of her options.

    a. If the woman has an IUD in place at the time of the rape or is on birth control pills, she should be considered protected against pregnancy.

    b. If no birth control is being practiced, it is necessary to calculate the probability of pregnancy as a result of the rape. A pregnancy test is indicated to determine if the patient was pregnant *before* the rape. If there is risk of pregnancy and you are certain the woman is not pregnant, the clinician can consider recommending the following options:

       i. "Morning-after" estrogen preparations have been used. We discourage their use because of significant side-effects (nausea, vomiting, menstrual changes) and increasing evidence of later problems secondary to these drugs.

      ii. Post-rape IUD insertion may be offered within 48 hr of the rape if hormones are contraindicated. The effectiveness of this therapy has not been well established.

     iii. Menstrual extraction within 2 weeks of a missed period.

     iv. Legal therapeutic abortion (D&C) 6 weeks after the last missed period should the woman become pregnant. The Beta Sub-Unit assay for human chorionic gonadotropin is now available to determine pregnancy after 3 days of gestation.

Medical Follow-up

The woman is to be given a follow-up appointment in 6 weeks. At that time she should be examined and informed of her physical condition. She should be encouraged to take advantage of rape counseling services if available.

The following lab work should be done at the 6-week follow-up visit:

1. Cervical culture and sensitivity
2. Repeat of the serologic test for syphilis
3. Pregnancy test
4. Blood typing if necessary for legal purposes

Of course, any injuries sustained during the rape experience should be followed in "appropriate ways."

References

Amir, M. *Patterns in forcible rape.* Chicago: Univ. of Chicago Press, 1971.
American College of Obstetrics and Gynecologists. *Technical Bulletin No. 14.* Chicago: Author, 1970.

Beth Israel Hospital. *Rape crisis intervention fact sheet: Rape a crime of violence.* Boston, Mass.: Author, 1979.

Brownmiller, S. *Against our will: Men, women and rape.* New York: Simon & Schuster, 1975.

Burgess, A., and Holmstrom, L. The rape victim in the emergency ward. *American Journal of Nursing,* October 1973, *73,* 1741–1745.

Burgess, A., and Holmstrom, L. Rape trauma syndrome. *American Journal of Psychiatry,* September 1974, *131,* 981–986.

Burgess, A., and Holmstrom, L. Coping behavior of the rape victim. *American Journal of Psychiatry,* 1976, *133,* 413–418.

Burgess, A., and Holmstrom, L. Rape: Sexual disruption and recovery. *American Journal of Orthopsychiatry,* 1979, *49*(4), 648–657.

Chappell, D. Forcible rape: A comparative study. In J. Henslin (Ed.), *Studies in the sociology of sex.* Meredith, 1971.

Federal Bureau of Investigation. *Uniform crime reports for the United States.* Washington, D.C.: U.S. Govt. Printing Office, 1978.

Groth, A. N., and Burgess, A. Rape: A sexual deviation. *American Journal of Orthopsychiatry,* 1977, *47*(3), 400–406.

Hilberman, E. *The rape victim.* Washington D.C.: American Psychiatric Association, 1976. Pp. 22–28.

Kilpatrick, D., Vernon, L., and Resnick, P. The aftermath of rape: Recent empirical findings. *American J. of Orthopsychiatry,* 1979, 49(4), 658–669.

Lindemann, D. Symptomatology and management of acute grief. *American Journal of Psychiatry,* 1944, *101,* 141–156.

McCombie, S. Characteristics of rape victims seen in crisis intervention. *Smith College Studies in Social Work,* 1976, *46*(2), 137–158.

McCombie, S. L., Bassuk, E., Savitz, R., and Pell, S. Development of a medical center rape crisis intervention program. *American Journal of Psychiatry,* 1976, *133*(4), 418–421.

Notman, M. T., and Nadelson, C. C, The rape victim: Psychodynamic considerations. *American Journal of Psychiatry,* 1976, *134,* 408–413.

Rabkin, J. G. The epidemiology of forcible rape. *American Journal of Orthopsychiatry,* 1979, *49*(4).

Schultz, L. G. (Ed.). *Rape victimology.* Springfield, Ill.: Charles C Thomas, 1975. Pp. 634–647.

Silverman, D. First do no more harm: Female rape victims and the male counselor. *American Journal of Orthopsychiatry,* 1777, *47*(1), 91–96.

Silverman, D. Sharing the crisis of rape: Counseling the mates and families of victims. *American Journal of Orthopsychiatry,* 1978, *48*(1), 166–173.

Sutherland, S., and Scherl, D. Patterns of response among victims of rape. *American Journal of Orthopsychiatry,* 1970, *40,* 503–511.

Fertility, Infertility, and Sexuality

Malkah T. Notman

Pregnancy and Sexuality

Pregnancy is a complex experience, with many personal, societal, and economic implications. It can be a confirmation of adulthood or a fulfillment of childhood wishes and fantasies. It can represent a mature wish for a child, an expression of creative desires, or an accidental, unanticipated, or denied result of sexual relations. Sometimes all of these elements are present to some extent. Pregnancy can also be a maturational experience and has been considered a normal "developmental crisis" (Benedek, 1959, 1970, Bibring, 1959). This chapter will consider some of the motivations, psychological concomitants, and consequences of pregnancy and the postpartum period and their effects on sexuality.

Although it is obvious that pregnancy results from sexual intercourse, many adults who know this consciously may deny to themselves the possibility that a particular sexual act may lead to a pregnancy. Residues of old and repressed childhood ideas and fantasies exist even in the minds of rational adults. Childrens' fantasies about conception and birth include oral impregnation, such as by eating or kissing or impregnation by other routes. These can remain in the minds of adults as unconscious ideas along with realistic information. These unconscious fantasies can influence a person's feelings about sexuality and pregnancy. For example, confusion of fatness with pregnancy, a common misperception of childhood, can persist into adulthood and affect a woman's eating patterns.

Motivation for Pregnancy

Motivations for becoming pregnant are complex (Benedek, 1959; Jessner et al., 1970; Deutsch, 1945). One fundamental wish is to reproduce oneself, to extend ones'

Malkah T. Notman • Department of Psychiatry, New England Medical Center, Tufts University School of Medicine, Boston, Massachusets.

existence beyond the limits of ones' own life and leave a legacy of immortality. One can thus feel one has an influence on the future. Identification with parents is important as well. To be an adult means in part to be like ones' own parent and, therefore, to have children. Although not every individual feels this way, these are important underlying themes for many.

Pregnancy confirms gender-role expectations for both women and men. For a woman, a pregnancy can represent an important component of her success as a woman. Whether or not she actually chooses to have children, it is meaningful for most women to feel they have the potential for a choice (Benedek, 1959). Many women who have made a deliberate decision not to have children nevertheless have mixed feelings when they find out that they no longer are fertile or that childbearing is no longer likely because of the direction their lives have taken. The knowledge that one can have children is part of femininity for most women (Deutsch, 1945; Stoller, 1976). For a man, an important component of masculinity is the knowledge that he can impregnate a woman. So that for both men and women, pregnancy helps establish their knowledge about their sexual maturity and functioning and thus potentially contributes to self-esteem.

Although pregnancy can represent the fulfillment of deep-seated creative wishes for both men and women, this is probably perceived more intimately by the woman, because she is carrying the baby within her. Many women also feel that having a baby finally gratifies wishes that have been postponed from childhood. As girls and boys develop, they are curious about their genitals and wonder about their normality. A boy can see his genitals; he can compare himself with others and check out his body. To some degree, he can answer his questions by simple inspection. Girls notice the differences between their genitals and those of boys. If they ask questions about these anatomical differences, why they seem to have ''less'' than boys, they may be told: ''You have internal genitals that can produce a baby.'' It may be difficult for a girl to gain much more direct information or reassurance about her internal or external genitals. They are often mislabeled, so that if she inspects herself she sees her vulva rather than the vagina or uterus which she has been told about. There is also no immediate way of checking out her inner anatomy comparable to the way a boy can (Lerner, 1976). Pregnancy can, therefore, represent affirmation that she has a normal female body with normal genitals, which is reassuring.

Wanting to be pregnant and wanting a baby are not synonymous. Even though everyone knows that a baby results from a pregnancy, some motivations that lead a woman to become pregnant or cause a man to impregnate a woman do not fully represent a conscious wish for a real child (Bibring, 1959; Deutsch, 1945). They derive from some of the other meanings of pregnancy, such as demonstrating that one can become pregnant, an act of rebellion against parents, a wish to hold on to a relationship, or sometimes a defense against moving into the next phase of life (Jessner et al., 1970; Deutsch, 1945; Bernard, 1944; Schaffer and Pine, 1975). Pregnancy may also be a response to a loss, a death, divorce, separation, or the breaking up of a relationship. The connection may be conscious, or more often, unconscious. Sometimes women become pregnant when their oldest child goes to college or when they consider going to work. Problems arise when the person or couple must then deal with the reality of a child and the changing needs and demands of this new person. Some of these problems may be particularly true for teenagers who may become pregnant because they are angry with their parents, want to be close to them, show that they are adults, or are acting out some other related feelings (Schaffer and Pine, 1975; Lidz, 1978).

Feelings about a pregnancy may be mixed. Sometimes a pregnancy is unwanted because the couple is not married, they are too young, the timing is wrong for having a child, or other reasons. Then the couple may choose to have an abortion, or they may try to adapt to the situation in spite of initial ambivalence. A more puzzling situation arises when a pregnancy appears to be wanted and planned and then engenders ambivalence or even stronger feelings of distress, which appear unexpected (Bibring, 1959; Friedman, 1978). Actually, some degree of ambivalence is usual.

Psychological Changes of Pregnancy

With pregnancy responsibilities are increased, and new tasks, roles, and conflicts are expected. For most people who want children, these are acknowledged and some accomodations are made. For some, the negative feelings are so strong that the individual may feel guilty and confused about them. It is important to recognize the ambivalence and periods of doubt, depression, anxiety, or inadequacy are really usual and occur in the course of most pregnancies. These feelings obviously influence sexual responses and may lead to hostility toward the partner or withdrawal but also to greater needs for support (Bibring, 1959; McCauley and Ehrhardt, 1980).

Women frequently experience some emotional lability and increased dependency during pregnancy. This in itself can be a source of confusion and conflict for someone used to being stable and independent, although if it is possible to acknowledge those needs, this can lead to potentially rewarding closeness (Klein et al., 1950). Sometimes it is at the time of pregnancy that a woman feels permitted to express her dependent feelings.

A pregnancy may revive a woman's feelings about her relationship with her own mother, as well as repressed dependent feelings. Caring for a baby or thinking and fantasizing about it can be a way of gratifying ones' own dependent yearnings through identifying with the baby who is helpless and needy and being cared for. Girls are socialized to expect to do this and to feel that this is an important part of their own development. Men are not usually so comfortable with their dependent feelings.

If a woman cannot tolerate her dependent feelings, she may find it difficult to ask for the support and help she needs or even to accept it without feeling "weak." Professional women, especially those who are interested in their careers, find these feelings are made more complicated by the responses of their environment, which may not encourage taking time off or paying attention to changing needs or interests. Support, affection, and flexibility in sexual relationships can be very important.

How Pregnancy Influences Sexual Behavior

For some couples, some of the most meaningful and fulfilling sex is when they are trying to conceive and create a baby (Grover, 1978, 1979). For some the procreative function of sexual intercourse relieves guilt attached to sexuality. For others, the stress of trying to conceive activates performance anxiety (Mazor, 1978). During pregnancy, intercourse can also be very enjoyable. Mutually satisfying sexual relations during most of pregnancy are potentially possible for the majority of couples. Yet, because of anxiety, misinformation, and negative attitudes, many people feel restricted during pregnancy. Research on sexual behavior during pregnancy indicates that "there is a gradual decline in sexual activity as pregnancy progresses with a marked decline during the third trimester for most women: sexual desire and behavior usually returns to prepregnancy levels about six-to-eight weeks after delivery" (McCauley and Ehrhardt, 1980). Masters and Johnson (1966) found differences between nulliparous and multiparous women. Accurate studies have yet to be done (McCauley and Ehrhardt, 1980).

One of the most prevalent negative feelings relates to the belief that sex after conception is "dirty" or "forbidden." Obviously if sex is considered to be only for procreation, then intercourse is no longer necessary after conception. Feelings of guilt may occur, reflecting concerns about sexuality that may be expressed in fear of harming the pregnancy. A common misconception is that coitus in early pregnancy may cause miscarriage or induce fetal anomalies. Some believe this is especially likely if coitus occurs at the monthly "anniversary"—the missed period. When couples feel the pressures of these anxieties during pregnancy, they often are reluctant to seek advice from physicians or nurses, fearing embarrassment or confirmation of their worst fears (Grover, 1978, 1979).

Before considering the physiological changes of pregnancy and their influence on sexuality, it is important to remember that many other complex issues affect the pregnant couple. These may directly or indirectly alter the relationship itself as well as their sexual function. Pregnancy itself also often exacerbates other problems in the life of the couple.

The earliest physical changes resulting from the pregnancy begin as soon as the first missed period. The breasts become tender and full, the abdomen may feel full, urinary frequency develops, and fatigue is common. Pelvic structures become more vascular, engorged, and sensitive. Vaginal secretions increase. The vagina becomes more moist with more mucous. Engorgement of the pelvic blood vessels takes place long before the uterus begins to enlarge. This engorgement generally increases vaginal lubrication and may make a woman more comfortable during intercourse. Some women will notice more intense arousal or more rapid arousal when they are pregnant, based on the effects of the engorgement of the pelvic vessels. The vagina may also be softer to touch and more sensitive. Later in pregnancy there are physiologic changes due to the effect of the mass of baby in the pelvis. Under certain conditions this can interfere mechanically and even cause pain.

Complications of the Pregnancy

There may be sexual problems due to some complications of pregnancy. Beyond the normal changes and their effects, pathologic problems of pregnancy obviously also influence sexual function (Grover, 1978, 1979; Mann and Armistead, 1976). When they occur, sensitive and adequate explanations and treatment are necessary if the couple is to maintain equilibrium and function.

One simple problem is implantation bleeding. This consists of a small amount of bleeding that derives from the trophoblast as it begins to obtain blood supply from the mother and occurs in 50% of pregnancies. It can be frightening and appear to be a signal of a potential miscarriage. Implantation bleeding can stir up these anxieties and certainly be inhibitory to sexual activity. This can produce considerable anxiety in the couple if no one has prepared them, and they may think they are doing some damage. The fear of hurting the pregnancy, whether it is based on the occurrence of real symptoms such as bleeding or on some misinformation, can certainly inhibit sexual response in both men and women.

Other physical problems that occur during pregnancy can cause sexual difficulties. The hormonal and secretory changes in the vagina secondary to pregnancy foster monilial and other vaginal infections, which are irritating and painful. Treatment should be direct and effective for the woman and her sexual partner. Herpes ulcers, though not confined to pregnancy, are painful when they occur and may be a contraindication to pelvic delivery if present at the time of labor.

Later in pregnancy, the growing abdomen may make intercourse awkward. Changing positions can be helpful and should be encouraged. Vulvar varicosities can be severe in late pregnancy, particularly in multigravidas and require sympathetic supportive treatment. In general, it may be advised that coitus can continue during pregnancy unless there is bleeding, pain, or ruptured membranes. Late in pregnancy, this advice may be modified, depending on the results of careful vaginal examination, and other assessments, and then advice can be given individually.

If it is necessary during the pregnancy to avoid vaginal penetration, the couple can be encouraged to satisfy each other by sexual stimulation if it is acceptable to them. These methods may run counter to religious beliefs or personal preferences, and sensitivity to these issues is necessary when counseling.

Some sexual problems relate to psychic as well as somatic aspects of pregnancy. The bodily changes have various psychological effects on both the woman and the man. Some women feel embarrassed at the visible evidence of their sexuality; this effects not only their sexual relationships but all their other relationships as well. Even though it is certainly socially acceptable to be having sex when one is married and, therefore, to be pregnant, the pregnancy still constitutes a public announcement about what one has been doing. Sexual taboos and inhibitions leave many women embarrassed to some degree to be demonstrating their sexuality. The enlargement of the abdomen and breasts are experienced by some men and women as positive, and attractive, but they can be seen by others as gross and distorting. Sometimes these views represent associations with unresolved experiences. An example of this kind of situation follows.

> Mary M had a boyfriend who insisted she stay extremely thin. Although she was slim by any standards, he became upset with her any time that she appeared to eat more and was very conscious of her eating behavior. He had been very unhappy when his younger brother was born and recalled his mother's pregnancy as her becoming fat. Subsequently he linked any wom-

an's fatness with the idea of pregnancy. This was especially true for a woman with whom he was sexually intimate. Without being conscious of it, he then set limits on any possibility of her getting fat. Consciously he knew that getting fat did not mean pregnancy, but the unconscious connection and the accompanying sense of distortion and ugliness that was associated with fatness was strong.

Some of the physiological changes later in pregnancy have important sexual consequences. The uterus becomes progressively more irritable as the pregnancy proceeds. The uterus is a contractile organ, and early in pregnancy the fetus is preserved from being expelled from the uterus by the suppression of uterine contractions. Later on in pregnancy, as the uterus is stretched, these begin to return, mildly at first, but in the last trimester of pregnancy Braxton–Hicks contractions become more prominent. They are harmless and are thought probably to be helpful in the normal course of pregnancy by contributing to cervical dilatation at term (Grover, 1978, 1979). However, a pregnant woman in the last trimester, or perhaps even earlier, may notice a series of three or four strong uterine contractions, sometimes occurring during sexual arousal or more often occurring after orgasm or initiated by the orgasm. This can produce considerable anxiety in the couple if no one informed them, and they may think they are going to precipitate labor.

Spontaneous miscarriage may occur in at least 10% of diagnosed pregnancies, usually before the 12th week of gestation, and is unrelated to any kind of trauma. The most frequent cause of pregnancy failure is thought to be the death of the embryo at an early stage of development, several weeks before the actual miscarriage. Other causes implicated are physical conditions, such as an incompetent cervix, which is thought to account for about 13% of abortions, and psychological factors (Babikian, 1976). The psychological consequences of miscarriage have often not been sufficiently attended to. The sense of loss and depression can be quite severe, greater than associated with an induced abortion. Women experience feelings of helplessness and grief with attendant mourning. Family or physicians who remind a woman who is saddened by a lost pregnancy that she can have another and replace it are overlooking the woman's immediate needs for an acknowledgment that something important has occurred to her, which cannot be dismissed by the thought of replacement.

Ectopic pregnancy occurs in about 1 pregnancy in every 200. It is often associated with pelvic pain and abnormal vaginal bleeding. Intercourse becomes quite painful, and medical treatment is necessary early in these potentially disastrous pregnancies. An ectopic pregnancy can result in an acute surgical emergency, with loss of the fallopian tube if the pregnancy is tubal. The psychological consequences combine those of miscarriage and those of coping with an acute illness (Grover, 1979, 1979).

As the pregnancy nears term, women report many increased anxieties and fears. They may be concerned about the realities of becoming a mother and the consequent changes in their lives or with the process of labor and potential problems with delivery. These can be related to changes in one's body and self-image, leading a woman to feel uncertain about herself and her competency. Fears of loss of control and one's adequacy during labor can emerge. Many women are worried about possible damage to themselves or the baby. These worries can add to the physical stresses of the end of the pregnancy and affect sexual interest or comfort.

Delivery

There have been many recent developments encouraging informed participation . by both parents, preparation, early contact with the baby, and early nursing. Information about the importance of early infant care and maternal–infant contact in the development of bonding is sometimes applied in the newer rooming-in programs. In many such programs, maternal medication is kept to a minimum, fostering alertness of the infant and encouraging early mother–child interaction (Seiden, 1978; Bradley, 1965; Mead and Newton, 1967; Wolff and Langley, 1968).

Pain in childbirth is affected by preparation and understanding of the process involved, the personality and maturity of the mother, and also by the entire context of the experience, including the real variations in the obstetrical situation and the difficulty of delivery. Pain from most stimuli is experienced quite variably and delivery is no exception. In addition, the woman's feelings about her pregnancy and approaching motherhood are important.

A sense of mastery about the experience of childbirth can make the pain seem something to be managed and overcome, such as an athlete's feelings of accomplishing a strenuous task successfully, rather than being associated with humiliating dependency that begs to be relieved, which has been the prevailing attitude (Seiden, 1978).

Bradley (1965) has observed that women may be made more vulnerable to obstetric pain because of the way they are socialized. A woman's critical views about her body and its functions may discourage her from being sufficiently insistent on their own comfort or make her feel ashamed of bodily exposure or function.

Since the discomfort of labor is potentially intensified by stress and fear, it may be relieved to some extent by measures aimed at removing these (Nadelson, 1973). Childbirth preparation has occupied much attention in recent decades. The experience of pain appears to be diminished by familiarizing the pregnant woman with the process of childbearing and delivery and encouraging self-confidence and active mastery.

The major approaches to "prepared" or "natural" childbirth do reduce the need for analgesic medication during normal births, and studies indicate that the preparation itself, and not merely the selection of women or their general education about birth, is an important factor (Bradley, 1965; Dick-Reid, 1944/1972; Enkin et al., 1972; Doering and Entwisle, 1975). These approaches may be especially important for those women who are higher risk by virtue of age, illness, or ambivalence about pregnancy or womanhood.

Involvement of the Father

The involvement of the father in the whole process of labor, delivery, and infant care has been an important trend in the last decade (Jessner et al., 1970; Bradley, 1965). Some obstetricians support this more actively than others. Some women and their doctors feel strongly that fathers can and should be involved throughout the pregnancy, in the preparation for childbirth, and in the labor and delivery process and available to share and witness the birth. They feel that this sets a more comfortable ground for the father's participation in the later care of the baby. Others are uncomfortable with what seems like an intrusion into the "medical" situation. Although there may be problems, such as competition with the mother in the care of the baby, on the whole, for many fathers it is a very important beginning to the relationship with their children (Seiden, 1978).

The postpartum period is a time of many changes, especially for parents with their first child. Both physical and psychological conditions affect sexual relationships.

There are physical sequelae to having a first child that can affect sexuality although in a normal first pelvic delivery with no complications, the vagina will virtually return to normal. The stretching due to delivery is visible on examinations but does not generally affect sexual functioning. Control of the pelvic muscles, which provide an important aspect of sexual response, is maintained. All the other genital structures are the same and do not usually provide any problems.

Some postpartum effects are not directly the result of physical changes but are indirectly related to these. Fatigue is an important factor. Most new mothers experience fatigue. To some extent this is related to the endocrine changes but is also due to the changes in life patterns and new demands. Fatigue that results from getting up at night and from absorption with the baby does affect libido for many people.

Sometimes the mother's preoccupation with the baby excludes the father and can foster a competition between the baby and the father for the mother's attention. The mother needs to arrive at a balance between her own sexual feelings and many other priorities, including the new role and responsibilities of taking care of an infant. This balance assumes a different form for each woman. Some degree of ambivalence and possibly depressive feelings is normal at this time; this is not necessarily the same as a clinical depression, but some sense of letdown usually occurs. The reorganization of feelings can be very gratifying but also very anxiety-provoking (Jessner et al., 1970). This certainly affects sexual interest and sexual response. Many women also need reassurance at this time that their bodies have not deteriorated and that they are still sexual and desirable.

This postpartum sense of depletion is often not sufficiently emphasized. A range of responses is also the rule, one can be positive but also experience annoyance, irritability, and lack of interest. Women experiencing these feelings may wonder about themselves and are relieved to learn that this is a normal response.

During the pregnancy and the postpartum period, some women have the feeling that there are sexual components to delivery or in taking care of the baby. A woman who is nursing a baby may describe erotic (Grover, 1978, 1979) feelings she has at that time, which she may find disturbing. These are fairly common since genital sexuality and labor are very closely physically related and the same anatomical organs are involved.

A question often asked is how soon after delivery one can resume sexual intercourse. Restrictions in the past have been far too strict. Current practice is to tell patients that it is permissible as soon as they are comfortable. Usually this period is about 3 weeks after the baby is born, sometimes somewhat longer after a first baby and shorter after a second or later baby. If things are going well and the bleeding has stopped, it is generally not possible to create a uterine infection by having intercourse at that time. If there has been an uncomplicated episiotomy, it has usually healed within 2 weeks and is no longer painful (Friedman, 1978; Grover, 1978, 1979).

One problem that is important to explain to patients, particularly those who are nursing, is that there may be a postpartum period of atrophy of the vagina and vaginal structures because of the suppression of ovarian activity by lactation. Because of this suppression of ovarian hormones, women who are nursing may not have periods for some time. There is an estrogen deficiency similar to that in a postmenopausal woman (Grover, 1978, 1979).

The usual nonpregnant cyclic pattern of hormonal interactions involves the hypothalamus, the pituitary, and the ovary. Pituitary hormones under the influence of the hypothalamus stimulate the development of the ovarian follicle (by follicle-stimulating hormone) and ovulation. The ovarian follicle in turn produces estrogen. High estrogen levels at midcycle result in a surge of luteinizing hormone from the pituitary that causes ovulation to occur from the mature follicle. Further development of remaining cells from the follicle form the corpus luteum and produce progesterone. Both inhibit the hypothalamus and in turn the pituitary hormones. If fertilization and implantation do not occur, progesterone and estrogen levels drop, causing the corpus luteum to deteriorate and menstruation begins. The low levels of estrogen allow the hypothalamic pituitary activity to increase again, and the cycle resumes. If pregnancy occurs, the continuing high level of estrogen and progesterone inhibit pituitary activity until the hormonal drop postpartum (McCauley and Ehrhardt, 1980).

In menopause, ovarian function declines and the resulting diminished estrogen levels affect skin and vaginal mucosa, leading to dryness and sometimes dyspareunia. In lactation, suppression of cyclic hormonal activity in ovulation also usually occurs. If this is sustained, similar mucosal changes may occur temporarily. Intercourse in those circumstances may be painful and sensitive. This can be treated by lubricants.

Responses on returning to having intercourse can be intense. The fulfillment of resuming a sexual relationship after a period of deprivation is important. The couple must also consider birth control again; they must adapt to the changes in their relationship and integrate altered body image and self-concept after having produced a child. Researchers agree that women who valued sexual activity before pregnancy usually return more rapidly to prepregnancy levels of activity after childbirth than those who had less positive attitudes about sex before pregnancy (McCauley and Ehrhardt, 1980).

Work and Depressive Reactions

In the current societal context where women are working and returning to work early after childbearing, the effect of leaving work to have a baby and the relationship of this change in life pattern to postpartum reactions must be considered, as well as the "appropriate" time to return, the meaning to the individual, and availability of care. For many people, work is drudgery, and some period of relief and special care and attention is welcome. For others, after a period of recovery and establishment of a relationship with the baby and regularity in the baby's pattern, return to work is important.

Sometimes postpartum depression is the result of the isolation of being alone with an young infant, especially a demanding one, without other adults and without the support and stimulation of work.

Most women who have been working at jobs they like or in professional settings have felt active and competent. The process of pregnancy and the delivery can evoke some feelings of helplessness by virtue of being a patient or not being in control. The stresses of this period can be expressed by specific demands on the husband or others, which strain the relationship, and can also be expressed sexually. This period can be very trying, not only because of the physical aspects of the childbearing but because of the feelings of uncertainty about one's feelings and unfamiliar dependency.

Psychological Postpartum Reactions

There is considerable controversy about the nature and causes of postpartum reactions (Notman and Nadelson, 1980). Unsettled questions include whether the relatively severe postpartum depression is a specific syndrome, a reaction to the psychological and physical changes of childbirth, or a disturbance that happens to occur at that particular time. The incidence of severe emotional illnesses following childbirth is approximately 1 or 2 per 1000 births (Norman, 1967). Less severe postpartum emotional disorders, referred to a *transient mild depression* or *postpartum blues,* are said to occur in over 50% of parturient women (Pitt, 1973).

Most often these disorders develop in the period beginning with the childbirth and ending with the involution of the uterus. Some investigators include disturbances associated with the stresses of early infant care. Confusion of definition abounds so that one is often unclear about the terms used and conditions discussed.

Although pregnancy and childbirth are undoubtedly associated with major endocrinological changes, there is relatively little clear evidence to explain why some women develop these syndromes and others do not. Specific vulnerability and factors responsible have not been clearly delineated nor is the endocrine relationship conclusive (Pitt, 1973).

Postpartum Neurotic Reactions

The most common neurotic symptomatology reported in the postpartum period are obsessive–compulsive reactions. These often take the form of rumination about the safety of the baby or an intense preoccupation with the details of his or her care. These concerns may evolve into a schizophrenic or depressive psychosis. Neurotic depressive reactions occur in approximately 10% of women. They generally last weeks or months and must be distinguished from the more common and benign postpartum blues often known as the *3-day blues*.

The prognosis of this heterogeneous group of disorders depends upon the clinical picture, the amount of time that has elapsed postpartum before the episode develops, and the previous history of mental illness. Generally women who develop postpartum illnesses shortly after childbirth have a poorer prognosis than those who develop symptoms later in the postpartum period. Women with a history of treatment for psychiatric illness prior to their pregnancies also have a poorer prognosis (Wilson et al., 1972). Women who have had a postpartum reaction are at risk for reactions following future pregnancies. It is estimated that approximately one out of four women with a history of postpartum psychosis will develop a similar disorder after subsequent pregnancies.

The early immediate depression is probably in part an endocrinological response and partially related to the emotional anticlimax of having delivered the baby and the "loss" of the baby which has been inside in an intimate way. This early depression can be helped by educating the couple about the likelihood of its occurrence. Expectation of an initial letdown and of emotional volatility permits the couple to adapt to it more effectively (Klein et al., 1950).

Contraception and Sexuality

This section will focus on the general description of the major contraceptive methods and their relation to sexuality. A detailed discussion of the various forms of contraceptives from a gynecological point of view can be found elsewhere.

It is important to be aware of the range of available contraceptive methods and to consider their advantages, disadvantages, and risks for a given individual or couple as well as the effectiveness of the method itself and its side effects. Tailoring contraceptive methods to the means and attitudes of the people involved is important. Emotional as well as physiological and other realistic reasons for using or not using any particular method are important. The method with which one is satisfied is the method that will be used best and, therefore, potentially most effective. Error and inconsistency of use are far more commonly the cause of contraceptive failure than those due to the method itself (Sandberg, 1976).

It is also important to consider the significance of fertility for a given individual or couple. Controlling fertility is not always unambivalently desired, even when realistic reasons abound against the appropriateness of becoming pregnant (Lidz, 1978). For some people, preventing pregnancy undermines their sense of masculinity or femininity, and they may feel less sexual desire when pregnancy is not a possibility. If resistance is based on cultural values or unconscious determinants, it is difficult to reach it with simple information about contraceptive techniques. It is, therefore, important to understand the individual's values and context before counseling and information can be effective.

In considering the emotional aspects of each method, one important issue concerns the determination of which partner has the initiative and control. For many women, having control and, therefore, choosing a contraceptive that a woman uses, such as the diaphragm or the pill, is a very positive experience. For others, it produces anger that it is they who have to take the risks and the responsibility. Both feelings can be present in the same person at the same time or at different times, so that it is possible to feel positive knowing that there is some way of effectively asserting control and at the same time feel some resentment at being the person who has to accept this responsibility.

Risks, benefits and side effects are important to present accurately, yet without an alarmist approach. The manner of presenting these is important. One can be frightening by compulsively mentioning all the possible side effects and warnings, or one can present this information in a way that emphasizes its importance and informs the patient's choice. Assessing the individual gives some clues. For example, people who are disorganized are very unlikely to be effective users of methods that require daily or regular attention. As with a couple, effectiveness for an individual must be thought of not only in relation to the method but the appropriateness of "fit" of the contraceptive and the individual (Sandberg, 1976; Grover, 1978, 1979). The most effective contraceptive, for example, the pill, is not effective if the woman cannot remember if she has or has not taken it. Someone who is paranoid, somewhat suspicious, or concerned about what she eats is likely to become concerned about taking the pill and may attribute any symptoms to it—even those that are not considered usual side effects. Emotional symptoms or those related to a concomitant illness can be attributed to the contraceptive and its use discontinued, often without substituting any other method.

Fear of side effects can interfere with contraceptive use. Good communication is extremely important in ensuring effective contraception.

The effect of the contraceptive method on coitus is important. Whether the method is constant or coitally dependent is one important area of choice. This will also vary with the particular sexual practices. "Messiness," excessive lubrication of foams and creams, and unpleasant taste, if oral sex is practiced, have been deterrants to diaphragm use as well. Pain with intrauterine devices (IUDs), and loss of full sensation with condoms have also created problems.

In evaluating risks and side effects, one must consider what are the alternatives. Contraceptive risks are sometimes compared with each other, yet another contraceptive may not be available or acceptable (Jaffe, 1977), and risks of mortality from any method of fertility control, except for older women who smoke and use contraceptive pills, are less than the risk of mortality in childbirth (Rosenfield, 1978).

Methods Which Are Not Related to Coitus

Contraceptive Pills

The contraceptive pills are the most reliable methods of preventing conception when used correctly (Jaffe, 1977). The development of the pill and the IUD created a major change in contraceptive use in the United States. Previously the diaphragm had been in use more by middle and upper-class individuals (Jaffe, 1977). The pill also interferes least with sexual intercourse and has met the needs of millions of sexually active women.

There has been considerable publicity and concern about its safety. The risks of long-term use are still in the process of evaluation. The paucity of research in this area has also been a matter of concern (Jaffe, 1977).

The side effects attributed to the pill have been numerous. Currently the potentially serious ones are thromboembolism, neuroocular disturbances, and protracted anovulation (Sandberg, 1976). Less serious ones are nausea, symptoms mimicking pregnancy, and breakthrough bleeding.

There has been ongoing controversy about the side effects of oral contraceptives.

Research findings have been inconclusive and are sometimes difficult to interpret (Warnes and Fitzpatrick, 1979). Diminished sexual interest and depression have been among the emotional side effects attributed to contraceptive pill use. Fleming and Seager (1978) surveyed these studies and also conducted a study of one population taking the pills and compared this group with a group of women who had previously used the pill and a group that had never taken the pill. They found that users did not have a higher incidence of depression than matched controls, although depression was correlated with age, personality, occupation, and several indices of "neuroticism."

The effect of oral contraceptives on sexual activity itself has also been a matter of concern. Currently the relationship of sexual activity to endocrine-related aspects of the menstrual cycle is inconclusive (McCauley and Ehrhardt, 1980; Adams et al., 1978), however, much of the data are obtained on questionnaires and retrospective. For example, Adams et al. (1978) found that in their study married women who used other contraceptives did show a significant increase in the sexual behavior that they initiated at ovulation, whereas women using oral contraception showed no increase. However, these behaviors are hard to measure and generalize, and these authors also hold that the majority of women do not lose sexual desire after adopting the use of oral contraceptives.

Some women are reluctant to use a noncoital-dependent substance, particularly the pill, which must be taken daily, if they are having intercourse sporadically. They also may forget, rendering the pill ineffective.

Immediate common side effects are likely to be worse the first few months of use, and a patient who persists may be able to overcome them. Recent research identified high-risk groups who should not use oral contraceptives; the clearest group are women over 35 who smoke, who are at risk for emboli. It is also not recommended for use in the presence of a variety of circulatory problems and occular abnormalities (Sandberg, 1976).

Sorting out the contribution of hormonal effects, the psychological consequence of changes in menses, the effects of changes in contraceptive safety, the effects of being regulated by a "foreign" substance that is ingested daily, and the effects on sexual behavior have not been easy. For adolescents, social, psychological, and family factors are as important as information (Morgenthau, 1977) in determining whether contraception will be used or not, as are peer pressure and other motivations for pregnancy. Effective methods of teaching contraceptive responsibility and planning have not been developed for the teenage population.

The IUD

When a device is place inside the uterus, it prevents pregnancy for reasons that are not completely understood. It may be due to mechanical prevention of implantation, and there is some evidence to support the idea that the device elicits a response in the uterine cavity that affects the sperm as they move up to the uterine cavity; possibly it is a combination of effects. Some devices have a third component that is biologically active material.

The IUD is somewhat less effective than the pill. Although different devices have different failure rates, IUDs have been concluded to have a standardized 12-month failure rate two times greater than that of the pill (Jaffe, 1977).

There are also physical problems. There is the possibility of discomfort, heavier menstrual flow, an increased risk of endometritis, and, rarely, uterine perforation. IUDs can also cause pain, discharge, and odors, all leading to sexual dissatisfaction (Grover, 1978, 1979).

One major advantage of the IUD is that once it is correctly inserted it may remain in place indefinitely, if untoward side effects do not occur. It requires no further attention and remains effective. For some people, IUDs are very satisfactory and do not produce side effects nor interfere with their sexual relationships.

Methods Used in Relation to Coitus

The Diaphragm

The diaphragm combined with contraceptive cream or jelly has regained popularity because of its relative effectiveness and safety. However, to use it one must be able to plan and have it available. This may make for major inconvenience and constitutes a significant impediment to effective use.

One problem with its use that sometimes becomes manifest is the taboo against masturbating or touching one's genitals. This makes inserting the diaphragm an uncomfortable experience. For a woman who has difficulty looking at her genitals, touching, or exploring, it is difficult to use a diaphragm effectively. There may be considerable inconsistency in this. A woman may talk freely about sex with apparent openness, but when it is a matter of her own behavior, early taboos about sex or touching can emerge as real blocks. Some women have considerable difficulty understanding their own genital anatomy, also complicated by childhood prohibitions and by the less visible and more internal female genitals. This further interferes with checking the diaphragm and assuring its proper placement fit.

Rhythm

Rhythm is widely practiced although not very reliable. It requires periodic abstinence and some knowledge of the fertile time of the cycle. The menstrual period calculations are not sufficiently accurate indications of when ovulation occurs. A period can occur several days early or several days late, and sperm can survive for a long enough period of time so that fertility is possible even though abstinence is practiced longer than the recommended time. However, it provides an important method where religious barriers to other approaches exist.

Withdrawal

Withdrawal is also common. Its effectiveness is limited because of the problems of control and the occasional presence of sperm before ejaculation.

The Condom

The condom, although not as effective as the pill and the diaphragm, is accessible without a great deal of difficulty and without having to go to a physician or birth control counselor. This makes it particularly available for teenagers. It is, therefore, the most widely used of any kind of effective method of contraception. It also gives the male the choice, which for some couples is important. Another contribution it offers is some protection from venereal disease.

A further area that is of recent interest, although still in the experimental stage, is the possible development of reversible, effective, and safe contraceptives for men. Although in well-established couples there is evidence that men participate strongly in fertility decisions (Lidz, 1978), it is difficult for teenagers or those first exploring relationships to take responsibility for contraception equal in effectiveness to those available to women. However, many men do express a wish to participate more in the process.

Abortion and Sexuality

There have been enormous changes in this country in the past decade in the process of obtaining an abortion and the experience of having one, since the Supreme Court decision in 1973 that struck down constraining laws interfering with the right of a woman to decide about an abortion in the first trimester of pregnancy (Roe, 1973). Prior to this, an abortion could be obtained in a number of states only to save the woman's life or possibly health or if the pregnancy followed incest or rape. In some regions and facilities, this ruling was interpreted more strictly than in others, and, thus, it was very difficult for some women to obtain a legal or safe abortion. Psychiatric indications, such as the stress a pregnancy would produce and the possibility of depression and suicide, were used to justify an abortion. Many illegal abortions were done under variable medical conditions, sometimes resulting in infections, bleeding, and even death. For obvious reasons, the extent to which illegal abortions were done prior to the Supreme Court decision was not known accurately. Current estimates are that more than a million abortions are done in the United States or that one out of four pregnancies is terminated by an abortion.

In the years since abortion became legal and the incidence of abortion increased, research data and clinical experience have demonstrated that many previously held ideas about the effects of abortions are not true but are beliefs and stereotypes that reflect other concerns, such as opposition to abortion on religious or other grounds.

Abortions are obtained by women of all ages, religions, classes, and beliefs. In spite of conservatism and opposition from some sources, opinion surveys repeatedly have indicated that the population is generally in favor of women having the option to choose to have an abortion. Since this is an issue about which there is a great emotion, many of the past studies were performed to demonstrate a preconceived point of view (Payne et al., 1976; Peck and Marcus, 1966). Many also were not methodologically sound, containing errors in sampling and poor design. More recent research has indicated some relatively consistent findings about abortions.

Medical Reactions to Abortions

The incidence of serious medical complications from abortions varies considerably depending on the skills of the person performing the procedure, the adequacy of the setting, and the stage of pregnancy. The fewest complications occur early in pregnancy, when it can be terminated by dilation and curettage or dilatation and suction. Late abortion, performed in the second trimester, is usually done by means of an intrauterine injection of an abortifacient agent, such as hypertonic saline or prostaglandins. Delaying the procedure increases the risk of complications. On rare occasions, a hysterotomy (an opening of the uterus) is required but increases complication rates further. The incidence of serious complications ranges from 1 to 20% with fewest in early pregnancy. Midtrimester abortion increases the complication rate threefold, and hysterotomy increases it an additional threefold (Friedman, 1978). The prostaglandins have reduced the risks associated with saline injections, primarily serious blood-clotting defects. Infection and hemorrhage must still be considered, although these are much reduced by proper medical care. Presently, under optimal conditions the overall morbidity and mortality from abortions is lower than the risk of death from oral contraceptives for certain high-risk women, such as women over 35 who smoke (Beral and Kay, 1977; Vessey et al., 1977). When considering any intervention, it is necessary to examine the alternatives and their relative risks and availability.

The Emotional Effects of Abortions

In the past, it was generally held that an abortion was a serious and psychologically damaging procedure with almost inevitable severe depression and other psychological symptoms. Depression was thought to recur at menopause for women who had abortions. High incidence of guilt, shame, and regret were also described. From current research, it is clear that severe or clinical depression is not an inevitable outcome of abortion, nor does depression occur or recur at the time of menopause in women who had abortions (Payne et al., 1976; Notman and Nadelson, 1980). In evaluating results from earlier research, the reaction to doing something that was socially stigmatized or performed in secret was not sufficiently separated from a woman's reaction to the procedure itself or in a context in which it is considered an acceptable or even preferred choice.

It would be equally erroneous to assume that there are no effects of an abortion. An unwanted pregnancy and a subsequent abortion are real experiences with inevitable psychological impact. As one might expect with any important experience, reactions will vary and depend on the individual and her situation (Payne et al., 1976; Belsey et al., 1977; Freeman, 1977; Mester, 1978). Women with a history of psychiatric problems are more vulnerable to postabortion depression or other psychological sequelae (Payne et al., 1976). Women with religious or other beliefs strongly in opposition to abortion are more likely to feel it is wrong and to suffer guilt even though they may decide to proceed with the abortion. A woman in such a position may feel that it is nevertheless the most responsible solution, both considering her own needs and also in relation the potential future of a child born in such circumstances (Gilligan, 1977). Sometimes the motivation for abortion is primarily from the father of the baby, even if the couple is married, since he may feel unable to provide for or cope with a child or an additional child.

A small number of abortions are performed for medical reasons, possibly 1% currently. Advances in medical technology have made it possible to manage a pregnancy coexisting with many potentially serious medical conditions, such as diabetes and heart and renal disease, which used to preclude pregnancy. Women who have abortions because of medical indications tend to have more depressions. Women who become pregnant in the face of serious illness do want to have a child, and although they understand the reasons for the abortion, they still feel conscious regret and considerable loss (Payne et al., 1976).

Insufficient attention has been paid to the psychological effects of having a spontaneous abortion, i.e., miscarriage. In this situation as well as in the case of a woman with medical illness, the pregnancy is usually desired but is aborted, usually because of some defect. It is common to see a fairly severe, if relatively short-lived, depression. The woman's self-esteem is damaged, and her sense of loss may be acute and is often met by a lack of understanding by people around her including her physician, who minimize the loss and tend to immediately raise the possibility of a future possible pregnancy as a replacement.

Irrational responses to an abortion do occur and can create problems. The guilt that many women do feel can be translated into an expectation of some punishment, such as the expectation that they will become sterile. This may be a conscious concern or misinformation about consequences of abortion; sometimes it is much less conscious, and the idea surfaces later when the woman raises this question with her physician. The sense of shame, wrongdoing, or guilt can also cause a woman to project, that is, to perceive criticism from others when it is not present, and sensitively interpret comments about herself as if they were judgmental. At the same time, support that is offered is readily responded to.

The personnel who work in an abortion clinic and those physicians who perform abortions often have difficulty particularly over time, because they are confronted with the actual fetus (Marder, 1970). Some of these personnel have a tendency to be critical of the patient, especially if a woman has had several abortions and seems to be casual about her sexuality and her contraceptive practice. Usually the nurse bears the major portion of the care of the patient even though the physician performs the procedures, and she sometimes find that a prolonged exposure stirs up feelings in herself that are difficult to handle (Adler, 1980). There have been studies that indicate that the negative attitudes on the part of hospital personnel, as well as inadequate counseling of the patient, contribute directly to the incidence of postabortion guilt, remorse, and depression in the patient (Marder, 1970; Adler, 1980).

Such charged situations as abortion or sterilization can create a conflict in the physician between his or her own values and what is considered to be the best care for the patient (Adler, 1980). Sometimes the physician feels that he or she knows better than the patient what would be right or what is appropriate and feels it is his or her prerogative to "let" or not "let" the patient do something that the patient may request. This is a very sensitive issue, which must be thought about carefully and a balance found between the kind of advice that helps the patient assess future possibilities and thus choose among alternatives and the kind of advising that really constitutes telling the patient what to do from one's own viewpoint. Some decisions that seem to be medical ones are actually value responses. For instance, an attitude that was common in the past was for the physician to agree to do an abortion but to suggest that the patient be sterilized at the same time, which often represented a punitive response.

Effects on Sexuality

One important effect of a woman's first pregnancy, even if it is expected and wanted, is to confirm for both her and her partner that pregnancy is possible, and they are fertile. There are indications that postabortion contraceptive use increases for some people (Tietze, 1975; Margolis et al., 1974). However, after becoming pregnant and having an abortion, a woman may be afraid of getting pregnant again, even when using contraceptives, and this can obviously interfere with sexual relationships. Probably the most significant disturbances in sexual function postabortion arise because of problems in the relationship and the feelings toward the partner that may be related to the pregnancy and abortion or may surface under the stress of coping with the crisis.

The pregnancy may also evoke feelings that were not previously present or recognized. Many women report feeling angry and let down by the way in which the man responds, particularly if they are left alone to handle the abortion, or feeling deserted. Others describe feeling supported and gratified by the sharing of the experience. The relationship with the man does not inevitably fall apart, as used to be thought. When it is disrupted, it is usually because of the issues that are precipitated by the pregnancy and abortion and not because of the abortion itself. If the woman remains angry or disappointed with the man who impregnated her, she is likely to express this in some sexual dysfunction or withdrawal as well.

Infertility and Sexuality

Infertility is usually defined as a failure to achieve a successful pregnancy following a year of regular sexual activity without contraception (Mazor, 1978). Primary infertility refers to a condition where a pregnancy has never occurred. Secondary infertility refers to those situations where there are one or more living children. Sterility is defined as absolute infertility, for instance, after a hysterectomy, a vasectomy, or other condition that makes it impossible for the male to produce sperm. About one in ten couples who want to conceive find that they have difficulty (Behrman and Kistner, 1975). Infertility may possibly be increasing. The postponement of marriage and childbearing, the possibly greater prevalence of certain illnesses and contaminants, the side effects of contraceptive methods, and increasing numbers of pelvic infections have all been implicated (Mazor, 1978; Menning, 1977). In an infertility problem the difficulties may reside in either partner or both. About 50% of the problems are related to some difficulties with the male and 50% involve the female. Some estimates attribute about 50% of the problems to the female partner, 30% to the male, and the remaining 20% as a combined problem in which each partner is relatively infertile. In approximately 70% of couples who have had a thorough physical investigation, some organic problem can be found (Grover, 1979).

Fertility is a relative process; two individuals with low fertility might not achieve a pregnancy, whereas with high fertility they would. In males, the major causes of infertility are related to trauma and infection (Grover, 1979). Problems may arise from the production of inadequate sperm in either number or motility, in transport of sperm through the reproductive organs, or in the deposition of sperm in the vagina. Since the genitals are external, the urethra is also largely external, and since males have tended to be physically active, they are exposed to many traumas with consequent damage to reproductive organs. Venereal diseases can also cause problems. The most common infection problem causing sterility is gonorrhea. Problems in sperm production can also result from childhood mumps, which can produce permanent damage to the testes.

Some structural problems in males are causes of infertility. An example of these is a varicocele, in which there are varicose veins in the testes accumulating blood, and this alters sperm formation. Removing or ligating the varicocele can result in a return of sperm function. Some congenital endocrine abnormalities, such as Klinefelter's syndrome, result in male sterility.

Sterility may be produced by certain drugs or chemicals, exposure to radiation, and other illnesses. Autoimmune responses have also been implicated, in which a man produces antibodies to his own sperm (Mazor, 1978).

Problems in the female can be grouped roughly into mechanical barriers to fertilization (Behrman and Kistner, 1975), endocrine disorders (Menning, 1977), and structural disorders of the reproductive tract (Mazor, 1978; Grover, 1979). Mechanical problems, which present a barrier to the sperm reaching the ovum, include nonpatent fallopian tubes due to either infection and scarring, such as from pelvic inflammatory disease, postsurgical infections, or adhesions. Endometriosis is a condition in which endometrial tissue grows in areas other than the uterus, such as in the tubes, the ovaries, or around the uterine ligaments, and this tissue bleeds at each menstruation and causes scarring and adhesions.

Anovulation for any reason can obviously be a cause of sterility. There are a number of endocrine conditions that cause irregular or diminished ovulation. Research is currently underway about the implications for fertility of the endocrine changes caused by anorexia or vigorous sustained physical exercise, which results in interruption or delay in normal menstrual functioning. Other endocrine disturbances can also interfere with ovulation or other phases of the process.

Structural problems are fibroids and some cervical problems.

Some couples have intercourse in a way that minimizes the likelihood of pregnancy or makes it impossible. Sometimes couples are not able to have intercourse at all. For some, the particular position may not be optimal, or they may have some misconceptions about what sexual intercourse consists of, with failure of penetration and ejaculation of sperm into the vagina.

Infertility Examination

In an infertility workup, it is important to include both partners and explore any potential problems in each. The initial investigation must include a thorough medical, social, and sexual history, a physical examination, and appropriate laboratory and radiological tests. Examining the cervix after intercourse to see whether sperm are present is an important component of the workup. For the man, a semen analysis permits visualization of the sperm, their motility, and an assessment of their normality and quantity. To assess the woman's ovulation, a couple is often advised that the woman keep a temperature chart. The basal temperature measured before she gets out of bed in the morning is charted. If she is ovulating normally, a lower basal temperature will occur in the preovulatory phase of the cycle. After ovulation the temperature rises half a degree, and this high level is maintained until just before the next menstrual period begins. If the woman does not ovulate, the chart may show a variable pattern. If she is pregnant, the high temperature is sustained beyond the time of the next cycle.

Psychological Effects

The awareness of infertility constitutes an important life crisis for the couple (Mazor, 1978). Although some couples are not interested in having children, involuntary infertility is generally stressful. Coming in for an infertility workup may be very stressful, since it challenges the normality of the genital functioning of each individual and thus questions masculinity and femininity. Particular parts of the workup, such as masturbating to produce sperm for the semen analysis, may be particularly distressing because of conflicts about masturbation. The temperature charting is not in itself difficult, but maintaining sexual interest in such a way as to have intercourse during fertile periods may be difficult. It is not easy to "perform" on command, and some couples describe impotence related to this performance anxiety. This can create mutual blame and tension.

Involuntary infertility profoundly affects the relationship of the couple, including their sexual relationship. It can be a devastating experience. The tension that is produced by month after month of inability to conceive is an enormous strain. Latent feeling about each person's adequacy are awakened. Feelings of helplessness are experienced by most couples. Sometimes a couple who has used contraception for many years decides that they want to have a baby, discontinues contraceptives, and then are surprised and shocked that a pregnancy does not result right away. The tendency to cast blame is considerable, and each person blames the other, feeling that he or she is not the cause of the problem but it is really the other one. Sometimes another pattern develops, and a person inappropriately assumes blame and feels that he or she is the total cause of the problem. It is not uncommon during this period for impotence to develop or unresponsiveness in the woman. For a couple who has postponed childbearing, each month takes on a particularly acute meaning, and the question as to whether they will be able to have children at all becomes more pressing.

Sometimes patients have magical expectations of their physicians and believe that when they come for an examination the problem will be immediately resolved. The physician is perceived as a magician who then becomes the target of anger if the magic doesn't work. The entire situation reactivates old conflicts in each individual, which play an important role in how the problem is handled and resolved. Many couples become intensely involved in the anticipation of the next cycle. If the woman menstruates or perceives a period approaching, she becomes depressed. Sometimes the inability to produce a baby makes a couple, particularly the woman, feel that she is unable to produce anything that is worthwhile, and the depression spreads to all other life activities. Other patients may be able to compensate by becoming invested in other aspects of their lives and activities.

The couple who does not succeed in conceiving has several choices (Mazor, 1978). Adoption is still possible but increasingly difficult. If the problem is the man's, the woman may be able to become pregnant with sperm from a donor. There are infertility programs with access to carefully screened donors. Sometimes the husband's sperm is pooled and added to the donor's sperm to introduce the possibility, however remote, that the baby would actually be his. Artificial insemination is a complex experience, with many psychological ramifications and in some cases legal complications as well. It can offer the possibility of a baby that is a least half genetically derived from that particular couple. Before reaching that kind of solution, the couple may need to mourn their inability to have their own children. This process may be important before the couple is able to come to some other solution and restore a sense of confidence in themselves and in each other. Unconscious feelings of anger, defectiveness, and helplessness may complicate the adaptation and can sometimes be displaced onto other people outside the family or those involved in the process of arranging for the procedure. Nevertheless, this offers a solution that has been very satisfactory for many couples.

A couple who achieves a pregnancy either during or after an infertility workup is usually enormously relieved. Self-esteem is increased and the sexual relationship usually improves. However, sometimes a paradoxical result occurs and the couple finds that they have actually adapted to not having a child, and the shifts that are entailed in having a child mobilize a considerable amount of conflict and tension.

Intrapsychic conflicts have been implicated in infertility particularly when an organic cause cannot be found. In the past, this diagnosis was sometimes made without an adequate workup and can be difficult for a couple to respond to without feeling criticized. There are problems involved in sexual relationships that interfere with fertility—such as impotence, vaginismus, and infrequent intercourse for emotional reasons (Mozley, 1980). Conflicts about femininity, pregnancy, and motherhood have been suggested as affecting somatic responses, leading to failure to become pregnant or habitual spontaneous abortion (Deutsch, 1945; Benedek, 1952). Since the reproductive system is sensitive to neuroendocrine influences (Mozley, 1980), this does seem plausible for some individuals. Others demonstrate considerable conflicts about the same issues but this does not interfere with repeated unwanted pregnancies. In one study of married childless women who elected sterilization, fears of inadequacy as mothers and avoidance of life commitments were found on psychological tests (Kaltreider and Margolis, 1977).

Counseling and psychotherapy can be extremely helpful for infertility, including counseling during the process of the workup and afterward. Counseling needs to address the couple's attitudes and sources of conflict. The narcissistic injury caused by not being able to conceive, which then extends to all feelings of adequacy and competence, is an important therapeutic issue. Feelings of defectiveness, helplessness, concerns about body image, and adequacies are prominent. Many people feel relieved and less responsible and guilty if the causes of infertility are found to be organically based, and, therefore, it is easier to determine how to correct them or whether they are correctible.

One important assessment is to determine those individuals in whom infertility may indeed be a defense against severe conflicts about pregnancy and motherhood. In some cases, these defenses need support since having a baby would be severely taxing and possibly decompansating (Sandler, 1968).

Support and understanding, as well as clarifying the emotional issues involved, can be very effective in helping an infertile couple deal with their concerns and choices.

Hysterectomy and Sexuality

The number of hysterectomies done in the United States has been increasing; the frequency of this procedure is now greater than any other major gynecological operation. The National Center for Health Statistics estimates that in 1973, 690,000 hysterectomies were performed in the United States. Bunker (1976) estimated in 1976 that this represented a rate of 647.7 per 100,000 and might result in the loss of the uterus by half of the female population by the time they reach 65 years if that rate were to continue. The hysterectomy rate for the United States was twice that of England and Wales, reflecting different approaches to gynecological problems. The indications for this procedure are obviously not firmly established nor universally agreed upon. Although there may be recent changes, it continues to be a common procedure.

The psychological impact of hysterectomy has been a subject of some concern and is complex. In part, it is a consequence of the biological reality and its personal significance; for a premenopausal woman, it precipitates the ending of menses. If the ovaries are removed also, it initiates other menopausal changes and the woman may then respond to an abrupt and often early menopause with its implications for her self-concept, feelings about her body, stage of life, and other meanings. Another aspect of a woman's response to hysterectomy is a result of cultural factors that influence the way a woman without a uterus is regarded. In contemporary middle-class American society, this is not a major concern, but it is in some other cultural groups where a woman is devalued if she does not have a uterus or the possibility for producing children.

An important component of a woman's response to hysterectomy derives from the symbolic and unconscious significance of the uterus (Roeske, 1978). There are certain universal aspects to this as well as individual personal meanings. Important sources of women's identity have been connected with the function of the uterus: femininity, motherhood, and sexuality. It is difficult at this point to assess the effects of the shifting emphasis away from the childbearing and domestic roles for women as the central source of their status and self-esteem.

For some women a hysterectomy seems to mark the end of their "youth" and the beginning of middle age, with its impact on their sense of their options and life plans. For others the hysterectomy is a less major event. Some may already be menopausal, and the surgery may provide welcome relief for someone who has had irregular and uncomfortable bleeding. Hysterectomy can also bring relief from concerns about becoming pregnant, particularly if, for any reason, contraception has not been permissible, possible, or effective.

The literature on the emotional effects of hysterectomy is somewhat inconclusive and complicated by methodological problems in the research (Meikle, 1977; Meikle et al., 1977; Richards, 1973) In some studies, women who had hysterectomies for varying indications were all grouped together so those with serious illness were considered together with relatively less serious illnesses. It is also difficult to evaluate some of the symptoms that are seen as resulting from hysterectomy, because at times pelvic symptoms, particularly pelvic pain, may represent a displacement from other problems, such as sexual conflicts, problems about femininity, and childbearing (Castelnuevo-Tedesco and Krout, 1970). When the uterus is removed, these symptoms may emerge as depression or some other form of emotional distress. Some individuals also tend to somatize more, that is, express their emotional problems through physical symptoms. This is particularly true for depression (Lipkowsky, 1975). These symptoms change and become more manifest as emotional problems if the organ that is initially the symptomatic one is removed. Some studies indicate depression is present presurgically (Moore and Tolley, 1976).

However, there does seem to be an important difference between the loss of the uterus and other surgical experiences, and posthysterectomy depression is a frequently mentioned entity, even though it has been difficult to evaluate accurately. All through life an individual must master losses. Loss of a part of one's body must be mastered by the process of mourning as with any other loss. Losing the menses may also be perceived as a loss (Morgner, 1978), since menstruation is part of normal feminine functioning. It usually affects a woman's sense of her physical intactness, completeness, or sexual desirability. The loss can also produce a general feeling of defectiveness (D'Esopo, 1962). Prevailing societal attitudes may reinforce this sense of being "damaged goods." Some men really do feel this way about a woman who has lost her uterus and find they are not sexually attracted or interested. To some extent this represents the absence of a possibility of impregnating her, at least theoretically; to some extent it is the feeling of "damage." The support of self-esteem and the reassurance provided by ongoing active sexual life after hysterectomy is very important.

Although posthysterectomy depression may represent the emergence of preexisting depression, the reaction to loss of an important part of the body, the loss of reproductive function, and a response to feeling devalued and injured, it is by no means inevitable. Many women experience a sense of well-being when they recover from the surgery and return to normal life and functioning.

Another component of the response to hysterectomy is related to the experience of undergoing surgery, including the way the procedure is described by the surgeon and the preparation the woman has for it. The surgeon may not discuss the implications for sexuality or may not be explicit about what the procedure will and will not do. Even with explicit preparation, the woman may be confused. The terminology may be more appropriate for the physician than the patient. Often anxiety relating to the anticipated procedure may cloud her capacity to really integrate the information given. It may be helpful to have her repeat what she thinks is going to happen.

The hidden nature of the uterus itself lends itself to fantasy, which is difficult to test. Concepts and ideas that one might have been damaged are not possible to correct by one's own observations without the help of a physician or another trained individual. Wherever possible, it is important to involve both partners in the preparation for surgery and to explore the attitudes of the man both toward the surgery and toward his partner.

One additional point to consider is the effect of any surgery on a patient. There are regressive aspects to any illness. Being a surgical patient involves conditions that are perhaps more regressive than other experiences with illness. Basic bodily functions over which an individual has maintained control since early childhood are taken over by the medical system. Control of urination, bowel movements, eating, and sometimes breathing is surrendered. This requires an extraordinary amount of trust and stirs up a considerable amount of anxiety.

Sometimes the demands placed on family members and sexual partners affect the relationships and later sexual functioning.

Sexuality does not have to be affected by a hysterectomy if a woman's general health is good. Sometimes the vagina is shortened in the surgical process and will produce changes that affect sexual satisfaction, but most often this is not so. However, there are many misconceptions women have as to what the procedure has actually done. The profundity of it is indicated by some of the colloquial descriptions in which a woman talking about her hysterectomy will say that "everything was taken out" or "I lost my 'nature.'" Since sexual functioning is multidetermined, it is difficult to sort out all the components affecting it that arise from the experience of a hysterectomy. Self-esteem, the attitude of the partner, the actual effects of the surgery, the effect on sexuality of some depression, and some postsurgical fatigue all need to be considered.

In spite of reassurance, women may be anxious about their own sexuality after a hysterectomy. They express a fear of losing sexual desire and responsiveness and are anxious about remaining attractive to men. The course of her relationships with men and others who are close to her have a considerable bearing on her feelings of depression or well-being.

References

Adams, D., Gold, A., and Burt, A. Rise in female-initiated sexual activity at ovulation and its suppression by oral contraceptives. *New England Journal of Medicine,* 1978, *299*(21), 1145–1150.

Adler, N. Psychosocial issues of therapeutic abortion. In D. Young and A. Ehrhardt (Eds.), *Psychosomatic obstetrics and genecology.* New York: Appleton–Century–Crofts, 1980. Pp. 159–177.

Babikian, H. Abortion. In B. Saddock, H. Kaplan, and A. Freedman (Eds.), *The sexual experience.* Baltimore, Md.: Williams and Wilkens, 1976. Pp. 349–357.

Behrman, S., and Kistner, R. *Progress in infertility* (2nd ed.). Boston: Little, Brown, 1975.

Belsey, E., Greer, H., Lal, S., Lewis, S., and Beard, R. Predictive factors in emotional response to abortion: Kings Termination Study IV. *Social Science and Medicine,* 1977, *11*, 71–82.

Benedek, T. Infertility as a Psychosomatic Defense, *Fertility and Sterility,* 1952, *3;* 527–541.

Benedek, T. Sexual functions in women. In S. Arieti, *American handbook of psychiatry.* New York: Basic Books, 1959. Vol. 1, p. 37.

Benedek, T. The psychobiology of pregnancy. In J. Anthony and T. Benedek (Eds.), *Parenthood: Its psychology and psychopathology.* Boston: Little, Brown, 1970.

Beral, V., and Kay, C. R. Mortality in women on oral contraceptives. *The Lancet,* 1977, *2;* 1276–1277.

Bernard, V. Psychodynamics of unmarried motherhood in early adolescence. *Nervous Child,* 1944, *4;* 26.

Bibring, G. Some considerations of the psychological processes in pregnancy. *Psychoanalytic Study of the Child,* 1959, *L4;* 113.

Bradley, R. *Husband-coached childbirth.* New York: Harper & Row, 1965.

Bunker, J. Elective hysterectomy: Pro and con. *New England Journal of Medicine,* 1976, *295*(5), 64–72.

Castelnuevo-Tedesco, P., and Krout, B. Psychosomatic aspects of chronic pelvic pain. *Psychiatry in Medicine* 1970, *1*(2); 109–126.

D'Esopo, D. Hysterectomy when the uterus is grossly normal. *American Journal of Obstetrics and Gynecology,* 1962, *83;* 113–122.

Deutsch, H. *Psychology of women,* Vol. II; *Motherhood.* New York: Grune & Stratton, 1945.

Dick-Reid, G. *Childbirth without fear* (4th Ed.). New York: Harper & Row, 1972. (Originally published, 1944.)

Doering, S., and Entwisle, D., Preparation during pregnancy and ability to cope with labor and delivery. *American Journal of Orthopsychiatry,* 1975, *45;* 825–837.

Enkin, M., Smith, S., Dermer, S., and Emmett, J. An adequately controlled study of the effectiveness of PM training. In M. Norris (Ed.), *Psychosomatic medicine in obstetrics and gynecology, Proceedings.* Basel: Karger, 1972.

Fleming, O., and Seager, C. Incidence of depressive symptoms in uses of the oral contraceptive. *British Journal of Psychiatry,* 1978, *132*(43); 430–440.

Freeman, E. Influence of personality attributes on abortion experience. *American Journal of Orthopsychiatry,* 1977, *47*(3); 503–513.

Friedman, E. The psychological aspects of pregnancy. In M. Notman and C. Nadelson (Eds.), *The woman patient,* (Vol. I). New York: Plenum, 1978.

Gilligan, C. In a different voice: Women's conception of the self and morality. *Harvard Education Review,* 1977, *47*(4), 481–517.

Grover, J. Personal communication, 1978. Lectures given in Human Sexuality course, Harvard Medical School, 1979.

Jaffe, F. The pill: A perspective for assessing risks and benefits. *New England Journal of Medicine,* 1977, *297*(11); 612–614.

Jessner, C., Weigert, E., and Foy, J. The development of parental attitudes during pregnancy. In J. Anthony and T. Benedek (Eds.), *Parenthood: Its psychology and psychopathology.* Boston: Little, Brown, 1970. Pp. 209–244.

Kaltreider, N., and Margolis, H. Childless by choice: A clinical study. *American Journal of Psychiatry,* 1977, *134;* 179–182.

Klein, H., Potter, H., and Dyk, R. *Anxiety in pregnancy and childbirth.* New York: Hoeber (Harper), 1950.

Lerner, J. Parental mislabeling of female genitals as a determinant of penis envy and learning inhibitions in women. *Journal of the American Psychoanalytic Association,* 1976, *24*(5); 269.

Lidz, R. Conflicts between fertility and infertility. In M. Notman and C. Nadelson (Eds.), *The woman patient* (Vol. I). New York: Plenum, 1978.

Lipowsky, Z. (Ed.). *Psychiatry in medicine,* Vol. 5, *Current trends in psychosomatic medicine I.* 1974.

Lipowsky, Z. (Ed.). *Psychiatry in medicine,* Vol. 6, *Current trends in psychosomatic medicine II.* 1975.

Mann, E., and Armistead, T. Pregnancy and sexual behavior. In B. Sadock, H. Kaplan and A. Freedman, (Eds.), *The sexual experience.* Baltimore, Md.: Williams & Wilkins, 1976. Chap. 8, pp. 238–248.

Marder, L. Psychiatric experiences with a liberalized therapeutic abortion law. *American Journal of Psychiatry,* 1970, *126,* 1230–1236.

Margolis, A., Rindfuss, R., Coghland, P., and Rochat, R. Contraceptive practice after abortion. *Family Planning Perspective,* 1974, *6*:55–60.

Masters, W. H., and Johnson, V. E. *Human sexual response.* Boston: Little, Brown, 1966.

Mazor, M. The problem of infertility. In M. T. Notman and C. Nadelson (Eds.), *The woman patient.* New York: Plenum, 1978.

McCauley, E., and Ehrhardt, A. Female sexual response. In D. Youngs and A. Ehrhardt (Eds.), *Psychosomatic obstetrics and gynecology.* New York: Appleton–Century–Crofts, 1980. P. 53.

Mead, M., and Newton, N. Cultural patterning of prenatal behavior. In S. Richardson and A. Guttmacher (Eds.), *Childbearing, its social and psychological aspects*. Baltimore, Md.: Williams & Wilkins, 1967.

Meikle, S. The psychological effects of hysterectomy. *Canadian Psychological Review*, 1977, *18*(2), 128–139.

Meikle, S., Brody, H., and Pysh, F. An investigation into the psychological effects of hysterectomy. *Journal of Nervous Mental Disorders*, 1977, *164*(1), 36–41.

Menning, B. *Infertility: A guide for the childless couple*. Englewood Cliffs, N.J.: Prentice–Hall, 1977.

Mester, R. Induced abortion and psychotherapy. *Psychotherapy and Psychosomatics*, 1978, *30*, 98–104.

Moore, J. T., and Tolley, D. Depression following hysterectomy. *Psychosomatics*, 1976, *17*, 86–89.

Morganthau, J. E. *Adolescent health care*. Westport, Conn.: Technomics, 1977.

Morgner, S. Sexuality after hysterectomy and castration. *Women and Health*, 1978, *3*(1), 5–9.

Mozley, P. Emotional parameters of infertility. In D. Youngs and A. Ehrhardt (Eds.) *Psychosomatic obstetrics and gynecology*. New York: Appleton–Century–Crofts, 1980.

Nadelson, C. Normal and special aspects of pregnancy. *Obstetrics and Gynecology*, April 1973, *41*, 4.

Norman, W. Postpartum disorders. In A. Freedman and H. Kaplan (Eds.), *Comprehensive textbook of psychiatry*. Baltimore, Md.: Williams & Wilkins, 1967.

Notman, M., and Nadelson, C. Reproductive crisis. In A. Brodsky and R. Hare-Mustin (Eds.), *Women and psychotherapy*. New York: Guilford, 1980.

Payne, E., Kravits, A., Notman, M., and Anderson, J. Outcome following therapeutic abortion. *Archives of General Psychiatry*, 1976, *33*, 725–733.

Peck, A., and Marcus, H. Psychiatric sequelae of therapeutic interruption of pregnancy. *Journal of Nervous and Mental Disorders*, 1966, *143*, 417–425.

Pitt, B. Maternity blues. *British Journal of Psychiatry*, 1973, *122*, 431–433.

Richards, D. Depression after hysterectomy. *The Lancet*, 1973, *2*, 429–433.

Roe, V., 1973, Wade: U.S. Supreme Court 93:705.

Roeske, N. Hysterectomy. In M. Notman and C. Nadelson (Eds.), *The woman patient*. New York: Plenum, 1978.

Rosenfield, A. Benefits still outweigh risks with OC's and IUD's. *Modern Medicine*, March–April 1978, *91*.

Sandberg, E. Psychological aspects of contraception. In B. Sadock, H. Kaplan, and M. Freedman (Eds.), *The sexual experience*. Baltimore, Md.: Williams & Wilkins, 1976.

Sandler, B. Emotional stress and infertility. *Quarterly Journal of Psychosomatic Research*, 1968, *12*, 51.

Schaffer, C., and Pine, F. Pregnancy, abortion and the development tasks of adolescence. *Journal of Child Psychiatry*, 1975, *14*, 511–536.

Seiden, A. The sense of mastery in the childbirth experience. In M. T. Notman and C. Nadelson (Eds.), *The woman patient*. New York: Plenum, 1978. Pp. 87–107.

Stoller, R. Primary feminity. *Journal of the American Psychoanalytic Association*, 1976, *24*(5), 59–78.

Tietze, C. Contraceptive practice in the context of a non-restrictive abortion law. *Family Planning Perspective*, 1975, *7*(3), 197–202.

Vessey, M., McPherson, K., and Johnson, B. Mortality among women participating in the Oxford Family Planning Association Contraceptive Study, *The Lancet*, 1977, *2*, 731–733.

Warnes, H., and Fitzpatrick, C. Oral contraceptives and depression. *Psychosomatics*, 1979, *20*(3), 187–194.

Wilson, J., Barglow, P., and Shippman, W. The prognosis of post-partum mental illness. *Comprehensive Psychiatry*, 1972, *13*, 305–316.

Wolff, B., and Langley, S. Cultural factors and the response to pain. *Journal of American Anthropological Society*, 1968, *70*, 494–501.

Sexual Dysfunctions in the Physically Ill and Disabled

Ernest R. Griffith and Roberta B. Trieschmann

Definition of the Problem

Any approach to the treatment of sexual dysfunctions in the physically ill and disabled requires a clear understanding of the distinction between those dysfunctions with an organic etiology and those with a psychogenic etiology during the evaluation of the problem. A delineation of these aspects of dysfunction is essential since treatment strategies will differ. Psychologically based dysfunctions have received the most attention in the literature, and multiple intervention strategies have been developed. Most of the patients seen for treatment by the average sexual counselor have psychogenic dysfunctions, and the patient initiates the referral, usually after suffering with the dysfunction for quite a while.

Organically based dysfunctions have neurological, endocrinological, urological, gynecological, musculosketal impairments, etc., as their etiological base. Until recently, these dysfunctions have received little attention by either researchers or therapists, and the literature regarding therapeutic interventions is far from complete. In addition, most sexual therapists in private practice screen out anyone with an organic dysfunction, and they, therefore, have little or no experience with psychosocial problems of the physically ill and disabled. This is unfortunate, since in our experience, most of these disorders have a psychosocial component, and successful treatment requires understanding and attention to both.

For the purposes of this chapter, we have labeled as primary those dysfunctions that derive from an alteration in the normal physiology of sexual function. We will label the psychological and behavioral aspects of a sexual dysfunction as secondary,

Ernest R. Griffith • Institute of Rehabilitation Medicine, Good Samaritan Medical Center, Phoenix, Arizona.   Roberta B. Trieschmann • Consulting Psychologist, Phoenix, Arizona.

TABLE 1 Primary and Secondary Dysfunctions

	Primary dysfunctions with secondary components	Secondary dysfunctions
Etiology	Physical and behavioral	Behavioral
Goal of therapy	Remedy or amelioration of physical problem, behavior change, or both	Behavior change
Method of therapy	Medical (pharmacological, local modalities, surgery, etc.), information and instruction, counseling, behavior therapy, or all of these	Counseling and behavior therapy
Qualifications of therapists	Specialized medical expertise and expertise in psychological treatment strategies, such as counseling and behavior therapy; team approach is recommended	Expertise in counseling and behavior change techniques
Detection of the problem	The professional, the patient, or both; patient may not identify it as a problem	The patient

not because they are less important, but because they often derive from the very presence of the primary disorder or may occur independent of organic dysfunction. Furthermore, it must be emphasized that many people who acquire primary sexual dysfunctions may have had a premorbid history of secondary sexual dysfunctions in the past.[1] This practically ensures that secondary sexual problems will complicate the evaluation and treatment of the primary sexual disorder.

This chapter addresses itself to primary dysfunctions with secondary components (Table 1). The etiology of the problem is physical with behavioral components (premorbid attitudes toward sexuality along with anxieties and fears about the primary disorder itself). The goal of therapy will be the remedy or amelioration of the physical problem, behavioral change, or both. The method of therapy will be physical (pharmacological, local modalities, surgery, etc.), information and instruction, counseling, behavior therapy, or any combination of these. Few therapists acting alone can deal with the diagnostic and therapeutic complexity of these cases since they often require specialized medical and sophisticated psychological interventions. Consequently, the team approach of medical specialist and psychologist or psychiatrist is usually desirable and, at times, necessary. Because of the complexity of many of these cases, the contributions of the physiatrist, internist, or surgeon in the management of these primary and secondary dysfunctions may be essential.

The sexual problem may be identified by a professional, by the patient, or both. Until recently, many professionals and patients have assumed that sexual functioning is impossible following severe illnesses and disabilities. Although the professional community is reversing its opinion gradually, many patients are not. Therefore, referral for treatment may be initiated by a professional rather than the patient, a reversal of the pattern for sexual problems that are exclusively secondary in nature. This may have major implications for treatment. Since the referral of the sexual dysfunction may be initiated by the medical specialist in charge of the case, the patient may have reservations about seeing a psychiatrist or psychologist. From the patient's point of view, he or she has a physical problem and may be exceedingly threatened by the arrival of a "shrink" on the scene. Exquisite sensitivity to this issue will be a determining factor in the success of treatment. Thus, the patient should be reassured that he or she is experiencing very *normal* anxieties and concerns regarding the illness, disability, and sexual dysfunction and that to see a psychiatrist or psychologist does not in any way imply abnormality or psychological sickness.

Secondary Components to the Sexual Dysfunction

The secondary components of primary sexual dysfunctions include the psychosocial and learned attitudes toward sexuality, which influence everyone. Cultural, ethnic, and religious factors may have a significant impact on sexual functioning following an illness or disability if previously defined "proper" sex acts are no longer available and alternative methods of sexual gratification are considered to be taboo.[2,3] Early experiences with parental figures and peer groups influence attitudes toward relationships and sexuality and may become a problem only after onset of the physical problem. Past social experience and general self-confidence are crucial in determining the patient's reaction to a disability and are critical in creating a social life as a disabled person.[4,5] One has to be able to interact comfortably with people in order to form a sexual relationship. Secondary dysfunctions that predate the onset of the illness or disability will further complicate postdisability sexual functioning.[1] For example, the male with a premorbid history of intermittent secondary impotence may have a exacerbation of the problem following a myocardial infarction. Wabrek and Burchell [1] found that two-thirds of males hospitalized with an acute myocardial infarction acknowledged sexual problems prior to the infarct. Kolodny et al.[6] report that impotence may be one of the first signs of diabetes even before other clinical symptoms are evident, which means that these men have developed a great deal of anxiety regarding performance and masculinity by the time the problem is diagnosed correctly. Thus, return to pre-illness level of sexual function may not always be the appropriate goal. Obviously, a pre-illness sexual history is mandatory.

Following the onset of the illness or disability, the individual is vulnerable to secondary responses. Devaluation and desexualization of the patient by himself and others occur frequently.[5,7,8] The person who suffers a physical disability may tend to devalue himself because of the change in physical attractiveness or physical ability, and this sense of devaluation may be communicated to others he or she meets.[9,10] Society prizes attractiveness, youth, and physical ability, and, thus, the disabled person's self-devaluation may be confirmed by the reactions of others.[8] Devaluation is often correlated with desexualization; the community may not recognize the person as a suitable sex partner and may believe that because a person is disabled, sex is no longer important in his or her life.[2] Consequently, there is a great potential for loneliness and feelings of isolation from others after a major illness and disability. As a result, most disabled persons complain, "Why can't people see me as someone who *has* a handicap rather than someone who is handicapped?"[11] Therefore, all of the person's premorbid social experience and self-confidence will be required to combat the devaluation and desexualization phenomena, and therapists should be aware of these influences on sexual functioning.

Anxiety and fear about the illness or handicap itself may also inhibit sexual satisfaction. Individuals with cardiovascular disease, diabetes, renal disease, cancer, etc., are faced with a serious illness that may be life threatening. Onset of these conditions in the sixth decade of life may produce fears of aging, loss of vocational status, financial worries, and significant depression. Rumination about one's entire life in terms of successes and failures (with an emphasis on failures) is not uncommon. The partner may equally share all of these concerns, but the healthy partner may cover up these fears in order to be supportive to the loved one. The onset of these conditions in the fourth or fifth decade of life becomes particularly unsettling for the entire family. Financial security usually has not been achieved since the person is often in midcareer and in the process of advancement. Worries about money and self-image vocationally need to be resolved. If the person has already been in personal crisis regarding goals, values, and success, as often happens sometime in the late thirties and early forties,[12,13] the onset of a major illness or disability can be devastating. These concerns may be as prevalent in women as in men. A sexual problem needs to be considered within the context of the profound impact of the illness or disability on the person's entire life, since anxieties about sexual functioning will be compounded by anxieties about other parameters of life.

The teenage years and the twenties are dominated by concerns of socialization, physical attractiveness, and physical capability (the primary factor in obtaining a first date in college is physical attractiveness)[14] and the initiation of steps (educationally or vocationally) leading to a life career. Thus, the onset of a major disability or illness during these years is a major social problem. Furthermore, since one's identity is so vulnerable in these years, a major illness or disability can interrupt the process of self-actualization, which is so important for adult adjustment.

The person who is disabled congenitally or early in life is vulnerable to most of the secondary components outlined earlier.[15,16]

However, particular attention should be given to the influence of early experiences on adult functioning.[7,17] For example, the disabled child may receive less mothering behavior (cuddling and other sensory stimulations), may be overprotected (fewer opportunities to develop self-confidence), and may be socially isolated (fewer opportunities to learn normal peer group and heterosexual behaviors). Devaluation, desexualization, cultural attitudes toward sexuality, and fears about the illness and disability may also influence sexual functioning.

A major problem may be the parent's tendency to avoid the issue of sexual functioning in their disabled or ill child. Parents of disabled teenagers see the issue of their child becoming independent as more important and pressing a concern than sexuality; therefore, they tend to avoid dealing with the issue of sex, hoping that it will not arise. Furthermore, parents may worry that sex education for their disabled or ill child will foster false expectations and hopes that may never be realized.[16] Hence, the parents of disabled or ill teenagers must often be a primary focus for the treatment interventions so that they will permit their child to experience many of the normal hurts and happinesses of life.

Evaluation of the Problem

To evaluate a sexual problem in a person with a major illness or physical disability, one must consider premorbid daily function, present function defined by the illness or disability, future expectations regarding life's activities, prognosis of the illness or disability, and characteristics of the spouse–partner relationship.

A thorough medical history of the current illness or disability must be obtained. Any associated medical conditions (cardiac disease, hypertension, pulmonary disease, diabetes, etc.) that might interfere with sexual function should be evaluated. The physical examination should review the neurological, musculoskeletal, urological, gynecological, and cardiovascular systems. In certain cases, measures of physical capacity may be indicated, such as monitoring of the cardiac patient with electrocardiograms, blood pressure, or pulse during sexual activity. Hypertensive patients may require blood pressure monitoring during or after sex. Objective measures of strength, range of motion of the joints, and endurance are of importance in arthritic patients. The physical assessment should include the various forms of mobility (walking, wheelchair, transfers to and from bed, capability of positional changes in bed) and self-care activities (dressing and undressing, bowel and bladder management, personal hygiene, and contraceptive use). These physical functions are best determined by actual observations by the physical or occupational therapist. Such functions should be adapted to the specifics of sexual activities, including precoital preparations—transfers to the bed, bowel and bladder management, positioning, etc. Urological assessment of the neuropathic bladder, as in spinal cord diseases or injury, and brain disorders is often required. X rays may be required to determine the structural integrity of bone in metastatic cancer or osteoporosis. Heterotopic bone formation inhibiting joint motion may be discovered by bone scan or X ray. Respiratory function should be evaluated if necessary and a pharmacological history should be obtained.

In order to assess the impact of the illness or disability, a thorough life history must be obtained to estimate self-perception and social skills prior to the onset of the disability or illness. Attention should be given to success and failure experiences with family, friends, school, work, and leisure activities. A sexual history should include attitudes toward various kinds of sex acts, "proper" sex roles for male and female, likes and dislikes, degree of experience, value system, and occurrence of secondary sexual dysfunctions in the past, particularly just prior to onset. Cultural, ethnic, and religious sanctions or prohibitions should be elicited. Sexual orientation should also be considered, so that preference for heterosexual or homosexual relationships could be understood and taken into account when a therapeutic plan is recommended.

Given a thorough background on premorbid functioning, a review of present physical, psychological, social, and vocational status will help to define the degree of change that the disability entails. This includes what has been lost and what assets and liabilities remain. The greater the impact, the greater the change from premorbid activities that the illness or disability requires and the more stress that will persist until the changes required by the medical condition are incorporated into the person's lifestyle. People exhibit stress in various ways but the stress will not always be as obvious as in patients who present themselves for psychological treatment in traditional settings. Thus, the clinician needs to be sensitive to the person's concerns that if he/she admits to fears and anxieties it is tantamount to admitting to being abnormal. Reassurance that these feelings are normal reactions to major life changes should be given during the evaluation stage of the process, since this will help to develop rapport for further interventions.

Cultural, ethnic, and religious influences should be carefully evaluated. This is particularly important in those cases in which the ill or disabled person is not the one to request assistance with a sexual problem. For example, those with fundamental religious beliefs may be exceedingly conservative and hesitant to discuss sexual problems with someone who is not of their faith. Regional differences can also be very important in the United States. Even within major metropolitan areas, there may be great variations among the attitudes of various groups regarding sexuality.

The spouse–partner relationship should be a prime area for evaluation. If there were tensions in the relationship prior to the onset of the illness or disability, these will be aggravated by the medical crisis and will become a factor requiring intervention in order to remedy the sexual dysfunction.[5] A sexual history from the partner is very helpful, with special emphasis on areas of satisfaction and dissatisfaction prior to the primary dysfunction. The partner often has many fears and concerns that have not been shared with the ill or disabled person in order to protect them from worry. The evaluation process becomes a convenient time to elicit these concerns and may be the first time that anyone on the professional team has given serious attention to the partner as an individual rather than as an adjunct to the patient. Fears about hurting the disabled person during sexual interactions or of precipitating another medical crisis are frequently found, and, therefore, the extent and accuracy of the partner's information concerning the nature of the illness and disability should be explored.

Knowledge of normal sexual functioning should be an additional area to be evaluated in both the ill or disabled person and the partner. Many people are not well informed regarding the anatomy and physiology of male and female sexual response, and, therefore, gaps in basic knowledge must be identified before intervention begins.[18] Furthermore, "there are vary few *un*informed teenagers but there are a great many *mis*informed ones who liberally share their impressions with one another."[16] Information about the impact of the illness or disability on the physiology of sexual functioning should be determined since often the mere giving of information and instruction may solve the problem.

The clinician, however, should remain wary of this as the only intervention strategy. For example, many women report that they had received information regarding sexual activities with their ill or disabled husbands, and this information did not alleviate their anxieties nor necessarily remedy the sexual disturbance.[19] Moreover, it has been demonstrated that giving of information alone is not a very effective way of changing behavior.[20] Nevertheless, this remains one of the major modes of intervention in most medical settings.

The congenitally disabled person should be evaluated along the same dimensions as just described, except that the emphasis is not on loss or change but on who the person has learned to be and on what the person has learned to do.[16] A sexual history must detail the behaviors in his or her repertoire, attitudes, preferences, and cultural taboos. The question of social skills should be carefully evaluated because the congenitally disabled and those disabled in childhood may have had a different kind of social life than others.

In summary, the focus of the evaluation process is to define what sexual behaviors were in the couple's or person's repertoire prior to the illness or disability, how many of these are no longer appropriate or possible, what sex acts are feasible now, how willing the individuals are to try new methods, and which sex acts they are willing to practice. The sexual problem must be viewed within the context of the impact of the illness or disability on the person's entire life.

Principles of Treatment

The timing of treatment will be influenced by the initiation of the referral for evaluation and treatment. It should be remembered that the patient often does not request the referral, nor may the sexual problem be identified by the person as a major problem given the multiplicity of issues surrounding the onset of a significant illness or disability. If the sexual dysfunction is identified soon after the onset of the disability or illness, the treatment may be initiated during the inpatient phase. However, the person may not be completely aware of all the parameters of living with the disability at that point. Treatment may also be initiated after discharge from the hospital after the person's life has stabilized somewhat.

Sometimes referral may be made to a therapist who is skilled in handling sexual dysfunctions at a time when the person is more aware of the impact of the medical problem on sexual functioning. Since sexual counselors can have a variety of backgrounds, we would emphasize the necessity of obtaining the essential physical–medical data from a qualified specialist in the relevant areas: urology, cardiology, physiatry, internal medicine, orthopedics, gynecology, etc. Furthermore, a thorough understanding of the specific psychosocial problems of the physically disabled is essential.[5]

Ideally, we would recommend a team approach to treatment based on professional discipline and sex, as advised by Masters and Johnson,[21] if this is feasible. For the more complicated cases, a team composed of a physician and psychologist has been our preference, since no member of any one discipline has all of the knowledge and skills required to manage these cases alone. Furthermore, the partner may have conflicts about role reversal and reactions to the illness and disability itself that influence the sexual and personal relationships. Thus, a therapeutic team representing both sexes is often beneficial but not mandatory. If treatment of the sexual problem occurs in the rehabilitation milieu, the question of who treats the patient is less well defined since many rehabilitation centers do not have formal sexual counseling programs. Nevertheless, counseling can be given, in uncomplicated cases, by those members of the rehabilitation team who are (1) comfortable with their own sexuality, (2) knowledgeable about the psychosocial and learned components of sexuality, (3) aware of the various religious and cultural prohibitions of certain sex acts, and (4) familiar with the relevant medical–physical factors of the individual case. It is essential that medical rehabilitation personnel be aware of the principles of counseling and the complexity of the psychosocial aspects of sexual behavior.[22] However, we continue to recommend the team approach and would suggest that complex cases be treated in this manner.

Within the context of the rehabilitation setting, the topic of sexual functioning may be introduced in a general manner following the acute phase of treatment. An acquired disability may be accompanied initially by a period of psychic and physical shock where the focus of the intervention is survival. Following this phase, the professional may discuss with the patient the various components of a rehabilitation program, sexual functioning being one.[2] This dialogue should be aimed at giving the patient permission to initiate questions about sexual functioning when he or she is ready and affirming that sexual functioning is a relevant aspect of postdisability living.[23] Even when granted such permission, many patients will not initiate discussion about sexuality. Those treating the patient should be aware of subtle cues that patients communicate. Not only should clinicians be aware of the patient's desire to discuss sexuality but should be equally sensitive to cues from the patient that he is neither ready for nor interested in sex at this point.[2] Some disabilities may provide the individual with a convenient excuse to avoid sexual contacts. This wish should also be respected.

In proceeding with treatment, ideally both patient and sexual partner should be included, if possible. A partner, however, may be unwilling to participate, inaccessible, or nonexistent. In these circumstances, the possibility of a surrogate partner may be considered. Although this is controversial and complicated, we believe that if the circumstances and conditions of such an arrangement are completely understood and acceptable to all responsible parties, it offers a further valuable dimension to the treatment process.[21]

Most disabilities do not affect the sex drive any more than they would affect hunger or thirst. The disability may influence the *type* of sex acts that would be feasible or advisable, but few disabilities preclude all sex acts.[2] Therefore, implicit in any discussion of the management principles is the meticulous appreciation of the value systems of the patient and the partner.[22] No form of intervention that is inconsistent with these values should be imposed, no matter how compatible with the best judgments of those treating the patient and partner. Value systems should be elicited as part of the evaluation process, and the professional should be clearly aware of his or her own values regarding sexuality in the severely ill or disabled. When the patient prefers not to engage in alternate sexual acts, other than genital–genital intercourse, the goal of treatment should be to advise what methods of sexual satisfaction are available. This may result in the decision to abstain from sex acts (other than kissing) and this choice should be respected.

Based on the results of the evaluation, minimal or extensive intervention might be indicated. We have found that the PLISSIT Model is helpful since it conceives of treatment at four levels: Permission, Limited Information, Specific Suggestions, Intensive Therapy.[24]

Level 1, Permission, becomes relevant in medical and rehabilitation patients since the person may harbor fears, concerns, misinformation, and myths that need to be discussed, but the person may feel uncomfortable about initiating such a discussion. The clinician can introduce the topic of sexuality indirectly and acknowledge that it is normal to be worried and that sexual functioning is a legitimate focus for discussion and treatment. For example, an individual or couple may have adjusted to a primary sexual dysfunction by turning to alternative sexual acts, but lingering taboos about these sex acts may create a climate of discomfort that needs to be dispelled with reassurance. Permission should take account of religious, cultural, and ethnic values that are important to the person and partner.

Level 2, Limited Information, provides the person with specific factual information directly relevant to his or her particular sexual concern. It may result in the person deciding to continue existing practices, or it may result in a behavior change. This is one way to dispel sexual myths regarding the illness or disability. For example, fears of producing another stroke or heart attack are common after such an event. Consequently, information regarding the health of the person is necessary along with information on the amount of exertion which is appropriate at various stages of recovery. It is very important to limit the information to that which is needed to answer specific questions or deal with the delimited problem, since evidence shows that patients often do not remember complex information or that which extends beyond the scope of the problem.[24]

Level 3, Specific Suggestions, involves more direct problem-oriented strategies, which include behavior change or specific medical interventions. Suggestions may relate to the prevention of pain or symptoms during sexual activity, or they may involve the use of alternative sex acts to achieve sexual satisfaction. Follow-up and feedback sessions are recommended in order to assist patients with details of managing the behavior changes recommended. Griffith and Trieschmann [25,26] have used a private hospital room located near the rehabilitation ward to teach sexual behaviors to persons with disabilities. Specific suggestions should be followed by the opportunity to practice the new behaviors and report back on progress and problems. Most of the information in the remainder of this chapter will provide the basis for level 3 interventions.

Level 4, Intensive Therapy, would involve the use and adaptation of principles and techniques described elsewhere in this book to the sexual dysfunction of the disabled person and partner. Such therapeutic interventions are required by a minority of disabled or ill persons and would be appropriate in those with significant psychosocial sexual dysfunctions.

Diseases and Disabilities That May Influence Sexual Function

Diseases and Disabilities of Children, Adolescents, and Young Adults

Generally, children with congenital defects, such as phocomelia, meningomyelocele, cranial–facial defects (hairlip or cleft palate), deafness, and blindness, have reached or passed puberty at the time of consultation. Hence, sexual dysfunctions related to the specific disability will be superimposed upon the stresses of adolescence and a learning history that has precluded many normal social experiences of childhood.

Phocomelia

The phocomelic child will have been fitted with one or more prostheses depending upon the nature and the degree of limb deficits. Upper extremity deficits may profoundly limit caressing, fondling, and masturbation of self or another. Lower extremity deficits may reduce mobility and balance. The cosmetic effects of residual limb segments may be overwhelming to even the casual observer and contribute to distortion of self-image and self-esteem. Fortunately phantom pain or sensation is virtually nonexistent in these children.[27] With or without their prosthesis, they should be offered the means of exploring their bodies and those of others.

The double upper-extremity amputee usually develops superb prehensile function of the feet and toes and extreme hip mobility. Thus, he or she can perform nearly all upper-extremity functions with the lower limbs. However, intimates must become desensitized to the aesthetic aspects of such adaptive use of the lower limbs. Adaptations, such as sponge rubber inserts to the terminal devices of the upper-limb prostheses, allow their safe use for manual masturbation.[28] Lower-extremity amputees may require modifications of position and pillow support to prevent loss of balance and toppling from the bed during sexual activities with partners.[2] Limited mobility influences the mechanics of sex acts and reduces opportunities to participate in the usual range of social and sexual experiences of childhood and adolescence. The altered appearance of these individuals has a profound social impact.

Meningomyelocele

The child with meningomyelocele has sexual dysfunctions that closely resemble, but are somewhat less frequent than those of the spinal cord-injured individual.[29,30] The type and degree of neurological disruption of sexual responses will depend upon the level of the spinal cord lesion as well as its degree of completeness. Girls usually achieve menarche and become fertile. Most boys will have erections although their ejaculations, if present, may be retrograde into the bladder. Unlike girls, their chances for fertility are reduced. Nevertheless, both boys and girls with meningomyelocele as well as their parents require genetic counseling since their progeny is at increased risk of having the same deficit.[31]

Orgasms in both sexes may be altered, infrequent, or absent. Many of these children have had ileal loop diversion procedures and thus have a urinary stoma. Others with neurogenic bladders require indwelling catheters or diapering. Boys may be using external urinary drainage systems. These various methods of management all render the child susceptible to incontinence, leakage of apparatus, and problems of uriniferous odor, which require meticulous management in everyday social life and as a preliminary to sexual activities. If the social–personal costs of a catheter-free existence are significant, then the use of an indwelling catheter should be considered if possible. Neurogenic bowel problems are handled in a manner similar to those of the spinal cord-injured patient.[23]

Unfortunately, the cosmetic problems in the meningomyelocele child are manifold and attention to these problems must be a primary focus of intervention. These youngsters are often delayed in their physical as well as psychosocial maturation. Their height may be greatly reduced. Their limbs are not only atrophied but often deformed by contractures and dislocations of lower limb segments. They frequently develop kyphosis and/or scoliosis, which in addition to cosmetic effects may produce severe restrictive lung disease. Many of these children have accompanying hydrocephalus with its characteristic craniofacial deformities. They bear multiple scars of surgeries including repair of the back defect, shunt procedures, urinary tract diversions, and various orthopedic procedures.

Additional sexual dysfunctions arise from the effects of the hydrocephalus itself. Over 50% of the hydrocephalic meningomyelocele children demonstrate some degree of intellectual deficit.[31] These deficits range from a very mild spotty deficiencies to profound and more generalized defects. Among the commonest of these are perceptual deficits. These children may also have involvement of the motor system, which can further impede lower-extremity function as well as produce various disabilities in upper-extremity function. Such brain dysfunctions may require a general habilitation approach much like that for the cerebral palsy child.

Sexual dysfunctions consist of partial or total neurological disruption of erection, ejaculation, orgasm, lubrication of the vagina, and fertility in the male. In addition, social and sexual immaturity, which derives from the altered learning experiences of children and adolescents, may be present. Furthermore, the children may deviate from some of the customary standards of physical attractiveness, which becomes a crucial issue in adolescence when "being different" ensures rejection. Mobility and intellectual deficits further interfere with social acceptance.

Case Report

A. J. was a 14-year-old white female with meningomyelocele and hydrocephalus. Her spinal and cephalic defects had been repaired at birth. Mildly retarded, she was a sixth grader in a special education class. While hospitalized for revision of long leg braces, she experienced her first menstrual cycle, much to her shock and horror. Her mother admitted that she had never discussed this with her daughter. A. J. was unable to attain a regular bowel program, which resulted in frequent constipation and occasional fecal incontinence. She had a lower motor neuron bladder, which caused overflow incontinence, necessitating the use of diapers and rubber liners. She was socially immature, bereft of friends, and without experience in social interaction.

While still hospitalized she was placed on a suppository regimen along with stool softeners to control her bowels. She was taught effective Crede–Valsalva techniques so that she could dispense with diapers. Since she was overweight, she was given a weight reduction diet. The occupational therapist stimulated her interest in dressing more attractively, better personal hygiene, and the use of cosmetics and helped her to improve her social skills.

In physical therapy, forearm crutches were introduced as a substitute for previous axillary crutches. New leg braces were fabricated of a combination of plastic and metal to make them more attractive in appearance and lighter in weight. The nursing service focused on specific instructions for management of her menses and they provided an educational program concerning basic sexual facts. Separate counseling sessions were held with her mother to discuss these issues and to review the mother's knowledge. After discharge, further follow-up was ensured through the nursing service at the meningomyelocele clinic and at school.

Blindness and Deafness

Congenital deafness or blindness produces sexual dysfunctions that are more profound and pervasive than those produced by adventitious blindness or deafness.[32] The early loss of all visual experience often produces major distortions of body image regardless of the accuracy of the customary forms of sexual information. These adolescents may perceive the genitalia to be located in unusual sites or even of unusual size or proportions. Without visual clues, they have lost a fundamental means of communication in social situations. They cannot have eye contact with others nor can they utilize the myriad gestures and body attitudes that are so important in interpersonal relationships. They may have developed peculiar motor activities, such as nodding of the head and/or grimacing, which are distracting and may be misinterpreted as purposeful movements.

As with all forms of education, sexual information must be conveyed by substituting existing sensory input for that which has been lost. Lessons on sexual anatomy and physiology may be confusing if models are used whose size and texture does not conform to the patient's perception. Thus, there are those who advocate the use of human models for educational purposes to eliminate such misperceptions. Congenitally blind individuals may also assume that they are in private when they are not. Therefore they may require training in assessing whether they are alone before proceeding with intimacies.

The congenitally deaf have difficulties due to auditory communications.[33] They either obtain no sexual information or, like those with visual handicaps, receive distorted information, leading to major misconceptions. Their concept of abstract features of sexuality may be particularly limited by their receptive and transmissive deficits. These people are often more socially isolated than the visually handicapped, and they may be more ill at ease in dating situations. The speech of the congenitally deaf may also be unusual and present aesthetic as well as communicative problems.

Educational and counseling approaches should accent substitution of other inputs for the missing modality. Educators and counselors must have expertise with these disabilities and be capable of communicating effectively through whatever modality the person has learned. In addition, one must find ways to introduce abstract concepts despite language deficiencies.

Both visual- and hearing-deficient children are often institutionalized for special training. Frequently, these children are not educated sexually by either school or parents, with each expecting the other to assume that responsibility. Additionally, they are more isolated from the non-sensory-impaired population because they are institutionalized. Thus, their social maturity and sexual experience may be limited, and their innocent attempts at exploration may be misinterpreted as aberrations of sexual behavior. In these cases, a major educational effort must be directed toward personnel of the institution as well as the parents.

For both the congenitally deaf and blind, deficits relate to potential lack of or misinformation about sexuality along with the impairments in social maturity. The acquired deficits of infancy and childhood that are most likely to affect sexuality are listed in Table 2.

Cerebral Palsy

By definition, the child with cerebral palsy has one or more motor deficits. Of these deficits, spastic hemiparesis, paraparesis, quadriparesis, ataxia, or athetosis may compromise mobility to such a degree that the usual self-exploration and sexual discoveries of childhood are denied.[34] Later social activities and sexual contacts may be severely compromised as well. Spasticity is often accompanied by contractures, subluxations, and dislocations, which have cosmetic as well as functional impact. Visual, auditory, and other sensory functions may be involved. Communication problems, including aphasia and dysarthia, are frequently encountered. Seizures are also common. Intellectual deficits may range from none to profound. Thus, the management of

TABLE 2 Some Acquired Defects of Infancy and Childhood Affecting Sexuality

1. Trauma
    a. Cerebral palsy
    b. Brain injury
    c. Spinal cord injury
    d. Burns
2. Infectious sequelae
    a. Meningitides
    b. Encephalitides
    c. Disseminated intravascular coagulopathies
    d. Deafness
    e. Blindness
3. Hereditofamilial disorders
    a. Muscular dystrophies
    b. Hereditary neuropathies
    c. Juvenile diabetes mellitus
4. Tumors
    a. Leukemias
    b. Soft-tissue and bone sarcomas
    c. Malignant tumors of the brain
    d. Wilm's tumor
5. Connective tissue disorders
    a. Juvenile rheumatoid arthritis
    b. Dermatomyositis
    c. Lupus erythematosus
6. End-stage renal disease
    a. Glomerulonephritis
    b. Diabetes mellitus
    c. Polycystic kidney disease
    d. Pyelonephritis

sexuality cannot be isolated from the total physical–psychosocial maturation and development of the individual.

Sexual dysfunctions are related in the kinesiology of sex acts. These are largely correctable or modifiable by physical–medical modalities such as spasticity management, motor retraining, alterations of positioning in sexual activities, adoption of a passive sexual role, and assistance in preparation for sexual activities. Many of the sexual dysfunctions in these children, however, arise from their intellectual and social deficits. These children are often socially isolated, psychosocially retarded, and regarded as asexual beings. More often than not, their sexual education has been neglected. Even those with superior mental function may be socially naïve and unskilled. Their sexual habilitation must proceed as part of a total psychosocial restoration program. Educational and counseling services regarding sexuality must be geared to their level of cognitive, emotional, behavioral, and perceptual capabilities. The British film *Like Other People*[35] has eloquently addressed the sexuality of the cerebral palsy individual in its most elemental terms, namely, the right to love and be loved.

Brain Trauma

The sexual dysfunctions of the brain-traumatized youth may be quite different from those of the cerebral-palsied child. The greatest frequency of brain injuries occurs in the teen years and early twenties and is most frequently associated with vehicular accidents. Thus, the majority of these persons are adolescents or older at the time of their injury and, consequently, have had the opportunity to experience the typical social and sexual joys and traumas of childhood or adolescence. Although the physical aspects of sexual dysfunctions may be quite similar to those of the child with cerebral palsy, the emotional components are in many ways distinctive.

Characteristically, as these children proceed through stages of recovery from coma following severe head injury, there are periods of agitation and disorientation accompanied by aggressive, assaultive behavior and coprolalia. These periods are often followed by inappropriate sexual activities, such as open masturbation, attempts to seduce various hospital personnel, ludic sexual behaviors, or utter disinterest in all matters relating to sexuality.

More profound sexual dysfunctions may evolve after return to the community. Due to persisting intellectual deficits, these individuals may remain childish and inappropriate in their social behaviors, resist the effective establishment of interpersonal relationships, as well as create tensions in family members.[37] Their loss of interest in sexual activities may persist. Alternatively, they may become obsessive and persistent in their sexual interests, often in an inappropriate, childish, selfish, and demanding way. At the same time there may be dependency, passivity, and lack of responsibility, which produces a caretaker relationship with those closest to them.[38] These young people, in effect, can become different persons, hardly recognizable to those who were closest to them before their injuries. There is a high incidence of alienation, a feeling of abhorrence, and a disruption of former close relationships or marriages. Once again, management of sexuality must be incorporated through a rehabilitation program that emphasizes the reintroduction of the individual to society.

Case Report

D. J. was a 21-year-old white male who received multiple injuries, including a closed head trauma, in an automobile accident. He was hospitalized for some 4 months for a fracture of the right femoral shaft, a right facial nerve injury, which produced nearly total paralysis of the entire right side of the face, and a right hemiparesis and mild aphasia, which resulted from the head injury itself. He was discharged from the rehabilitation unit with residual cognitive and emotional deficits.

There was very little recovery from the facial nerve injury, which resulted in a marked cosmetic defect. He became fully independent physically and elected to move to an apartment with his girlfriend. This relationship developed after his injury. While hospitalized, he had a number of weekend passes during which he was able to enjoy sexual activities with the young woman. Although he was generally of good humor and cooperative with all the hospital personnel, he became moody and occasionally verbally abusive to his family and his girlfriend. These episodes mounted in intensity after discharge.

The couple continued to be followed by the rehabilitation psychologist for counseling regarding this problem. Despite her satisfaction with their sexual relationship and her acceptance of his physical status, she grew increasingly intolerant of the behavioral outbursts and finally decided to leave him because of them.

Spinal Cord Injury

Spinal cord injury is also a disability occurring with greatest frequency in the teens and early twenties, due to its association with vehicular accidents, falls, sports events, and violence. The sexual dysfunctions of this disability are similar to those discussed in the section on meningomyelocele. Unlike meningomyelocele patients, however, the spinal cord-injured patient may have severe spasticity that interferes with mobility and positioning during sexual acts. The spasticity may respond well to antispasmodic drugs, but these drugs may produce side effects, one of which is impotence. Those with lesions at or above the sixth thoracic level are prone to autonomic dysreflexia, which may be triggered during sexual activities.[23] This condition is potentially life-threatening and, therefore, must be properly treated. All possible stimuli, including bladder and bowel distention and sexual activity, should be reduced or eliminated. Rapid acting ganglionic blockaders, such as trimethapan, may be given intravenously. These drugs also may be given orally as prophylaxis.

Teenage girls who have spinal cord injury should be assured that they are capable of normal pregnancies and deliveries, although there are certain hazards with both.[39] Pregnancy may produce increasing difficulty with mobility leading to decubitus ulcers or falls. There is increased likelihood of urinary tract infection and anemia. Labor may be premature and precipitous, although usually caesarean section is unnecessary.

Contraceptive considerations should include avoidance of hormones because of the proclivity to thrombophlebitis. Intrauterine devices may dislodge without being detected due to sensory deficits. Diaphragms may be difficult to place in the case quadriplegics and become readily dislodged without a woman's awareness.

With spinal cord-injured men and women, sexual activities must be preceded by preparations that include assurance that bowel and bladder functions will not interfere. Assistance of a third person may be necessary in positioning and other preparations of quadriplegics. A number of techniques are described that may facilitate erections.[40] Men with low-level cord injuries or with incomplete injuries may respond to psychic stimuli; otherwise, multiple local stimuli, such as cold, heat, and various forms of friction including electrical vibrators, are often effective. If the male remains impotent beyond a year following injury, among the alternatives is penile prosthetic implantation.[41]

Other sexual activities, such as manual or oral stimulation of the female partner, should be considered if erection and penile–vaginal intercourse are not vitally important to the person and his partner.

Other problems with sexuality in the spinal cord-injured individuals often proceed from prevailing myths. They believe that absent genital sensation and flaccid genitalia allow no options for sexual activity. They may equate motor prowess and strength with youth and beauty. The early introduction of hospital educational and counseling programs for these patients, their families, and significant others, as well as the education and training of the hospital staff who rehabilitate these patients has done much to dispel these myths.[42]

Burns

Burns produce devastating disabilities in children. In addition to the obvious cosmetic problems of scarring of face and other exposed parts of the body, there is a cosmetic effect of the equipment that must be worn for long periods of time including masks, elastic gauntlets, splints, etc.[43] These children frequently have amputations and musculoskeletal deformities such as contractures. They are prone to polyneuropathies, which cause weakness and decreased sensation of limbs. Although they ordinarily have no problems with sexual performance on an organic basis, they are often beset with psychosocial problems.

Meningitis and Encephalitis

The sequalae produce primary and secondary sexual disabilities, which are quite similar to those of cerebral palsy. Disseminated intravascular coagulopathies produce multiple amputations and often severe scarring of skin due to multiple focal necrosis.[44] The amputations are often of terminal digits. If amputation occurs after the age of 2 to 3, phantom sensations usually result.

Hereditary Familial Disorders

Muscular dystrophies and neuropathies such as Charcot–Marie Tooth disease stand out as examples of progressive muscular weakness which affect sexuality. With aggressive pulmonary care, individuals with progressive muscular dystrophy (Duchenne dystrophy) often survive into their late twenties.[45] These individuals are confined to wheelchairs and may eventually require respiratory equipment in their homes. Their limbs become so weak as to prohibit manual masturbation. Yet they retain normal sexual responses and often unabating sexual interest. By providing an electrical vibrator, the one available expression of that interest may be continued. Unlike Duchenne's dystrophy, other forms of dystrophy may allow for a sufficient life span so that it is possible to consider marriage and a family. The progressive immobility of these individuals may make modifications of positions necessary. Genetic counseling is of utmost importance in these cases.

Hereditary polyneuropathies, such as Charcot–Marie Tooth disease, produce problems related to progressive sensory loss as well as weakness. These individuals may eventually function much like incomplete spinal cord-injured quadriplegics; however, they are flaccid rather than spastic in muscle function. Eventually, sensory disturbances may interfere with genital function and some cases of impotence have been observed.

Benign and Malignant Tumors

The common malignant tumors of early life impinge upon sexuality mainly by causing secondary dysfunctions. However, chemotherapy, radiation therapy, or surgery may have direct effects upon the sexual apparatus.[46] Certain of the chemotherapeutic agents, notably alkaloids, profoundly depress sperm production. This effect is usually reversible. Radiation produces a similar effect and may cause sterility, depending on the dosage and site irradiated. Other prominent side effects of chemotherapy and X-rays, including hair loss, nausea and vomiting, skin pigmentation, anorexia, and bleeding, may be ameliorated to the degree that they will not directly interfere with sexual function. Occasionally, leukemias may be associated with priapism, which in turn results in organic impotence.[47] Retroperitoneal dissection of lymph nodes as a treatment for testicular tumors may disrupt ejaculatory function.[46]

Many children with these disorders experience delays in physical and psychosocial maturation. Corticosteroids contribute to the cosmetic and maturation problems. Children surviving brain tumors may have significant intellectual, motor, and sensory deficits. However, the chief sexual disabilities consist of the challenges to body image and self-esteem in addition to the fear of all cancer patients: the fear of death, recurrent disease, pain, progressive disability, and dependence.

Connective Tissue Disorders

The most frequently encountered connective tissue disorder of youth is juvenile rheumatoid arthritis.[48] Since this is a systemic disease, fatigue and weakness, chronic pain, delayed physical–psychosocial maturation, inordinate dependence upon family, and despair over physical appearance are frequently seen. Neither the disease nor its treatments directly affect the sexual responses. The chief threat to sexual activities in a female is the painful, contracted hips, which may preclude intromission.[49] With the failure of conservative measures, such as analgesics, heat, limbering-up exercises, diathermy, and stretching, prosthetic joint replacement may be the definitive solution.

Case Report

B. C. was an attractive professional woman in her mid-twenties with prominent residua of juvenile rheumatoid arthritis. Her hips were nearly fused in a fairly neutral position, allowing her to walk in a mincing, painful gait. She would swivel on each foot to substitute for the lost rotary motion of the hips. The other stigmata of her disease were less prominent, mainly in the form of contractures of her fingers, wrists, and elbows. These deformities were inconspicuous as she sat conversing at social events. Whenever she caught the eye of an apparently admiring male observer, she would invariably arise and exhibit her peculiar gait as she approached another point of the room. This was her calling card, her announcement ''before you come any further, please be aware of this.'' Eventually she had bilateral hip replacements, which obliterated pain and increased her mobility. The impact on her social and professional life was momentous.

Renal Disease

End-stage renal disease is often a disease of youth. Like other severe systemic illnesses, it produces many symptoms that directly and indirectly affect sexuality.[50,51] Generalized weakness, malaise, nausea and vomiting, mental obtundation, edema, skin pigmentation, anorexia, and sensory disturbances of the limbs are all likely to decrease interest in sexual matters. In addition, these people develop impotence, ejaculatory difficulties, and orgasmic dysfunction at least in part secondary to progressive neuropathy. Although many of these symptoms improve on dialysis, the sexual dysfunctions usually do not. Males may eventually develop testicular atrophy with reduced sperm count, decreased testosterone secretion, and gynecomastia. As with so many disabilities, there is less information concerning women, although amenorrhea and infertility occur.

Diseases and Disabilities of Middle to Late Adulthood

Diseases and disabilities affecting sexuality in the middle to late adult years are presented in Table 3. Although the incidence of spinal cord injury and head trauma decreases after the thirties, there is another moderate peak in the late fifties. Those that survive the catastrophic injuries are often more severely physically and psychologically disabled.[52] They may be less mobile and less physically independent than their younger counterparts with the same degree of physical injury. However, they are more likely to be married, frequently with a long and stable relationship. They are also at an age where sexual activities may have already been curtailed or even discontinued. Thus, the partner may be content with physical closeness in the form of caressing or kissing without specific genital activities. However, a fair number of these couples may have been quite sexually active and, therefore, the guidelines discussed earlier regarding spinal injury apply. The presence of coexisting medical disorders must also be assessed.

TABLE 3 Some Diseases and Disabilities Affecting Sexuality in Middle to Late Adulthood

1. Trauma
   a. Head injury
   b. Spinal cord injury
   c. Multiple fractures and soft-tissue injury
2. Hereditofamilial diseases
   a. Diabetes mellitus
   b. Friedreich's ataxia and other degenerative neurological syndromes
3. Tumors
   a. Breast
   b. Prostate
   c. Gynecological
   d. Bladder
   e. Gastrointestinal
4. Musculoskeletal and connective tissue disorders
   a. Degenerative arthritis
   b. Juvenile rheumatoid arthritis
5. Degenerative diseases
   a. Peripheral vascular disease
   b. Coronary artery disease
   c. Stroke
   d. Hypertension
   e. Parkinson's disease

Diabetes

Juvenile-onset diabetes is often a progressive systemic disorder whose complications eventually produce sexual dysfunctions of various sorts. Fibrosis from multiple injections and fatty necrosis create unsightly deformities. Polyneuropathies result in atrophy of peripheral limb muscles as well as decreasing sensation of the extremities. Autonomic neuropathies result in impotence and ejaculatory difficulties.[6] Peculiarly, autonomic neuropathy in women diabetics is not associated with equivalent sexual dysfunctions as a rule.[53]

Other eventual complications of diabetes include severe peripheral vascular disease leading to amputations and Leriche's syndrome, the latter a prominent cause of organic impotence. Diabetic retinopathy may eventuate in blindness. Other later manifestations include coronary artery disease and end-stage renal disease. Lest too a dark picture be portrayed, it should be stressed that these outcomes are not inevitable nor should genetic counseling preclude marriage and children. Unfortunately, there is no certain evidence that strict control of diabetes prevents most of these complications.

Although less dramatic in its onset and progression, late-onset diabetes can produce the very same complications as the juvenile form. Impotence is the most common symptom, affecting approximately 50 to 60% of diabetic males.[54] In fact, impotence is often the first symptom of diabetes and may appear before other clinical signs occur. Prosthetic penile implantation has become a major modality in dealing with this form of impotence in selected cases.

Neuromuscular Disorders

Hereditofamilial disorders, such as Friedreich's ataxia,[55] are often progressive and involve motor functions predominantly. Thus, mobility may be impaired. Furthermore, Friedreich's ataxia may at times involve intellectual functions and may produce sensory deficits. Perhaps the most critical area of counseling in these diseases is the offering of accurate genetic information. With most of these disorders, there are no screening tests to discern carriers before the symptoms begin. These clinical symptoms may not appear until well after middle age.

Recent reports indicate that primary sexual dysfunctions are extremely common in multiple sclerosis patients.[56,57] Impotence, ejaculatory disorders, and anorgasmia occur in males. Equivalent difficulties are present in women. In certain instances, these dysfunctions are reversible, corresponding with the remissions of other neurologic signs and symptoms. Such primary dysfunctions are closely related to other neurologic findings including absence of sweating of the lower torso and lower extremities and decreased or absent sensation in the genitalia and adjacent regions. These problems and concurrent bowel and bladder dysfunctions should be managed in much the same fashion as with spinal cord injury dysfunctions. Indeed it appears that the basis for these neurogenic dysfunctions of multiple sclerosis is spinal cord lesions.

Benign and Malignant Tumors

Malignant tumors of the breast, ovary, uterus, bladder, testes, prostrate, and penis pose a direct problem for sexual functioning. Although radical mastectomy has been largely supplanted by modified mastectomy, the procedure is still viewed by patients as mutilating. Mammoplasty may be performed immediately after the mastectomy or within 3 to 6 months, provided that no contraindications exist, and may be important for improved body image and self-esteem.[58] Prompt fitting with a temporary prosthesis, to be followed by a permanent one, is a major consideration in early management of these patients. The unsightly problem of lymphedema can often be prevented by early measures offered by the physical or occupational therapist. These women should be counseled to avoid undue pressure on the chest wall soon after surgery. With this precaution, sexual activities may be resumed after discharge from the hospital. More advanced disease may require further extirpative surgery, hormone therapy, chemotherapy, or radiation. The use of testosterone may be associated with the expected masculinizing effects and it may produce increased libido. Metastatic disease to the bones may produce pain and pathological fractures, which often respond to combinations of radiation therapy and orthopedic stabilization or back support in the case of vertebral metastases. Sexual dysfunctions is usually related to loss of self-image and self-esteem, as well as to the general concerns of the cancer patient.

Carcinoma of the cervix may be treated by hysterectomy or radiation therapy. Generally, hysterectomy produces very little physical disability. However, radiation therapy can cause stenosis, adhesions, and coaptation of the vaginal walls producing dyspareunia or precluding vaginal intercourse entirely.[59] Early vaginal dilatation and resumption of sexual intercourse often prevents these complications. Radical pelvic exenteration (Werthheim's procedure) often produces a double ostomy plus shortening of the vagina.[60] Vulvar cancer results in a radical vulvectomy including loss of the clitoris and often stenosis of the vagina. Clitorectomy need not abolish orgasms. Creation of a neovagina is a possible option in such cases.

Bladder cancer is often treated with cystectomy and prostatectomy, vesiculectomy, and urethrectomy. Most men will lose erectile function but will retain orgasm without ejaculation.[61] After total prostatectomy for cancer, erection occurs only in exceptional cases. Transurethral resection of the bladder for benign prostatic hypertrophy often does not cause impotence but rather produces retrograde ejaculation. When erectile difficulties occur, organic and functional causes may coexist. The study of rapid eye movement phases of sleep with the penile tumescence monitor may further clarify whether an organic or functional cause is paramount.[62] Carcinoma of the prostate is frequently managed by orchiectomy and estrogen therapy. The side effects of estrogen include decreased libido, impotence, feminizing secondary sexual characteristics, such as decreased genital and body hair, gynecomastia, and changes in voice.

Case Report

A 76-year-old black male was found on biopsy to have adenocarcinoma of the prostate gland. Because of spread beyond the confines of the gland, it was advised that he have bilateral orchiectomy and initiation of oral estrogen. When these suggestions were discussed with the patient, he immediately voiced strong objection and indicated that he fully realized the potential consequence of not proceeding with the measures advised. He then stated that he was accustomed to having sexual intercourse each evening with his wife and that he would do absolutely nothing that would interfere with that activity. He was particularly concerned that the mechanism of ejaculation remain intact.

Case Report

A 35-year-old white married male was hospitalized with a carcinoma of the penis, which required radical penectomy and creation of a new urethra ventral to the site of the amputation. The operating urologist avoided contact other than routine postsurgical medical monitoring. The nursing staff recognized the man's need for counseling regarding self-image and sexual function and prevailed upon the urologist to refer him for consultation.

The consultants explored his feelings about the surgery and self-image, his previous sexual preferences, and his attitude toward masturbation. He seemed capable of using his imagination in order to create an orgasm-like experience in the current circumstances. Therefore, the consultants suggested that he practice rubbing the surgical area and, at the height of his excitement, try to mentally recreate as much of an orgasm as possible. After several practice sessions, he reported that his current orgasms were approximately 75% of the intensity of presurgical orgasms.

Tumors of the colon and rectum may require colostomy and, in the latter case, abdominal–perineal resection. The resection frequently results in impotence in males.[63] The colostomy itself may be perceived as a desexualizing and mutilating procedure; however, sexual functioning may be resumed. Many patients or their partners are understandably anxious concerning possible injury to the stoma during sexual activity. They can be reassured that a healthy stoma will tolerate such activity without problems and that there is no leakage or odor. Some patients report that the stoma itself becomes an erogenous zone.[64]

Joint Disease

Degenerative joint disease may interfere with sexual activities in several ways. The hips may be a focus of disease, causing severe pain and contractures. With women, this may be a major limitation, at times making penetration impossible.[49] In some instances, the disability is less severe and alternate positions, such as penetration from the rear, prove satisfactory. At other times, prosthetic joint replacements will be necessary. Arthritis of the cervical and lumbosacral spine produces chronic stiffness and pain, which may interfere with positioning during sexual activities.[65] The application of heat, presexual limbering-up exercises, and modifications of positions so as to avoid painful movements, often reduce discomfort during sexual activities. Furthermore, sexual activity acts as a potent analgesic in some instances, often allaying discomfort for a number of hours.

There have been reports of marked increase in impotence associated with chronic low back pain produced by disc disease.[66,67]

There is conjecture about whether such pain is organic in nature, secondary to sacral root involvement. More likely, it is functional in most instances. Availability of the penile tumescence monitor should clarify the basis of the impotence.

Amputation

The amputee in later life is most often the victim of peripheral vascular disease, unlike the younger amputee who generally loses a limb secondary to either trauma or tumor.[27] Most of these amputees have lower-limb deficits, which often become bilateral. Thus, their mobility and balance are usually more severely impaired than those functions in younger amputees. Additionally, amputees with diabetes or Leriche's syndrome may be impotent.

Sexual dysfunctions are often those associated with aging, the perception of castration imposed by the amputation in men, and concerns about altered physical attractiveness in women. Phantom pain may severely impede sexual activities. However, the cause of pain should be investigated since it may be due to organic factors, such as stump neuroma.

Stroke

The stroke victim has associated medical problems that may contribute to sexual dysfunctions.[68,69] Frequently hypertension, diabetes, and cardiac disease are antecedents to the stroke. The stroke itself may produce a variety of problems. A right hemiplegic often has severe communication deficits, such as apraxia or aphasia. Speech may include profanities or obscenities, which are shocking to the partner. In addition, what is usually the dominant upper extremity is frequently rendered insensate and immobile. Body mobility and balance may be profoundly affected. Hemianopsia may limit vision. Mental deficits, including memory, quality control, judgment, and emotional lability, may contribute to the sexual dysfunctions.

The left hemiplegic often has accompanying perceptual deficits, left-sided neglect, as well as significant problems with judgment and impulsivity. Victims of posterior circulation lesions often have quadriparesis, dysfunction of one or more cranial nerves, and ataxia. These patients will require extensive motor and sensory retraining with specific regard to sexual activities. In addition, they must often be taught appropriate times and places for sexual behaviors. They may profit by repositioning techniques that allow their still-functioning extremities to be uppermost. Hemianesthesia should result in redirection of stimulatory foci to the unaffected side. The sexual partners of these patients should be reassured that resumption of sexual activities will not result in a stroke provided there is good medical control of hypertension and cardiac disease. However, a major source of sexual difficulty often arises because of the caretaker role that one partner may assume.

Case Report

A previously healthy 39-year-old white male incurred a cerebral infarct over the distribution of the left cerebral artery. No contributory disease could be found. After several months of hospitalization, he was discharged to his home. He had residual hemiparesis and nearly global aphasia. By means of hand signals, he could indicate his desire for sexual activities. Despite this system of signals, he occasionally attempted to initiate foreplay with his wife in the presence of the children. Specific attention was given to this problem in counseling sessions with both parents. His wife was reluctant to discuss the details of sexual intercourse. She indicated that he was extremely satisfied and seemed to function essentially as he had before the stroke. However she derived less enjoyment, particularly because of increasing responsibility for his care and the need to return to work while he cared for the household.

Myocardial Infarction

The survivor of a myocardial infarction who has no medical complications may resume sexual activities approximately 6 weeks after infarction.[70] Since intercourse with one's customary partner rarely raises the pulse above 120 per minute, a patient who can tolerate other activities at that level should have no problems. Pulse or electrocardiogram (EKG) can be monitored for 24 to 48 hr. Submaximal stress testing with the EKG monitoring will give a more precise picture of activity tolerances for cardiac patients.

In the earlier literature, much was made of alternate positions as a means of conserving energy during sexual activity. A more recent study indicates that whether the healthy male is supine or prone makes very little difference in this regard.[71] However, similar studies of cardiac patients do not exist, and, thus, this report should be interpreted with caution. For men and women, the cardiac cost of masturbation is substantially less than for sexual intercourse.[72] Anginal attacks during sexual activities may be prevented by use of nitroglycerin before anticipated activity. Other precautions include avoidance of activity after ingestion of heavy meals and alcohol, at temperature extremes, and during emotional and physical fatigue. Concern about the frequency of occurrence of ventricular arrhythmias during sexual intercourse, early postinfarction and revascularization surgery remains[73] despite an earlier report suggesting that arrhythmias of submaximal stress testing are more frequent than arrhythmias in postinfarction patients.[74] Generally, coitus has no deleterious effect on the patient prone to atrial arrhythmias.[75] Coronary bypass patients should probably wait 4 to 6 weeks postsurgery before resumption of sexual activities. Similar to the stroke patient, cardiac patients and their sexual partners have unspoken fears that sexual activity may result in death. Actually cardiac deaths during intercourse appear to be extremely rare.[76]

Hypertension

Disabilities associated with hypertension are predominantly related to side effects of antihypertension drugs.[77] Most, but not all, of these drugs interfere with sexual functioning to some degree. The thiazide drugs reportedly inhibit vaginal lubrication and decrease libido. Propranolol has been reported, in rare instances, to cause impotence. Hydralazine probably has not been responsible for any sexual dysfunction. Prazosin causes impotence much less frequently than other antihypertensive drugs. Of the remaining drugs, the most potent, such as ganglionic blocking agents, cause frequent impotence and ejaculation difficulties. Additional side effects may include gynecomastia in the case of spironolactone, methyldopa, and clonidine hydrochloride. Spironolactone also produces menstrual irregularities and inhibition of vaginal secretions. Methyldopa may produce breast enlargement in women. These side effects may be reduced by carefully choosing combinations of drugs and reducing the individual doses.

Chronic Obstructive Pulmonary Disease

Chronic obstructive pulmonary disease, usually in the form of chronic bronchitis or emphysema, is associated with dyspnea, coughing, and wheezing on attempted vigorous activities, including sexual ones.[78] The use of low-flow oxygen with portable tanks and nasal cannulas may facilitate continuing intimate activities. Presexual pulmonary toileting such as postural drainage, intermittent positive pressure breathing, bronchodilator aerosols, and chest percussion may improve respiratory functions. Many of these patients should be advised to avoid compression of the chest wall. As with hypertensive patients, careful positioning of the head with respect to the feet may be beneficial. Systematic physical conditioning may benefit the pulmonary patient as it does the cardiac patient in improving endurance and capacity for tolerating sexual activities.

Management of Sexual Dysfunctions

The management of the dysfunctions caused by the diseases and disabilities discussed can be summarized according to the chief modalities of treatment.

Transfer Activities

In considering the kinesiology of sex acts, training and preparation often must include transfer activities for patients with severe motor disabilities. Such activities may often be shared by the partner or a third party who thus require training in movements to bed, couch, floor, wheelchair, or other suitable sites.

Preparations for Sexual Activity

Similarly, the disabled partner may require assistance for other preparations, such as undressing, positioning, bowel and bladder care, and placement of contraceptives. The arthritic may benefit from the application of local superficial heat or a shower or bath followed by limbering-up exercises. Preliminary postural drainage, chest tapping, and other methods as mentioned in the previous section may well improve respiratory function for the chronic obstructive pulmonary patients. If neurological diseases have reduced the control over bowel and bladder functions, routine emptying before sexual activity assures continence during intercourse. There are no deleterious effects of leaving an indwelling catheter in place. Conversely, it may be removed temporarily and then reinserted following sexual activities. Placement of a diaphragm may require assistance by the able-bodied partner when upper-limb function is reduced, as with peripheral neuropathies or quadriplegia. Local lubrication with a water-soluble substance should be provided in conditions where vaginal lubrication is inadequate, such as Sjogren's syndrome and spinal cord disabilities.

Stimulation of Erection

For those neurological disorders in which erections are not under cerebral control, a variety of regional stimuli may be applied in attempts to achieve erection. Tactile stimulation of the penis, particularly in the region of the glans and frenulum may be adequate. Other regional trigger points may be discovered in the perineal, perianal, and adjacent areas. Light touch, tapping, scratching, pinching, massaging, pulling of hair, vibration, heat, cold, oral stimulation, and digital rectal massage may be effective for this purpose. Women respond to similar stimuli with resultant vaginal lubrication and clitoral erection. Erogenous sites throughout the body should be sought. Where sensation remains intact, the breasts of these women become exquisitely responsive as do skin segments directly above the dermatomal level of involvement.

Erections may sometimes be elicited as a component of the mass reflex produced by scratching of the sole of the foot in spinal cord patients with upper neuron lesions. By use of the stuffing technique, a semiturgid penis may further engorge. The sexual partner may enhance this process by rhythmic grasping of the penis in contracting the perivaginal musculature, a technique best learned by performing the Kegel exercise.[79] The exercise consists of contracting and relaxing the pelvic musculature repeatedly as in shutting off and resuming urinary flow. An electrical vibrator may be more effective than any other methods as a stimulus to erection, ejaculation, and orgasm, as well as the equivalents in the female. Erections may be enhanced by the application of a rubber band around the base of the penis. However, this tourniquet should be released within a half-hour of its application. Fantasy and transposition of stimuli from sensate to insensate erogenous zones has proven effective.

Positions for Sexual Activity

Positional variations must be considered for a number of disorders discussed previously.[80] Severely immobilized patients usually assume the supine or side-lying position, often requiring support with pillows or padding. Above-knee or bilateral lower-extremity amputees may require support to maintain a level pelvis, whereas a single below-knee amputee rarely has difficulty with balance. Some amputees insist upon wearing their prosthesis for sexual activities. Paraplegics are usually capable of assuming the prone position during intercourse although this is virtually impossible for the complete quadriplegic. A sitting position in a wheelchair or supine, oblique, or side-lying positions with adequate support may all be attempted to learn which is most comfortable. Unilateral upper-extremity amputees and hemiplegics may prefer a side-lying position with the unaffected extremity uppermost.

Cardiac and hypertensive patients should avoid positions that require sustained isometric contractions. Therefore, relatively more comfortable positions than the classic missionary position should be considered. Sexual partners of women with severe arthritis of the hips may be limited to a posterior approach to intromission. For patients with discogenic and other spinal disabilities, as well as recent chest surgery, the posterior approach may offer the greatest comfort. By elevating the head of the bed, hypertensive patients may minimize rises in blood pressure. Lowering the head of the bed may facilitate drainage of bronchial secretions in chronic obstructive pulmonary patients and may prevent orthostatic hypotension in hypertensive patients.

Positioning techniques must take into consideration the potential hazards of fractures in those with osteoporosis. Postmenopausal women, patients with any disorder producing significant muscle weakness, individuals with hormonal inbalances, such as hyperparathyroidism (as in end-stage renal disease), and those on long-term corticosteroids are all likely to develop significant osteoporosis and, therefore, are vulnerable to pathological fractures. Such fractures also occur in individuals with metastatic bone disease. Direct weight bearing or undue leverage on these susceptible limbs must be avoided.

Variety of Sex Acts

Alternate sex acts should be considered for those who for any reason are unable to perform penile–vaginal intercourse.[23] A spectrum of other activities are available provided that there are no psychological constraints upon either sexual partner. These activities may range from gentle caressing and kissing to various types of masturbation, including oral–genital activity, as well as the application of penile–shaped objects, such as dildoes, electrical vibrators, and vaginal douche nozzles. One must consider this entire repertoire for homosexual as well as heterosexual activities.

Precautions in Sexual Activity

Precautions in sexual activities must often be specifically discussed during the educational training procedures. Patients with osteoporosis and metastatic bone disease should avoid direct weight bearing or sudden leverage as described earlier. Patients with recent surgery, such as radical vulvectomies, may not tolerate sexual activity until full healing has occurred. However, the recent mastectomy patient may proceed with sexual activity provided that minimal or no pressure is placed on the chest wall. Individuals with limited mobility or reduced sensation are prone to decubitus ulcers and must periodically alter positions so as to relieve skin pressure over major bony prominences. Spinal cord injury patients with lesions above the midthoracic level may experience autonomic dysreflexia during sexual activities. Patients with neurologic disorders should be instructed about the eventuality of occasional fecal or urinary incontinence. Their partners should be aware of the possibility of these events. Meticulous hygiene with frequent cleaning and deodorizing of urinary and fecal collection devices is important. Stomal collection devices are currently chemically treated so as to be free of odor.

The side effects of antihypertensive drugs were discussed earlier. Tranquilizers, sedatives, narcotics, antidepressants, anticholinergics, male and female hormones, antihistamines, corticosteroids, digitalis, nicotine, and alcohol have all been implicated as possible inhibitors of sex drive, erections, or ejaculation. Cardiac patients should be warned about the stresses during intercourse occasioned by anxiety or guilt, physical fatigue, extremes of humidity or temperature, recent heavy meals, alcoholic excess, and hyperventilation. Those with acute heart diseases, congestive heart failure, or functional classification IV (New York Heart Association) are best advised to abstain from sexual intercourse. Patients with prosthetic hip replacements should avoid forceful abduction or adduction to prevent hip dislocation. Those with chronic back disabilities should be cautioned about the painful effects of sudden turning, twisting, or hyperextension of the body.

Penile Prostheses

In selective cases of organic impotence where there has been very careful neurological and psychological screening plus inclusion of the sexual partner in both psychological screening and counseling, penile implantation devices may be considered.[41] The neurological disorder should be stable for a considerable period of time. For example, patients with multiple sclerosis may experience impotence, which is usually reversible. The patient and his partner should be emotionally stable and have realistic expectations and understanding of the effects of the prosthesis. They should be willing to continue follow-up for an extended period of time after the surgical procedure. The major current choices of devices are the Small–Carrion semirigid plastic prosthesis and the Scott–Bradley hydraulic implant. Both devices are highly acceptable to their recipients although the hydraulic device appears to be somewhat more acceptable to the partners.[81] The incidence of complications is somewhat less with the semirigid device. However, it occasionally produces cosmetic problems because of the persistent semierect state, and it is somewhat less lengthy than the hydraulic device.

Drug Management

In considering pharmocological management of sexual dysfunctions, one must conclude that sex hormone therapy has rarely been beneficial for any of the dysfunctions, including impotence. Comfort[82] mentions the occasional efficacy of Mesterolone in improving the impotence and well-being of the elderly male as well as increasing or initiating spermatogenesis. Male hormones have been used in recently injured male spinal cord-injured patients to treat gynecomastia and testicular atrophy. More recent evidence indicates that the reduction of endogenous androgen levels in spinal cord-injured patients is limited to quadriplegics and may be temporary.[83,84] There is no evidence that testosterone will modify sexual performance or affect eventual testicular function. There are no diseases other than the endocrine-deficiency states where male or female hormones are specifically indicated. The timing of administration of various drugs in relation to sexual activities may be of utmost importance. Use of analgesics in chronic pain situations may be timed so as to minimize pain during sexual activities. Antispasmodic drugs may be scheduled so as to have their maximal affect on reducing spasticity during sex acts.

Temporal lobe seizures occasionally produce bizarre sexual behavior.[85] These may be controlled by antiseizure medication. Sedatives, tranquilizers, and a protective environment may reduce impulsive or inappropriate sexual behaviors of patients with cerebral dysfunctions, such as brain injury, stroke, or degenerative diseases. Carefully timed combinations of antihypertensive drugs may have maximal effects on controlling blood pressure during activities that normally tend to elevate it. At the same time, it is possible to reduce side effects by combining selected agents so as to lower the dose of those that are most likely to cause sexual dysfunctions. The combination of drugs least likely to cause side effects include thiazides, hydralazine, and prazosin or propranolol.

Sperm Banks

Men who are about to embark upon extensive or prolonged chemotherapy and radiation therapy may wish to store their sperm.[86] Shortly after spinal cord injury, men may have a similar option although the method of sperm collection must be either by electrical massager, installation of intrathecal prostigmine, or intrarectal electrical stimulation.[23] When ejaculation is retrograde, the sperm must be collected from the bladder.

Exercise

Exercise programs have proven to be beneficial for sexual performance in certain chronic diseases and disability states. Those with coronary artery disease improve sexual function following general conditioning activities.[87] Similar programs may improve physical endurance during sexual activity in other cardiovascular, pulmonary, or neuromuscular states. Therapeutic exercise may improve range of motion of contracted hip or knee joints sufficiently to allow intercourse, which had previously been painful or mechanically impossible. Disorders of the neuromuscular and musculoskeletal systems may be accompanied by disuse atrophy and weakness, which can be improved by strengthening programs. Similarly, mobility skills can be enhanced by specific training in transfers and bed mobility. Spasticity may be inhibited at least temporarily by therapy techniques of prolonged stretch, local application of heat or cold, and inhibitory positioning. Such techniques may be transferred to a home setting to be used by the patient or partner prior to sexual activities. Gentle stretching and range-of-motion exercises for afflicted joints are often helpful in reducing stiffness and pain in various arthritic states. Patients with back disabilities may be subjected to various positions and maneuvers so as to determine whether or not pain will occur under similar conditions during sexual activities. As a form of exercise, sexual intercourse produces several unique effects. It may produce pain relief in patients with various musculoskeletal disorders for periods of several hours. At times it reduces spasticity for similar durations.

The assessment of physical capacities of patients with pulmonary or cardiovascular disease may involve several types of monitored exercise.[70] The Holter electromagnetic tape is a method of continuous EKG recording during daily activities. Recording of EKG, blood pressure, pulse, and respiratory rate may all be monitored during various types of submaximal or maximal stress testing on a treadmill or using bicycle ergometry. The Master's two-step test, a rapid ascent of two flights of stairs, use of the treadmill at 4 miles per hour, or bicycle ergometry at 600 kilopon meters a minute are all equivalent to 6.1 kilocalories per minute of energy consumption, the approximate level of energy expenditure at orgasm. Hence, if these tests are accompanied by no major signs or symptoms of distress, sexual intercourse can safely be recommended.

Surgery

Surgical interventions may be appropriate in certain cases. Musculoskeletal deformities interfering with sexual performance may be present in a variety of musculoskeletal or neurological disorders. Major difficulties arise from contractures of the lower limbs, particularly of the hips. Adduction contractures secondary to various forms of spasticity may be corrected by tenotomies, whereas joint contractures or pain secondary to arthritis may require prostheses.[49] Heterotopic bone may cause fusion of the hips in conditions such as spinal cord injury, head trauma, poliomyelitis, and occasionally in other neuropathic states. Once the bone formation is mature, surgical exision may be the treatment of choice. Lower-limb spasticity may be reduced or ablated by such procedures as peripheral neurotomies, anterior rhizotomy, myelotomy, dorsal cord electrical stimulation, or cerebellar electrical stimulation.[88]

Organic impotence may be treated by penile implant prostheses. Other plastic procedures include reconstruction of the vagina after radical cancer surgery of the pelvis or vulva, and penile reconstruction following penectomy for cancer. Mammoplasty is a major consideration for management of the woman following mastectomy. Upper-extremity function may be considerably improved by plastic surgical procedures in the case of rheumatoid arthritic or traumatic quadriplegic. Among the improved functions may be those associated with caressing, fondling, and masturbation. Women with pelvic deformities secondary to meningomyelocele, juvenile rheumatoid arthritis, scoliosis, arthrogryposis, and other neuromuscular skeletal disorders may require cesarean section because of cephalopelvic disproportion. Unremitting incontinence of the neuropathic bladder may occasionally be a primary indication for a modified Bricker ileal loop procedure, especially in the female. Impotence accompanying the Leriche syndrome may improve by corrective vascular surgery. An alternative to contraceptive techniques is either tubal ligation or vasectomy.

Adaptive Devices

Adaptive devices may be useful to those with a variety of disorders. Modifications of upper extremity prostheses, particularly in the double-upper-extremity amputee, provide capabilities for masturbation and other sexual activities without danger of inadvertent injuries. Upper extremity splinting or bracing will enhance similar functions in the quadriplegic, rheumatoid arthritic, poliomyelitic, or dystrophic individual. Electrical vibrators are potentially useful as stimulators to self or others for patients with upper extremity disabilities or neurogenic disorders, such as spinal cord injuries.

Contraceptives

The type of contraceptive used will depend upon the individual's motor ability and anticipated side effects. Women with malignant tumors of the pelvis or breast, hypertension, or vascular disorders with proclivities to thromboembolic or vasoconstrictive disease should be cautioned against the use of cyclic sex hormones. Women with significant deficits of sensibility, for example, those with spinal cord injuries, may have difficulties with intrauterine devices. These women may be unaware of perforations, expulsions, and pelvic infections. Similarly, such patients may have difficulties positioning a diaphragm or be unaware of its displacement. For similar reasons, the condom may be difficult for quadriplegic males to apply.

Timing of Sexual Activity

The timing of sexual activities may be a major consideration in certain instances. Many patients with chronic disease perform better in the early part of the day rather than the evening. Arthritic patients may feel best in the middle part of the day as opposed to the early morning or later evening. Pain and morning stiffness may be negating elements in the early hours, whereas fatigue and pain may amplify as the day reaches its end. With patients who are taking drugs causing side effects, such as lethargy and drowsiness, sexual activities may be regulated so that peak effects are past. Certain drugs may be critical in facilitating sexual activity, for example, analgesics, antispasmodics, bronchodilators, and coronary dilators.

An Integrative Approach to the Management of Sexual Dysfunctions

The principles of treatment that focus on psychogenic sexual dysfunctions have been discussed elsewhere in this book and should be considered to be basic to any approach to the management of those dysfunctions that are primarily organically caused. However, all of the fears, concerns, and anxieties associated with the physical illness and disability must be considered in defining the parameters of the sexual problem and in choosing the treatment strategy.

If treatment is begun while the patient is hospitalized, a specific room may be assigned for practice, but privacy must be assured.[25,26] Only so much can be accomplished through counseling alone. The opportunity to practice the suggested alterations in sexual routine is essential for treatment success, especially to reduce the anxiety associated with performance and physical attractiveness. The attitudes of the staff will influence those of the patient, and, therefore, all efforts should be directed at creating a comfortable and accepting atmosphere regarding a sex education or reeducation program. Passes from the hospital into the home environment provide a natural and more comfortable milieu for practicing sexual activities. However, if the couple have had an opportunity for some private time prior to a visit home, the pass will provide the opportunity for a more relaxed atmosphere during sexual interactions. Patients may be instructed specifically or generally before the practice session and time for feedback should be scheduled. The number of structured practice sessions depend on the needs of the individual case. Persons with compromised intellectual function may need specific instruction in the appropriate time and place for sexual activities; the behaviors of dating and courting; the mechanics of foreplay and lovemaking; the mechanics of sex acts with special reference to balance, coordination, energy conservation, and pain prevention; and means of reducing anxiety and fear. Brain-injured or developmentally disabled persons are more likely to profit from highly structured sessions in which specific behaviors and consequences are outlined.

Treatment strategies may include individual or team counseling with patient and partner. Although there may be occasions for the former, we concur with Masters and Johnson[21] that there is no uninvolved partner. Group sessions may assist individuals by hearing of others' difficulties and by learning from their successes and failures in coping with postdisability problems.[18] Groups may be structured around couples or disabled persons without the partner present. These sessions can be particularly useful for the presentation of audiovisual materials and didactic information (Multi-Media Resource Center). We are convinced, however, that the mere presentation of information alone is not usually sufficient to lead to behavior change and the resolution of sexual dysfunctions. Although these counseling and group sessions may be focused on the issues of sexuality, this topic must always be placed within the context of the broader issues of adjusting to the primary illness and disability. Without this broader emphasis, treatment will be much less successful.

Masters and Johnson[21] discussed the issue of surrogate partners, and we agree that surrogates may be helpful in certain situations. The disabled individual may not always have a partner, but this should not preclude this important part of a rehabilitation program. Ethical and political issues must be considered along with the values and religious principles of the disabled person before a surrogate partner should be suggested. There are instances in which a surrogate program should be possible. Ethical considerations become acute when one finds a disabled teenager who desperately wants to learn about sexual activities in order to gain some self-confidence before approaching an actual dating situation. Close consultation with the parents in these situations is mandatory.

State-of-the-Art Management of Sexual Problems in the 1980s

Our presentation of the parameters of sexual dysfunctions associated with major illnesses and disabilities is brief and superficial considering the tremendous complexity of sexual problems in these cases. Unfortunately, our truncated approach may lull professionals into believing that the usual consultation techniques are applicable in these situations. However, there is no simple behavioral or medical approach that can be used to assess or treat these types of sexual difficulties. Nor can the consultation be a "one shot" venture with the consultant spending an hour with the patient, making recommendations in the chart, and leaving the scene. Rather the assessment and treatment requires a considerable investment of time on the part of members of several disciplines who will work together to integrate evaluation data and plan a team approach.

One of the most deceptive aspects of these cases is the apparent simplicity of the sexual dysfunction. Focus inadvertently is placed on managing the medical aspects of the difficulty and the psychosocial aspects are assumed to resolve easily once the medical problem has been treated. This is not so. It is the *interaction* of these factors which creates the complexity in the evaluation and treatment process. They cannot be separated and treated in isolation. The sexual dysfunction should be placed within the context of the person's overall adjustment to the illness and disability and not viewed as an isolated phenomenon. Therefore, a team concept is essential, since no one discipline has the necessary background and information to assess and manage these cases alone. Furthermore, the members of the team need to know, understand, and respect the areas of knowledge and skill of each other in order to work together effectively.

The individual who chooses to work with these patients needs to be available for multiple meetings with the patient and partner and with other team members in order to share information and implement the treatment interventions.

Development of the Sexual Management Team

All effective sexual treatment programs begin with the education of the members of the sexual management team. This education process provides an opportunity to evaluate personal values and attitudes and to "desensationalize" the concept of sexuality.[89] One format for accomplishing this is the Sexual Attitude Reassessment Workshops (SAR) in which able-bodied and disabled persons are faced with a variety of sexual stimuli in an intense fashion and given the opportunity to discuss and consider personal feelings and beliefs about sexual behavior for themselves and others.[90]

Didactic sessions that provide information about details of normal sexual anatomy and physiology and the changes that are associated with various disorders must be offered to the rehabilitation team. The dual process of desensationalization of sexuality plus the presentation of complete information helps to create an atmosphere of acceptance and comfort among the staff, which is very definitely but subtly communicated to patients in the department. Educational resources include audiovisual aides of the Multi-Media Resource Center and a handbook entitled *Who Cares?* which is a compendium of information and resources necessary for an education program.[91]

Summary

This chapter has defined the problems of sexual dysfunctions associated with physical disabilities by differentiating between organic and behavioral dysfunctions. Both types of dysfunctions are usually present when sexual difficulties occur in physical states. Treatment of these problems is often best accomplished by a professional health care team knowledgeable in the medical–physical modalities and behavioral and counseling techniques.

Secondary factors that were discussed include premorbid psychosocial influences and attitudes in addition to mechanisms of personal devaluation and desexualization, fears, and anxieties about the primary disability. The problems are compounded when disability occurs in early life or congenitally since normal social learning is frequently lacking.

The evaluation process must include an assessment of the individual's premorbid, present, and future expectations of physical, psychological, vocational, and educational function. The sexual difficulty must be placed within the context of the overall adjustment process to the primary illness or disability. Thus, the evaluation will be more complex than in cases in which sexual difficulty occurs without a primary disorder.

The principles of management have been considered from the viewpoint of when to initiate treatment, who is best qualified to treat, how to introduce the subject to the patient, the importance of including the sexual partner in treatment, and the need to recognize and respect the value systems of the sexual unit.

References

1. Wabrek, A. and Burchell, R. Male sexual dysfunction associated with coronary heart disease. *Archives of Sexual Behavior*, 1980, *9*, 69–75.

2. Griffith, E., Trieschmann, R., Hohmann, G., Cole, T., Tobis, J., and Cummings, V. Sexual dysfunctions associated with physical disabilities. *Archives of Physical Medicine and Rehabilitation, 1975, 56,* 8–13.

3. Pfeiffer, E., and Davis, G. Determinants of sexual behavior in middle and old age. *Journal of the American Geriatric Society,* 1972, *20,* 151–160.

4. Trieschmann, R. Coping with a disability: A sliding scale of goals. *Archives of Physical Medicine and Rehabilitation,* 1974, *55,* 556–560.

5. Trieschmann, R. *Spinal cord injuries: The psychological, social, and vocational adjustment.* Elmsford, N.Y.: Pergamon, 1980.

6. Kolodny, R., Kahn, C., Goldstein, H., and Barnett, D. Sexual dysfunction in diabetic men. In A. Comfort (Ed.), *Sexual consequences of disability.* Philadelphia: Stickley, 1978. Pp. 89–97.

7. Wright, B. *Physical disability: A psychological approach.* New York: Harper & Row, 1960.

8. Haring, M., and Meyerson, L. Attitudes of college students toward sexual behavior of disabled persons. *Archives of Physical Medicine and Rehabilitation,* 1979, *60,* 257–260.

9. Goffman, E. *Stigma,* Englewood Cliffs, N.J.: Prentice–Hall, 1963.

10. Ford, A., and Orfirer, A. Sexual behavior and the chronically ill patient. *Medical Aspects of Human Sexuality,* 1967, *1,* 51–54.

11. Zola, I. Communication barriers between 'the able-bodied' and 'the handicapped.' *Archives of Physical Medicine and Rehabilitation,* 1981, *62,* 355–359.

12. Sheehy, G. *Passages: Predictable crises of adult life,* New York: Bantam Books, 1974.

13. Levinson, D., Darrow, C., Klein, E., Levinson, M., and McKee, B. *The seasons of a man's life.* New York: Knopf, 1978.

14. Berscheid, E., and Walster, E. Physical attractiveness. *Advances in Experimental Social Psychology,* 1974, *7,* 157–215.

15. Brown, C. *Down all the days.* New York: Stein & Day, 1970.

16. Robinault, I. *Sex, society, and the disabled.* Hagerstown, Md.: Harper & Row, 1978.

17. Harlow, H. *Learning to love.* New York: Ballantine Books, 1971.

18. Romano, M., and Lassiter, R. Sexual counseling with the spinal cord injured. *Archives of Physical Medicine and Rehabilitation,* 1972, *53,* 568–572.

19. Papadopoulos, C., Larrimore, P., Cardin, S., and Shelley, S. Sexual concerns and needs of the post coronary patient's wife. *Archives of Internal Medicine,* 1980, *140,* 38–41.

20. Bandura, A. *Principles of behavior modification.* New York: Holt, Rinehart & Winston, 1969.

21. Masters, W., and Johnson, V. *Human sexual inadequacy.* Boston: Little, Brown, 1970.

22. Hohmann, G. Considerations in management of psychosexual readjustment in the cord injured male. *Rehabilitation Psychology,* 1972, *19,* 50–58.

23. Griffith, E., and Trieschmann, R. Sexual function in patients with physical disorders. In J. Meyer (Ed.), *Clinical management of sexual disorders.* Baltimore, Md.: Williams & Wilkins, 1976. Pp. 206–223.

24. Annon, J., and Robinson, C. Behavioral treatment of sexual dysfunctions. In A. Sha'Ked (Ed.), *Human sexuality and rehabilitation medicine: Sexual functioning following spinal cord injury.* Baltimore, Md.: Williams & Wilkins, 1981. Pp. 104–118.

25. Griffith, E., and Trieschmann, R. Sexual function restoration in the physically disabled: Use of a private room. *Archives of Physical Medicine and Rehabilitation,* 1977, *58,* 368–369.

26. Griffith, E., and Trieschmann, R. Use of a private room in the treatment of sexual dysfunctions in the physically disabled. *Journal of Sex and Disability,* 1978, *1,* 179–183.

27. Friedmann, L. Rehabilitation of amputees. In S. Licht (Ed.), *Rehabilitation and medicine* (Vol. 10). New Haven, Conn.: Licht, 1968.

28. Comfort, A. (Ed.). Miscellaneous medical and surgical conditions. In A. Comfort (Ed.), *Sexual consequences of disability.* Philadelphia: Stickley, 1978. Pp. 227–232.

29. Wabrek, A., Wabrek, C., and Burchell, R. C. The human tragedy of spina bifida: spinal myelomeningocele. *Sexuality and Disability,* 1978, *1* (3), 210–217.

30. Shurtleff, D., and Sousa, J. The adolescent with myelodysplasia: development, achievement, sex and deterioration. *Delaware Medical Journal* 1977, *49* (11), 631–638.

31. Curtis, B. H., Butler, J. E., and Emerson, C. C. In *Symposium of myelomeningocele,* American Academy of Orthopedic Surgeons. St. Louis, Mo.: Mosby, 1972.

32. Hamilton, T. Sexuality in deaf-blind persons. *Sexuality and Disability,* 1979, *2* (3), 238–246.

33. Fitz-gerald, D., and Fitz-gerald, M. Sexual implications of deafness. *Sexuality and Disability*, 1978, *1* (1), 57–69.
34. Freeman, R. Psychiatric problems in adolescents with cerebral palsy. *Developmental Medicine and Child Neurology*, 1970, *12*, 64–70.
35. *Like other people*. Ravinia Highland Park, Ill.: Perennial Education, Inc. (Film)
36. Weinstein, E. Sexual disturbances after brain injury. *Medical Aspects of Human Sexuality*, 1974, *1*, 10–31.
37. Rosenbaum, M., and Najinson, T. Changes in life patterns and symptoms in low mood as reported by wives of severely brain injured soldiers. *Journal of Consulting and Clinical Psychology*, 1976, *44* (6), 881–888.
38. Lezak, M. Living with the characterologically altered brain injured patient. *Journal of Clinical Psychiatry*, 1978, *39*, 592–598.
39. Ohry, A., Peleg, D., Goldman, J., David, A., and Rozen, R. Sexual function, pregnancy and delivery in spinal cord injured women. *Gynecologic and Obstetric Investigation*, 1978, *9*, 281–291.
40. Griffith, E., and Trieschmann, R. Sexual training of the spinal cord injured male and his partner. In A. Sha'Ked (Ed.), *Human sexuality and rehabilitation medicine: Sexual functioning following spinal cord injury*. Baltimore, Md.: Williams & Wilkins, 1981. Pp. 119–133.
41. Melman, A. Surgical management of impotence. In A. Comfort (Ed.), *Sexual consequences of disability*. Philadelphia: Stickley, 1978. Pp. 167–176.
42. Eisenberg, M., and Rustad, L. Sex education and counseling program in a spinal cord injury service. *Archives of Physical Medicine and Rehabilitation*, 1976, *57*, 135–140.
43. Bowden, M. L., Feller, I., Tholen, D., Davidson, T., and James, M. Self-esteem of severely burned patients. *Archives of Physical Medicine and Rehabilitation*, 1980, *61* (10), 449–452.
44. Reinstein, L., and Govindau, S. Extremity amputation: Disseminated intravascular coagulation syndrome. *Archives of Physical Medicine and Rehabilitation*, 1980, *61* (2), 97–102.
45. Bach, J. Alba, A., Pilkington, L., and Lee, M. Long-term rehabilitation in advanced stage of childhood onset, rapidly progressive muscular dystrophy. *Archives of Physical Medicine and Rehabilitation*, 1981, *62* (7), 328–331.
46. Lamb, M., Woods, N. Sexuality and the cancer patient. *Cancer and Nursing*, 1981, *4* (2), 137–144.
47. Belt, B. Some organic causes of impotence. *Medical Aspects of Human Sexuality*, 1973, *7*, 152–157.
48. Herstein, A., Hill, R., and Walters, K. Adult sexuality and juvenile rheumatoid arthritis. *Journal of Rheumatology*, 1977, *4* (1), 35–39.
49. Erlich, G. Sexual problems of the arthritic. In A. Comfort (Ed.), *Sexual consequences of disability*. Philadelphia: Stickley, 1978. Pp. 61–84.
50. Levy, N. The sexual rehabilitation of the hemodialysis patient. *Sexuality and Disability*, 1979, *2* (1), 60–65.
51. Milne, J., Golden, J., and Fibus, L. Sexual dysfunction in renal failure: A survey of chronic hemodialysis patients. *International Journal of Psychiatry in Medicine*, 1977/1978, *8* (4), 335–345.
52. Jennett, B., and Teasdale, G. Prognosis after severe head injury. In B. Jennett and G. Teasdale (Eds.), *Management of head injuries*. Philadelphia: Davis, 1981. Pp. 317–332.
53. Ellenberg, M. Sexual function in diabetic patients. *Annals of Internal Medicine*, 1980, *92* (2), 331–333.
54. Krosnick, A., and Podalsky, S. Diabetes and sexual function: Restoring normal ability. *Geriatrics*, 1981, *36* (3), 92–100.
55. Tyler, A. Marriage, sex and counseling in Huntington's chorea. *Sexuality and Disability*, 1980, *3* (3), 159–161.
56. Vas, C. Sexual impotence and some autonomic disturbances in men with multiple sclerosis. In A. Comfort (Ed.), *Sexual consequences of disability*. Philadelphia: Stickley, 1978. Pp. 45–60.
57. Lundberg, P. Sexual dysfunction in patients with multiple sclerosis. *Sexuality and Disability*, 1978, *1* (3) 218–222.
58. Harvey, R. Breast reconstruction following mastectomy. *Frontiers in Radiation Therapy and Oncology*, 1980, *14*, 90–103.
59. Adelusi, B. Cortal function after radiotherapy for carcinoma of the cervix uteri. *British Journal of Obstetrics and Gynecology*, 1980, *87* (9), 821–823.
60. Donahue, V., and Knapp, R. Sexual rehabilitation of gynecological cancer patients. *Obstetrics and Gynecology* 1977, *49* (1), 118–121.

61. Boyarsky, A., and Boyarsky, R. Prostatectomy, sexual disabilities and their management. In A. Comfort (Ed.), *Sexual consequences of disability*. Philadelphia: Stickley, 1978. Pp. 133–152.
62. Karacan, I. Advances in the diagnosis of erectile impotence. *Medical Aspects of Human Sexuality*, 1978, *12*, 85–97.
63. Kirkpatrick, J. The stoma patient and his return to society. *Frontiers in Radiation Therapy and Oncology*, 1980, *14*, 20–25.
64. Wise, T. Effects of cancer on sexual activity. *Psychosomatics*, 1978, *19* (12), 769–775.
65. Rubin, D. Sex in patients with neck, back, and radicular pain syndromes. *Medical Aspects of Human Sexuality*, 1972, *6*, 14–26.
66. LaBan, M., Burk, R., and Johnson, E. Sexual impotence in men having low back syndrome. *Archives of Physical Medicine and Rehabilitation*, 1966, *47*, 715–723.
67. Shafer, N., and Rosenblum, J. Occult lumbar disk causing impotency. *New York State Journal of Medicine*, 1969, *69*, 2465–2470.
68. Fugl-Meyer, A., and Jaasko, L. Post stroke hemiplegia and sexual intercourse. *Scandinavian Journal of Rehabilitation Supplement*, 1980, *7*, 158–166.
69. Bray, G., DeFrank, R., and Wolfe, T. Sexual functioning in stroke survivors. *Archives of Physical Medicine Rehabilitation* 1981, *62*, 286–288.
70. Mackey, F. Sexuality and heart disease. In A. Comfort (Ed.), *Sexual consequences of disability*. Philadelphia: Strickley, 1978. Pp. 107–120.
71. Nemec, D., and Mansfield, L. Blood pressure and heart rate responses during sexual activity in normal males. *Circulation*, 1974, *49–50* (Suppl. III), 254–260.
72. Scheingold, L., and Wagner, N. *Sound sex and the aging heart*. New York: Human Sciences Press, 1974.
73. Johnson, B., Fletcher, G. Dynamic electrocardiographic recording during sexual activity in recent post-myocardial infarction and revascularization patients. *American Heart Journal*, 1979, *98* (6), 736–741.
74. Kavanaugh, T., and Shephard, R. Sexual activity after myocardial infarction. *Canadian Medical Association Journal*, 1977, *116* (11), 1250–1253.
75. Regenstein, A., and Horn, H. Coitus in patients with cardiac arrhythmias. *Medical Aspects of Human Sexuality*, 1978, *2*, 108–121.
76. Ueno, M. The so-called coition death. *Japanese Journal of Legal Medicine*, 1963, *17*, 535–541.
77. Papadopoulas, C. Cardiovascular drugs and sexuality. *Archives of Internal Medicine*, 1980, *140* (10), 1341–1345.
78. Kass, I., Updegraff, K., and Muffly, R. Sex in chronic obstructive pulmonary disease. *Medical Aspects of Human Sexuality*, 1972, *6*, 32–42.
79. Kegel, A. Exercise in restoration of perineum. *American Journal of Obstetrics and Gynecology*, 1948, *56*, 238–242.
80. Mooney, T., Cole, T., and Chilgren, R. *Sexual options for paraplegics and quadriplegics*. Boston: Little, Brown, 1975.
81. Furlow, W. Sexual consequences of male genitourinary cancer: The role of sex prosthetics. *Frontiers in Radiation Therapy and Oncology*, 1980, *14*, 104–107.
82. Comfort, A. Drug therapy and sexual function in the older patient. In A. Comfort (Ed.), *Sexual consequences of disability*. Philadelphia: Stickley, 1978. Pp. 183–192.
83. Naftchi, N., Vrau, A., Sell, G. H., and Lowman, E. Pituitary-testicular axes dysfunction in spinal cord injury. *Archives of Physical Medicine and Rehabilitation*, 1980, *61* (9), 402–405.
84. Claus-Walker, J., Scurry, M., Carter, R., and Campos, R. Steady state hormonal secretion in traumatic quadriplegia. *Journal of Clinical Endocrinology and Metabolism*, 1977, *44*, 530–535.
85. Blumer, D. Hypersexual episodes in temporal lobe epilepsy. *American Journal of Psychiatry*, 1970, *126*, (8), 1099–1106.
86. Chapman, R., Sutcliffe S., and Malpas, J. Male gonadal dysfunction in Hodgkin's disease. *Journal of the American Medical Association*, 1981, *245* (13), 1323–1328.
87. Stein, R. The effect of exercise training on heart rate during coitus in the post myocardial infarction patient. *Circulation*, 1977, *55* (5), 738–740.
88. Rosenthal, M., Griffith, E., Bond, M., and Miller, J. D. (Eds.). *Rehabilitation of the adult with traumatic brain injury*. Philadelphia: Davis, 1983, in press.
89. Cole, T. Personal communication, January 23, 1978.

90. Cole, T., and Cole, S. *A guide for trainers: Sexuality and physical disability*. Minneapolis: University of Minnesota Medical School, Multi-Resource Center, Inc., 1976.
91. Chipouras, A., Cornelius, D., Daniels, S., and Makas, E. *Who cares? A handbook on sex education and counseling services for disabled people. The sex and disability project*. Washington, D.C.: George Washington University, 1979.

13

Human Sexuality and the American Minority Experience

Adela G. Wilkeson, Alvin F. Poussaint, Elizabeth C. Small, and Esther Shapiro

Introduction

Each of the coauthors has been asked to contribute to this chapter both because of our expertise in minority mental health issues and because of our personal ethnic backgrounds. Dr. Poussaint is a Black American; Dr. Small, Chinese American; Dr. Shapiro, Cuban American; and Dr. Wilkeson, Puerto Rican American. We appreciate the sensitivity of our editors in recognizing that materials related to minority persons can be most accurately portrayed by those of us who know and personally esteem the various cultural groups to be described. Primarily because of this shared conviction, we have decided not to attempt to present material on other groups. We trust that the reader will recognize that there is a marked diversity between and within different cultural groups and will understand the importance of acquiring specific knowledge of the cultural backgrounds of all patients.

Ours is a country of many nationalities. Earlier concepts and hopes that life in America would be a melting pot, where persons of different ethnic backgrounds could live and work side by side as equals without emphasis on our differences, have been replaced by an upsurgence of cultural pride. With this, there is a new hope for and commitment to the experience of coexistence, with equal valuation and recognition of the different norms and attitudes of our distinctive heritages.

Adela G. Wilkeson • Harvard Medical School, Boston, Massachusetts.   Alvin F. Poussaint • Harvard Medical School, Boston, Massachusetts.   Elizabeth C. Small • Departments of Psychiatry and Obstetrics and Gynecology, Tufts University School of Medicine, Boston, Massachusetts.   Esther Shapiro • Department of Psychiatry, Beth Israel Hospital, Boston, Massachusetts.

Our principal goals in the preparation of this chapter are twofold. First, we want to attempt to sensitize clinicians to the pervasive and powerful influence of a person's cultural background on all aspects of individual self-concepts and interpersonal behavior. Concepts of health and illness, patient–doctor interaction, and sexual stereotypes are particularly germane. Second, we hope to stimulate interest in continued learning. Ultimately, the therapeutic orientation of learning from one's patients is paramount. Interacting with persons from different cultures, either by living in a foreign country or by close working relationships over time, can greatly enhance our awareness of the multitude of assumed cultural attitudes that form the social fabric of what is considered normal, admirable, and accepted behavior.

There is a paucity of validated clinical information available regarding minority group mental health issues in general and even less recorded on any of the particular aspects of human sexual experiences. A number of concepts relative to the consideration of culture and to the particular experiences of designated minority groups in the United States will be presented in the following section. In each of the three major sections that follow, an orientation to the general cultural attitudes of Asian, Black, and Hispanic Americans will be combined with a more focused discussion of available information on sexual issues.

Culture and the American Minority Experience

Anthropologists, whose discipline is devoted to the study of different cultures, have provided voluminous data on how differently (yet with equal success) diverse societies have met the various interpersonal needs of their members. Aspects of human sexual experiences and of health maintenance are only two of the many societal functions encompassed by the concept of culture. Concepts of disease and of mental health, expressions of subjective distress caused by either physical or emotional illness, health care and help-seeking behavior, expectations of health care providers by persons in need of assistance and the expectations providers have regarding persons who seek their services, and acceptance and response to treatment are all culturally determined phenomena. When dealing with individuals from different ethnic backgrounds, a clinician's capacity to interact successfully with a patient and/or family will depend largely upon the clinician's awareness of how the patient's cultural attitudes and expectations differ from his/her own culture.

In his introductory chapter to a recently published textbook on *Cross-Cultural Psychiatry,* Leighton (1981) provides the following definition of culture:

> Culture is a label for the total way of life exhibited by society. This includes material objects, or as they are called by anthropologists, "artifacts," and the relationship between patterns of livelihood and environmental resources. Our emphasis, however, is on what Hallowell has termed "psychological reality." This means shared patterns of beliefs, feelings and adaptation which people carry in their heads as guides for conduct and for interpreting reality. Besides concerning all aspects of human life, social relationships, economics, and religion, for example, culture as a totality contains patterns of interconnections and interdependencies among objects and events.

Leighton emphasizes the following aspects of what is defined as culture. First, culture is learned, not innate or instinctual. Second, a culture is a logically integrated, functional, and sense-making whole. Within this whole, however, there can be considerable individual variation. This is important to emphasize because of the fairly common tendency to think of members of different cultures in rather narrowly defined stereotypic ways. Third, cultures change and different parts of the culture may change at different rates. An important corollary to the foregoing is that the degree to which any particular subgroup of a culture (e.g., women or minority groups) can change is contingent upon the nature of the reactions and degree of accomodation of other subgroups in the system, particularly those that are immediately affected by the change. The two final aspects of culture emphasized by Leighton are that every culture has a "value system" and that the symbolic representation of this system is transmitted from one generation to the next by families. Recognition of the psychological reality of symbolic meaning and processes, where certain attributes, attitudes, ideas, and behaviors are valued, whereas reciprocal ones are devalued, are common ground between anthropologists and mental health professionals. As each individual identifies with parental values, they become integrally interwoven into each one's personality. Winnicott (1953) has in fact suggested that cultural value systems are substituted for earlier transitional objects and thus play an important developmental role in allowing for gradual decreased attachment to parental figures. As an infant attempts to maintain a sense of object constancy in its relationship with principal objects in its environment, ambivalent, intense, primitive, sexual, and aggressive feelings are split: aggressive, potentially destructive affects are projected onto external bad objects, whereas affiliative, positive, libidinal affects are projected and introjected in relation to good objects. Transitional objects symbolically replace the soothing presents of libidinally cathected parental figures providing a mechanism for assuring a sense of basic security. Pinderhughes (1970) summarizes these points as follows:

> There is a need in the child part of human personality for constancy in relationship to the principal object relied on, whether this be a mother, a transitional object, a family or a social group or some component of culture. Attachment to parents and to transitional objects weaken as cultural attachments develop. Whether they be adaptive or not and whether developing within one's group or imposed by outsiders, important cultural elements are clung to by adults with the same intensity with which children cling to mothers, lollipops and teddy bears.

Since societal values involve such an integral part of an individual's assumptive world, they are ordinarily not questioned or considered consciously. In fact, consideration of differing values can evoke marked resistance since it is experienced as a threat to a person's psychological integrity (threatened loss of object constancy is associated with fears of disintegration or annihilation of the self).

It is important to integrate consideration of a patient's illness and his/her interactions with health care providers into the process of clinical evaluation. Consideration of *the context of* a patient's presentation including asking the question Why now? is an important aspect of initial and ongoing assessment. For instance, the diagnostic assessment of a patient presenting with feelings of depression, frequent weeping, and refusal to take in food is clearly dependent on whether these symptoms have occurred in the context of a recent bereavement. The following vignette highlights the distinctive manner an unacculturated Chinese-American would experience and present concerns about a recent loss (Gaw, 1981):

> An elderly Cantonese woman who presented with the symptom of belching, which on upper GI series revealed no abnormal physical findings. She was depressed and openly teared when she mentioned her recently deceased husband. Using DSM-II diagnostic scheme, she appeared to be suffering from an acute grief reaction with features of neurotic depression. She denied, however, the presence of a depressive affect. She was very preoccupied with the fact that on realizing her husband was dying, she had touched him before he died. When she found him dead a few hours later, she was afraid his vital energy called "CHI" had entered her body. Her belching, which occurred frequently in the morning when she thought of him, was her way of expelling excessive "CHI" (gas) in her body. She was given some minor tranquilizer in an attempt to control her symptom of belching, but developed drug allergy in the form of urticaria. Her interpretation of the cause of urticaria was that bad "CHI" was escaping from under her skin. She interpreted her whole illness experience in terms of traditional Chinese belief in "CHI" or vital energy as causing her illness.

Knowledge of traditional Chinese beliefs about medical illness would eliminate clinical concerns of a psychotic reaction in this individual and guide decisions regarding potentially effective interventions.

Ascertaining a patient's age, sex, educational background, occupation, religion, social economic status, marital status, and place of residency are all familiar contextually relevant questions. Arriving at a diagnosis in essence requires careful delineation of *which patterns of disorder* are being manifest by a patient. Reciprocally, this involves *distinguishing normal behaviors and feelings*. Again, it is a person's cultural background that *provides the contextual definition of normality*.

Although learning specific culturally related material about any patient's particular background is of obvious importance, the capacity to openly listen to a patient's subjective life experience is a skill of generalizable value. Attempting to work with patients from different cultural backgrounds provides invaluable experience for therapists in their effort to learn to listen to patients from a nonprojective, empathic perspective and to explore inevitable countertransference reactions. A clinician's efforts to consciously review heretofore assumed attitudes about his/herself and others may be accompanied by transient distressful psychological reactions (anxiety, depression, withdrawal, defensive anger, etc.) depending on the particular significance of a given concept for the individual. A number of authors have noted potential countertransference pitfalls for cross-cultural work (Bradshaw, 1973; Ticho, 1971; Ruffin, 1973; Cohen, 1974; Boyer, 1964; Bernard, 1953; Wittkower, 1974; Calnek, 1970). Bradshaw (1976) summarizes a number of such reactions: They include a "potpourri" of overidentification, over compensation, condescension, and flight, all linked together by countertransference involving warded off aggression and compensatory mechanisms against feelings of inferiority and badness. Such reactions almost always occur vis-à-vis the recognition of descriminatory attitudes as these are in conflict with the altruistic motivations of most health care professionals.

Ticho, an Austrian woman analyst who practiced initially in Europe but also in Brazil and later in the United States, provides several clinical examples of countertransference reactions in cross-cultured work (Ticho, 1971). In one case, a young

Brazilian male had entered analysis secondary to the emergence of diffuse anxiety as he became engaged and anticipated marriage. Approximately 9 months into the analysis during which time the patient had focused on concerns about his betrothal and work issues, he spent one session being notably disturbed about a recent minor auto accident. Just at the end of this hour, he revealed that the accident occurred when he was returning from his weekly visit to a brothel. Dr. Ticho describes her countertransference reaction to this revelation in noting that a temporary breakdown in empathy occurred for her toward the patient and caused her to review her clinical impression of her diagnosis believing she may have missed evidence of sociopathy. This suspiciousness she realized was based on her cultural background and values that established expectations that a person would be in conflict and feel guilty about regular contact with prostitutes. However, as she further reconsidered the situation, she recognized that a much greater dichotomy between the good woman and the bad woman exists in Latin American countries. Linked with this is a marked double standard regarding sexual activity: Young men are encouraged to become sexually active before marriage and are often introduced to prostitution by family, members; young women are expected to have no sexual experiences until they marry. Reviewing these cultural values, Dr. Ticho recognized that her patient's involvement with prostitution had not been mentioned earlier because it was egosyntonic for him. She was then able to reestablish a sense of empathy with him and continue work on the emerging oedipal conflicts.

Studying the cultural attitudes of different minority groups can provide a major stimulus for clinicians to begin considering their own cultural values, which may not otherwise be subject to conscious reflection. A review of the predominant attitudes of our middle-class American culture, with its Protestant and Western European roots, can be facilitated by learning the comparative and contrasting attitudes of other cultures. Such a review could lead to further consideration of how prevailing American values influence current psychiatric evaluation and treatment (Sabshin et al., 1970; Thomas and Sillen, 1972; Willie et al., 1973), as well as the influence of such values on the presentation of psychic distress and dysfunction of white Americans (Draguns, 1974). Once accustomed to asking about a patient's ethnic background, one will find that it is a rare person who does not readily talk of his ethnic heritage with quite varied but unequivocal associated affect. Also learning how minority individuals have dealt with the pressures of change implicit in the process of acculturation and assimilation may help clinicians respond more meaningfully to contemporary American patients who are having to deal with rapidly changing cultural values. Values and attitudes toward sex are particularly noteworthy in this regard.

Utilization of one's capacity to learn from the patient of his or her particular life experience cannot be overemphasized with regard to patients who are members of designated minority groups in the United States. As mentioned earlier, the ubiquitous tendency to think of minority individuals in stereotypic ways must be continuously guarded against. Lack of familiarity with a culture tends to limit a person's awareness of the vast diversity within each cultural group. Thus, it is not uncommon for Americans to assume that oriental cultures are very similar, though, in reality, the cultural and historical differences between Asian countries (Japan, China, Korea, and Vietnam) are far greater than the differences between various English-speaking countries (New Zealand, Australia, Canada, United States, and England). Similarly, since there was a greater intermixing of Spaniards with endogenous Indians and Africans (initially brought to the New World as slaves) in Latin American countries, they are both as distinctive one from the other as the just-mentioned English countries and probably more distinctive with regard to what is maintained of their common Spanish heritage. Regional differences also exist within the countries of origin of American minority groups that are at least as distinctive as the deep South, New England, the corn belt, California, etc., in the United States.

The particular historical experience of each minority group since its arrival in the United States, with regard to the group's effect on contemporary cultural attitudes also must be considered (Bernal and Flores-Oritz, 1981; Alvarez, 1971). Particularly noteworthy in this regard is the experience of American blacks who were not only stripped initially of their freedom but also of all but the most privately guarded aspects of their original cultural identity during their years of enslavement.

Pinderhughes (1964, 1969a, 1971) describes the processes of adaptation (with their profound psychological impact) to the denigrative reality of slavery, de facto racism, and segregation that characterize the Black American's historical experience. Describing the underlying group dynamics of projective paranoia, he notes how American blacks have had to conform to false beliefs about themselves, beliefs that define them as less worthy and less human, as persons who must surrender themselves, defeat themselves, accept persecution, and seek direction from others. Transmitted within families, school systems, and the larger segregated communities, these beliefs have been incorporated into the Black American's self-concept. The difference between this Black American cultural experience and that of Black Africans is clear. The more recent World War II concentration camp experience of Japanese Americans is a more recent example. Enacted with this imprisonment is the realization that the rights of American Japanese are not guaranteed by the white majority. The inevitable scars of bitterness and hatred as well as mistrust and insecurity will continue to influence Japanese Americans for many generations much as the psychological consequences of the Holocaust affect Jewish people around the world.

The degree and particular mode of acculturation and assimilation any individual minority has experienced is yet another variable that requires consideration (Padilla, 1977). The cultural issues and conflicts of a first-generation immigrant differ from cultural struggles of second-generation adolescents that again are different from the cultural concerns of fourth-generation members of the same minority group. The distinction between assimilation and acculturation is important. *Assimilation* refers to the process of successful adaptation to the predominant culture without necessarily relinquishing or changing cultural attitudes and value identifications. The term *acculturation* is used to describe the process of changing value orientation, that is, substituting and adopting majority American cultural norms in place of one's original ethnic group values. Struggling with biases, experiencing overt and covert discrimination because of one's ethnic background (usually for the first time), and being unfamiliar with a new set of cultural values are all part of the stress new immigrants must grapple with. Simultaneously, leaving one's country of origin involves substantial loss. There is at least a transient threat to a person's identity, as each person's identity is in part maintained by the experience of continuity and consistency of one's self within a social network. The degree to which each immigrant either holds to their cultural identity in an effort to minimize the experience of loss or more readily relinquishes aspects of what was left behind in the hope of feeling accepted into the new group is quite individually determined. Szapocsnik's (1981) research with Cuban immigrants suggests that biculturalism, or the fluid integration of aspects of both the culture of origin and the new culture, offers the best adaptation to immigration.

Acquisition of a second language is a particularly important component of the process of acculturation. Clinical work with bilingual and/or monolingual non-English-speaking patients presents particular difficulties. Immigrant families also experience language-related strain. Children generally learn English more quickly than their parents. Becoming more accustomed to an English-speaking environment can lead to children losing full communication access with their parents. In some families, children become the mediators between their parents and the outside world, which sometimes presents a reversal of the traditional family roles and an undermining of parental authority.

The aforementioned examples of distinctive historical experiences also highlight the phenomenon of discrimination and prejudice that impact each American minority group. Discriminatory prejudicial attitudes are part of our culture and as such have had a profound effect on all members of our society as the previously mentioned attitudes toward human sexuality and health care maintenance. Discrimination and prejudice are actually intracultural experiences. They relate to how any given culture distinguishes and attaches different values to various human attributes and activities. Ethnocentric biases are in actuality not a rare occurrence. Many authors have noted that the denigration of a minority group and simultaneous aggrandizement of a majority group (or more powerful group) is a ubiquitous pattern of human behavior (Wilkeson, 1981b). Person (1969) summarizes this point as follows:

> History as the story of mankind chronicles largely the resolution and non-resolution of group conflicts. The group may be defined by a distinction of race, religion, language, culture, class or geographical boundaries but the distinction is jealously guarded and is usually prized at about the value of common humanity. Prejudice, national supremacy, manifest destinies, wars and genocide on behalf of such group distinctions span the centuries and continents and seem almost universal.

Though a discussion of the ubiquitous and pervasive processes that perpetuate racial discrimination is beyond the scope of this chapter, it is apparent that clinical sensitivity to their impact is warranted. The following references are particularly valuable for further reading (Pinderhughes, 1964, 1969a, 1969b, 1970, 1971, 1974, 1979; Kovel, 1970; Willie et al., 1973, Allport, 1954; Jones, 1972).

The fact that discrimination and prejudice do exist means that ethnic minorities are to a greater or lesser extent barred from access to the goods and privileges most Americans take for granted. Stereotypic prejudicial attitudes are integrally interwoven into all facets of our daily interactions and greatly reduce the chances of minority individual's advancement. Majority and minority individuals alike share the responsibility for perpetuating the problem. Denial and consciously expressed good intentions are pitfalls for members of the majority culture. Projection and attribution of blame for difficult circumstances to the felt oppressor are problems for individuals who are the objects of discrimination. Though majority and minority individuals share the cultural identity of being Americans, it is important clinically to recognize that interaction between physician and patient of different ethnic backgrounds will inevitably evoke stereotypic, racially laden projections. Based both on their social/historical experiences and on the underlying emotional insecurities that have prompted seeking professional assistance, minority individuals will fear racial bias on the part of the majority clinician. It is unlikely that a therapeutic alliance can be created without clinicians being aware of and responsive to both the external and internal determinations of such apprehensions.

All persons have fears of not belonging as well as feelings of inadequacy and insecurity. Parental values and attitudes provide labels and categories for a child's continuous struggle to create some sense of order and continuity in his/her inner world. Minority individuals who have grown up in a culture where they and their families for any number of generations have been the objects of discrimination do have to eventually personally struggle with their devalued early introjects and question any way these ethnically linked self-concepts may contribute to the evocation and propagation of discriminatory processes (i.e., seeking punishment for what is considered bad). Majority individuals reciprocally must struggle with the guilt associated with their utilization of aggrandizement and aggression as a means of warding off similar feelings of inadequacy.

Finally, with regard to the phenomenon of discrimination, it is important to recognize that discriminatory practices are pervasive in psychiatry as well as other fields (Sabshin et al., 1970; Thomas and Sillen, 1972; Willie et al., 1973). The prevalence of stereotypic biases is one of several factors limiting available information on the mental health and sexual concerns of minority ethnic groups. From the perspective of the psychotherapist working through transferential distortions, the problems of subjective bias are familiar. Biases are at times blatant and at other times more subtle. Examples of the latter are studies that present data correlating low self-esteem with minority group identification without ascertaining relative degrees of self-esteem or asking culturally sensitive questions that would tap feelings of ethnic pride (Dworkin, 1965, 1971).

Overall, relatively little has been written about ethnic minorities. In part, this is attributable to the fact that many were not provided any accessible mental health care until the Community Mental Health (CMH) Act of the early 1960s. Underrepresentation of minorities within mental health professions, inattention to minority concerns, and lack of adequate recording of basic demographic data have also limited available knowledge. With the establishment of the CMH system and the gradual accumulation of experience, community psychiatrists have begun to replace uniformed myths with clinical data. Failure to distinguish the impact of low socioeconomic status on minority individuals has further compounded the problems of obtaining adequate data (Casavantes, 1971; Guerray, 1971). There have, however, been a number of reports that ascertain distinctive sexual experiences between members of low and middle socioeconomic classes. Since a high percentage of impoverished Americans are of minority backgrounds, these reports will be summarized separately as aspects of the "culture of poverty."

Briefly summarizing what is described earlier is an integration of the conceptualization of culture into all aspects of a clinician's work. A definition of culture is followed by noting the interrelationship of cultural value systems and individual personality development.

Each American minority individual's experience is distinctive in a number of ways from that of his/her majority counterpart. Ethnic heritage is deeply interwoven with an individual's self-concept and invariably esteemed as the original in-group of a child's world. The degree of adherence to the values of one's culture varies from generation to generation and substantially between individuals. Similarly variable is the manner by which each minority individual wrestles with the biased sterotypic perception and discriminatory behavior that form integral parts of his/her daily life. For many, segregating processes are the principal factors in the propagation of a life of poverty, with concomitant feelings of futility, lack of access to adequate education, etc. These societal issues are external realities that impinge on a minority individual's life and have been psychologically incorporated into aspects of their self-concepts. Ultimately, their influence is worthy of consideration during the evaluation of sexual concerns of minority patients. Clinicians who work with minority individuals and who have sufficiently worked through their own countertransferential conflicts with the distinctive experience of cross-cultural work, in the context of a culture where racial discrimination persists, will be able to add much needed data on how culturally determined attitudes and values impact on the more intimate realm of sexual experience.

Black Sexuality: Myth and Reality*

Introduction

There are numerous stereotypes and at least as many myths about so-called "black sexuality" that have been generated in an American society permeated to a great degree by white racist practices. Allport writes in his classic, *The Nature of Prejudice,*

> There is a subtle psychological reason why Negroid characteristics favor an association of ideas with sex. The Negro seems dark, mysterious, distant—yet at the same time warm and potentially accessible. Sex is forbidden; colored people are forbidden; the ideas begin to fuse. It is no accident that prejudiced people call tolerant people "nigger-lovers." The very choice of the word suggests that they are fighting the feeling of attraction in themselves. (Allport, 1958, p. 351)

This ambiguous national environment has had a significant social and psychological impact on the Afro-American's sexual behavior and has profoundly distorted sexual relationships between blacks and whites (Grier and Cobbs, 1968; Halsell, 1972; Day, 1972; Gutman, 1976). Its effects have even been seen to hamper efforts to create a functioning community of interests between the races.

*Alvin F. Poussaint

Historical Background

Current issues in black sexuality can be traced to slavery and its aftermath. Blacks who were first brought to America's shores were stripped almost completely of their cultural heritage (Frazier, 1961). Slaves were torn from their families and communities in Africa and deposited in this country without consideration for kinship ties or social relationships. No respect or understanding of African concepts of what was normal and acceptable in sex was shown by the slaveholders. Instead, the white masters, from their often hypocritical Puritan perspective, construed black sexual behavior as savage, bestial, and immoral. They were unable or unwilling to recognize what now has become obvious fact: The sex life of Africans from childhood to marriage followed a well-defined social arrangement. Sex was not generally viewed in moralistic terms but as one aspect of the function of social groupings. Many African sexual practices naturally differed from those of Western nations, but a social system for sexual function was very much in evidence (Hambly, 1961).

In the New World, without the structure of their own societies, black people had to find new avenues for sexual expression. Raw sexual impulses were apparent, because new rules had been crudely imposed under conditions in which blacks were enslaved and abused. Slavery was hardly the setting in which to develop sexual attitudes and behaviors to replace those that were well integrated into established family structures and cultural mores.

Plantation life as well as the haphazard sale of slaves often prevented the formation of new family institutions, which would then influence the sexual styles of these unwilling new inhabitants. According to historical reports, sexual relations on the slave plantations were very casual and could be ended when a partner was sold or when the white master decided to break up a slave liaison that displeased him. In addition, there was considerable sex between adolescents, which led to many so-called "out-of-wedlock" pregnancies, further convincing some whites that blacks were "hot-blooded." The truth, however, is that European customs and morality were not assimilated; furthermore, slaves often did not even have the right to formally marry.

However, Gutman (1976) reports in his well-documented study of the black family during slavery that although premarital intercourse was common among the slaves, it was not an indication of indiscriminate mating. Most women, he reports, had all of their children by a single father. He argues that sexual activity among slaves was not "casual" as other historians have suggested. Sexual fidelity was an expected standard among married slaves. He concludes that "no aspect of slave behavior has been more greatly misunderstood than sexual mores and practices" (Gutman, 1976).

Current Issues

Be that as it may, today the black community is coping with value conflicts and the legacies of slavery, which are reflected in nonnormative sexual practices. A recent report indicates that the percentage of children under 18 in single families is about 14% for whites and 45% for blacks (National Research Council, 1976). Some social science observers in low-income black communities report a strong sexual awareness among black children of elementary school age, which is not typically the pattern of middle-class youngsters, black or white (Bernard, 1966; Reiss, 1975; Silverstein and Krate, 1975). Black males, in particular, engage in a great deal of verbal sexual repartee often called the *dozens*. The following observation was made of black female teenagers in Harlem:

> Many ghetto daughters and mothers regard a pregnancy outside marriage as a mistake that is regrettable, but the baby is usually accepted as a member of the girl's family without stigma. Black teenage girls generally regard having a baby as a symbol of womanhood. (Silverstine and Krate, 1976, p. 116)

Although the out-of-wedlock birthrate among white teenagers is on a steep rise, the attention paid to black illegitimacy rates gives the widespread impression, originating from slave times, of black sexual promiscuity. Joyce Ladner, a respected sociologist who conducted a study of low-income black female teenagers concluded

> Still, their attitudes and behavior toward premarital sex emerge out of a value context within the black community. . . . They are also informally socialized in a tradition that places high value on the positive features of sexual involvement—within or without marriage. The moral stigma is not nearly so strong as in middle-class society because sex is considered a very human act. . . . (Ladner, 1971, p. 215)

Many whites did not see blacks as having *different* morals but instead labeled them as "loose morals," an accusation that generated other black sexual stereotypes, which were passed down and today still have a significant impact on the black experience. White preoccupation with fantasies of animalistic black sexual prowess have come to profoundly influence sexual–racial politics in America (Thomas and Sillen, 1972).

The actual sexual behavior of blacks has been so misrepresented that it is difficult to obtain an objective scientific impression. In fact, one is struck with the lack of critical sociological and psychological studies of black sexual behavior. Kinsey's classic survey of sexual behavior in the human male and female three decades ago scarcely mentions the black population (Kinsey et al., 1948, 1953). More recently, the pioneering work of Masters and Johnson (1966) in *Human Sexual Response* does not report on the small number of black subjects in their study. Similarly, the extremely popular bestseller, *Everything You Wanted to Know about Sex but Were Afraid to Ask* refers to blacks only in stereotypic comments about their affinity for venereal diseases (Reuben, 1969). Although blacks do have higher rates of venereal disease, those figures result from poverty and poor health care rather than from race *per se* (Pettigrew, 1964). Scientific neglect of black sexual behavior is particularly surprising when one considers the widespread popular attention that has been focused on sexual themes in black stereotypes and in black–white relationships.

It is difficult, therefore, to discuss black sexuality analytically and then support it with carefully evaluated scientific data. It is difficult (and perhaps impossible) to categorize the sexual behavior of a whole race. In addition, statistical differences between races or groups tend to blur the extent to which races and groups behave similarly. Thus, it is not legitimate to refer to white sexuality and black sexuality (though we do so here for the sake of convenience). Sexual behavior of a particular black individual will depend on many variables, prime among which are socioeconomic and class factors. Reports indicate that blacks suffer from the same type and range of sexual problems, such as impotency and orgasmic dysfunction, as whites. Rates of homosexuality and other alternative forms of sexual release are felt to be similar among the white and black populations (Staples, 1981). However, it is clear that sexual exploitation and sexual stereotypes remain serious issues in the behavior and psychology of black Americans.

Clinical Implications

Dr. Kenneth Clark, a prominent black psychologist, suggests that in U.S. society, sex is a prime measure of personal success and feelings of self-worth, and, therefore, sexual images have had an especially important impact on the black psyche (Clark, 1965).

Many whites have viewed blacks as genetically inferior and have frantically condemned interracial marriage or the "mongrelization" of the white race. At the same time, white men considered illicit and abusive sexual contact with black women as appropriate to their position of power. Many white men arranged to have both black and white women available to them while denying the black male access to white women. Additionally, black men often could not withhold or protect their women from white men. Not surprisingly it followed that black males were emasculated not only sexually but economically, socially, and politically. The theme of powerlessness is central to the black experience in America and intrudes significantly in black sexual activity as it would with any racial or ethnic group in similar circumstances.

Whenever an entire racial group is degraded and oppressed, compensatory attitudes and behavior usually develop in its members. For example, it has been observed by clinicians that because of societal images of blacks as sexually animalistic, many blacks, particularly those in the middle class, have reacted by adopting strong Victorian attitudes about sex (Kardiner and Ovesey, 1955). Some black parents overcompensating for negative sexual images raised their children to be erotically restricted. Young middle-class black females especially were taught to follow strict moral codes in order to project an image in contradiction to the prevailing stereotypes.

Today, many black women are overly sensitive to any attitudes that suggest that they are sexually promiscuous (Karon, 1975). This is only one example of the psychological price black people have had to pay and continue to pay because of demeaning sexual images. Kardiner and Ovesey concluded that

> the most surprising fact about the sex life of the Negro of all classes—lies in its marked deviation from the white stereotypes that exist on the subject. The Negro is hardly the abandoned sexual hedonist he is supposed to be. (Kardiner and Ovesey, 1955, p. 69)

The Black Woman

The black woman, like the black man, occupies a lurid sexual image in the unconscious of many whites. But the black woman, sought after by white men for sexual gratification, was otherwise degraded as ugly and socially undesirable. Blackness itself was viewed as dirty. The prevailing, idealized standards of beauty and grace were and continue to be focused on white physical characteristics. So-called "Negroid" features and hair were not seen as attractive. Thus, an additional effect of racism was to cause many blacks (particularly those of darker complexion) to feel sexually unwanted as well as a sexual threat to the whole society (Grier and Cobbs, 1968).

Black women, in a society where men do the courting and male chauvinism prevails, have not only felt the pain of being rejected by white males as mates but have often been denied approval and admiration from black men as well. Within the black community, there has been a color hierarchy that incorporates racist feelings and contributes to group self-hatred. Lighter-skinned black women with straight hair were frequently preferred by black men. Black women who did not fit that image often became demoralized, depressed, and bitter. Grier and Cobbs summarize

> . . . depreciated by her own kind, judged grotesque by her society, and valued only as a sexually convenient laboring animal, the black girl has the disheartening prospect of a life in which the cards are stacked against her and the achievement of a healthy mature womanhood seems a very long shot indeed. (Grier and Cobbs, 1968, p. 41)

The black woman has had to endure the additional burden of the "superwoman" image—strong and self-sufficient. Because of the responsibilities she had to share outside in employment and in managing a marriage and a household, she was often labeled as a "matriarch" and a "mammy." These images usually connoted an overweight, unattractive, loud-talking, aggressive woman who, by American standards, was sexually unattractive (Herskovits, 1958; Staples, 1981). Grier and Cobbs (1968) have speculated that many black women give up trying to be attractive and become obese and unkempt, because they feel no hope of being attractive under standards that do not apply to their racial characteristics. Black women usually seen as attractive in America have to be overwhelmingly fair-skinned, mulatto types with straight hair, but darker women have become more popular recently.

In our society, attractiveness for a woman still remains a significant aspect of her self-image and feelings of sexual desirability. Therefore, there is no doubt that the pressures on black women have contributed significantly to various forms of sexual dysfunction and incompatibility.

The Black Man

Historically, the presumed hypersexuality of blacks was seen as evidence of their bestiality. Since white men first began to explore Africa, they have returned with wild tales about the large size of black male genitalia. Currently, there is no controlled scientific study that presents data on the size of the black penis versus the white penis. However, it is known that penises in both groups range widely from very small to very large. In any case, it is widely accepted among sex researchers that the size of the penis *per se* has little to do with the sexual satisfaction of one's partner (Masters and Johnson, 1966). Yet the imagined enormous dimensions of the black male's penis remain a preoccupation of many whites. Often, pornographic literature reflects such preoccupations. The author came across one salacious booklet entitled *Black Power,* which showed a black male with a large organ "taking care of" a bevy of white women. During the late 1960s a number of white psychiatry colleagues suggested that many whites were frightened of the slogan "Black Power," because unconsciously they heard "Black Penis" (personal communication). A number of psychoanalysts have explored the unconscious sexual aspects of racism (Kovel, 1970).

Since sexual prowess has a close association with aggressive behavior in any form, white control of potential black male aggression has been profound. Black male violence, particularly against whites, was met swiftly, harshly, and often with a disregard for law and due process. Many black males through history have been summarily lynched, executed, or given overly severe prison penalties (Pettigrew, 1964). As a result, many black males adopted a manner of docility and compliance in order to survive and be accepted in the white world. So-called "racial etiquette" required that black males bow, shuffle, and act like "boys" (Poussaint, 1979). In its worst form, conformity and emasculation was expressed in the "Uncle Tom" syndrome. Today, there remains undue fear of black male aggression even in clinicians and often that fear has obvious sexual connotations.

Black men have felt rejection both in and outside the group, but most severely in the taboo against social and sexual relations with white women. The white man's fantasy of such possible contact led them to develop a rape complex—a paranoid fear of black male aggression (Dollård, 1949). Historically, some black men were lynched for "rape" when they merely glanced at a white woman. From 1930 to 1961, 90% of men receiving the death penalty for rape were black even though they accounted for less than 50% of the rapes. The death penalty was much more likely to be the punishment if the female victim was white. During the same period no white man was sentenced to die for raping a black woman, although such rapes were quite common (Pettigrew, 1964). Clearly, black men were not only emasculated but had to live in a state of fear and apprehension in their contact with white women. In fact, the rape issue became such a profound symbol of the oppression of the black male that in the late 1960s some black militants elevated the rape of a white woman by a black male to an "insurrectionary act" (Cleaver, 1968). Such twisted thinking can pervade relations between blacks and whites even in the sanctity of the bedroom.

Interracial Sex

Black males have also resented the generalized notion in white society that they are all yearning to sleep with or marry a white woman. Yet it is clear that a number of black men and women have rejected their own race and seek social and sexual relations exclusively with white partners. With the removal of many social barriers since the civil rights movement of the 1960s, however, there has been no rush to intermarry. There are approximately 125,000 interracial, black–white marriages, and about 90,000 are black male–white female (Porterfield, 1978; Bureau of the Census, 1978). This figure represents only about 2% of black married men. Nevertheless, the bottom line appeal of ardent racists to their liberal white counterparts is often "Would you want your daughter to marry one?"

There remains today some degree of the "forbidden fruit syndrome" in the interactions of black men and white women and also to some extent between white men and black women. Kardiner and Ovesey, in their 1951 psychoanalytic study of a small sample of black patients wrote "sex relations with white women have a high demonstrative value in terms of pride and prestige" (Kardiner and Ovesey, 1955). Grier and Cobbs present an alternative interpretation of black male interest in white women:

> If he cannot fight the white man openly, he can and does battle him secretly. Recurrently, the pattern evolves of black men using sex as a dagger to be symbolically thrust into the white man. (Grier and Cobbs, 1968)

The theme of sex as a weapon of revenge in black–white relations emerges repeatedly in the popular literature. Black–white sex has also remained a titillating subject for the popular media but was treated with seriousness by Halsell (1972) and Day (1972). It is only in recent decades that antimiscegenation statutes have been struck down by the courts; this attests to the widespread and profound fear of black–white copulation. These authors as well as others point to the intense paranoia that underlies whites' fear of interracial sex. These issues have become so complex that professionals have wondered and postulated whether most interracial sexual–romantic liaisons are pathological or "sick" (Poussaint, 1980). This speculation itself places a stigma and an additional burden on the interracial couple.

Although black–white psychological dynamics have certainly been modified since the legal demise of segregation and the "black-is-beautiful" movement of the 1960s, it is certain that black–white sex relationships continue to suffer from the intrusion of psychological issues generated by racism.

Black Male–Female Relations

In recent years there has been an increased interest in and analysis of the effects of racism on the romantic interactions between black men and women. Several areas of strain, particularly white beauty standards, have already been alluded to. However, some investigators believe the the black experience has differed so significantly from white norms that black men and women sometimes have difficulty (both socially and psychologically) relating to each other free of the taint of defensiveness and ambivalence. Kardiner and Ovesey (1955) bluntly stated that the black male uniformly has bad relations with black females on an emotional level. They attribute this difficulty to the frustrated dependency and hostility that many black males develop in female-dominated households. Currently about 35–40% of black families are female headed (National Research Council, 1976). Many authors suggest that black males cannot feel securely masculine because of their powerlessness and frequent socioeconomic failure. Thus, the black male may feel more vulnerable and at the mercy of the black woman, which in turn may create a degree of dissonance in their relationship. Grier and Cobbs (1968) express similar views about the emasculation of the black male but add that a significant problem in black male–female interactions is that the black male devalues the black woman because of her low caste status. They and others further suggest that the black woman may also devalue the black male for similar reasons. Mutual respect, so crucial for a romantic partnership, may be lacking. On the other hand, social scientists, such as Billingsley (1968) and Hill (1971), argue that these categories are biased, stereotypic, and belie the essential strength of the black family. Hill, for example, suggests that one of the strengths of black families lies in the ability of its members to adapt comfortably to unusual and changing family roles. Billingsley also reports that black men and women have evolved relationships that demonstrate shared responsibility and egalitarian family roles quite different from the basic patriarchal structure of the normative white family.

These questions are constantly being debated in the black community and have been the subject of conferences and seminars on black male–female relations. Part of this crisis has been precipitated by the women's movement and blistering attacks on black male chauvinism (Wallace, 1978). Furthermore, many black women feel threatened by the shortage of black males who are lost to the armed services or, prison or who die at an early age from homicide, accidents, and suicide (Staples, 1981). Black men have also been involved in interracial dating on a large scale, whereas black women have been more reluctant to date interracially. The problem of added stress in black male–female relations will continue to exist and evolve into new forms as a consequence of changing racial patterns in America.

Summary

Black Americans have been deeply affected in their sexual behaviors in a variety of ways, which can be traced to the legacies of slavery and racism. As a result, distortions often appear in black erotic encounters with each other as well as with whites. Human sexual behavior is heavily influenced by class and socioeconomic factors; this makes it impossible to scientifically distinguish "black sexuality" or "white sexuality."

Clinicians should be cognizant of their own prejudices and the dynamics that may be unique in the sexual activities and values of their black clients. At the same time, they must avoid any well-meaning attitudes and interpretations that are based on myth and stereotypes about black sexual inclinations.

Racial issues are only one factor among a host of others that must be taken into consideration when formulating clinical judgments about any individual's sexual behavior.

Psychosexual Issues in Asian Cultures*

Introduction

Under the rubric of Asian American there are several distinctly separate ethnic groups, including Chinese, Japanese, Koreans, Filipinos, Pacific Islanders, and, most

*Elizabeth C. Small

recently, several groups of Indochinese refugees: Vietnamese, Cambodian, Laotian, and Thai. In the American environment, other differences occur among generations, ages, socioeconomic levels, etc. Scientific research into specific psychosexual issues among Asians is sparse. The data for this section come primarily from Chinese and Japanese groups, with a few additional data from Korean and East Indian groups. As there are certain cultural factors in common emanating from the influence of Chinese society on the cultures of the Far East, a cautious attempt at generalization will be made to connect the influence of ethnicity with Asian sexual attitudes and practices. The influences of Buddhism and Islam on Southeast Asians and the Japanese Shinto-ism practices will not be elaborated.

The Asian American Population in the United States

Early Immigration

Immigration laws have determined the immigration patterns of Asian subgroups entering the United States. The earliest Asian immigrants were Chinese males who in the late 1800s formed a substantial component of the work force in western states and Hawaii building railroads, working in mines, and doing farm work. Chinese women did not initially accompany their husbands but received from them financial support for themselves and their family. Unmarried men remained bachelors, observing laws of miscegenation, which prohibited marriage to white women. A few of them married Indian or Mexican women. Though Chinese women remained in their homeland ini-tially, secondary to customs prohibiting women from traveling, from 1884 to 1930 restrictive immigration laws even prohibited wives of men in the United States from joining their spouses. Thus, a marked disruption in the maintenance of family structure occurred for the first generation of Chinese Americans. More affluent husbands did visit their families in China, often conceiving additional children during each visit. For all, however, the eventual reunion of these couples involved a sense of estrangement and hardly knowing the spouse (Lee, 1960).

The second largest group to arrive were Japanese. At the beginning of the 20th century the first generation (the Issei) were young men who also had the "sojourners" outlook, intending to work in America and to return to Japan with accumulated funds. Performing similar jobs to the Chinese (Lyman, 1970b), both work forces began to be experienced as potential economic threats. The immigration restrictions evoked by such concerns differed for Japanese in that men were allowed to bring their wives. Married men did eventually send for their wives, whereas bachelors arranged be-throthal with "picture brides" who met their intended spouses at the time of disem-barkment (Gee, 1971). Eventually, in 1922, issuance of passports for picture brides was discontinued, but by this time the number of Japanese women actually exceeded the number of men who had immigrated.

Different from the Chinese or Japanese, a few Koreans immigrated in the early 20th century. The Hawaii Sugar Planters' Association recruited mainly Korean work-ers to Hawaii until 1905, when the Korean government ended a liberal emigration policy. From 1911 to 1923, Korean picture brides immigrated to Hawaii and to the

U.S. The current immigration to the United States from Korea, since the Korean war of the 1950s, greatly overshadows the small number of Koreans who came early this century (Pian, 1980).

Recent Immigration

The most important recent immigration act is the Act of 1965, which has allowed a large influx, particularly from the Philippines. Although most European immigration occurred before the 1960s, about half of all the Asian immigrants have arrived since 1961. The second largest group to arrive are Koreans. The highest rate of Chinese entry occurred in 1967, at the height of the Cultural Revolution, and since then the numbers have decreased. The rate of Japanese immigration has been low.

Since World War II, women from Asia arriving as wives of military and nonmilitary personnel has significantly increased. Many women are married to white or black servicemen, beginning with Japanese women who met and married the occupational forces in Japan during the 1950s (Pian, 1974). Since the 1950s, Asian wives have immigrated primarily from Korea, Japan, the Philippines, and more recently from Vietnam, Cambodia, Laos, Thailand, and Taiwan.

Though Vietnamese refugees are not the first Asian refugees to seek asylum, the fall of the South Vietnamese government and the massive evacuation of nearly 130,000 Vietnamese refugees and 5000 Cambodian refugees represents the largest single entrance of refugees from Asia at any time in U.S. history. The increase of the Vietnamese and the Southeast Asian population has increased this population in size to be the fifth or sixth largest Asian American population in the United States. Whereas earlier immigrants were predominantly Asian wives and children of U.S. servicemen, this refugee population is a balanced group with equal proportions of men and women (Pian, 1980).

Asian Culture and Family

Cultural Factors

Using the Chinese model to discuss the basic cultural and philosophical features of the countries affected by China in the Far East, the contrast to Western civilization is noted. Rather than having concern with ontological issues, such as the existence of God or the ultimate fate of the human race, the two dominant Chinese philosophical traditions, Taoism and Confucianism, are both focused in efforts of delineating the Tao (The Way): the proper way of conducting a social and personal life. Taoists have devoted attention to searching for the optimal way for harmonious living in relation to nature and the cosmos (Ishihara and Levy, 1970), whereas Confucianists have been mostly concerned with the proper way of conducting social and political life to maintain order. The setting of these philosophies is in an agrarian situation, and, through the ages, the Confucian attitudes have dominated family life and influenced the rules on sexual behaviors in order to enhance productivity of the agrarian and feudal economy.

Before proceeding further, the concept of Yin and Yang (Female and Male) should be addressed to understand the general philosophical attitude of harmony. *Yin* and *Yang* are a pair of polar terms that describe contrasting aspects of phenomena in the universe. The terms are dynamic, functional, and relative. Invariably, using the terms infers a comparison. Although they are at the same time contradictory, they are also complementary and interdependent with each other. For example, in order to understand darkness, it is necessary to have brightness. The interaction of Yin and Yang serves as a basis for all change in the universe, both macro- and microcosmic. Due to their interaction, and the changes that result, temporary imbalance is unavoidable, but ultimately if balance cannot be achieved, the result will be a situation of dysfunction (Lin, 1981). Yin signifies the passive, inhibited, inward, retrogressive, cold, dark, soft, unaggressive, material, and concrete (female) elements. Yang signifies the apparent, active, excited, external, upward, aggressive, volatile, hard, bright, hot, abstract, and functional (male) elements. Both elements coexist and are in dynamic operation at all times. In this setting, the harmony between male and female elements obviates the concept of conflict. Thus, in the Asian family, search for order and harmony is established by strict Confucian rules governing male and female roles.

Marriage

The Western concept of romantic love does not take precedence in mating. Marriages are arranged to meet the economic and political needs of the respective families. The patrilineal descent of property and surname that demonstrates woman's social and legal inferiority to men was institutional and persisted unchanged over the centuries, even as actual behaviors and values that it expressed had changed. The woman was subordinate to her father and elder brothers before marriage, her husband and father-in-law during marriage, and her sons in her widowhood. The woman took her basic social position from her husband and had no real independent existence. She was expected to be subordinate and submissive and the relationship between husband and wife was comparable to that between an elder and a junior within a kin line. In customary law, a husband issues orders to the wife, and it was her duty to obey. Ill treatment or punishment of the wife was not actionable in court, no matter how arbitrary or unreasonable it might have been unless it went as far as serious injury or death. On the other hand, if injury or death is caused to the husband, a wife's punishment would be excessive since she had also violated the socially and legally defined relationship between herself and her husband.

The officially approved marriage was theoretically monogamous but was in fact often polygamous. Under Ch'ing Code, to have more than one principal wife was a crime. The only exception was that a man could marry a second principal wife as a "stand-in" for a deceased brother to ensure that his brother's line would not die out (McGough, 1981). Secondary wives (concubines) were permitted. Supposedly, these were taken only if the first wife was infertile, however, a man could take as many concubines as he wanted or could afford. The concubine had a definite and legally guarded status in the household and family but was inferior to the principal wife. Children of the concubine were legitimate, but their family rights to the estate were inferior to the heirs of the principal wife (McGough, 1981; Chipp and Green, 1980; von Siebold, 1841/1973). A recent report from Mainland China notes that concubinage still exists (*Parade,* 1981). Wives were expected at all times to maintain fidelity to their husbands. Transgressions were punishable by shame, death, or suicide. Though mutual support was not clearly defined, by custom the husband was bound to support wife and concubine as well. If he was unable to do so, then the wife had the duty to support him. Divorce is not condoned and considered to be a disgrace (Tseng and Char, 1974).

Sexual Attitudes

Sexual attitudes from ancient times unenlightened by accurate knowledge of anatomy and physiology of sexual and reproductive functioning still influence the Asian peoples of today. It was believed that during sexual intercourse, a man absorbs the female (Yin) essence, which strengthens his vital powers and life. Ejaculation, however, results in the debilitating loss of the vital (Yang) essence. Thus, too frequent intercourse so drains the male's vital essence that he is vulnerable to several serious diseases. For this reason, numerous techniques are recommended that enable men to avoid ejaculation. Women are in no danger for their supply of Yin essence is inexhaustible. Under Taoist thinking, women were portrayed as having a right to sexual pleasure, with foreplay being extensively discussed and the goal of the act itself, each time with orgasm of the woman, whereas the man rejuvenates himself to maintain health and longevity (Ishihara and Levy, 1970). However, under Confucian edict, eroticism became subordinate to the goal of procreation, and sexuality had no value outside of breeding. Later, Confucianists embarked on an all-out attack on any demonstration of heterosexual behavior, and eroticism was relegated to pornographic and bordello status. Although Confucius had written that "sex and appetite are the natural desires of human nature," sexuality was not acceptable *per se* and had no value of its own. Though not associated with sinfulness since the philosophy did not encompass a concept of evil and original sin, public display of affection or sensuality was unacceptable as proper behavior. Even in marital intercourse, wives participated in coitus while fully clothed. This denial of sexuality persists to present day and has resulted in the poor status of research into the psychosexual disorders of the Asians, since it is nearly impossible for an Asian to comfortably divulge his sexual experiences even for research's sake.

Though it was emphasized that homosexuality is rare in China (van Gulik, 1971), it may be more accurate to say that homosexual practices are rare if seen in isolation. Homosexual practices can be incorporated into heterosexual experiences as the realm of "normal" sexuality includes whatever is pleasurable. Thus, one can engage in homosexual, sadistic, or masochistic activities without being defined as a sadist or a homosexual (Ishihara and Levy, 1970). Nonmarrying pacts for women and same-sex institutionalized marriages for men have been described (McGough, 1981).

In Chinese society, women are regarded as both unclean and dangerously powerful and are thus barred from certain activities because of the harm they threaten to inflict on others. Principally, the body fluids, menstrual blood, and postpartum discharge are believed to be of the same substance and considered unclean. These fluids are associated with dangerous power, with menstrual blood being the most directly powerful since it is believed that it creates babies. Some of the menstrual blood produced during delivery is lost, whereas the rest becomes the body of the child; "It creates flesh and bones" (Ahern, 1975). Semen, on the other hand, merely begins the growth of the child. Thus, the female role in procreation is very substantial. Menstrual blood is also thought to be bad for the body. There is a distinction between good blood, i.e., blood in the general circulation, which is essential to health, and the menstrual blood, which is harmful. Both kinds of blood escape during childbirth. The woman hopes to replace the good blood by eating proper foods after parturition and allows the bad blood to escape. Contact with menstrual blood by male or female will bar the individual from worship of the gods, and a period of cleansing is required.

Children are highly valued, with male children of the highest value since they increase the family fortunes and can bring wives into the household who will procreate for the family. With children, there is also a hierarchical order with age and with gender, the males being superior. Girl children are not considered assets but liabilities, since after nurturing, they are lost to another family. The strength and solidarity of the Asian family extends from the nuclear family to the extended family and beyond to kinships involving individuals of the community so that an entire village may derive its economic, social, and political identity as a clan.

Care of the children resides in the sphere of the woman, and from the beginning, the child develops a close physical and emotional attachment to the mother. Breast-feeding is expected and adds to the close physical (oral) gratification of children. If a mother's milk is inadequate, wet nurses in the household provide the needed nourishment (Tseng and Hsu, 1974). However, even in this area, physical modesty is practiced. For example, the Ainu women of Japan, when nursing a child in the presence of men do so covertly, only exposing enough of the breast to allow the child to take the nipple (Ford and Beach, 1951). Children are carried on the backs of women and share the same bed with parents. Toilet training is permissive, and, in the agrarian setting, the use of night soil as a valuable fertilizer precludes a negative attitude toward bodily excretions. Mothers tend to be sensitive to the child's biologic rhythms and train themselves to facilitate the children's excretory behavior rather than training the child to meet their needs. Early gratification in infancy tended to lay the foundation for continued gratification from other members of the family group. Feeding and food, a major modality for communication and interpersonal relationship, reflect the importance of oral needs well recognized in the culture. Instead of concern for sphincter control, more attention was paid to neuromuscular control and control of hostility. Binding an infant's limbs to avoid the development of violent behavior was common, and the skill of brush painting also offered character training in sitting in a quiet, controlled fashion. Younger children were subordinate to the older and were discouraged from displaying aggressive or hostile behavior toward seniors. Rules governing dress, work, and social behavior of boys and girls followed gender lines and no sexual behavior was allowed before marriage. Children are taught not to misbehave outside the family, and family secrets or shameful factors are never revealed to outsiders. Sin and guilt are not characteristics of Chinese ethics, but the sense of shame is a powerful punitive element (Tseng and Hsu, 1968; Lyman, 1970a).

Fertility Control

There is very little known data on the frequency of contraceptive or abortion practices among Asians in earlier times; however, it may be deduced that such practices were infrequent, due to the lack of understanding of the physiology of reproduction and appropriate techniques. Furthermore, the high priority on having many children, with the added support of extended families to raise children, would not allow for strong motivation to avoid reproduction except in dire circumstances of pregnancy out of wedlock. Even in these cases, the societal structure allows for support of these children as in concubinage. Even in modern times, there are no national statistics on contraception or abortion in the Far East. However, with modern technology and the economic incentive to control population, all known methods of contraception and abortion are known to be practiced. Abortion by acupuncture anesthesia, for example, is performed by midwives and barefoot doctors in the People's Republic of China and is done particularly in women who have already had two children. Sterilization is easily available for both men and women (Adey, 1974; Bowers, 1973).

For those Asian Americans living in the United States, the attitudes toward both contraception and abortion will depend on the individual's acculturation and to what degree the influence of Old World customs has upon the couple (Goldscheider and Uhlenberg, 1969).

Psychological Aspects of Traditional Medical Beliefs

Chinese and Asian medical concepts reflect the central theme of Chinese culture, characterized by a dynamic interaction between the idea of Tao and a strong pragmatic material focus (Lin, 1981). In the search for the optimal way to live a harmonious life relating to nature and social realities, traditional Chinese medicine and folk healing demonstrate the same orientation toward harmony with nature and pragmatic factors. The theory of Yin–Yang has broad application in Chinese medicine and is used to describe anatomy, physiology, and pathological conditions. It encompasses the etiology, staging, and medicinal treatment of diseases, which includes dietary and other therapeutic modalities. The primary concern in diagnosis is to recognize and treat the imbalance between Yin and Yang. One outgrowth of the Yin–Yang balance theory is that through its relationship with "hot" and "cold" and other opposites, diet and herbs are dichotomized. Attention in eating proper foods based on balancing these opposites affects illness and health maintenance.

The most psychiatrically relevant aspect of traditional Chinese medicine is its unwillingness to differentiate between psychological and physiological functions. This does not obviate a psychological approach, since there is ample evidence of psychic factors in all aspects of health and illness, but the tendency toward somatization may be qualitatively different from other cultures.

Psychological factors are clearly indicated in all major classics of Chinese medicine as one of two major causes of imbalance and disease, but the psychological features are dealt with differently from other etiologies. The excess of seven kinds of emotions are regarded as pathogenic. These emotions are identified as happiness, anger, worry, desire, sadness, fear, and fright. In contrast to the Western tradition, which emphasizes the emotional value of catharsis, the Chinese direct efforts to avoid excesses of emotion and attempt to place emotions into a natural and social milieu. Since excess rather than emotions themselves are considered pathogenic, high value is given to moderation and inhibition of expression of affect. To prevent psychosomatic and somatopsychic imbalance, Taoist medical tradition evolved methods of training Chinese not to respond to threatening stimuli with excessive emotions. These included techniques in mental exercise and meditation. Confucians also taught that maintaining harmony in familial and other social relationships necessitated inhibition and avoidance of affectivity. These combined traditions reinforce Chinese and Asian legitimization of suppression as a psychoculturally adaptive coping mechanism, resulting in the impression that Asians are not psychologically oriented.

The reverse emphasis of the Chinese psychosomatic model on somatopsychic effects is difficult for the Western-style psychotherapist to manage. Once physiological functions are disturbed, the logical approach to treatment becomes physiological or pharmacological, even if emotions are considered to be in excess. Training body–mind together is basic as a tradition of psychological intervention, and its value is held to be greater for prevention than for therapeutics. Interestingly, the principle of moderation is applied not only to negative emotions but also the positive one of happiness. Thus, psychological health was believed to be maintained through this culturally approved system of somatopsychic training of moderation and leaves very little room for the classic Western style of psychologically dominant approach to theory.

Psychosexual Issues

It is in this setting that addressing psychosexual phenomena through a psychiatric approach has led to very little elucidation of the status of psychosexual disorders in the Asian population. Though psychosexual disorders do exist, they may present mainly through physiological symptoms and appear first to general practitioners, internists, gynecologists, urologists, or surgeons (Tseng and Char, 1968). Furthermore, classical medical texts make no mention of women nor are there illustrative demonstrations of a female body in which to discuss female pathology. The Yellow Emperor's Treatise on Internal Medicine makes no mention of women (Veith, 1949); acupuncture charts do not use females as models. Until 1911, the physical examination of the female was performed by the extension of a woman's hand through a curtain for examination by the physician. (Data obtained from individuals who lived in China during the period before the Revolution of 1911.) In current practice, it is still not uncommon for an Asian woman to refuse physical examination by a male physician.

Although research data are sparse, studies of anxiety (Tan, 1981) have revealed psychosexual dysfunctions that range from masturbatory guilt, guilt following contact with prostitutes, impotence, premature ejaculation, nocturnal emission, and spermatorrhea to delayed ejaculation (disorders of the male). The preoccupation with sexual function as a manifestation of emotional conflict is widespread in Asia, with the focus on the belief that sexual excess in men leads to emaciation and eventually death. An industry of sexual potions and commodities support this myth by reinforcing it in advertisements that attempt to sell these products in all of Asia and on a worldwide basis. Feminine concerns about sexuality and sexual dysfunction, understandably, are yet to be systematically discovered and researched.

It is relevant at this point to describe several culture-bound psychosexual disorders that have been identified, dealing mainly with male dysfunction. The syndrome of *Koro* consists of a sudden onset of complaints of the sensation of penile retraction into the body. Psychodynamically, it is akin to castration anxiety, usually associated with some feelings of guilt related to sexual or other misbehavior, and the syndrome is believed to be a prime example of excess of Yin (Gwee, 1963). Its treatment is based on the avoidance of foodstuffs that contain excess of Yin: cold drinks and raw fruits and vegetables. For balance, Yang foods are encouraged: genseng root, alcohol, and lean meat. As a form of acute management, it has been suggested (Tan, 1981) that an intravenous infusion of calcium gluconate will give the patient a sense of warmth throughout the body. Once anxiety and panic is reduced, the patient can be sedated for the night and psychotherapeutic treatment dealing with conflicts can take place the following morning. *Koro* has also been described in women who experience sensations of nipple, breast, or labia retraction (van Wulfften Palthe, 1936).

Spermatorrhea has been described as a pathological entity. With the widespread Asian belief that sexual dissipation and excessive loss of seminal fluid can lead to emaciation and death, any involuntary seminal loss generates anxiety and urgency (even normal physiological events). Spermatorrhea includes excessive masturbation and nocturnal emissions. Patients who complain of multiple symptoms relating to sexual functioning may have other hypochondriacal complaints. Lack of scientific information on the part of patients as well as some of their health providers as to the normal physiology of seminal emissions perpetuates the mythology and maintains the anxiety states. Apparently in some women, the anxiety over vaginal secretions also exists (Tan, 1981), and, again, the need for clarification of normal physiology for both men and women is obvious. Delayed or retarded ejaculation is noted to be common among Asians. It is understandable that if seminal loss is culturally feared, unconscious or conscious factors may well lead to a withholding of the ejaculate.

Problems of Asian Wives of American Servicemen

Although not strictly in the area of psychosexual disorders, comment should be made on the psychosocial stresses of the Asian wives of U.S. servicemen who have specific problems that may well be addressed by psychiatric and social agencies. Intermarriage of Asian women with American men began in numbers after World War II. The largest percentage of war brides came from Japan as a result of the postwar occupation. A few Chinese wives also came in the late 1940s as well as Korean wives who returned with U.S. servicemen after the Korean war. Intermarriage, for the most part, was not condoned by Asian families. However, the fact that some couples already had pregnancies or children while abroad forced the reality that economic survival was much better in America. Full acceptance in the American culture did not occur for these Eurasian families. Often, the women were from a lower socioeconomic strata (many had been working in bordellos) with limited education, skills, and ability to speak English.

With the Vietnamese War, Vietnamese, Cambodian, and Thai immigrant families as well as brides have come to the United States and are now being integrated into American society with stress and conflict, internal and external. Women who arrived as "boat people" and intermarry with Americans share similar cultural stresses with war brides.

Common problems encountered by these wives include lack of ability to communicate, social and personal isolation, lack of survival skills, and lack of extended family support (Kim, 1975; Kim, 1976). They may be unable to carry out routine tasks, like shopping and maintaining the household. This increases dependency on the husband and his family, which may become burdensome. She is often not accepted by her in-laws because of racial and cultural differences. This increases her sense of isolation, helplessness, and alienation. Husband–wife conflicts occur frequently. Whereas the relationship often began as a customer–entertainer arrangement; conversion to a marital relationship requires substantial adaptation. The husband may devalue his wife's different cultural background as he struggles with the adaptational problems of reentry into nonmilitary life. Such stress further limits his tolerance of her maladaptation. Often the husband becomes involved in alcohol and drug abuse. Jealousy (evoked by his preferred social position) and rage lead some wives to threats of self-destruction or provocation of their husbands to violent acts of physical abuse. Since she has few survival skills, the woman feels that she cannot seek a divorce unless she works in areas that are not affected by her limited fluency in English and education, such as in the entertainment industry (go-go girls, barmaids, masseuses), on farms (as fruit and vegetable pickers or poultry cleaners), or as seamstresses in the garment factories. More recently, groups of Asian wives have formed "extended families," where restoration of a sense of identity, mutual assistance in finding employment, and elevation of self-esteem seems to occur.

Children of these families require special attention, although discussion of this subject is not in the purview of this chapter.

There is a distinction between the war brides and those women and men of Asian background who intermarry in the United States. The acculturated Asian appears to have less social difficulty, is more educated, and has the language and occupational skills for survival. Intermarriage among Asians and non-Asians becomes increasingly more common with each generation, with females more likely than males to intermarry (Fujitomi and Wong, 1973; Tseng and Char, 1974).

Conclusion

The foregoing discussion of Asian cultural influences on sexual attitudes and behavior is based on the Chinese and Japanese elements that have had the strongest overall influence in the Far East. The current paucity of data on sexuality in Asian culture precludes more detailed and differentiated discussion of the various Asian subgroups now residing in the United States. Further systematized studies of Asians in their homeland and in the country are needed. It may, however, take time to gather clinical information because both Asian patients and Asian professionals are still strongly influenced by the general attitude of Asians to avoid open discussion and demonstration of affect and sexuality.

Hispanic Americans

Recent estimates of the total number of Hispanic Americans range from 13.3 to 27.8 million (*Report to the President's Commission on Mental Health*, 1978; Bernal and Flores-Ortiz, 1981). Mexican Americans are the largest subgroup (59%); Puerto Ricans living in Puerto Rico and on the mainland represent 16% of the total. Cuban Americans make up another 6 to 7%. The remaining 18% includes indivduals from other Latin and South American countries. Due to a higher birthrate and continued immigration, it is predicted the Hispanics will become the largest U.S. ethnic minority group well before the year 2000.

All Latin American countries share a common heritage which involved the development of a *mestizo* race (mixed European, predominately Spanish, and indigenous Indian). A similar life philosophy evolved combining Spanish traits of pride, passion, and emotional expression with the Indian world view harmony and coexistence with nature. A sense of community interdependence exists. Generosity, concern, and a willingness to sacrifice for others, respect for elders and persons in authority (manifest by politeness and deference often misinterpreted by non-Latins as a tendency toward submissive passivity), and a high value on family ties are characteristic. There is a distinctive love of life and a belief in joy and happiness (McWilliams, 1968; Wilkeson, 1981a; Murrillo, 1971). Good times are enhanced with music, bright colors, *fiestas* (parties), and other socialization, whereas bad times are shared, lightening the burden for any one individual.

The Hispanic Mental Health Research Center at UCLA provided a thorough literature search on the various topics covered in this book. Only 2 of the 104 citations dealt with specific sexual topics (21 citations discussed family planning; 20, aspects of Latin family life; and 14 reports dealt with marriage patterns and marital relationships). We have, therefore, decided to combine a brief historical cultural summary of Mexican American, Puerto Rican, and Cuban people with a discussion of family life, sex-role stereotypes, and developmental issues that are related to attitudes about sex and sexual identity.

Mexican Americans

When Spanish explorers first entered Mexico, they encountered the highly developed Aztec society. Immediate destruction of the Aztec nation was motivated by the Spaniards desire to claim land and riches for their then faltering Spanish crown. Being the first land conquered by the Spaniards, Mexico became the base for further Spanish exploration of Latin America. The fact that the New World was viewed as uncivilized delayed the arrival of Spanish women until Mexican settlements were well developed. This delay increased the initial involvement of Spanish men with Indian women, contributing to Mexican people being the most racially intermixed of all Latin American countries.

McWilliams (1968) begins his excellent account of Mexican American history by describing the early-1500s Spanish settlement of the later-to-be-annexed "borderlands" of the Southwest. McWilliams emphasizes the fact that the actual history of this part of the United States and of its inhabitants is quite distinctive from the initially romanticized and later devalued stereotypic notions that have characteristically been presented by American educators and social scientists. Their motivations were not primarily that of chivalry, adventure, and conquest. They were actually quite pragmatic people, who gradually explored areas north of Mexico City seeking reasonable land to settle. They brought with them animals, plants, and tools that were readily adaptable to the region. The borderlands remained relatively isolated until quite late in the 1800s. It is, thus, only in the last 100 years that Mexican Americans have not directly experienced their cultural heritage as being exclusively imprinted and rooted in the land of the Southwest.

Recent authors have emphasized (Guerra, 1971; McWilliams, 1968; Romano, 1968; Alvarez, 1971) that much Mexican American history has been ignored by social scientists and the majority culture in general, thereby allowing for the propagation of quite distorted stereotypic portrayals of Mexican American individual and collective character. Many Mexican Americans are not immigrants but the offspring of an earlier established culture that was defeated and dominated by Yankees, who were motivated by the philosophy of Manifest Destiny. Further defeats have characterized interactions of Mexican Americans and Anglos since that time. Shortly after the signing of the Treaty of Guadalupe, a process began whereby Mexican land ownership was challenged and removed through technical legal loopholes. From the initial migration of Anglos into the Southwest, an attitude of racial superiority has been maintained toward Mexican Americans and used to rationalize discriminatory behavior including very low pay for agricultural work, separate and less well-financed schools and housing, and, periodically, overt violence.

Though lacking historical perspective, Grebler's (1970) text on *The Mexican American* is a valuable comprehensive summary of the socioeconomic experience of the Mexican American experience over the past century. Awareness of the historical and contemporary heritage of Mexican Americans is important for clinicians who hope to evaluate sexual concerns of Chicano patients. A principal result of the disharmonious relations between Mexican Americans and the majority culture is the ongoing prevelance of stereotypic notions held by majority individuals toward Mexican Americans and by Mexican Americans toward Anglos. Clinical familiarity with this complicated set of expectations, Mexican American patients bring to their initial encounter with non-Latin clinicians is necessary to prevent patients from dropping out during the early phases of their evaluation.

Simmons (1971) interviews study the Anglo-Americans and Mexican Americans in a small Texas city and provide a meaningful (though stark) summary of such attitudes. Basically, Mexican Americans are seen by Anglo-Americans to be inately inferior, intolerant, irresponsible, imprudent, uncleanly, and prone to drunkenness, delinquency, and criminality. Mexican Americans hold some favorable notions about Anglo-Americans including such traits as taking initiative, ambition, and industriousness, but the preponderance of their attitudes toward Anglos are negative, cold, mercenary, exploitive, conceited, inconsistent, and insincere.

Neither the history of Mexico nor the history of Mexican Americans is consistent with these notions. Seen from within the culture, despite oppression, the combined Spanish/Indian values of pride, honor, respect, dignity, and enjoyment of life have been maintained. Particularly respectful and deferential toward persons in authority, Mexican Americans are unlikely to express any sentiments of animosity or mistrust unless expressly asked and encouraged to do so. Even subtle differences in the professional style of a non-Latin clinician from interpersonal behavior characteristic of Latin professionals may be misinterpreted by an anxious patient and cause them to flee treatment. Sensitive yet explicit questioning regarding such potential impasses will facilitate the formation of an initial sense of trust and alliance.

A fairly substantial proportion of the mental health literature on Mexican Americans has addressed the observation that Mexican Americans underutilize mental health treatment (Padilla and Ruiz, 1973; Wilkeson, 1981b; Karno, 1966; Karno and Edgerton, 1969; Sue et al., 1978; Barrera, 1978; Miranda and Kitano, 1976; Keefe, 1978). Many possible reasons for this apparent lack of interest in professional help have been postulated but a recent study by Keefe (1978) has shown no correlation between mental health contact and ''social economic status, the presence of an integrated extended family, commitment to the folk medical system, attitudes toward mental health services or the reliance on relatives, doctors, clergymen, Mexican American community workers or 'curanderos' (folk healers) for emotional support.'' Since 1970, a number of mental health facilities that were specifically designed to provide mental health services for Latinos have demonstrated that Mexican Americans, in fact, are interested in and will seek professional help as readily as other ethnic groups (Flores, 1978; Heiman et al., 1975; Heiman and Kahn, 1975; Karno and Morales, 1971; Long et al., 1977; Martinez, 1977; Phillippus, 1971).

Another unsubstantiated myth about Mexican Americans and mental health is an alleged absence of ''psychological mindedness.'' Karno and Edgerton (1969) dispelled this notion. Interviews of 444 Mexican Americans and 200 Anglo controls showed the former more frequently identified symptoms of depression and psychosis as elements of mental illness, were more optimistic about the curability of mental illness via psychiatric intervention, and believed the origin of mental disorders begins in childhood. Fabrega and Metzger (1978) found Mexican villagers believed psychological factors as well as physical and spiritual forces cause mental illness. Among other psychological factors noted was the belief that either insufficient or excessive sexual contact and masturbation can cause mental illness.

Reports on the prevalence of continued adherence to folk beliefs and reliance on the folk healing methods of *curanderos* (folk healers) are quite contradictory (Wilkeson, 1981a). As with other cultural beliefs, it would be advantageous for clinicians to become familiar with the predominant ideas of these more primitive disease concepts which incorporate beliefs in supernatural forces with hellenic concepts of body harmony and humors brought to the New World by 16th-century Europeans (Kiev, 1968). For the purposes of this chapter it is important to note that included in these beliefs is the notion that both jealousy and envy are particularly powerful emotions and are considered as potential precipitants of two disorders. One, *Susto* (fright) is caused by any sudden dramatic experience and is a magical state of fright or soul loss. It is a state of anxiety and fear, which in some cases involves catatonic symptoms; other associative symptoms may be anorexia, insomnia, hallucinations, weakness, and various painful sensations. The other, *mal puesto,* is a hex, an evil put on someone willfully by another. It involves major psychiatric and/or neurologic symptoms including uncontrolled urination, sudden attacks of screaming, crying, and singing, and in some instances bodily exposure and convulsions.

Interpersonal relationships are highly valued by Mexican Americans as an orientation toward interrelatedness is central to their world view. These sentiments are actually extensions of the central place the family plays in Mexican American (and Mexican) life. Murillo's (1971) fairly recent description of the Mexican American family is of the most sensitive and accurate portrayal currently available. He emphasizes the highly important role of the family: It is "at the core of thinking and behavior and the center from which his view of the rest of the world stems." Strong bonds of loyalty and unity exist within the nuclear and extended family. They extend beyond as well to *compadres* (unrelated godparents), friends, neighbors, and the community. Each family has its own particular history, which is highly valued by its members. This is important to emphasize, for, as Murillo sums up, there is a marked diversity of background among Mexican American people:

> The reality is that there is no Mexican American family "type." Instead there are literally thousands of Mexican American families all different significantly from one another along a variety of dimensions. There are significant regional, historical, political, social, economic, acculturational and assimilational factors. . . . There are families where Spanish is the exclusive language spoken in the home and others where it is never spoken. There are families who trace their ancestry back to their Spanish forefathers and others trace their ancestry back to their Mayan, Zapotec, Toltec or Aztec forefathers. Some families were living on land which is now the Southwestern part of the U.S. before the pilgrims landed at Plymouth Rock while others have immigrated to the U.S. in recent years. (Murillo, 1971)

The family is the primary source of an individual's sense of security (Muriel, 1971; Bernal and Flores-Oritz, 1981). Family members (including *compadres*) provide for each other's emotional, social, and economic support and are almost exclusively turned to for any type of problem solving. Psychologically an individual's identification as part of a given family has greater importance than his/her individual identity. Respect and obedience for elders and male dominance are characteristic. Children are highly valued and the home environment is child centered during the early years of childbearing. Child-rearing patterns are strict as the behavior of any and all family members is seen as a reflection on the honor of the entire family.

The father's authority in the family is not questioned, but his male or masculine image in the community is based in part on his fairness and justice in the authority role. The fathers are described as warm and permissive toward their children until puberty and thereafter are distant and authoritarian. The wife–mother has a subservient, though highly respected, role and continues to be giving to all family members even when children have reached adulthood. Distinctive roles and responsibilities are taught to boys and girls, though all children are given tasks that are valued functions of the entire family from an early age. In adolescence, there is an expectation that young men gain worldly knowledge through experience, whereas young women are expected to remain close to their mothers and have few social contacts beyond the family.

In their review of literature relevant to "Latino Mental Health," Padilla and Ruiz (1973) note that there exists an "impressive unanimity" in the extant descriptions of Latin families but that "very little confirmatory data exists." Goodman and Berman's (1971) well-designed perspectives of children living in a typical Mexican American barrio neighborhood does provide some substantiating data for the foregoing descriptions of familial and culture values. In a manner noted to be quite distinctive of white and black children who value peer relationships, Mexican American children value relationships with parents, grandparents, siblings, aunts, uncles, and *compadres* more than friendships outside the family. Fathers earn money, are the final authority figure, and are experienced as available to respond to questions and emotional needs by girl children but are distant to boys. Mother's primary involvement, even if she works, is the domestic role. Despite being the day-to-day disciplinarian, she is valued and experienced with feelings of warmth and closeness by both girls and boys. Elders are respected and treated with deference. Work is valued as a contribution to and participation in family life.

Most of the unsubstantiated descriptions of Mexican and Mexican American family life emphasize a particularly strong role segregation between men and women with men being considered unquestionably superior and dominant and women being forced to assume a role of absolute subservience and self-abnegation. Two 1950s studies by Ramirez and Parres (1957) and Dia-Guerro (1955) of prototypic and *mestizo* families in Mexico are often referenced in providing collaboration of these segregated roles. Though these authors do present some interesting demographic data, their analytic interpretations are based primarily on the analysis of 11 subjects considered to be typical Mexicans. Their main emphases are twofold. First, there is in the culture an overevaluation of "the feminine relationship in its maternal aspects and a (devaluation) of the emotional and sexual living with a husband." An intense valuing of the maternal role and the maternal–child bond is elaborated. The male role is described as that of provider and authority figure who is granted absolute supremacy but is generally distant and uninvolved with children. Masculinity for the Mexican male is primarily associated with sexual prowess. The masculine self-image is maintained by ongoing participation in group activities with males outside the family plus frequent involvement in sexual experiences outside the marital relationship (these behaviors are what is referred to by the term *machismo*). A definitive sexual double standard is emphasized. Virginity and purity are expected of women who as children are taught that their destiny includes three areas: superlative femininity, the home, and maternity. The young woman's femininity is admired and reinforced only during the years before marriage. Once married, a maternal and subservient role is assumed. For the male from adolescence on, sexual activity with numerous partners is encouraged.

Validation of the earlier descriptions of Mexican and Mexican American family life awaits clinical confirmation. Stereotypic biases may be an influencing factor (Montiel, 1970, 1973; Alvarez, 1971; Romano, 1968; Senour, 1978). The starkness of the absolute role segregation and polarized opposite view of men and women seems rather incongruent with the dominant cultural valuing of compassion and concern for others. A few studies do exist that in fact do not substantiate the earlier characteristics. Two anthropological works by Lewis (1949) and MacCoby (1971) did not find that the earlier role descriptions existed in the subjects of the two Mexican villages investigated. MacCoby's more recent work involved interviewing the entire population of a typical Mexican village. He found that only 11% of the men demonstrated any significant pattern of compulsive "masculinity," whereas 30% showed some *machismo* traits. Seventy migrant-worker Mexican American couples interviewed by Hawkes and Taylor (1975) actually demonstrated unequivocally equalitarian marital relations. Cromwell's (1976) study of 134 married Chicano, Black, and Anglo couples from Kansas City found no support for the primary hypothesis of that study that the degree of patriarchy would be greatest among Chicanos.

The impact of the processes of acculturation and assimilation on Mexican American family life and marital relations is not clear. Two relatively small studies (Tharp et al., 1968) reported a substantial difference among English-speaking (high acculturation) wives versus Spanish-speaking Mexican American married women (low acculturation) with the former having much more equalitarian, complementary, and mutual marital sex-role expectation. The much more extensive review of Borah and Cook (1966) that provides a detailed description of both Mexican and Mexican American marriage and legitimacy patterns from precolonial times until the present finds no such distinction between Mexican and Mexican American couples. Reports on the relative incidence of marital instability are contradictory (Eberstein and Frisbie, 1976; Hayner, 1954; Uhlerberg, 1972) but a fairly high rate of intermarriage has consistently been found (Bean and Bradshaw, 1970). Not unlike the contemporary majority American marital experience, marital discord has been found to correlate with increased availability of resources and exposures to different ideologies. Also, two authors report a correlation between involvement of men in male peer groups and/or extramarital affairs and spouse alienation (Stoker et al., 1968–1969; De Huyos and De Huyos, 1966).

A number of articles have been written attempting to evaluate the consistently reported high fertility rate among Mexican Americans (Lopez and Sabach, 1978; Browning, 1974; Uhlenberg, 1973). The distinctive patterns of marriage, marital stability, and fertility reported by Uhlenberg (1974) in his analysis of the 1970 census data support Browning's contention that ethnic group membership is an influential factor in these trends independent of social economic status, education, occupation, etc. However, Uhlenberg also notes that there is considerable variation of fertility rates within the Mexican American population and that middle-class Mexican Americans have similar family sizes as other whites. Johnson (1976) also found in evaluating 1970 census data that employment of Mexican American women corresponded with smaller family size. It remains to be determined whether adequate education and full availability of birth control to lower-class Mexican Americans will affect the higher Mexican American birthrate. A dramatic decrease in the black birthrate did occur once black women were fully informed of the given options (Browning, 1974). Bullough's (1972) finding that underutilization of family planning services is the type of preventive health care most influenced by alienation warrants further consideration in this regard.

If at all comparable to attitudes of Mexican American women, the 1971 survey of Vankeep and Rice-Wray (1973) on ''Attitudes toward Family Planning and Contraception in Mexico City'' provides some interesting findings. The attitudes of 250 women who have chosen to avail themselves to free family planning services is compared with 500 randomly selected married women. It was found that the clinic sample was less likely to agree with statements suggesting that the desirability of large families; within both groups younger women tended to disavow this standard more often. Only 25% of the clinic sample feel contraception interferes with intercourse, whereas 50% of the random group held such beliefs. Over three-quarters of both groups felt it was not for the husband alone to decide whether contraception should be practiced, and 50% of both groups felt it should only be utilized secondary to medical indications. The clinic sample was much less inclined than the city sample to regard God or the Catholic Church as determiners of family size or contraceptive practice. Fifty percent of the city sample actually indicated that the church should allow all methods of contraception.

Williams' (1973) article on the "Cultural Patterning of Role Response to Hysterectomy" is one of the few reports on specific sexual issues. This brief article evaluates interviews of 32 Mexican American and 32 Anglo women convalescing from hysterectomies. The author suggests Mexican American women experience greater conflict vis-à-vis the decision to have a hysterectomy than Anglo women, but the difference in the small sample groups does not reach statistical significance.

Carrier's articles (1971, 1976, 1977) on Mexican male homosexuality suggest specific cultural influences on the sexual behavior and attitudes of these men. It has not been determined whether similar patterns exist among Mexican American men.

Puerto Rican and Cuban Americans

The historical and political backgrounds of the Hispanic countries had differed in ways that have affected their present cultural circumstances. Puerto Rico, colonized by the Spanish, was invaded by the United States during the Spanish–American War of 1898, becoming a U.S. territory thereafter. Intermixing of Spaniards, native Americans, and Africans in Puerto Rico led to a distinctive blending of these three cultures (Banks, 1979; Bernal and Flores-Ortiz, 1981; Rogler and Hollingshead, 1965; Wagenheim, 1975). The Spanish conquerors were almost completely successful in imposing the Spanish language on the native population of the colonies. Catholicism was similarly vigorously transmitted to the native groups and was integrated as a blending of Catholic religious imagery and ideology with indigenous religious practices and beliefs. To some degree, Catholicism has represented the repression of sexuality and control of emotions, while African and indigenous cultures have represented sexual and emotional expression (Beales, 1961). Throughout the Caribbean and Latin America, the *mulatto* or person of *mestizo* (mixed) racial background has been mythologized as having greater virility and sexual interest.

Puerto Ricans are citizens of the United States, so that technically their movements from the island to the mainland are relocations within their native country. However, this citizenship status belies the enormous cultural transitions involved in these migrations. Because of the ease of the migration, Puerto Ricans may underestimate or deny the experience of loss of homeland or culture that typically accompanies leaving the island. Any immigration is to some degree experienced as a loss of the native land and its culture, as well as a loss of the roots in community and often in family relationships. Puerto Ricans have access to their home culture in ways that to some degree ease the sense of loss, because within financial limits one can go home again. Paradoxically, though, this accessibility sometimes makes it difficult for Puerto Ricans to acknowledge the grief and loss that often accompany coming to the mainland. Puerto Ricans are found to be in the lowest socioeconomic groups, in spite of the fact that migrations are most often motivated by interest in economic improvement.

Puerto Ricans in the United States have tended to settle in the East Coast cities. At the present time, a steady flow of immigrants from the island move to the mainland for economic opportunity and to join relatives who have made the move. Among Puerto Ricans who have been in the United States for several generations, some speak little or no Spanish, whereas others remain monolingual Spanish. In addition, increasing numbers of United States-born, English-speaking Puerto Ricans are migrating to the island and establishing communities of "New Yoricans" and others who are in cultural transition within Puerto Rican culture.

Cuba was also colonized by the Spanish. The indigenous population was almost completely decimated, so that Cuban culture evolved as a blend of primarily Spanish and African cultures (Bernal and Flores-Ortiz, 1981; Casal and Hernandez, 1975). The United States invaded Cuba during the Spanish–American War of 1898. Cuba achieved its independence from the United States in 1902, although the United States remained involved in the internal politics of Cuba until the Cuban revolution in 1959. At that time (in response to the socialist political changes initiated by the Castro government), a large migration of the upper social classes of the Cubans began. The social and political motivations of Cuban immigrants are atypical among immigrant groups who most often hope for economic advancement in the United States. Also, until recently, Cuban Americans could not return to Cuba under any circumstances. Many Cubans in the United States still remember and preserve a culture steeped in the ambiance of pre-Castro Cuba, even though Cuban culture on the island has changed enormously in the last 22 years. The "freezing in time" of the culture of origin is typical of immigrant groups and can lead to value conflicts within the majority culture and to value conflicts within family generations (Szapocsnik, 1981; Bernal and Flores-Oritz, 1981).

Cubans have tended to migrate primarily to the southeast Florida and Miami areas, with some significant groups settling in the cities of the northeastern United States. Cubans have had a significant impact in Miami. There is a large section of the city described as "Little Havana," where Cuban culture has been dramatically transplanted. In the last year, a large new wave of immigrants from Cuba has caused enormous conflict between Cubans and Americans and within the Cuban immigrant community.

Large Hispanic neighborhoods exist within a number of American cities. Spanish is the principal language spoken in these neighborhoods, which are sufficiently extensive to allow a certain percentage of Hispanics to exist entirely within their confines, eliminating the necessity to acquire fluency in English. However, these individuals and families are more fragile if any necessity for contact outside of the community emerges. The problems of learning a new language are an important dimension of any immigrant's transition. Language limitations clearly influence Hispanic individuals' economic possibilities and potential for mobility.

Another important aspect of Hispanic experience in the United States is racism. Caribbean cultures, because of the *mestizaje* or blending of European, indigenous, and African groups, do not dichotomize race into black and white groups, rather, race is seen as a continuum (Beales, 1961). A substantial number of people in Cuba and Puerto Rico who are defined as light skinned in their native countries would be treated as blacks in the United States. When migrating to the mainland, many Hispanics of *mestizo* background are shocked by the United States' system of "either black or white." Longres (1970) describes the painful family situations that can arise when couples who migrate from Puerto Rico are suddenly defined as an "interracial marriage." Light-skinned spouses or children may become ashamed of their darker-skinned relatives, who are treated as blacks while they can "pass" as whites. Further, the majority American culture tends to see Spanish-speaking, Spanish-surnamed Americans as a distinct minority group devalued for their culture status, regardless of their racial characteristics. The shock of American racism and entry into minority status are important aspects of Hispanic experience in the United States.

Family relationships and gender roles are organized similarly in Caribbean and Latin American cultures. Family roles and authority are delineated along age and sex lines, with the greatest power and respect offered to the adult male. Sex roles, in general, and sexual behavior, in particular, are at least in public terms and in cultural mythology defined by a rigid double standard. The terms *machismo* and *marianismo* capture the sexual- and gender-role definitions of male and female functioning. *Machismo* is such a powerful image of men, both within and outside of Hispanic culture, that is has become incorporated into American culture as the symbol of a particular type of aggressive, sexually active masculinity. *Marianismo* is the image of women juxtaposed with the *machismo* of men, in which women are ideally seen as having "Virgin Mary" qualities of sexual purity and fidelity, spirituality, and complete self-sacrifice for the sake of others (Gomez, 1976, 1977; Mattei, 1977; Stevens, 1973). The reality of male and female behaviors may vary enormously, but these stylized images of male and female characteristics have substantial impact on the self-esteem and self-evaluation of Hispanic men and women.

Although many images of gender characteristics are reflected through aspects of the larger society, the most profound gender socialization takes place within the family. Gender roles are socialized vigorously and consistently within the family at a very young age. From the earliest age, boys are seen as active and impulsive and are permitted far greater freedom of movement outside the home. They are encouraged to be more adventurous, explore, and gain exposure to the public world outside of the family. In contrast, girls are far more restricted in their social contacts. They are taught to be passive, obedient of parental authority, and serve the needs of men, such as their fathers and brothers, in preparation for their roles as wives and mothers. The highest praise for a woman is to describe her as *casera* (of the home).

During courtship, girls are closely observed and supervised, since girls' passivity and boys' sexual aggressiveness creates a situation that in the girl's family's mind is volatile and dangerous to their daughter's virtue. The girl's socialized acquiescence to the wishes of others is seen as a reason for mandating strict supervision and enforcement of sexual standards of chastity. Girls are assumed to be either sexually unavailable and potential marital partners or sexually available and not considered for a marital commitment. It is socially assumed that the male will constantly test the female's resolve to maintain her chastity. Although the chaperonage system is disappearing under the influence of modern ideas of sexual freedom, the importance of female chastity continues to be emphasized, although men are encouraged to become sexually active at an early age.

For women, preparation for courtship becomes an enormously central aspect of her life, since marriage and childbearing is the role for which she has been prepared. Courtship and marriage become the socially acceptable means of escaping the sometimes tyrannical control of family of origin and establishing an independent adult identity. In contrast, men often appear to be more reluctant to enter marriage, although they see marriage as a means of establishing order and organization in their lives and providing for and enjoying a comfortable home life. Although freedom of movement outside the parental home is greater for men, for both men and women, adult status is not conferred until an individual establishes their own home. Until marriage, men and women are seen as governed by the authority of their parents.

Hispanic men and women have different expectations of marriage than Americans. Obedience to parents and establishment of a respectful, hierarchically organized home take precedence over romantic love. Although American social scientists tend to be critical of parental control exercised over courtship and marital choice among Hispanic families (Hill, 1972), the rituals and traditions of family relationships in this and other areas of Hispanic family life can be seen as offering order, continuity, meaning, and relief from what can be seen as the burden of overwhelming choices.

Marital relationships are affected by social prescriptions for male and female gender-role behavior. Men are assumed to enter marriage as sexually experienced and interested and knowledgeable of the world outside the family and home. Women, in contrast, go from the supervision of their parent's home to the supervision of their husband's home, with little privacy or freedom of movement. Often, women find it difficult to make the transition from the sexual control and inhibitions of courtship to the relative sexual freedom of marriage (Rainwater, 1971; Wagenheim, 1975). *Respeto* (respect) and modesty restrict the discussion of sexuality among women, so that women often have little opportunity to expand their learning of sexuality. Both men and women tend to see male sexual interest as a physical necessity rather than as a form of expression or marital communication. For women, there's an aspect of martyrdom and self-abnegation in sexual compliance with their husband's physical needs.

In marriage, women are defined as the emotional and social caretakers of husband and children, whereas men are seen as the economic providers. Women are expected to *aguantar* (tolerate) any whims or idiosyncracies on the part of their husbands in exchange for support of the family. Physical violence against women is socially more acceptable in some Hispanic groups, although it may not, in fact, be statistically more prevalent than in other American households.

The supposed devaluation of women in an authoritarian family represents only one aspect of family relationships. In fact, among Hispanic families the maternal role is central to the point of reverence. The wife and mother is perceived as the most important emotional and relational member of the family. Whether this division of family roles is a fair division of labor or an unfair exploitation of either sex has been argued by many writers and cannot be succinctly settled.

Changing economic situations and family organization have affected the marital relationships and power structure in Hispanic families. An extremely high percentage of Hispanic women are in the work force (Banks, 1979). Menial or service-related jobs are often more accessible to women than to men, so that many women find they can get jobs when their husbands cannot. Some writers suggest that economic circumstances have helped undermine the male's traditional position of provider and authority in the family (Cooney, 1975; Cromwell et al., 1973).

The welfare system also rewards absent men. Women can earn a larger income from the welfare department as mothers of children if they declare themselves as abandoned by their husbands. Although census figures report a large proportion of

Hispanic households in the United States have female heads, it is thought that these figures are at least somewhat inflated by the economic necessities of poverty that force families to report themselves as abandoned by their men.

Women's greater economic and family power is viewed ambivalently in minority as well as in majority cultures. *La mujer que se pone los pantalones* (the woman who wears the pants) is implied to be unfeminine and castrating of her husband. Richmond (1976) suggests that the wife's contribution of income alone does not affect decision-making power in the family. The couple has to adhere to an egalitarian ideology before the wife's contribution of income has an impact on family decision making. Several authors (Tharp et al., 1968; Alonso, 1976) suggest that the more acculturated the woman, the more likely she will be to value an egalitarian–companionate marriage or what Rainwater (1971) calls a shift from a segregated to a joint conjugal role pattern.

Hispanic families see childbearing as an important aspect of marital and family life. Children have many different meanings and functions in a marriage. For men, children establish virility and are expected to be an economic help. Children become especially central in the lives of women, whose life is organized around the principle of sacrificing herself out of love for her children. Children are viewed as a form of social power for parents, since they are seen as extensions of the parents who will respond to parental authority with obedience. They are also seen as essential to the cohesion and functioning of the family (Heath et al., 1974). The use of contraception is a psychologically complicated process under any cultural circumstances. For Hispanics, children have a special meaning in a marriage and family, which may take precedence over emphasis on careful family planning.

Implications for Psychiatric Intervention

Underutilization of mental health resources is typical of minority populations. As noted with Mexican Americans, research suggests that services appropriate to the population are more likely to be utilized if culturally sensitive staff were present in community agencies (Bernal and Flores-Ortiz, 1981; Derbyshire, 1967; Szapocsnik et al., 1978).

The different world view and value orientations of Hispanics can lead to misunderstandings in the therapeutic relationship with non-Latins. Initially, majority mental health practitioners tend to have difficulty understanding Hispanic valuation of the extended family. An active extended family may be labeled as "intrusive" or "symbiotic" with an implied sense of a pathologic lack of separation. Though some individual autonomy is relinquished, the presence of a close, supportive family offers a great deal of security and confirmation to its individual members. Only with appreciation and respect for this deep embeddedness in family relationships can therapists help Hispanic individuals establish appropriate independence and autonomy.

It is also important for practitioners to respect Hispanic family organization around sex and age hierarchies in order to engage a family in therapy. It is often necessary to affirm the existing family roles in initiating family therapy, even if the eventual goal is to change family patterns. Bernal and Flores-Ortiz (1981) thus suggest that the father should be addressed first in introductions and treated as the authority because undermining his position can disturb the family's equilibrium and make therapeutic interventions impossible. The devluation of women and of the feminine role, which is often seen as characteristic of Hispanic cultures, is as controversial a topic among Hispanic groups as it is in mainstream American culture. The traditional role of Hispanic men and women within the family can be seen as having both negative or limiting aspects and positive or adaptive aspects (Garcia-Bahne, 1977).

Even when an individual rather than the family is the participant in psychotherapeutic treatment, consciousness of family issues and loyalties is important in preserving the therapy relationship. Whereas mainstream American patients often enter mental health settings with the preface "I waited until now because I thought I should be able to handle these problems myself," Hispanic patients more often say "I waited until now because I thought we should be able to handle these problems within the family." Speaking with a therapist about marital or family conflicts can sometimes be experienced as disloyalty to the family, by both patient and family members. It is often useful for the therapist to meet the spouse or parents of an individual in psychotherapy and establish an acceptance of the family as a unit, even if the therapy will take place with the individual. In a project providing educational and supportive services to the Hispanic teenage mothers in Boston, this author has found that both the grandmothers and the teenage fathers needed to become familiar with the program before the young mothers were given "permission" to actively participate in the program.

The family's level of acculturation or adaptation to the majority culture is also an important variable in working with a Hispanic family in the United States (Bernal and Flores-Ortiz, 1981; Padilla, 1977; Szapocsnik, 1981). Some families value a quick Americanization, whereas others remain more involved in their native culture. Generational differences in assimilation can create extremely complex and sometimes conflictual family situations, especially in areas of gender roles and sexual expression or behavior. Hispanic families in the United States often find that their children are exposed to a barrage of drastically different values and expectations in the very areas of family and intimate relationships where the family has traditionally exercised the greatest control. Since children learn a new language much more quickly than adults and through peers and school come into contact with and integrate the American cultures more completely, they often assimilate the majority culture more rapidly than their parents.

In some families, enormous discrepancies between the cultural values of parents and children can lead to serious family problems (Bernal and Flores-Ortiz, 1981; Szapocsnik, 1981). Some parents from extremely impoverished or traumatic backgrounds find it difficult to identify or sympathize with the relative affluence and ease of the Americanized childhoods that their children are enjoying. This can lead to parent's ignoring symptoms of psychological distress in their children, or labeling them as the *malcrianza* (of bad upbringing, a misbehaving child).

Szapocsnik (1981) has developed a family therapy model from his work with Cuban families in Miami, based on his observation that a significant number of families with problem adolescents had a wide discrepancy between the cultural identifications of parents and children. Although the parents rigidly adhered to extremely traditional views retained from Cuba, the children had become very completely identified with American culture. Szapocsnik has successfully treated these families by helping them develop biculturalism so that both generations have greater, more fluid access to aspects of both Cuban and American culture.

Rendon (1974) reviews epidemiological studies of Puerto Ricans in New York and reports that mental illness is especially high in this group and most often affects Puerto Rican adolescents. Rendon suggests that in addition to poverty, crowding, illiteracy, lack of employment, and other sources of stress, Puerto Rican adolescents in New York face problems of transculturation that affect their identity development and social functioning. Rendon suggests that cultural conflicts may lead to the presentation of symptoms, such as dissociation, which can sometimes be misdiagnosed as schizophrenia because of lack of understanding of the cultural context.

In working with Hispanic patients on sexual issues, traditional modesty about sexuality, especially on the part of women patients, can make it difficult to talk directly. For example, sexual self-exposure to a male physician or discussion of sexual acts or fantasies with a male may seem unacceptable.

The "Culture of Poverty"*

Rainwater's (1966) study of lower-class sexual behavior exemplifies the replacement of myth by fact. In his introductory comments, he provides some background for the widely held myth that the sexual behavior among members of the lower class involves a great deal more sexual gratification than occurs for more restrained, respectable members of the middle class.

> Confounded in the complex myths which express this belief are natural virtue, innocence, honesty, love, fun, sensuality, and taking pleasure where and how one can find it. Natural man as hero can be constructed by any selection of these characteristics. But to our Puritan minds natural man can also be evil; we have myths of naturalness that emphasize immorality, hatefulness, sexual avarice, promiscuity and sensual gluttony. Whatever the evaluative overtones to a particular version of these myths, they add up to the fact that the lower classes (like racial and ethnic minorities, primitive peoples, Communists and others) are supposed to be gaining gratifications which more responsible middle-class people give up or sharply limit to appropriate relationships (like marriage) and situations (like in bed at night).

Culturally determined sexual myths, such as the hypersexuality of black males, the Don Juanism (*machismo*) of Latin males, and the sexual mystique attributed to Asian women, are further examples.

Rainwater (1966) studied marital sexuality by interviewing 409 individuals, 152 couples and 50 men and 55 women not married to each other (total of 257 couples thus being represented). His subjects lived in three large American cities and were chosen to include a social class range of whites from upper-middle to lower-lower and blacks from low-middle to lower-lower class levels. The subjects were asked to discuss their sexual relations in marriage, the gratification and/or dissatisfaction they had, the meaning of sex to their marriage, and its importance to themselves and their spouses. A

*Esther Shapiro

continuance of interest and enjoyment, which ranged from great interest and enjoyment to strong rejection, was found with a broad range among women subjects, some of whom, unlike men, expressed strong feelings of disgust and rejection of sex. One major finding in this study is the fact that the degree of interest and enjoyment varied directly with economic status; this is, that the amount of sexual pleasure was greater for the more affluent subjects. Also this pattern existed for both black and white subjects, whereas no differences between the reports of sexual interest and enjoyment was found between black and white subjects of the same economic class. Earlier studies by Kinsey (1948, 1953) produced similar findings.

In discussing these findings, Rainwater summarized his more extensive evaluation of the nature of the marital relationships of his subjects. He describes a continuum with regard to how couples organize their activities and share the responsibilities of daily living, which involves the degree to which the spouses jointly participate in activities around the house and share activities outside the home versus couples where the role relationships emphasized a separation of functions and interests of husband and wife. The latter corresponds to a lessoned experience of commonality and greater interpersonal distance since less time is spent together. Highly work-segregated relationships were found to be much more characteristic of lower-class couples, whereas more conjointly organized and integrated relationships typified the middle class. Evaluating couples on this continuum, Rainwater found that the degree of interest and enjoyment of sex highly corresponded with the degree of nonsegregated marital organization, thus, the finding of greater joint marital relatedness and greater sexual pleasure for middle-class couples and lesser sexual interest and pleasure among lower-class couples who had segregated job relations. Conversely, middle-class couples who utilized segregated roles reported less sexual interest and lower-class couples who had jointly organized marriages reported greater interest than the mean range for their class.

Reviewing a number of studies on sexual attitudes and behavior of impoverished Puerto Rican, Mexican, English, and American subjects, Rainwater (1971) notes that the tendency toward highly segregated role relationships is a consistent finding and may represent one component of the concept of a ''culture of poverty'' first described by Oscar Lewis. In this review, Rainwater also presents evidence substantiating his hypothesis that there are a number of attitudes and values regarding sex that are common to impoverished and illiterate people independent of their particular cultural background. Central to these attitudes is a deeply entrenched double standard that includes ''the dictum that sex is a man's pleasure and a woman's duty.'' Ficher's (1980) paper on the ''Treatment of Sexual Disorders in a Community Program'' also notes double standards in majority and minority working-class subjects. She highlights as well the fact that there is a greater tendency for lower socioeconomic class individuals to repeat the sexual patterns of their parents as the day-to-day struggle to secure basic needs markedly reduces the level of education and, therefore, exposure to the changing norms and attitudes of middle-class Americans.

The central attitude regarding sexual experiences is based on the concept that a man's nature demands sexual experience. Premarital and extramarital sexual activity for men is considered understandable and at least implicity condoned or even (within Latin cultures) encouraged as part of a man's learning and self-assertion. Correspondingly a dichotomy between bad women ("loose women," prostitutes) and good women exists. Good women are those sought for marriage who are expected to maintain virginity until matrimony. After matrimony, though not considered likely by either men or women, men often express the fantasy that sexual satisfaction might cause their wives to seek other relationships. This is a reason often given by a man for not stimulating his spouse too much or developing her sensual capacities through long or elaborate lovemaking.

A woman's sexual satisfaction is either considered optional or disapproved of with the corresponding belief that women either have no sexual desires or have much weaker sexual needs. Girls are not educated about sex. It is virtually not discussed at all unless sexual activity on the part of an unmarried woman is discovered. Thus, women describe being totally unprepared for sexual relations upon marriage and experience substantial initial "honeymoon trauma." A wife's reticence and modesty regarding intercourse is often valued by her spouse as evidence of premarital virginity and not being "oversexed." In an effort to minimize a husband's inclination to seek extramarital sexual gratification, women tend to seek a balance between apparent enjoyment and reticence. With this, a woman's intention is to communicate to the husband that her interest is solely due to her love for him and her enjoyment secondary to his right.

Lack of sexual pleasure for women often leads to various excuses to lessen the frequency of intercourse (feigning sleep or illness, arguing about the danger of pregnancy, welcoming menstruation, prolonging postpartum abstinence). However, these behaviors are risky as they may make the husband become violent and/or suspect infidelity.

Rosenberg and Bensman's (1971) report on "Sexual Problems in Three Ethnic Subcultures of an American Underclass" describes sexual attitudes and behaviors of white, black, and Puerto Rican adolescents that do generally correspond to the above norms. However, this excellent interview study also provides, in rich detail, aspects of these teenagers' differences in their culturally determined attitudes and sexual activities. The reader is particularly encouraged to review this article, as it highlights many of the concepts presented in this chapter.

References

Adey, E. Population control in China. *British Medical Journal,* 1974, *21,* 548.

Ahern, E.M. The power and pollution of Chinese women. In M. Wolf and R. Witkem (Eds.), *Women in Chinese society.* Stanford, Calif.: Stanford Univ. Press, 1975, Pp. 193–214.

Allport, G.W. *The nature of prejudice: A psychohistory.* Reading, Mass.: Addison–Wesley, 1954.

Allport, G.W. *The nature of prejudice.* Garden City, N.Y.: Doubleday Anchor Books, 1958.

Alonso, I. *A Critical Review of the Literature Relating to the Conjugal Roles and Social Networks of Middle Income Puerto Rican Families.* Qualitative paper, Harvard Graduate School of Education, 1976.

Alvarez, R. The unique psycho-historical experience of the Mexican American people. *Social Science Quarterly,* 1971, *2, 15.*

Banks, J. *Teaching strategies for ethinic studies* (2nd ed.). Boston: Allyn & Bacon, 1979.

Barrera, M. Mexican-American mental health service utilization: A critical examination of some proposed variables. *Community Mental Health Journal,* 1978, *4,* 35.

Beales, J. Sex life in Latin America. In A. Ellis (Ed.), *Encyclopedia of sexual behavior* (Vol. II). 1961.

Bean, E.D., and Bradshaw, B.S. Intermarriage between persons of Spanish and non-Spanish surname: Changes from mid-nineteenth to mid-twentieth century. *Social Science Quarterly,* 1970, *51,* 389.

Bernal, G., and Flores-Ortiz, Y. Latino families: Considerations in family therapy with Latinos having different Hispanic backgrounds. In M. McGoldrich, J. Giordano, and J.K. Pearce (Eds.), *Ethnicity and family therapy,* New York: Guildford Press, 1981, in press.

Bernard, J. *Marriage and family among Negroes.* Englewood Cliffs, N.J.: Prentice–Hall, 1966.

Bernard, V.W. Psychoanalysis and members of minority groups. *Journal of the American Psychoanalytic Association,* 1953, *1,* 256.

Billingsley, A. *Black families in white America.* Englewood Cliffs, N.J.: Prentice–Hall, 1968.

Borah, W., and Cook, S.G. Marriage and Legitimacy in Mexican Culture: Mexico and California. *California Law Review,* 1966, *54*(2), 946.

Bowers, J.Z. Observations on the politics of population control in China. *International Journal of Health Service,* 1973, *3,* 833–835.

Boyer, B. Psychoanalytic insights in working with ethnic minorities. *Social Casework,* November 1964, p. 519.

Bradshaw, W.H. Training psychiatrists for working with blacks in basic residency programs. *American Journal of Psychiatry,* 1973, *135*(12), 1520.

Browning, H.L. The reproductive behavior of minority groups in the USA. In W. Montagna and W.A. Sadler (Eds.), *Reproductive behavior.* New York: Plenum Press, 1974. Pp. 299–317.

Bullough, B. Poverty, ethnic identity and preventive health care, *Journal of Health and Social Behavior,* 1972, 347.

Bureau of the Census. *Perspectives on American husbands and wives* (Current Population Reports, Special Studies, Series P-23, No. 77). Washington, D.C.: U.S. Department of Commerce, 1978.

Calnek, M. Racial factors in the countertransferences: The black therapist and the black client. *American Journal of Orthopsychiatry,* 1970, *40*(1), 39.

Carrier, J.M. Participants in urban Mexican male homosexual encounters. *Archives of Sexual Behavior,* 1971, *1*(4), 279.

Carrier, J.M. Family attitudes and Mexican male homosexuality. *Urban Life,* 1976, *5,* 359.

Carrier, J.M. Sex role preference as an explanatory variable in homosexual behavior. *Archives of Sexual Behavior,* 1977, *6,* 53.

Casal, L., and Hernandez, A. Cubans in the United States: A survey of the literature. *Cuban Studies/Estudios Cubanos,* 1975, *5,* 2.

Casavantes, E. Pride and prejudice: A Mexican American dilemma. In N.N. Wagner and M.J. Haug (Eds.), *Chicanos: Social and psychological perspectives.* St. Louis, Mo.: Mosby, 1971. Pp. 46–51.

Chipp, S.A., and Green, J.J. (Eds.). *Asian Women in transition.* University Park, Pa.: Pennsylvania State Univ. Press, 1980.

Clark, K.B. *Dark ghetto: Dilemmas of social power.* New York: Harper & Row, 1965.

Cleaver, E. *Soul on ice.* New York: McGraw–Hill, 1968.

Cohen, R.I. Borderline conditions: Transcultural perspective. *Psychiatric Annual,* 1974, *4*(9), 7.

Cooney, R. Changing labor force participation of Mexican American wives: A comparison with Anglos and Blacks. *Social Science Quarterly,* 1975, *56*(2), 252–261.

Cromwell, R.E., Corrales, R., and Torsiello, P.M. Normative patterns of marital decision making power and influence in Mexico and the United States: A partial test of resource and ideology theory. *Journal of Comparative Family Studies* 1973, *4,* 175–196.

Cromwell, V.T. *A study of ethnic minority couples: An examination of decision making structures, patriarch, and traditional sex role stereotypes with implications for counseling.* Unpublished doctoral dissertation, University of Missouri, 1976.

Day, B. *Sexual life between blacks and whites: The roots of racism.* New York: World Publishing Co., 1972.

De Hoyos, A., and De Hoyos, G. The amigo system and alienation of the wife in the conjugal Mexican family. In B. Farber (Ed.), *Kinship and family organization.* New York: Wiley, 1966. Pp. 102–115.

Derbyshire, R.L. *Mental Health Needs and Resource Utilization among Mexican Americans in East Los Angeles,* Report No. IR11, MH-01539. Los Angeles: Welfare Planning Council, 1967.

Diaz-Guerrero, R. Neurosis and the Mexican family structure. *American Journal of Psychiatry,* 1955, *112*(6), 411.

Dollard, J. *Caste and class in a southern town.* New York: Harper & Row, 1949.

Draquns, J.G. Values reflected on psychopathology: The case of the protestant ethic. *Ethos,* 1974, *2,* 115.

Dworkin, A.G. Stereotypes and self-images held by native-born and foreign-born Mexican Americans. *Social Science Research,* 1965, *49*(2), 214.

Dworkin, A. *Woman-hating.* New York: Dutton, 1974.

Eberstein, I.W., and Frisbie, W.P. Differences in marital stability among Mexican Americans, Blacks and Anglos. *Social Problems,* 1976, *23*(5), 609.

Fabrega, H., Jr., and Metzger, D. Psychiatric illness in a small Latino community. *Psychiatry,* 1968, *31*(4), 339.

Ficher, I. Treatment of sexual disorders in a community program. In M. Andolfi and I. Zwerling (Eds.) *Dimensions of family therapy.* New York, Guilford Press, 1980. Pp. 109–122.

Flores, J.L. The utilization of a community mental health service by Mexican-Americans. *International Journal of Social Psychiatry,* 1978, *24,* 271.

Ford, C.S., and Beach, F.A. *Patterns of sexual behavior.* New York: Harper & Row, 1951.

Frazier, E.F. Negro, sex life of the African and American. In A. Ellis and A. Abarbanel (Eds.), *The encyclopedia of sexual behavior.* New York: Hawthorn Books, 1961. Pp. 769–775.

Fujitomi, I., and Wong, D. The new Asian-American woman. In S. Sue and N. Wagner (Eds.), *Asian-American: Psychological perspectives.* Palo Alto, Calif.: Science Behavior Books, 1973. Pp. 252–263.

Garcia-Bahne, 1977, The chicano family.

Gaw, A. Cultural aspects of mental health for Asian Americans: Chinese Americans. In A. Gaw (Ed.), *Cross-cultural psychiatry* Littleton, Mass.: Wright–P.S.G. Publishing Co., 1981. Pp. 1–29.

Gee, E. Issei: The first women. In *Asian women.* Berkeley: Univ. of California Press, 1971. Pp. 8–15.

Goldscheider, C., and Uhlenberg, P.R. Minority group status fertility. *American Journal of Sociology,* 1969, *74,* 361–372.

Gomez, A.G. Some considerations in structuring human services for the Spanish-speaking population of the United States. *International Journal of Mental Health,* 1976, *5*(2), 60–68.

Gomez, A.G. Hembrismo: Expression of a socio-cultural phenomenon in Puerto Rico. Paper presented at the Annual Meeting, Section of Psychiatry, Neurology and Neurosurgery, Puerto Rico Medical Association, San Juan, Puerto Rico, October 1977.

Goodman, M.E., and Beman, A.M. The child's-eye views of life in an urban barrio. In N.N. Wagner and M.J. Haug (Eds.), *Chicanos: Social and psychological perspectives.* St. Louis, Mo.: Mosby, 1971. Pp. 109–122.

Grebler, L., Moore, J.W., and Guzman, R.C. (Eds.), *Mexican American people: the nation's second largest minority.* Los Angeles: Free Press, 1970.

Grier, W.H., and Cobbs, P.M. *Black rage.* New York: Basic Books, 1968.

Guerray, G. *The Mexican-American* (Ethnic Differences Series No. 3). Washington: National Rehabilitation Association, 1971.

Gutman, H.C. *The black family in slavery and freedom, 1750–1925.* New York: Pantheon Books, 1976.

Gwee, A.L. Koro: A cultural disease. *Singapore Medical Journal,* 1963, *4,* 119–122.

Halsell, G. *Black/white sex.* New York: Morrow, 1972.

Hambly, W.D. Africans, the sex life of. In A. Ellis and A. Abarbanel (Eds.), *The encyclopedia of sexual behavior* (Vol. I), New York: Hawthorn Books, 1961. Pp. 69–74.

Hawkes, G.R., and Taylor, M. Power structure in Mexican and Mexican-American farm labor families. *Journal of Marriage and Family,* 1975, *3*(4), 807.

Hayner, N.A. The family in Mexico. *Marriage and Family Living,* 1954, *16,* 369.

Heath, L.L., Roper, B.S., and King, C.D. A research note on children viewed as contributors to marital stability: The relationship to birth control use, ideal and expected family size. *Journal of Marriage and Family,* 1974, *36*(2), 304–306.

Heiman, E.M., Burruel, G., and Chavez, N. Factors determining effective psychiatric outpatient treatment for Mexican-Americans. *Hospital and Community Psychiatry,* 1975, *16*(8), 515.

Heiman, E.M., and Kahn, M.S. Mental health patients in a barrio health center. *International Journal of Social Psychiatry,* 1975, *21*(3), 197.

Herskovits, M.J. *The myth of the Negro past.* Boston: Beacon Press, 1958.

Hill, R.B. *The strengths of black families.* New York: Emerson Hall, 1971.

Hill, R. Impediments to freedom of mate selection in Puerto Rico. In F. Mendez (Ed.), *Portrait of a society: Readings on Puerto Rico sociology* San Juan: Univ. of Puerto Rico Press, 1972.

Homma-True, R. Mental health issues among Asian-American women. In *Conference on the education and occupational needs of Asian-Pacific-American women,* Office of Educational Research and Improvement. Washington, D.C.: National Institute of Education, 1980. Pp. 65–87.

Hutchins, F.L. Teenage pregnancy and the black community. *Journal of National Medical Association,* 1978, *70*(11), 857–859.

Ishihara, A., and Levy, H.S. *The tao of sex: A Chinese introduction to the bedroom arts.* New York: Harper & Row, 1970.

Johnson, C.A. Mexican-American women in the labor force and lowered fertility. *American Journal of Public Health,* 1976, *66*(12), 1186.

Jones, J.M. *Prejudice and racism.* Reading, Mass.: Addison–Wesley, 1972.

Jones, R.L. (Ed.) *Black psychology.* New York: Harper & Row, 1972.

Kardiner, A., and Ovesey, L. *The mark of oppression: Explorations in the personality of the American Negro.* Cleveland, Ohio: World Publishers Co., 1955.

Karno, M. The enigma of ethnicity in a psychiatric clinic. *Archives of General Psychiatry,* 1966, *14,* 516.

Karno, M., and Edgerton, R.B. Perception of mental illness in a Mexican-American community. *Archives of General Psychiatry,* 1969, *20,* 233.

Karno, M., and Morales, A. A community mental health service for Mexican-Americans in a metropolis. In N.N. Wagner and M.J. Haug (Eds.), *Chicanos: Social and psychological perspectives.* St. Louis, Mo.: Mosby, 1971.

Karon, B.D. *Black scars.* New York: Springer,

Keefe, S.E. Why Mexican Americans underutilize mental health clinics: Fact or fallacy. In J.M. Kasas and S.E. Keefe (Eds.), *Family and mental health in the Mexican-American community.* Los Angeles: Spanish Speaking Mental Health Research Center, 1978. Pp. 91–108.

Kiev, A. *Curanderismo: Mexican American folk psychiatry.* New York: Free Press, 1968.

Kim, S.D. *Demonstration project for Asian Americans: An analysis of problems of Asian wives of U.S. servicemen,* Office of Research and Demonstration, Social and Rehabilitative Service. Washington, D.C.: U.S. Department of Health, Education and Welfare, 1975.

Kim, B.L. Asian wives of U.S. servicemen: Women in triple jeopardy. In *Report on the conference on the educational and occupational needs of Asian-Pacific American women* (August 1976). Washington, D.C.: U.S. Government Printing Office, pp. 359–379.

Kinsey, A.C., Pomeroy, W.B., and Martin, C.E. *Sexual behavior in the human male.* Philadelphia, Pa.: Saunders, 1948.

Kinsey, A.C., Pomeroy, W.B., Martin, C.E., and Gebhard, P.H. *Sexual behavior in the human female.* Philadelphia, Pa.: Saunders, 1953.

Kovel, J. *White racism: A psychohistory.* New York: Pantheon, 1970.

Kristeva, J. [*About Chinese women*] (A. Barrows, trans.). New York: Urizen Books, 1974.

Ladner, J.A. *Tomorrow's tomorrow, the Black woman.* Garden City, N.Y.: Doubleday, 1971.

Lee, R.H. *The Chinese in the United States of America.* Hong Kong: Hong Kong Univ. Press, 1960.

Leighton, A. Cultural issues in psychiatric residency training: Relevant generic issues. In A. Gaw, (Ed.), *Cross-cultural psychiatry.* Littleton, Mass.: Wright–P.S.G. Publishing Co., 1981. Pp. 199–236.

Lin, K.M. Traditional Chinese medical beliefs and their relevance for mental illness and psychiatry. In A. Kleinman and T.Y. Lin (Eds.), *Normal and abnormal behavior in Chinese culture.* Dordrecht: Reidel, 1981.

Lin, Y. (Ed.). *The wisdom of Confucius.* New York: The Modern Library, 1980.

Long, E.G., Horel, R., and Radinsky, T. *Transcultural psychiatry: Hispanic perspective* (Monograph 4). Los Angeles: Spanish Speaking Mental Health Research Center, University of California at Los Angeles, 1977.

Lopez, D.E., and Sabach, G. Untangling structural and normative aspects of the minority status-fertility hypothesis. *American Journal of Sociology,* 1978, *83,* 1491.

Lyman, S. Marriage and the family among Chinese immigrants to American 1850–1970. In *The Asian in the West* (Social Science and Humanities Publication, No. 4, Western Studies Center). Reno/Las Vegas: University of Nevada, 1970. Pp. 27–31. (a)

Lyman, S. The social demography of the Chinese and Japanese in the U.S. of America. In *The Asian in the West* (Social Science and Humanities Publication, No. 4, Western Studies Center). Reno/Las Vegas: University of Nevada, 1970. Pp. 65–80. (b)

MacCoby, M. On Mexican national character. In N.N. Wagner and M.J. Haug (Eds.), *Chicanos: Social and psychological perspectives.* St. Louis, Mo.: Mosby, 1971. Pp. 123–131.

Martinez, C. Psychiatric consultation in a rural Mexican-American clinic. *Psychiatric Annal,* 1977, *12,* 74.

Masters, W.H., and Johnson, V.E. *Human sexual response.* Boston: Little, Brown, 1966.

Mattei, L. *Psychology "Of" women: A look at Hispanic women.* Comprehensive examination paper, University of Massachusetts, Amherst, 1977.

McGough, J. Deviant marriage patterns in Chinese society. In L.A. Kleinman and T.Y. Lin (Eds.), *Normal and abnormal behavior in Chinese culture.* Dordrecht: Reidel, 1981. Pp. 171–201.

McWilliams, C. *North from Mexico: The Spanish speaking people of the United States.* Westport, Conn.: Greenwood Press, 1968.

Miranda, M.R., and Kitano, H. Mental health services in third world communities. *International Journal of Mental Health,* 1976, *5*(2), 39.

Mittelbach, F.G., and Moore, J.W. Ethnic endogamy—The case of the Mexican Americans. *American Journal of Sociology* 1968, *74*(1), 50.

Montiel, M. The social science myth of the Mexican-American family. *El Grito,* 1970, *4,* 56.

Montiel, M. The chicano family: A review of research. Social Work, 1973, *18*(2), 22.

Murillo, N. The Mexican-American family. In N.N. Wagner and M.J. Haug (Eds.), *Chicanos: Social and psychological perspectives.* St. Louis, Mo.: Mosby, 1971. Pp. 97–108.

National Research Council. *Toward a national policy for children and families.* Washington, D.C.: National Academy of Sciences, 1976.

Padilla, A., and Ruiz, R. *Latino mental health: A review of literature* (DHEW Publication No. (HSM). Washington, D.C.: U.S. Government Printing Office, 1973, pp. 73–143.

Padilla, A.M. Measuring ethnicity among Mexican Americans: Some questions for chicanos in mental health. In A.M. Padilla and E.R. Padilla (Eds.), *Improving mental health and human services for Hispanic communities.* Washington, D.C.: National Coalition of Hispanic Mental Health and Human Services Organizations, 1977. Pp. 23–34.

Parade magazine, Concubine comeback. June 28, 1981, p. 9.

Person, E.S. Racism: Evil or ill. *International Journal of Psychiatry,* 1969, *8,* 929.

Pettigrew, T.F. *A profile of the Negro American.* Princeton, N.J.: Van Nostrand, 1964.

Philippus, M.J. Successful and unsuccessful approaches to mental health services for an urban Hispano-American population. *American Journal of Public Health,* 1971, *61*(4), 820.

Pian, C. *A study of selected socio-economic characteristics of ethnic minorities based on the 1970 census.* Vol. II, *Asian Americans* (R.J. Associates, Inc., Office for Special Concerns), Washington, D.C.: U.S. Department of Health, Education and Welfare, 1974.

Pian, C. Immigration of Asian women and the status of recent Asian women immigrants. In *Report on the conference on the educational and occupational needs of Asian-Pacific-American women* (August 1976). Washington, D.C.: U.S. Government Printing Office, 1980. Pp. 181–212.

Pinderhughes, C.A. Effects of ethnic group concentration upon educational process, personality formation and mental health. *Journal of the National Medical Association,* 1964, *56*(5), 407.

Pinderhughes, C.A. The origins of racism. *International Journal of Psychiatry,* 1969, *8,* 934. (a)

Pinderhughes, C.A. Understanding black power: Processes and prospects. *American Journal of Psychiatry,* 1969, *125*(11), 106. (b)

Pinderhughes, C.A. The universal resolution of ambivalence by paranoia with an example in black and white. *American Journal of Psychotherapy,* 1970, *24,* 597.

Pinderhughes, C.A. Psychological and physiological origins of racism and other social discrimination. *Journal of the National Medical Association,* 1971, *63*(1), 25.

Pinderhughes, C.A. Ego development and cultural differences. *American Journal of Psychiatry,* 1974, *131*(2), 171.

Pinderhughes, C.A. Differential bonding: Toward a psychophysiological theory of stereotyping. *American Journal of Psychiatry,* 1979, *136*(1), 33.

Porterfield, E. *Black and white mixed marriages: An ethnographic study of black-white families.* Chicago: Nelson–Hall, 1978.

Poussaint, A.F. White manipulation & Black oppression. In *The Black scholar* (Vol. 10, Nos. 8, 9). 1979. Pp. 52–55.

Poussaint, A.F. Interracial relations and prejudice. In H.I. Kaplan, A.M., Freedman, and B.J. Sadock (Eds.), *Comprehensive textbook of psychiatry III*. Baltimore, Md.: Williams & Wilkins, 1980.

Rainwater, L. Some aspects of lower class sexual behavior. *Social Issues*, 1966, *22*, 96.

Rainwater, L. Marital sexuality in four cultures of poverty. In D.S. Marshall and R.C. Suggs (Eds.), *Human sexual behavior*. New York: Basic Books, 1971. Pp. 187–205.

Ramirez, S., and Parres, R. Some dynamic patterns in organization of the Mexican family. *International Journal of Social Psychiatry*, 1957, *3*(1), 18.

Reiss, I.L. Premarital sexual permissiveness among Negroes and whites. In R. Staples (Ed.), *The black family*. Belmont, Calif.: Wadsworth, 1975. Pp. 127–130.

Rendon, M. Transcultural aspects of Puerto Rican mental illness in New York. *International Journal of Social Psychiatry*, 1974, *20*(1–2), 18.

Report to the President from the President's Commission on Mental Health. Washington, D.C.: U.S. Government Printing Office, 1978.

Reuben, D. *Everything you always wanted to know about sex but were afraid to ask*. New York: Bantam Books, 1969.

Richmond, M.L. Beyond resource theory: Another look at factors enabling women to affect family interaction. *Journal of Marriage and the Family*, 1976, *38*(2), 257.

Rogler, L., and Hollingshead, A. *Trapped: Families and schizophrenia*. New York: Wiley, 1965.

Romano, V.O. The anthropology and sociology of Mexican-Americans: The distortion of Mexican-American history. *El Grito*, 1968, *2*, 13.

Rosenberg, B., and Bensman, J. Sexual patterns in three ethnic subcultures of an American underclass. In H. Thornberg (Ed.), *Contemporary adolescence: Readings*. Belmont, Calif.: Brooks/Cole, 1971. Pp. 94–107.

Ruffin, J.E. Racism as countertransference in psychotherapy groups. *Perspectives in Psychiatric Care*, 1973, *11*(4), 172.

Sabshin, M., Diensenhaus, H., and Wilkeson, R. Dimensions of institutional racism in psychiatry. *American Journal of Psychiatry*, 1970, *127*, 787.

Senour, M.N. Psychology of the Chicano. In J.L. Martinez (Ed.), *Chicano psychology* New York: Academic Press, 1978. Pp. 329–342.

Silverstein, B., and Krate, R. *Children of the dark ghetto: A developmental psychology*. New York: Praeger, 1976.

Simmons, O.G. The mutual images and expectations of Anglo-Americans and Mexican Americans. In N.N. Wagner and M.J. Haug (Eds.), *Chicanos: Social and psychological perspectives*. St. Louis, Mo.: Mosby, 1971. Pp. 62–71.

Staples, R. *The World of Black Singles: Changing Patterns of Male/female relations*. Westport, Conn.: Greenwood Press, 1981.

Stevens, E. Marianismo: The other face of machismo in Latin America. In A. Pescatello (Ed.), *Female and male in Latin America*. Pittsburgh, Pa.: Univ. of Pittsburgh Press, 1973.

Stoker, D.H., Zurcher, L.A., and Fox, W. Women in psychotherapy: A cross-cultural comparison. *International Journal of Social Psychiatry*, 1968–1969, *15*(1), 5.

Sue, S., Allen, D.B., and Conaway, L. The responsiveness and equality of mental health care to Chicanos and native Americans. *American Journal of Community Psychology*, 1978, *6*(2), 137.

Szapocsnik, J. *Biculturalism and family therapy*. Paper presented at a conference on minorities and family therapy, Judge Baker Guidance Center, Boston, 1981.

Szapocsnik, J., Scopetta, M., and King, O. Theory and practice in matching treatment to the special characteristics and problems of Cuban immigrants. *Journal of Community Psychology*, 1978, *6*(2), 112.

Tan, E.S. Culture-bound syndromes. In A. Kleinman and T.Y. Lin (Eds.), *Normal and abnormal behavior in Chinese culture*. Dordrecht: Reidel, 1981. Pp. 371–386.

Tharp, R.G., Meadown, A., Lennhoff, S.G., and Satterfield, D. Changes in marriage rules accompanying the acculturation of the Mexican-American wife. *Journal of Marriage and Family*, 1968, *30*(3), 404.

Thomas, A., and Sillen, S. *Racism and psychiatry*. New York: Brunner/Mazel, 1972.

Ticho, G.R. Cultural aspects of transference and countertransference. *Bulletin of the Menninger Clinic* 1971, *35*(5), 313.

324

Tseng, W.S., and Hsu, J. *Chinese culture, personality formation and mental illness.* Boston: Massachusetts Mental Health Center, 1968.
Tseng, W.S., and Char, W.F. The Chinese of Hawaii. In W.S. Tseng, J.F. McDermott, Jr., and T.W. Maretzki (Eds.), *People and cultures in Hawaii.* Honolulu: University of Hawaii, 1974. Pp. 24–33.

Uhlenberg, P. Marital instability among Mexican-Americans: Following the patterns of blacks. *Social Problems,* 1972, *20*(1), 49.
Uhlenberg, P. Fertility patterns within the Mexican-American population. *Social Biology,* 1973, *20*(1), 30.
Uhlenberg, P. The changing family patterns of blacks, chicanos, and whites: 1969–70. *Research Previews,* 1974, *21*(1), 1.

van Gulik, R. *La vie sexuelle dans la Chine ancienne.* Paris: Gallimard, 1971.
van Wulfften Palthe, P.M. Neuropsychiatry. In C.D. de Langen and A. Lichtenstein (Eds.) *Textbook of tropical medicine.* Batavia: Kloff, 1936.
Vankeep, P.A., and Rice-Wray, F.R. Attitudes toward family planning and contraception in Mexico City. *Studies in Family Planning,* 1973, *11*(4), 305.
Veith, I. [*The yellow emperor's classic of internal medicine*] (I. Veith, trans.). Baltimore, Md.: Williams & Wilkins, 1949.
von Siebold, P.F. *Manners and customs of the Japanese in the 19th century.* Rutland, Vt.: Tuttle, 1973. (Originally published, 1841.)

Wagenheim, K. *Puerto Rico: A profile* (2nd ed.). New York: Prager, 1975.
Wallace, M. *Black macho and the myth of the superwoman.* New York: The Dial Press, 1978.
Wilkeson, A. Cultural aspects of mental health care for Hispanic Americans: Mexican Americans. In A. Gaw (Ed.), *Cross-cultural psychiatry.* Littleton, Mass.: Wright–P.S.G. Publishing Co., 1981. Pp. 87–107. (a)
Wilkeson, A. Cultural issues in psychiatric residency training: A resident's perspective. In A. Gaw (Ed.), *Cross-cultural psychiatry.* Littleton, Mass., Wright–P.S.G. Publishing Co., 1981. Pp. 285–300. (b)
Williams, M.A. Cultural patterning of role and response to hysterectomy. *Nursing Forum,* 1973, *12*(4), 378.
Willie, V., Kramer, B.M., and Brown, B.S. (Eds.), *Racism and mental health: Essays.* Pittsburgh, Pa.: Univ. of Pittsburgh Press, 1973.
Winnicott, D.W. Transitional objects and transitional phenomena. *International Journal of Psychoanalysis,* 1953, *34,* 89.
Wittkower, E.D. Cultural aspects of psychotherapy. *American Journal of Psychotherapy,* 1974, *28,* 566.
Wolf, M., and Witkem, R. *Women in Chinese society.* Stanford, Calif.: Stanford Univ. Press, 1975.

14

Separation and Divorce: Crisis and Development

Toni E. Svéchin Greatrex

Introduction

This chapter will focus on problems that arise in the sexual sphere of the lives of people involved in marital crisis, separation, and divorce and in the reconstruction of new family units. Not only do the men and women playing major roles suffer disruption or distortion in their sexual lives, but their children are also subject to sexual tension and problems special to the stressful course of events.

The epidemic increase in the rate of separation and divorce in the past decade has led some social scientists to question the viability of the traditional nuclear family. Between March 1970 and March 1979, the ratio of all divorced persons per 1000 married persons rose by 96% (U.S. Bureau of the Census, 1979). There seems little doubt that changes in commitments to and expectations of marriage are occurring. The United States, with its current emphasis on self-realization, has the highest divorce rate in the Western world: 1,122,000 divorces occurred in 1979 compared to 2,243,000 marriages. Over 2 million adults and 1 million children under the age of 18 were involved directly and indirectly a multitude of friends, relatives, neighbors, and colleagues (U.S. Vital Statistics, 1978). At today's rate, one-third of first marriages and close to one-half of second marriages will end in divorce (Glick, 1975). Although verifiable statistics are difficult to establish, it is estimated that one-half of all separations lead not to divorce but to reconciliation. In turn, half of these reconciliations lead to further separation and ultimate divorce (U.S. Bureau of the Census, 1976). A rough projection based on divorce rates is that 30% of children growing up in the 1970s will experience parental divorce (Bane, 1979).

Toni E. Svéchin Greatrex • 115 Dean Road, Brookline, Massachusetts.

In addition to the termination of legally sanctioned relationships, very large numbers of adults and children are affected by the stress of the dissolution of relationships where individuals live together as couples, both homosexual and heterosexual, but without legal commitment. Although the 1979 Census reported that 1.3 million households were shared by two unrelated adults of the opposite sex (U.S. Bureau of the Census, 1979), it is estimated that today at least 6 million men and women live together without marriage ties. This chapter focuses largely on the traditional marriage unit. Similar stresses, however, are experienced by heterosexual unmarried couples and homosexual couples and by people in relationship to them.

We find ourselves in an era of flux in which a loosening of the fabric of society has resulted in changes of social customs, religious codes, economic influences, and basic laws that govern the status of men and women. Pertinent to our understanding of these events are (1) changes in the social, economic, and legal position of women; (2) changes in divorce and custody laws; and (3) growth in our knowledge and understanding of human sexuality. In recent years, the importance of sexuality has been increasingly recognized as contributing not only to the well-being of each individual but also to the healthy functioning of the family unit.

Multicausal Factors in Marital Crises

During this era of social change with its emphasis on individual rights and self-development, divorce is accepted as a reasonable alternative to an unhappy marriage. Marriage is seen increasingly as a source of individual support and nourishment rather than as a sacrament consummated for procreative purposes and social responsibility. No longer are roles of husbands (breadwinners) and wives (homemakers) simply complementary and clearly defined. This change from traditional social, religious, and economic ties of mutual dependency within the marriage to a position in which people make great demands on each other for sexual and emotional fulfillment places a heavy burden on marriage partners.

Primary care providers worked for years within the framework of the cultural expectations that most marriages were meant to endure except those severely stressed by such problems as (1) grossly abusive behavior, (2) psychopathy or criminality, (3) psychosis, (4) alcoholism or drug abuse, (5) persistent infidelity, or (6) desertion. Today the clinician must contend with these problems and, in addition, face the changing attitudes and expectations of our culture.

It is the common experience of all clinicians that although a patient's chief complaint is of a somatic nature, the underlying stress is emotional. He/she frequently encounters individuals in a state of marital crisis who need to consider whether their marriage is worth reaffirming, as well as those who are experiencing the distress of ending a relationship. Often the patients' complaints about the marriage are vague: estrangement, lack of communication, lack of fulfillment. These nebulous complaints will invariably be accompanied by statements indicating the erosion of the couple's sex life and frequently by concerns about the individual's sexual functioning. The clinician must keep in mind that the anxiety and depression that can disrupt and ultimately destroy harmony and compatibility may arise from within the family unit or may be only peripherally related to the marriage itself. Major life events, such as the birth of a child, a career change, a relocation of the home, a death of a family member, or retirement, create inner stress and may alter the sexual behavior of the partners. Other important problems that lead to estrangement and separation are (1) persistent economic difficulties, (2) infertility, (3) the discovery of extramarital sex, and (4) the discovery of homosexuality of a partner.

Sex and Family Life

Sex is basic to the functioning of the family unit as well as to the functioning of the couple. It is a vital aspect of all our primary relationships in causing fulfillment or frustration, self-enhancement or devaluation. It is the foundation upon which the structure of intimacy is built. In its best aspects, sexual fulfillment between two adults enhances their individual lives and provides an atmosphere of warmth and respect within the family. It nurtures healthy self-esteem in developing children and provides for them a model of mutual love, empathy, and trust. The sexual relationship between two individuals is an exquisite barometer that reflects the state of their union. Anger, resentment, fears, and desires can be camouflaged more easily at the dinner table than in bed. Sexual problems are often the first symptoms of the breakdown of family life. It is important for the clinician to be aware that patients' complaints, particularly about sexual issues, while appearing clear-cut and straightforward, evolve from multicausal stresses on the individual and on the family unit. The following history illustrates how a patient's manifest symptoms of retarded ejaculation evolved from a number of internal and external stresses, involving not only him but also his wife and child.

> The Browns, a couple in their early thirties, were caught up in a sexual struggle. Mrs. Brown had shown little interest in sexual contact with her husband since her mother's death the year before. As the anniversary of her mother's death approached, she became increasingly preoccupied. Mr. Brown did not address the problem openly, but his mounting frustration and anger made him withdraw. The Browns drank more at dinner, watched more television, and had little to say to each other. Their 3-year-old daughter became the focus of their attention and affection. She was allowed to stay up later and began experiencing bad dreams. As the opportunity for sexual encounters decreased, the daughter was placed in a more prominent role. For some time masturbation was a sexual outlet for Mr. Brown, but eventually he lost interest in self-stimulation. Their sporadic attempts at intercourse found him unable to ejaculate. Mr. Brown finally made an appointment with his physician and expressed concern about his general state of health and, in particular, his sexual functioning. The physician, as part of his/her evaluation, suggested a psychiatric consultation. During a separate interview with Mrs. Brown, the consultant noted that she had been struggling for some months to combat the symptoms of depression that she had tried to hide from the family. She experienced early-morning awakening, cried easily, was

generally irritable, and was unable to feel closeness to her husband. As the anniversary approached, these symptoms intensified and included undue sensitivity and feelings of unworthiness and rejection. Mr. Brown seemed unaware of how deeply troubled his wife was and had experienced her withdrawal and lack of enthusiasm as a rejection of him. Her sexual with-drawal triggered feelings of anxiety and hostility that ultimately manifested themselves in his sexual distress. The treatment plan for this family involved evaluating and treating Mrs. Brown's depression and helping the couple strengthen their ability to communicate so that they would be able to focus on one another instead of on their child.

Emotional and Physical Illness Resulting from the Stress of Separation and Divorce

It is clear that disease entities cannot be conceptualized as evolving from a single cause. Rather, complex etiological factors interrelate to give rise to what we recognize as illness. Furthermore, each patient must be considered in terms of his/her psychoso-cial and cultural background. For several decades researchers have been studying the proposition that "many if not all diseases have their onset in a setting of mounting frequency of social stress." In 1967, Rahe and co-workers developed the Social Readjustment Rating Scale (SRRS) (Holmes and Rahe, 1967). (See Chapter 16.) On the SRRS, separation and divorce rank only below death of spouse in terms of the impact on the individual. This scale was devised after sampling many kinds of life adjustment, but Rahe made no claim that it covered every possible life-change event. There is no unanimity of opinion among researchers today as to which life-change events are most representative and/or meaningful in a persons' life (Rahe, 1979). Nevertheless, a substantial amount of work using actual life stresses demonstrates both prospectively and retrospectively that the more stress people experience (including marital disruption) the more likely they are to become ill (Rahe, 1978; Masuda and Holmes, 1978).

Clearly, marital disruption and the transition to singleness are stressor events entailing a variety of psychic traumas that may manifest themselves as emotional or physical symptoms. The first study conducted by the National Center for Health Statistics of Differentials in Health Characteristics as a Function of Marital Status demonstrated the following: Generally, widowed, separated, and divorced persons have higher rates of disability than married or never-married persons. Separated and divorced individuals, particularly women, seem unusually vulnerable to acute condi-tions. The most vulnerable period appears to occur during separation (National Center for Health Statistics, 1976).

People who are separated or divorced have also been found repeatedly to be overrepresented among psychiatric patients, whereas those persons married and living with their spouses have been found to be underrepresented. Of all the social variables related to the distribution of psychopathology in the population, none has been more consistently found to be so crucial for the population than marital status (Cragu, 1972).

In both sexes, the automobile-accident fatality is higher among the divorced than among any other marital status group (National Center for Health Statistics, 1970). It has been found that the accident rate doubled during the period from 6 months before to 6 months after divorce (McMurray, 1970). It also appears that when there has been a definite loss of a loved person—spouse, parent, child, or lover, within the previous year (by death, divorce, or separation)—the potential for self-destruction is greater. The suicide rate is higher among the divorced than among people of any other marital status. Although people within the divorced/separated/widowed segment of the population are underrepresented among those who attempt suicide, they are overrepresented among those who successfully commit it (Schneidman and Farberow, 1961). Evidence is accumulating linking human loneliness, or a sense of separateness, to disease and to premature death. "Although marital status is not clearly indicative of the presence or absence of loneliness, a few comparative statistics in the premature death rates of white males reveal strikingly higher death rates among the unmarried." Besides statistics from the suicide and automobile fatalities, data demonstrate increased mortality rates from cirrhosis of the liver, pulmonary carcinoma, gastrointestinal carcinoma, CVA and cardiac disease among the divorced and widowed population (Lynch and Convey, 1979).

Phases of Separation and Divorce

Just as marital disruption indicates the disintegration of a family unit, so the personalities of the individuals involved are thrown into chaos. People in the throes of marital crisis may experience lowered self-esteem and may be more vulnerable to symptoms, including sexual ones. There is nothing unique in the sexual problems of people in this situation. The important factor is that the problems exist and are in danger of being overlooked.

Since marital disruption is such a common occurrence and follows a predictable pattern of events, it is important that clinicians be familiar with the repercussions. Although the ritual of mourning for the dead and support for the bereaved are culturally established, there are no social customs to help the individual and family experiencing the loss of separation or divorce.

Weiss delineates three phases in his study of men and women going through divorce: (1) the acute phase, (2) the transition phase, and (3) the recovery phase (Weiss, 1975).

The Acute Phase

The acute phase lasts approximately 1 month. During this time patients are at their most vulnerable and often seek help for physical and emotional illness. In the first few weeks after physical leave-taking, most people experience relief, intermingled with intense waves of emotions, such as disbelief, numbness, anger, longing, and fear that may border on panic. Only a small portion experienced a sustained sense of freedom or exhileration.

The inner panic state is similar to a small child's fear of abandonment. This can be better understood if we examine the nature of the bond that develops between two people. Weiss uses the term *attachment* to describe the deep binding of the selves that occurs in a union after approximately 2 years. By that time, the individual has integrated the new identity as husband or wife. The degree of panic during separation speaks to the degree of dependency between partners. The degree of pain speaks to the depth of the attachment. Contrary to the mythology of the Western movie, where the lone hero rides off into the distance, most men and women seek one-to-one relationships in which they can achieve and sustain closeness. Marriage creates kin by ceremony. In this culture, marriage is still considered the ideal goal for men and women. The attraction must lie in this most human of all needs, to interact with another at an emotional level where one is loved, accepted, and able to express one's deepest needs.

Sexual expression in such a relationship is unique because it involves both an emotional and physical exchange of nurturance and pleasure. As such, it renews the bond between the physical and symbolic levels of gratification and is the forum to which individuals bring not only their desires and hopes but their repertoire of past experiences. The only other time such intense physical closeness occurs is in the interaction between a young child and its parents.

Therefore, during the detachment process, people talk of losing part of themselves and of feeling anchorless. Their identity has been wrenched from its mooring. It is a state of crisis. The following case history serves as an illustration.

> Mrs. D. appeared at the psychiatric clinic without an appointment, disheveled and in obvious distress. Her salesman husband had left the family several days before, stating that this separation would have to be the final one. He no longer wished to be married or to attempt to work out marital problems. Mr. D. had always been a good provider and attentive father, but his lack of interest in sex with his wife began early in the marriage. Two years earlier, Mrs. D. had accidentally discovered a suitcase filled with pornography, particularly homosexual material. That incident had initiated the first separation. Although Mrs. D. displayed remarkably little curiosity about her husband's life outside the home, she had wanted the marriage to work out and had tried hard to please him. Sexual contact between them occurred rarely and always left her feeling angry and ashamed. During the appointment Mrs. D. cried unceasingly and manifested symptoms of acute anxiety and depression. She had not slept for several nights and had eaten little. She had spent the previous night drinking heavily, feeling inwardly disorganized and thinking of ways to harm herself. She felt abandoned, afraid, and unwomanly, stating that it was her fault that the marriage had not worked out.
>
> In evaluating Mrs. D., the therapist attempts to provide a forum where she can vent her feelings freely and receive the reassurance that the crisis, however painful, is temporary. This can best be accomplished through an attitude of empathy toward Mrs. D., in which the therapist responds with understanding and offers support that will help her regain perspective and

plan a course of action. It is helpful to keep in mind the question, "How do you wish or hope that I can be of help to you?"

The initial part of every evaluation involves an assessment of the patient's personality structure and coping mechanisms. Where there is evidence of psychosis or suicidal (homicidal) ideation, hospitalization is advised, so that further evaluation of the patient and family and the creation of an effective treatment plan can evolve in a protective setting. Where the evaluation can proceed on an outpatient basis, it is vital to investigate the marital situation, including its sexual aspect, and the level of distress that both patient and family members are experiencing. The patient's support structure, including relatives, friends, work, and community involvements, needs to be explored. Treatment includes reassurance and guidance of the patient in designing a short-term plan that will ensure he/she is secure in day-to-day functioning and has the maximum support from those involved in his/her life. Frequent appointments should be arranged along with the offer of telephone contact. On occasion medication (tranquilizers, hypnotics, antidepressants) is necessary and should be prescribed appropriately.

Depending on the outcome of the crisis, the therapist's evaluation and the patient's wishes, longer-term treatment for the patient and/or family may be indicated.

The Transition Phase

The transition phase of separation, which lasts from 8 to 12 months, is invariably associated with some depression of affect. Each person gradually moves from experiencing the self as part of a couple to being single again. The preexisting life patterns have been shattered and the disruption of the inner sense of self continues. Out of the separation shock, a new life pattern gradually evolves.

In an analysis of stresses associated with divorce, Bohannan (1970) identified six overlapping experiences faced by each spouse: (1) emotional divorce, which centers on the problem of the deteriorating marriage, (2) legal divorce usually based on specific grounds, (3) economic divorce dealing with money and property, (4) coparental divorce dealing with custody, single-parent homes, and visitation, (5) community divorce involving the changes of friends and community, (6) psychic divorce and the problem of regaining individual autonomy.

This categorization helps in understanding the intricate pieces of the divorce process that have to be negotiated. The transition period is generally a very active time. Much energy is consumed by the tasks of establishing a new domicile, struggling with financial matters, and dealing with children, kin, community, and colleagues. During this time, legal proceedings may be initiated and they are inevitably traumatic.

The panic of the first few weeks modulates into a less acute but deeper sense of loss. The mourning process peaks at 6 months postseparation and is experienced as an inner aching, a love void, and loneliness in bed at night when the missing person may be most yearned for. At the same time, anger has a place in the mourning process, anger at the wasted years and at the shambles of one's emotional, social, and economic life. Grievances against the missing spouse are recounted endlessly; painful events of the marriage are gone over repeatedly in ruminative fashion. The anger tends to become highlighted during the legal process. The previously gentle spouse remarks, ''I never knew I could hate so much!''

Separated people talk of feeling unattractive and helpless and of lacking identity. For many separated people, being a couple was a way of life for years. A housewife in her midforties, whose children had left home and who had no previous work experience and no readily marketable skills, felt listless and hopeless during this phase. She said of herself, ''I felt totally lost in the world. I always wanted to be married because I felt I had no worth except in my roles as wife and mother.''

Women, unless they have established ongoing careers, suffer a greater destruction of their identities during the divorce and often hit rock bottom during the first months of separation. Men, who more often have work roles to sustain them, may be able to suppress the sense of loss and incompleteness longer.

Even though divorced people are described as being ''single again,'' many men and women have never functioned as totally independent adults before. For example, many women move from dependency in the parental home to dependency in marriage, where the husband is both provider and decision maker. These women, even the ones who initiate the divorce, are often emotionally unprepared for the pressures and multiple discontinuities that follow divorce decisions. For them, the psychic divorce process as they struggle to become autonomous individuals is particularly difficult.

The magnitude of the impact of divorce on most men is a fact that most women (and many men) find hard to accept, in spite of the fact that statistically the relationship between marital disruption and psychopathology appears to be stronger for men than for women (Bloom et al., 1978). Separated men complain of a sense of rootlessness, a loss of purpose, and a lack of meaning in their lives. They seem to experience, more than women, a sense of personal failure at the ending of a marriage. Men can be even more frightened than women by the feelings of guilt, responsibility, helplessness, loneliness, and fear that erupt within them. They may be horrified by the reactions they are unable to control. One separated man awoke for several weeks from nightmares that left him with a feeling of inner panic. He lay curled up in his bed for hours each night shivering, waiting for dawn to arrive. During this phase, he dreaded weekends because, without structured work activities, he had great difficulty planning how to spend his time. He felt both ashamed and confused by his overwhelming feelings. He hesitated to disclose them to anyone. It seems socially more acceptable to many for women to seek professional help. Men often find it difficult to do so and wait.

Many men and women will request help from their primary care provider when the psychological distress has transferred itself into a bodily symptom. They complain of fatigue and general malaise, vague aches, headaches, sleeping disturbances, menstrual disturbances, etc. Sometimes a previous condition is exacerbated, such as ulcerative colitis, arthritis, low back syndromes, and asthma. Sometimes a new concern is mentioned. For example, symptoms may appear that frighten the patient and are reminiscent of serious illness in other family members. In addition to managing the physical disorder, the physician can be most helpful if he/she provides an atmosphere in which the patient can talk freely. Through an attitude of support and reassurance, he/she can identify the covert emotional issues underlying overt psychosomatic ones.

When symptoms are of mild depression—such as expressions of boredom, feeling burdened, and feeling gloomy—the physician may choose to monitor the patient by regular visits and possibly with medication or suggest a psychiatric consultation, realizing the patient might benefit from psychotherapy.

However, the mood disturbance may be chronic and resistant to help, or the physician may become aware of more serious symptomatology, such as strong feelings of guilt or worthlessness, suicidal thoughts, or hallucinations, or vegetative symptoms, such as sleep disturbances, loss of appetite, or psychomotor retardation. In such instances, the physician should make an appropriate referral to a psychiatrist or mental health professional. It is important to keep in mind that individuals function best when they have personal skills, stable work, financial security, support from friends and family, and a feeling of sexual attractiveness.

Over and over again men and women living alone say that conquering loneliness is the greatest challenge they face. Divorce in childless couples does signify the end of a relationship. The detachment process is more complete and reattachment is easier. Where children are involved, however, divorce ends the marriage but not the relationship with the children or, usually, with the exspouse. One divorced father said to a friend who was also in the process of separation, "You're so lucky; no burdens—no wife, no children, no past that just hangs over you. A clean break. You can get started again with no liabilities. My former wife thinks I've got it easy, but I'm still tied to them. At least she has the children. All I have is an empty room to go home to." Fathers in particular suffer from being displaced. Losing a spouse may overtly be viewed as a blessing, but the absence of children can cause severe emotional upset in the noncustodial spouse. Men rejected by their wives may fear equal rejection by their children. One overwhelmed father who had lost his child custody suit expressed his bitter feelings at the end of the divorce proceedings: "I'm through missing my children so intensely. But they're being cheated. I don't get to share the trivia of their daily lives. I wanted a family desperately. It was the part of the marriage I valued the most. Recently, I spent the holidays with friends up north. It was great to feel part of a family for the weekend. Monday night we returned and I went back to my place alone. I really crashed. It was awful."

The Recovery Phase

During the 2 to 4 years following the transition period, people find that the various stages of the divorce process are successfully negotiated and can be put behind them. They have developed a new life pattern that includes a new identity, a new living situation, a new style of relating to children, career changes, and a new pattern of friendships. These have become resilient and stable enough to withstand stress.

Just as marriage is a development stage, so, too, is divorce. In optimal circumstances, men and women will use the divorce process in the service of growth, self-exploration, and development. It is important to work through the pain, bitterness, and mistrust and to understand what went wrong in the old union. Otherwise, there is a great danger of remaining uninvolved in a new relationship or of repeating the old pattern. As one couple, both in their second marriage pointed out, "It's no good carrying the old baggage to a new relationship."

Sexual Patterns during Separation and Divorce

Ultimately for both men and women, the most important factor leading back to a positive self-image is a satisfying sexual relationship. People's sexual needs and responses vary greatly and include some of the following patterns during separation and divorce: (1) diminished sexual desire; (2) the immediate formation of a new, dependent relationship; and (3) multiple sexual encounters.

The diminished sexual desire that some people experience may be a reaction to the fear of being hurt and rejected; it may be an expression of anger at the opposite sex; it may also be a manifestation of mild to moderate depression. For example, they make few social contacts, refuse invitations, and feel awkward at social gatherings. They complain of low energy levels and chronic fatigue. They drag to work and drag home. They may spend evenings and weekends resting or sleeping. They are prone to overeating and at times to an increase in alcohol consumption and/or drug abuse. Other individuals may feel sexually dormant but experience a surge of energy, which they channel into new pursuits. For example, they may begin a new career, expand a circle of friends, reestablish old family ties, find new hobbies, or join new organizations. For some people, it is a time when they may be drawn more to members of their own sex for comfort, support, and companionship. Previously heterosexual individuals may experience their first homosexual relationship in the search for acceptance and intimacy.

Eventually most people will return to an active social life that includes the possibility of sexual intimacy. The process of reentering the single world is a difficult task for most people, who are surprised to find within themselves feelings of adolescent awkwardness. "Before every date I would pace up and down the hall of my apartment. I was petrified of the opposite sex just the way I had been as a teenager." Many people have had very limited sexual experiences in the past, frequently only with exspouses, and those frequently unsatisfactory. "My experience with sex is so limited, 12 years with one man (woman). I have no standard of judgment. I feel chronically deprived sexually and I cannot conceive of sex outside the context of a relationship. I don't know how to go about meeting men (women). I am scared to go out into the world. It has changed so."

Psychiatrists must realize that many patients are reluctant to reveal sexual problems because of their embarassment over their lack of knowledge and their fear of disapproval. In assessing any adult involved in a separation and divorce process, the individual's as well as the couples' sexual life must be addressed. A routine psychiatric evaluation should include questions about sexuality, level of satisfaction, discomforts, and expectations. Through the therapist's own attitude of ease and sympathetic concern, the patient can be encouraged to speak freely and to ask questions. Usually concerns over expectations and disappointments in the individual's sexual life will be expressed. Problems about sexual functioning may be revealed, and questions may be asked about pragmatic but potentially embarrassing issues, such as birth control methods, pregnancy fears, abortion, and venereal disease. Patients will be very grateful for specific information and advice. Simple facts about anatomy or physiology will help dispel myths. Many people are simply searching for permission to become sexually active and for reassurance that their sexual fantasies and feelings are appropriate.

A second pattern of handling separation is to leave the marriage and immediately to establish a new dependency relationship, especially a sexual one, where the individual feels valued as a man or a woman. Such relationships are usually temporizing and serve to insulate the people from the trauma of separateness. Some individuals experience rejuvenated sexual gratification that has been absent from their lives for a long time, along with a new-found sense of freedom and purpose. Others may be disturbed by confused feelings and begin to experience a variety of sexual difficulties, such as impotence, premature ejaculation, and vaginismus.

Yet a third group of individuals avoids the painful effect of separation by fleeing into an euphoric state that is reflected in boundless energy and includes multiple sexual encounters. These may vary in duration and include heterosexual and homosexual experiments. The experienced therapist will keep in mind the broad pattern of sexual behavior that his/her patients may follow but hesitate to discuss. Many may knowingly, or unknowingly, have been exposed to venereal disease (genital, oral). Frequent sexual activity in both men and women can be a way of avoiding or coping with depression and at the same time acting out anger at the person who has rejected them.

Children and Divorce

As noted previously, it has been estimated that of all children born in the 1970s, 30% will experience parental divorce (Bane, 1979). As the ranks of children involved in marital disruption swell, it becomes necessary to focus more sharply on the effects of this process on them. It has been said that children are the true victims of divorce; yet their role in this process has thus far been poorly explored. Currently, close to 60% of all divorces involve children under the age of 18. In 1979 over 1 million children were involved in divorce proceedings (Bane, 1979). What is it about divorce that troubles children?

We recognize that divorce is a time-limited disorganization and reorganization process of a family system. This time period, though bounded, may be substantial. Some authorities limit the time frame to 2 to 3 years. Others feel that the average disruption affecting children lasts from 5 to 6 years. For an adult, such disequilibrium may seem long enough, but for a child it is a significant proportion of his/her life span thus far and seems to last forever.

If it is true of children as it is for adults that life-event changes are stressors that produce emotional and physical illness, then the knowledge of the major changes that accompany the divorce process can enable us to make a more accurate prediction of its impact on children.

The body of research on children and divorce that has thus far been developed provides contradictory and inconclusive answers at best. Verification is lacking for statements such as "Divorce directly causes harmful consequences to children in the form of confusion over sex roles, juvenile delinquency, poor academic performance." There are a number of flaws in the research to date:

1. Oversimplification in an attempt to demonstrate direct cause/effect sequences. For example, a child's troubles may be attributed to a single event, such as the departure of the father, rather than to the complexity of change a child constantly negotiates. Some important factors in a child's adjustment to a divorce or separation are socioeonomic and environmental changes that coincide with the divorce; custodial parent's emotional well-being; the continuing relationship with the departed (visiting) parent; the relationship between the separated parents; the quality of the family's other interrelationships and outside support; the age, developmental level, and sex of the child; and the difficulties and differences when the absent parent is of the same sex as against the whole different range of problems if the absent parent is of the opposite sex.

2. Children of divorce have generally been compared to children of well-functioning families rather than to those from disturbed, tension-ridden, predivorce homes.

3. Except for a few studies, notably Wallerstein and Kelly (1974, 1975, 1976), systematic observation of children at the very time of divorce has been lacking. The literature usually assesses some aspect of the child's development at a later date and makes retrospective interpretations.

4. Most research is drawn from mental health clinic populations rather than from randomly selected normal populations.

5. In interpreting findings, most studies have failed to emphasize the meaning of age differences in children undergoing divorce. Consequently, the research suffers from the lack of a theoretical perspective that would enable us to interpret and to integrate the findings.

Two aspects of family relationships that have received attention in the past decade are conflict within the home and the quality of the parent/child interaction. Most authorities agree that parental conflict alone is sufficient to produce symptoms in children and that children function better in an atmosphere of contentment, whether in a two-parent home or in a single-parent situation. What is becoming clear also is that the quality of the parent/child relationship is crucial to the childrens' well-being. So it is not the divorce itself but the emotional situation in the home, with or without divorce, that is the determining factor in the children's development.

The best insurance for children is a well-functioning parent, with a healthy self-esteem and an ability not only to survive but also to negotiate life situations successfully, with confidence and positive expectation.

Developmental Perspective

As children grow and mature, their reasoning about the social and physical world changes. Thus, in order to understand and evaluate a child's response to divorce, it is important to consider a child's level of development, for this has implications as to how he/she perceives and processes the experience of divorce. Longfellow (1979) has reviewed the literature and reinterpreted some data in children's reactions to divorce using a social–cognitive developmental framework. She uses Wallerstein's (1974, 1975, 1976) observations of children whom they studied after dividing them into the customary age groupings: (1) preschool ages 3 to 6; (2) early latency ages 7 to 8; (3) late latency ages 8 to 11; and (4) adolescence.

They found that preschool children with their limited and egocentric reasoning ability tended to center explanations on themselves, e.g., Daddy left our home because I was a bad girl. Self-blame attitudes for illogical reasons frequently developed and were resistent to intervention by parents and counselors. These young children had difficulty expressing their feelings and were confused about the nature of families and interpersonal relationships. There was a lack of a firm sense of continuing family relationships after the divorce, since their conception of a family was based on those individuals who lived together in the same household. The findings to date suggest that long-term disruption is more probable in younger children. It has also been noted that a single parent is most vulnerable to depression when his/her children are under the age of 5.

By the age of 7, children were more aware of their feelings and better able to admit to sadness, although not much anger. They tended to blame themselves less, but experiences strong feelings of abandonment and rejection. These were coupled with the fear that their mother's anger could be strong enough to expel them from the family as well.

By the age of 9, children rarely felt at fault, but experienced profound rejection and abandonment by the departing parent. They acknowledged their intense feelings of anger toward one or both parents, but they tried to hide their own pain in order to present a more courageous front to the outside world. Within, they experienced intense loneliness. They were torn by anger and loyalty and betrayed by their parents' behavior and by the family dissolution. They were also troubled because they sensed the erosion in their relationship with a particular parent due to that parent's withdrawal of emotional support.

Adolescents seemed painfully aware of their feelings and were frequently able to express the anger, sadness, loss, betrayal, and shame that they experienced. Generally they seemed thoughtful about their parents as individual people and achieved much insight by reflecting about their parents' marriage and their own relationship to their parents. They demonstrated good understanding of their parents' incompatibility. However, they were extremely concerned about their own future marriages and the possibility of sustaining relationships based on mutual concern, respect, and interest. It appeared that those teenagers who were able to detach themselves from their parents' emotional turmoil early achieved a better long-term adjustment (Sorosky, 1977).

Thus, it is important to specify the impact of divorce on children by considering them as individuals at distinct stages of development during the major changes divorce produces. It is necessary to keep in mind the importance and to examine the quality of family relationships, the single parent's adjustment and well-being, social and economic and environmental changes, and the continuing relationship with the absent parent.

Long- and Short-Term Effects

One can only speculate that divorce, which is a severance of a relationship between two adults, is bound to have an emotional impact on children that will take years to unfold. If one interprets the increasing divorce rate and proliferating market for self-help books in America as a nationwide statement being made by one generation that as adult men and women they are unable to sustain a relationship with mutual love, respect, and trust; then that message, internalized by their children, will add another dimension of difficulty in the future struggle to define themselves in their roles as men and women. Teenagers of today appear cynical about the value of marriage for themselves and about the desirability and possibility of sustaining intimacy and interest in a potential partner. It is noteworthy that in this era of increased divorce and family fragmentation, two other phenomena have also occurred: (1) the median age of first marriage has risen; (2) the number of people living alone has grown by 60% in the past decade (U.S. Vital Statistics, 1978). Today's young adults are more frequently opting for an extended period of singleness and have established households for independent nonfamily living.

A child's loyalty is deeply rooted and undergoes enormous stress when he/she learns that parents are no longer committed to each other. Children suffer: They experience intense longing for the departed parent. Frequently their pain needs to be denied by one or both parents, who are struggling with emotions of their own. Children may fear that they will lose the love of their remaining parent if they continue to love the absent one. For youngsters, divorce implies loss that is difficult to assimilate because of the unresolved ambivalence about and the intense need for the absent parent. In reality for the child there is frequently the continued availability of the departed parent as an alive but only partially present figure who creates intense inner longing and conflict. Fantasies of reconciliation can last for years, even after one parent has remarried. One child expressed her scorn for the "false daddy" who was currently part of her daily household and her wish to be reunited with her "real daddy." It is vitally important to encourage the meaningful relationship between the child and the absent parent.

It is a major psychological accomplishment for a child to complete the process of mourning the loss of the predivorce family and to accept a new family constellation, which includes a new relationship with both the custodial and the visiting parent. During the divorce process, the child's daily routine will probably change and he/she will have to adapt to new economic burdens along with the rest of the family. This may include founding a new home and making new friends, adapting to a new school situation, and living with a custodial parent who will undoubtedly be preoccupied, overburdened, anxious, and depressed.

Divorce seems to have some short-term effects on all children's psychological, social, and cognitive behavior (Santrock, 1972). A variety of symptoms accompany the psychological states and, of course, reflect the child's developmental level. Symptoms include sleeplessness; nightmares; the inability to concentrate; decline in schoolwork; emotional instability, including crying and anger outbursts; regressive behavior, such as enuresis, thumb sucking, and compulsive masturbation; and behavior that is overtly sexual or aggressive. Children also experience a spectrum of functional complaints that attest to their troubled inner state—muscle weakness, physical exhaustion, change in appetite, stomach aches, headaches, general fears, and hopelessness. It is a time when a variety of psychosomatic disorders, such as asthma and ulcerative colitis, may begin or may be exacerbated.

Frequently a parent will worry about the child's physical health but will be unable to acknowledge the emotional distress within himself, the child, or the family in general. It is important for the physician to realize that the child may be the immediate problem, but that the parent and probably the family as a whole is struggling and in need of help. A most appropriate time of intervention for the child, as for the adult, seems to be the first 6 months of the separation period. This is the time when children worry about such questions as Who will take care of me? Will I be left alone? Where will I live? Will I still be with both of you? Will you still be my mommy and daddy? What should I tell my friends, teachers, etc.? The more children are prepared by explanations geared to their age and level of maturity, the more their fears and anxieties are listened to, the less will they be burdened by parental bitterness, anxiety, and depression. Their loyalty will be less vulnerable to manipulation the more they are allowed to retain their own relationship with each individual parent. Children have a tremendous capacity for adjusting to new situations, especially if they feel secure and loved. The best antidote to the chaotic emotional situation is a well-functioning parent. Otherwise children are in danger of losing their own developmental stride, internalizing a sense of low self-esteem, and losing their own internal sense of integrity.

The Single Parent

In 1979, 77% of all children under 18 in this country lived with both parents; 18.5%, or 11.5 million children, lived in a single-parent family largely because of a divorce situation (other contributing factors were death of a parent, long-term separation, or birth to an unwed mother), 16.9% of children lived with mothers only; 1.6% with fathers only; the remainder, 4.1%, lived with neither (U.S. Bureau of the Census, 1979).

Adaptation is required of all family members when a divorce occurs. The functions of the family remain the same, but a structural change has occurred. Tasks must be reassigned. It is necessary to continue providing emotional and physical care for children. The household must be kept in an acceptable state of order and repair. Usually the mother seeks employment, and the children are expected to assume more household and personal care responsibilities. Single-parent families often suffer from a sense of social isolation as a family unit and from a more erratic life-style (Klebanow, 1976). For many children, this includes the shuffle from weekday homes to weekend homes. In single-parent families, there is a great need for children to use other adults as male and female role models and support figures, be they teachers, relatives, or friends. Clearly, one adult's attempts to do what was previously done by two will lead to short-changing somewhere. "You're it. There is no buffer." Both men and women who are the sole heads of families complain of being chronically overburdened by housekeeping chores and childrearing responsibilities; they experience loneliness and isolation. Their emotional and physical well-being is in greater jeopardy and can cause, in turn, deteriorating relationships with their children. In such situations for both men and women, children are seen more as burdens than as joys. As has been pointed out: "It is not the divorce but the emotional situation in the home with or without divorce that is the determining factor in the child's development."

When a single parent is the mother, the economic burden becomes awesome. Divorce thrusts most families into a lower socioeconomic situation. Less than 50% of departed fathers provide financial support for their children and one can assume that they also lose an active contact with them (U.S. Bureau of the Census, 1978). Thus, the earning potential of female heads of family is crucial. The participation of divorced mothers in the labor force is higher than that of any other group of mothers. Most of these women suffer the effects of wage discrimination, occupational segregation, and lack of training. Usually they are concentrated in low-paying occupational groups. In 1976, 52% of children in female-headed families were in families living below the poverty line (U.S. Bureau of the Census, 1978). "The combination most productive of psychological distress is to be simultaneously single, socially isolated, exposed to burdensome parental obligations and poor" (Pearlin and Johnson, 1977).

At any stage, the offspring's sexuality is sometimes seductive for the parent who is ambivalent about his/her own sexuality. Within the framework of divorce, the single mother or father may turn to a child to assume some aspect of the role of the missing spouse. For example, a father who wins custody of his children may unwittingly set up a new household in which his oldest daughter becomes the caretaker of the family. She then has to struggle with her own wishes and fears about replacing her mother in her father's life. Not infrequently, a situation such as this results in adolescent acting out, such as pregnancy. Similarly, there is the danger that a visiting parent will establish a relationship with his/her children that is awkward and inappropriate. For example, the visiting father treating his teenage daughter more as a date than a child may be surprised that she does not wish to visit him for weekends unless she brings a friend with her. He has failed to recognize her awkwardness about her own sexuality and her need to provide a buffer for herself.

The psychiatrist will be asked to advise parents about dating, their own behavior, and ultimately about their concerns in regard to sleeping-over arrangements when the children are on the premises. It is important for the clinician to be aware of his/her own personal biases and to try to advise his/her patients in a nondogmatic fashion. Many adults are afraid to begin dating again, because they fear the children will resent sharing the parents with a newcomer. One 12-year-old boy had become so close to his mother who depended on him heavily that he flew into a rage whenever she brought a man home with her, and on one occasion broke down a door when his mother and a man were alone in a room. However, it is important for children to know that close relationships and sexual satisfaction are natural needs of all human beings, including their parents. Children generally approve of a parent's companion if they feel that this is not an individual who will displace them or with whom they must compete for love.

If a parent's own pattern of sexual behavior is manipulative, self-centered, or lacks qualities of respect, honesty, and empathy, then the child will be acutely aware of it and may learn to behave the same way. Certainly it will be very difficult for a parent who has one set of standards for him/herself and another for his/her child to exert firmness, consistency, and appropriate limit setting while keeping open the lines of communication. A 45-year-old father who introduces his pubescent daughter to his 25-year-old girlfriend can create intense inner turmoil within the child. She may choose the path of regressive dependent behavior with delayed entry into adolescence, or, on the other hand, she may catapult herself into pseudoadolescence and engage in premature and potentially harmful sexual activity. As another example, a mother who brings home a succession of lovers can subject her children not only to threatening stimulation as opposed to sexual intimacy, but she can also involve them in serial object losses that can lead children to develop a shallow style of relating and ultimately to difficulty in trusting and to chronic depression.

Adolescents of today are pressured to be more sexually active. Although the atmosphere of increased openness about sex at all levels and ages in our society has more advantges than disadvantages, the child may use sexuality in an angry attempt at independence or in a search for the love and approval that he/she can't find at home. The potential hazards of the new openness and even permissiveness about sex have not yet been adequately studied.

Remarriage/Stepparents

"To the extent that the marriage state—but not necessarily being married only once—is a preferred status, some available indicators portent a relatively optimistic future for married life. A high divorce rate coupled with a high remarriage rate appears to signal a strong desire for a compatible marriage and family life." Four out of five divorced individuals remarry, with younger individuals more likely to remarry than older ones, and men more likely to remarry than women. Current statistics show that only about half of these marriages succeed (Glick, 1975). People do seek a fulfilling life with one specific other human being, a stable partnership that involves good communication, a good sex life together, compatibility, a comfortable home life, and consistency of commitment.

By 1975, 15 million children under the age of 18 were living in stepfamilies in America and there was a minimum of 25 million husbands and wives who were stepmothers and stepfathers (Roosevelt and Lofas, 1976). There has been, to date, no clear definition of the role of the stepparent. Until now, the only social and legal model has been the natural parent role. Currently there is increasing interest in and research into the stresses that affect the life of a stepparent and of a new family unit. This will hopefully lead in time to a definition of the responsibilities and rewards specific to stepparenting and to role models that might give more suitable guidance to (and carry more realistic expectations of) stepparents and the rest of the family.

The original nuclear family is a tenacious, closed system that dissolves slowly. Frequently during the separation/divorce process, a survivor bond develops between parent and child, a bond in which the relationship becomes overcharged and overinvested. In most cases when a stepparent appears, he/she is a newcomer who is not welcomed into the existing system; he/she is experienced by the children as an intruder. Stepfamilies are likened by Visher and Visher (1978) to open systems with greater instability and lack of control than nuclear families. They list the popular myths about stepparents that need to be dispelled, namely, (1) stepfamilies are the same as nuclear families and if the stepparent were at all caring the newly reconstituted family would be the same as the original, natural family; (2) the death of a spouse makes stepparenting easier; (3) stepchildren are less burdensome when not living at home; (4) love of a partner guarantees love of the partner's children; and (5) every new stepparent will immediately love his/her stepchildren. As mothers, and, therefore, society's nurturers, women feel more pressure to achieve closeness with stepchildren and to avoid being cast in the role of "wicked stepmother." Women tend to experience more guilt than men if they do not succeed in this task. Mrs. V. was very eager to become the stepmother to Kevin, the 10-year-old son of her new husband. Kevin's parents had separated and divorced 3 years earlier. Kevin's mother waived custody rights and moved to another country to pursue her career, thereby virtually abandoning Kevin. Mrs. V. had always sensed Kevin's reserve but was surprised and bewildered by his mounting anger, directed at her specifically, and by his generally unruly behavior in school during the first months of the new marriage. Her initial responsiveness and warmth were severely tested as she experienced anger, disappointment, and resentment in reaction to the child's rejection of her. While trying to explain her situation to her therapist she complained overtly of feeling inadequate as a mother and guilty. She was aware that she had withdrawn in anger from her husband because he had been unable to protect and support her in her new role as Kevin's mother.

The rivalries which exist in nuclear families are magnified in stepfamilies. The early days of stepmarriage lack honeymoon tranquility. A new unit is plunged into "early shock" and unresolved feelings toward exspouses and toward lost parents are revived and stir up anger and competition. In nuclear families, children will exert pressure to keep parents together. In stepfamilies children may act to fragment the adults as a result of conscious or unconscious wishes to eliminate the intruder and reunite the original family. One girl of 12 had formed a relationship with her father in the 2 years since her parents' divorce that made her both housewife and confidante to him. She felt highly valued in her roles. He married unexpectedly and although Jennifer did not actively dislike her new stepmother, she experienced this woman's entry into her home as an intrusion into her territory. In attempting to control her feelings of betrayal and competition with her new mother, she withdrew into sullen depression, became moody and tense at home, and began to spend increasing amounts of time outside of the house with a newly acquired boyfriend. She felt misunderstood and excluded from the new relationship her father had formed. She managed to direct her father's active concern onto her by not returning home on a number of weekends. On the last occasion her father was summoned by the local police to take his daughter home because Jennifer had been found drinking in a car with several other teenagers.

The first 3 to 4 years of a new family unit are the most turbulent as the husband and wife struggle to create a rewarding marital relationship. A marriage that begins and continues with little privacy, with the need to devote much time and energy to children with a natural tendency of the system toward the exclusion of the stepparent from family intimacy, has a formidable array of stresses to overcome. The predominant reaction of stepparents is confusion. How should he/she act? For women, there is a fear of giving up newly found independence, the fear that giving to one's child or to a stepchild may involve depriving one's spouse, and the burdensome feeling that she ought to be the central nurturer of a family unit with responsibility for the emotional welfare of all its members. For men, there is frequently the fear of reexperiencing rejection by a woman who might be too independent and who won't "need him" or "trust him." Both husband and wife will not have the usual assets of time alone with spouse and will frequently each feel unsupported by the other in dealing with the stresses. Self-doubt, insecurity, and inferiority feelings are reactions to all the confusing demands and pressures. Not surprisingly, lowered self-esteem, feelings of helplessness, and depression are psychological risks of stepparents (Messinger et al., 1978).

Fathers are usually the partners who have to leave the old unit and step into a new one. It is hard to know how to act as disciplinarian, provider, and protector. Guilt may be stirred up in a man if he feels his own children are being neglected, and it may be hard for him to fully enjoy his stepchildren and unselfconsciously express joy, warmth, love, and concern. Stress may occur during those times when his own children come to visit, on weekends or over holidays, and he experiences tension over their acceptance into the new unit. Money conflicts are also frequent in these situations and create enormous stress. One father, pressurized by financial problems in caring for his old and new families, complained: "Too much is never enough. You can't get two pints out of a one-pint pot."

Sexual conflicts in stepfamilies are also a greater source of tension than in nuclear families. A variety of new, intimate living situations stir up wishes, fantasies, and fears in all the members of the new family, adults and children, which are not subject to the same degree of repression as in a nuclear family. One man of 35, who was in psychotherapy, made his first marriage to a woman of 40 who had two teenage daughters. It became clear to his therapist after the first few months of the marriage that considerable tension existed within the home that reflected the poorly repressed yet unacknowledged sexual fantasies stirred up in the patient. By acknowledging the problem and talking about the feelings in therapy, the patient was able to strengthen his alignment with his wife, including their mutual sexual gratification, and thus provide a model to the daughters of a healthy, adult, sexually based relationship. Because he and his wife were seen as united, warm, consistent, and limit-setting parents, they were able to appropriately guide the children through that developmental phase in which maturing sexuality is such an important factor.

Summary

Men and women are having a hard time being together. In the confusion and shifting attitudes of the past two decades, sexual mores have undergone much reexamination. As a result, we have experienced an upheaval in our views on and expectations of marital union. Sexual roles are no longer as clearly defined as they once were and the attitudes on sexuality have widened to allow more personal freedom and choice to women and men.

In these circumstances, marital ties are no longer the unbreakable bonds they once were. But with the freedom to end unworkable relationships have come an increase in the experiences of disappointment, rejection, and mistrust between men and women and within family units. The failure of intimacy, when a marriage ends, includes its sexual aspects, which can be profoundly shaking.

Separation and divorce, even within a climate of diminished social censure, are often seen as negative experiences. One must neither deny nor underestimate the stressful aspects of the decision to end a marriage or, indeed, any close, one-to-one sexually based adult relationship. Divorce is the repudiation of a relationship between a woman and a man, which in its fundamental nature was sexual; primary to the relationship, underpinning its social and psychological significances, was the joining together of the two sexes, the implicit sexual aspect of the union. To sever such a bond must inflict some crises of identity, potency, sufficiency, and sexuality. The total spectrum of psychological and physical consequences on each partner, as well as each family member involved, needs to be considered and dealt with at such a time. When properly negotiated, the experience of divorce can result in inner growth and development for all the individuals concerned.

Nevertheless, it is generally agreed that marriage and family life are the most satisfying parts of most people's lives, and being married is one of the most important determinants of being satisfied with life. So, in spite of past disappointments, marriage and remarriage rates speak to the strong basic desire of men and women to form stable sexual and emotional partnerships.

References

Bane, M.J. Marital disruption and the lives of children. In G. Levinger and O. Moles (Eds.), *Divorce and separation: Conditions, causes and consequences.* New York: Basic Books, 1979. Pp. 276–286.

Bloom, B.L., Asher, S.J., and White, S.W. Marital disruption as a stressor: A review and analysis. *Psychological Bulletin,* 1978, *85*(4), 867–894.

Bohannan, P. (Ed.). *Divorce and after.* Garden City, N.Y.: Doubleday, 1970.

Cragu, M.A. Psychopathology in married couples. *Psychological Bulletin,* 1972, *77*, 114–128.

Glick, P.C. A demographer looks at American families. *Journal of Marriage and Family,* 1975, *37*, 15–26.

Holmes, T.H., and Rahe, R.H. The social readjustment rating scale. *Journal of Psychosomatic Research,* 1967, *11*, 213.

Klebanow, S. Parenting in the single parent family. *Journal of the American Academy of Psychoanalysis,* 1976, *4*(1), 37–78.

Longfellow, C. Divorce in context: Its impact on children. In G. Levinger and O. Moles (Eds.), *Divorce and separation: Conditions, causes and consequences.* New York: Basic Books, 1979. Pp. 299–306.

Lynch, J.J., and Convey, W.H. Loneliness, disease and death: Alternative approaches. *Psychosomatics,* 1979, *20*(10), 702–708.

Masuda, M., and Holmes, T.H. Life events: Perception and frequencies. *Psychosomatic Medicine,* 1978, *40*, 236–261.

McMurray, L. Emotional stress and driving performance: The effect of divorce. *Behavioral Research in Highway Safety,* 1970, *1*, 100–114.

Messinger, L., Walker, K.N., and Freeman, S.J.J. Preparation for remarriage following divorce: The use of group techniques. *American Journal of Orthopsychiatry,* 1978, *48*(2), 263–272.

National Center for Health Statistics. *Mortality from selected causes by marital status* (Vital Health Statistics, Series 20, Nos. 8a, 8b). Washington, D.C.: U.S. Government Printing Office, 1970.

National Center for Health Statistics. *Differentials in health characteristics by marital status: United States, 1971–72* (Vital Health Statistics, Series 10, No. 104). Washington, D.C.: U.S. Government Printing Office, 1976.

Pearlin, L.I., and Johnson, J.S. Marital status and depression. *American Sociological Review,* 1977, *42,* 704–715.

Rahe, R.H. Life change measurement clarification (editorial). *Psychosomatic Medicine,* 1978, *40*(2), 95.

Rahe, R.H. Life change events and mental illness: An overview. *Journal of Human Stress,* 1979, *5*(3), 2–10.

Roosevelt, R., and Lofas, J. *Living in step.* New York: Stein & Day, 1976.

Santrock, J.W. Relation to type and onset of father absence to cognitive development. *Child Development,* 1972, *43*(2), 455–469.

Schneidman, E.S., and Farberow, W.L. Statistical comparisons between attempted and committed suicides. In N.L. Fawberow and E.S. Schneidman (Eds.), *The cry for help.* New York: McGraw-Hill, 1961.

Sorosky, A.D. The psychological effects of divorce on adolescents. *Adolescence,* 1977, *12,* 123–136.

U.S. Bureau of the Census. *Current population reports. Marital status and living arrangements: March, 1977.* (Series P-20, No. 323). Washington, D.C.: U.S. Government Printing Office, 1978.

U.S. Bureau of the Census. *Current population reports. Marital status and living arrangements: March, 1979.* (Series P-20, No. 349). Washington, D.C.: U.S. Government Printing Office, 1980.

U.S. National Center for Health Statistics. *Vital statistics of the U.S., Annual.* Washington, D.C.: U.S. Government Printing Office, 1978.

Visher, E.B., and Visher, J.S. Common problems of stepparents and their spouses. *American Journal of Orthopsychiatry,* 1978, *48*(2), 252–262.

Wallerstein, J.S., and Kelly, J.B. The effects of parental divorce: The adolescent experience. In E.J. Anthony and C. Koupernik (Eds.), *The child in his family,* Vol. III, *Children at psychiatric risk.* New York: Wiley, 1974. Pp. 479–505.

Wallerstein, J.S., and Kelly, J.B. The effects of parental divorce: Experiences of the preschool child. *Journal of American Academy of Child Psychiatry,* 1975, *14*(4), 600–616.

Wallerstein, J.S., and Kelly, J.B. The effects of parental divorce: Experiences of the child in later latency. *American Journal of Orthopsychiatry,* 1976, *46*(2), 256–269.

Weiss, R.S. *Marital separation.* New York: Basic Books, 1975.

Alcohol, Medications, and Other Drugs

Joseph Westermeyer

Folk Beliefs and Use of Drugs

Drugs have long been used to facilitate and enhance sexual experience. Alcohol in Europe and Asia, opium in Asia, and yohimbine in Africa have served that purpose for centuries and continue to do so today. Other traditional compounds have included cantharides (Spanish fly—a urinary tract irritant), strychnine in homeopathic doses, ginseng root, and various mammalian organs (e.g., rhinoceros or deer horn, water buffalo testes, bear bile). Depending on era, location, informant, and drug, these presumed aphrodiasiac agents have gained reputations as causing, allowing, and/or enhancing sexual function (Jarvik, 1977).

Certain compounds have served ancillary sexual purposes and have had major effects on sexual behavior or sex-related rituals. For example, belladonna was used a century ago by women in Europe and the Americas to produce pupil dilitation and facial blush. These physiologic characteristics were viewed as enhancing their physical attractiveness. Anovulatory medications and spermicidal agents have effectively reduced fear of pregnancy so that they have played a part in the recent changes in sexual behavior; fewer people avoid intercourse because of fear of pregnancy. Antibiotics have served the same purpose since they have reduced the incidence and complications of venereal disease. Tobacco, although not generally viewed as an aphrodisiac, is used in ritual fashion by many heavy smokers before and/or after intercourse, presumably for relaxation.

Folk beliefs regarding the effects of drugs on sexual performance have changed rapidly over the last decade and probably will continue to change. Numerous studies, both in North America and Europe, have identified cannabis as a favorite choice for

Joseph Westermeyer • Department of Psychiatry, University of Minnesota Hospital, Minneapolis, Minnesota.

enhancing sexual experience, although reports on the effects are not uniform, and the rationales for sexual enhancement differ widely among informants (Goode, 1972; Ewing, 1972; Gay and Sheppard, 1973; Robbins and Tanck, 1973; Koff, 1974; Parr, 1976). Methaqualone (Mandrax, Quaalude) has been touted as an aphrodisiac, especially among women (Parr, 1976). This is somewhat unexpected since barbiturates and other sedatives are not preferred for this purpose. Cocaine and amphetamines have been used, especially by men to sustain erection, delay ejaculation, and/or facilitate repeated orgasm (Gay and Sheppard, 1973; Parr, 1976). Amyl nitrate, a vasodilator prescribed for angina pectoris, has been described as potentiating or facilitating orgasm (Everett, 1972). Among some homosexuals it is used as a means to delay orgasms. Opioids have long been used as a means of delaying ejaculation, alleviating anorgasmia, and prolonging orgasm (Westermeyer, 1971). Besides differences in type of drug, there are also wide variations in doses, time relation between drug taking and sexual performance, and source of drugs. Individual expectation and previous experience with a given nostrum play major roles in the perceived effects of folk prescriptions.

Of all the available psychoactive substances, alcohol has perhaps been most widely employed to facilitate sexual performance. For example, in many societies alcohol intoxication is an integral part of marriage ceremonies. Alcohol drinking contributes to ritual celebration of the event and symbolizes an amelioration of the strangeness and latent hostility between the two families. It also presumably aids the couple in initiating their sexual life together, an often stressful process of engaging in behavior previously taboo, as well as overcoming concern with one's own sexual performance and one's own sexual attractiveness to the partner.

Available Knowledge Regarding Drugs and Sex

Physiologic Effects

The abundance of folk beliefs contrasts with the limited data available regarding the effects of recreational intoxicants on sexual function. Studies have been conducted on effects of alcohol on young men, using erotic films and penile strain gauges (Farkas and Rosen, 1976; Rubin and Henson, 1976). These have demonstrated that quite low alcohol doses (i.e., 1.0 ml alcohol/kg body wt or 25 mg% blood alcohol level) do not interfere with penile diameter, although such low levels do reduce the rate of tumescence. Above this level, even moderate alcohol doses (i.e., 1.5 ml alcohol/kg body wt or 50 mg% blood alcohol level) appreciably reduce maximum penile diameter and delay tumescence rate. At higher doses (i.e., 75 mg% blood alcohol level), penile diameter and tumescence rate continue to decrease at a linear rate. These studies have proven at least the second part of Shakespeare's aphorism that alcohol provokes desire but diminishes the performance.

Unfortunately, similar studies do not exist for other drugs nor for the alcohol effects on the sexual performance of heavy drinkers, older men, women, or alcoholics. So long as valid information is nonexistent, folk myths regarding the effects of drug and alcohol on sexuality can be expected to predominate.

Psychological Effects

Information on the specific psychological effects of drugs on sexuality is minimal. Even in relatively small doses, alcohol inhibits the ability to process numerous complex sensory inputs and precise sensorimotor output, such as are required to fly an airplane (Underwood, 1975). In doses up to a blood alcohol level of 50 mg%, alcohol interferes little with simpler tasks, such as driving an automobile. Alcohol may even facilitate certain tasks by impeding extraneous sensory inputs. As a sedative–relaxant drug, it can also alleviate moderate anxiety. These psychological effects, together with the delay of tumescence rate in the male, suggest that alcohol in moderate doses may well serve to facilitate sexual performance for anxious, hyperalert or highly stimulated individuals. Conversely, the same doses could conceivably impede sexual performance in depressed, fatigued, or bored individuals.

Narcotic and sedative drugs may function in a manner similar to alcohol, since their psychoactive properties are similar. Conversely, amphetamines may assist the depressed, fatigued, or withdrawn person to function sexually. Cannabis alters time perception and thus may enhance sexual experience by making orgasms seem to last longer (Milkman and Frasch, 1973).

Drugs affect the manner in which people assess themselves and their own behavior in a social context, as well as the manner in which they are viewed by others. Stated differently, drugs have effects on individuals aside from their physiological or psychological effects; they also may influence how people behave socially or how others view the drug-using person.

Most societies have specified times when the ordinarily social norms are suspended, often referred to as "time out." For example, during carnival time (pre-Lenten festivals) in parts of central Europe or the Americas or the New Year in parts of Europe and Asia, the usual social responsibilities are suspended, sex roles may be reversed, and authorities chided. Marital fidelity and premarital sexual strictures may be relaxed, either in association with drugs (e.g., alcohol and pre-Lenten carnivals) or without drugs (e.g., certain annual festivals in Oceania).

In the same way that societies permit time out at specific times, individuals may also associate time out from usual norms with drugs or alcohol use. Such time out from sexual strictures is encouraged by some ethnic groups that do not enculturate their members into socialized drinking during childhood but permit peer teaching of alcohol use during adolescence. This has been described for one American Indian group (Westermeyer, 1972) but probably prevails among other cultures as well. Groups that enculturate their members into alcohol use in childhood generally expect them to be equally responsible for their sexual behavior whether drinking or not. Laboratory studies further support the notion that experienced drinkers can better inhibit sexual response while drinking than can naive or infrequent users (Rubin and Hensen, 1976).

Effects of Alcohol and Drug Abuse on Sexuality

Chronic, heavy use of drugs has effects on sexuality that differ qualitatively and quantitatively from episodic light or moderate use of drugs. In many respects, the psychological and social concomitants of drug dependence vary little across drug type. Despite pharmacologic differences in drug types, the effects of drug dependence on sexual physiology are more similar than different.

Physiologic Effects

Among alcoholic men, secondary impotence is well known. Often it is reversible with abstinence, but it may be permanent when associated with neuropathy and testicular atrophy (Van Thiel et al., 1974). Alcoholic hepatitis and cirrhosis, as well as serum hepatitis associated with parental drug use, is generally accompanied by decreased libido in both men and women. Both alcoholic males and females report a diminished interest in sexual relations (Levine, 1955). The following case exemplifies this problem:

> A 53-year-old married man had been drinking 1 to 2 quarts of wine per evening over a 10-year period. He presented to his physician with complaints of headache and visual problems. A senior executive in a large corporation, he also had difficulty recalling recent events and decisions. Other problems included irritability, insomnia, weight loss, and difficulty obtaining and maintaining erections. Ophthalmologic consultation verified alcohol–tobacco amblyopia. He was able to maintain abstinence from alcohol, but symptoms of depression became worse. Following a course of antidepressant medications, his memory deficit improved somewhat, but his impotence persisted. Although his erections improved slightly, they were insufficient to use alternative sexual techniques and he had no ejaculations. Treatment consisted of aiding the couple to find other sexual outlets acceptable to both. At the same time, the couple required help in working through their feelings about the impotence (i.e., grief for the husband, anger and disappointment for the wife).

Many heroin addicts report premature ejaculation (from their own subjective frame of reference) prior to addiction and during drug-free periods (Mintz et al., 1974). Among a group of 31 heroin addicts, mean ejaculation time was increased from a previously reported 8.7 min to 44.2 min when using heroin (DeLeon and Wezler, 1973). Common problems reported by many male addicts after addiction to heroin are secondary impotence, retarded ejaculation, and inability to ejaculate (Cushman, 1973; Gossop et al., 1974; Parr, 1976). Decreased plasma testosterone has been observed among addicts while taking narcotic drugs (Mendelson et al., 1974). Amenorrhea has also been reported among female heroin addicts (Goulden et al., 1964; Santen, 1974). Both male and female heroin addicts report decreased libido and decreased sexual enjoyment during periods of addiction (Wieland and Yungur, 1970).

Less is known about effects of other drugs on sexuality. One study of amphetamine abusers indicated sexual problems prior to beginning drug use in many cases (Bell and Trethowan, 1961). The effects of amphetamine abuse on sexuality were mixed, with some people having increased drive and performance and others reporting decreased or no change. Those experiencing enhanced sexuality reported prolonged erection and delayed ejaculation (men), delayed orgasm (women), and increased drive (both).

Psychosocial Effects

These effects on sexuality are mainly manifest in the alcohol- or drug-dependent person's ability to obtain and maintain a stable sexual relationship. To continue and flourish, sexual relationships (like interpersonal relationships in general) must be reciprocal; that is, each partner must give to and receive from the other. As in other human relationships, reciprocity must occur in more than one sphere, not just in the sexual one.

The economic effects of alcohol or drug dependency severely impede the ability to reciprocate within a sexual relationship. Frequent intoxication and withdrawal leads to decreased work efficiency and productivity, absenteeism, and interpersonal problems with co-workers and supervisors. Loss of income can also occur because of drug cost itself; this can be high. Legal costs to attorneys and courts for drug-related offenses (from drunk driving to felonies) further undermine economic resources, as do medical costs (infectious disease, trauma, and certain other disorders are many times more numerous in chemically dependent people as compared to others). If the chemically dependent person is married, the spouse is often forced into protecting family resources. Few people are sanguine about an enduring sexual relationship with someone who is likely to become a liability.

The quality of the interpersonal relationships also suffers. "Blackouts" (i.e., periods of amnesia associated with alcohol and sedative abuse) make it difficult to communicate, and may include property destruction, vehicular accidents, child abuse, and spouse abuse. Alcoholic women are reported to be more apt than others to become rape victims (Rada, 1974). In the face of a deteriorating marital relationship, the alcohol- or drug-dependent partner and the nondependent partner are apt to seek extramarital sexual relationships. Venereal disease is frequently associated with addiction and heavy drug use (Leonida et al., 1972; Medhus, 1975). Social isolation also becomes a problem for the couple as former friends and relatives become alienated from the alcohol or drug abuser.

Financially destitute addicts or alcoholics may turn to prostitution as a means of supporting themselves and their drug habit (Holzner & Ding, 1973). Although alcohol- or drug-dependent women tend to be stereotyped as engaging in this activity, the proportion of addicted men selling themselves as homosexual prostitutes may also be high.

Alcohol or drug dependence often occurs by "contagion" within a sexual relationship or marriage (Bernstein, 1972). A large proportion of herion-addicted women were first introduced to drugs by a male consort or husband, and a large proportion of alcoholic women have alcoholic husbands (Freedman and Ilana, 1968). Although the reverse also occurs, in which women introduce men to alcohol or drug dependence, it is less common (O'Donnell et al., 1967).

Sexual partners or spouses of alcohol or drug abusers may become victims of alcohol–drug dependence, and, unwittingly, they also become perpetrators of the problem. By their alternately rejecting and accepting, enabling continued drug use, and rescuing their partner from drug-related problems, they further elicit and exacerbate drug abuse. Although many are not abusers themselves, they often come from families where alcohol or drug abuse was present.

Sexual dysfunction may afflict the nondependent spouse or partner. Dyspareunia, anorgasmia, impotence, and premature ejaculation are the most common problems. Surprisingly, the dysfunctional individual may not relate the problem to the spouse's drug abuse. The following case is fairly typical:

> A 34-year-old married woman came to her family physician complaining of vaginal pain associated with penile penetration. The mother of two children, she had never previously experienced this symptom and attributed it to organic causes. Physical examination including pelvic examination was entirely negative. Further history revealed that her husband had been drinking heavily in the last few years. He had become irritable and unpredictable with the patient and their two children and had recently been suspended from work. The psychosocial etiology of the symptom was explored and treatment alternatives for her husband were offered. Since he was not willing to seek treatment voluntarily, the wife was supported in her efforts to confront him and seek alternatives. Within a few weeks he sought residential treatment. During the first year he had two relapses but has been abstinent for 3 years at this writing. The wife's dyspareunia disappeared and has not recurred.

Diagnosis and Treatment

Amelioration of drug-related sexual dysfunction depends upon identification of the alcohol or drug dependence problem. Every case involving sexual dysfunction should be screened for alcohol or drugs.

This can be done effectively in most cases by simply asking about the person's use of alcohol and drugs during the last week. It is important to learn what intoxicants they have used and the doses and frequency. Alcohol- and drug-dependent people who are ambivalent about their use tend to provide vague responses. In such cases, the consultant should continue the questioning until some answers are forthcoming. In advanced cases, where the prognosis is poor, dependent people often lie about their use. Other informants can provide the relevant data in these cases. In taking an alcohol and drug history, neutral, nonjudgmental terms can be helpful, e.g., "use" instead of "abuse," "high" instead of "drunk."

Once the presence of potentially pathogenic use is suspected, a complete assessment should be made. This includes the following detailed information: (1) use of alcohol or drugs over the years; (2) legal, social, financial, marital, sexual, and health problems; and (3) current social functioning and resources. (See Westermeyer, 1976, for the kinds of questions and data needed for a thorough assessment.)

With regard to treatment, merely recommending abstinence is seldom worth the time it takes to do so, except in early cases. The patient, and wherever possible the sexual or marital partner, must be oriented and motivated to the need for treatment. With adequate medical, social, and psychological data, the patient's treatment need can be evaluated. These must then be integrated with treatment modalities available in the community.

> A 29-year-old physician was seen in crisis after having been involved in a car accident during an alcoholic "blackout." The son of alcoholic parents, he had experienced amnesic episodes while drinking and he had been convicted for driving while intoxicated. He recognized the need for abstinence, but his wife believed he was a "normal drinker" and insisted abstinence was "ridiculous" for him. Disulfiram (antabuse) was prescribed for the patient, and the couple was seen weekly for several evaluation sessions and referred to a weekly couples' group program. After maintaining abstinence for 3 years, he was able to return to limited social use of alcohol without difficulty over the last 2 years.

Although an extensive discussion of the treatment of substance abuse is beyond the scope of this chapter, it is important to emphasize that a large number of modalities have been employed. These include the psychotherapies as well as medication. Family involvement in the therapeutic process is central regardless of the specific therapeutic techniques employed. This support can enhance the motivation of the patient and facilitate progress. Moreover, since substance abuse may serve a purpose for other family members, the symptoms presented by the identified patient must be understood within the family system. On the other hand, symptoms such as depression, anxiety, or personality disorders may be etiologic in the development of substance abuse or they may be symptoms of a primary drug problem. These disorders must be recognized and treated when they occur.

Since substance abuse may also mask underlying sexual problems, some patients respond to the treatment of their abuse with the emergence of sexual problems. They may have sexual anxiety or inhibitions that are defensively dealt with by using drugs or alcohol. Thus, these basic problems when unresolved may emerge again as the abuse is treated. Recurrence of substance abuse or treatment failure may result if the patient, in experiencing this symptom again, finds it intolerable and for whatever reason is unable to work through a resolution.

Successful treatment of alcohol/drug dependence does result in improved sexual functioning including decreased impotence and ejaculation problems (Mintz et al., 1974) and increased frequency of sexual activity and participation in family activities (Clark et al., 1972).

Prescribed Medications

Psychotropic Drugs

Tricyclic antidepressant medications may effect an improvement in problems because they relieve the underlying depression, which often causes sexual dysfunction.

The tricyclics have been reported to cause sexual dysfunctions in some patients. In rare cases, monoamine oxidase inhibitors may be used in cases where prolonged tricyclic antidepressant regimens interfere with sexual function.

Antipsychotic medications similarly can impede erection and ejaculation in the male. Such effects tend to be dose-related and generally recede as dosage is gradually reduced after an acute psychotic episode. In addition to drug effect, people with psychosis often have decreased libido, secondary impotence or anorgasmia, and difficulty obtaining or maintaining a sexual relationship related to their illness and irrespective of whether they take antipsychotic medication.

Antianxiety drugs can impede normal sexuality by releasing the normal inhibition of hostility. By promoting behavioral expression of anger, they can disrupt the psychosocial aspects of a sexual relationship.

Antihypertensive Drugs

Numerous ganglionic blocking agents prescribed for hypertension have been reported to impair erection and ejaculation in the male (Money and Yankowitz, 1967). Their use in the treatment of hypertension can create a serious problem in compliance, since the patient may opt against longer-term morbidity and mortality and for shorter-term sexual function.

Resperpine, an effective antihypertensive in some cases, can precipitate depression, thereby leading to decreased libido and sexual dysfunction. Since permanent impotence can result from untreated or undertreated hypertension, the patient should be educated to the importance of a proper antihypertensive regimen.

Hormones

Treatment of certain sex-related cancers with hormones can produce sexual problems. Women with metastatic breast cancer treated with androgens sometimes experience a greatly increased libido. Men with disseminated prostatic cancer treated with estrogens complain of a decreased libido. Amelioration of these sexual complications consists of informing the patient ahead of time of their possible presence, providing opportunity for the patient to discuss them and facilitating expression of feelings both by patient and spouse.

Treatment

In some instances, some sexual dysfunction will persist even after alternate medications, regimens, and reduced dosages have been tried. Specific recommendations regarding sexual behaviors can assist in some cases. Partial impotence or partial inorgasmia may be alleviated by enlarging the couple's sexual repertoire, by setting aside a longer period of time for lovemaking, or removing the pressure for orgasm via sensate focus activities. Partners temporarily or permanently unable to have orgasm (usually with erection–ejaculation problems) accept their disability better if they can participate in their partner's orgasms.

References

Bell, D.S., and Trethowan, W.H. Amphetamine addiction and disturbed sexuality. *Archives of General Psychiatry,* 1961, *4,* 74–78.

Bernstein, D.M. Methadone in the family. *Proceedings of the Fourth National Conference on Methadone Treatment,* New York, 1972, pp. 367–368.

Clark, J.A., Capel, W.C., Goldsmith, B.M., and Stewart, G.L. Marriage and methadone: Spouse behavior patterns in heroin addicts maintained on methadone, *Journal of Marriage Family,* 1972, *34,* 497–502.

Cushman, P. Sexual behavior in heroin addiction and methadone maintenance. *New York State Journal of Medicine,* 1973, *72,* 1261–1265.

DeLeon, G., and Wezler, H.K. Heroin addiction: Its relation to sexual behavior and sexual experience. *Journal of Abnormal Psychology,* 1973, *81,* 36–38.

Everett, G.M. Effects of amyl nitrate ("poppers") on sexual experience. *Medical Aspects of Human Sexuality,* 1972, *6,* 146–151.

Ewing, J.A. Students, sex, and marijuana. *Medical Aspects of Human Sexuality,* 1972, *6,* 100–117.

Farkas, G.M., and Rosen, R.C. Effect of alcohol on elicited male sexual response. *Quarterly Journal of Studies on Alcohol,* 1976, *37,* 265–272.

Freedman, I., and Ilana, P. Drug addiction among pimps and prostitutes, Israel 1967. *International Journal of Addictions,* 1968, *3,* 271–300.

Gay, G.R., and Sheppard, C. "Sex-crazed dope fiends"—Myth or reality? *Drug Forum,* 1973, *2,* 125–140.

Goode, E. Sex and marijuana. *Sexual Behavior,* 1972, *2,* 45–51.

Gossop, M.R., Stern, R., and Connell, P.H. Drug dependence and sexual dysfunction: Comparison of intravenous users of narcotics and oral users of amphetamines. *British Journal of Psychiatry,* 1974, *124,* 431–434.

Goulden, E.C., Littlefield, D.C., Putoff, O.E., and Seivert, A.L. Menstrual abnormalities associated with heroin addiction. *American Journal of Obstetrics and Gynecology,* 1964, *90,* 155–160.

Holzner, A.S., Ding, L.K. White dragon pearls in Hong Kong: A study of young women drug addicts. *International Journal of Addictions,* 1973, *8,* 253–263.

Jarvik, M.E. Drugs and sexual functioning. *Journal of Family Practice,* 1977, *4,* 994–1006.

Koff, W.C. Marijuana and sexual activity. *Journal of Sexual Research,* 1974, *10,* 194–204.

Leonida, D.J., Modrijan, A.A., and Dogot, E. Trends in gonorrhea ecology. *Illinois Medical Journal,* 1972, *142,* 199–203.

Levine, J. Sexual adjustment of alcoholics: A clinical study of a selected sample. *Quarterly Journal of Studies on Alcohol,* 1955, *16,* 675–678.

Medhus, A. Venereal diseases among female alcoholics. *Scandinavian Journal of Social Medicine,* 1975, *3,* 29–33.

Mendelson, J., Mendelson, J.E., and Patch, V. Effects of heroin and methadone on plasma testosterone in narcotic addicts. *Federal Proceedings,* 1974, *33,* 232.

Milkman, H., and Frasch, W.A. On the preferential abuse of heroin and amphetamine. *Journal of Nervous and Mental Disease,* 1973, *156,* 242–248.

Mintz, J., O'Hare, K., O'Brien, C.P., and Goldschmidt, J. Sexual problems of heroin addicts. *Archives of General Psychiatry,* 1974, *31,* 700–703.

Money, J., and Yankowitz, R. The sympathetic-inhibiting effects of the drug ismelin on human male eroticism, with a note on mellaril. *Journal of Sexual Research,* 1967, *3,* 69–82.

O'Donnell, J.A., Besteman, K.J., and Jones, J.P. Marital history of narcotic addicts. *International Journal of Addictions,* 1967, *2,* 21–38.

Parr, D. Sexual aspects of drug abuse in narcotic addicts. *British Journal of Addiction,* 1976, *71,* 261–268.

Rada, R.T. *Alcoholism and forcible rape.* Paper presented at the annual meeting of the American Psychiatric Association, 1974.

Robbins, P.R., and Tanck, R.H. Psychological correlates of marijuana use: An exploratory study. *Psychiatric Research Reports,* 1973, *33,* 703–706.

Rubin, H.B., and Henson, D.E. Effects of alcohol on male sexual responding. *Psychopharmacology,* 1976, *47,* 123–124.

Santen, R.J. How narcotic addiction affects reproductive function in women. *Contemporary OB/GYN* 1974, *3,* 93–96.

Underwood Ground, K.E. Impaired pilot performance: Drugs and alcohol. *Aviation, Space and Environmental Medicine,* 1975, *46,* 1284–1288.

Van Thiel, D.H., Lester, R., and Sherins, R.J. Hypogonadism in alcoholic liver disease: Evidence for a double effect. *Gastroenterology,* 1974, *67,* 1188.

Westermeyer, J. Use of alcohol and opium by the Meo of Laos. *American Journal of Psychiatry,* 1971, *127,* 1019–1023.

Westermeyer, J. Options regarding alcohol usage among the Chippewa. *American Journal of Orthopsychiatry,* 1972, *42,* 398–403.

Westermeyer, J. *A primer on chemical dependency.* Baltimore, Md.: Williams & Wilkins, 1976.

Wieland, W.F., and Yungur, M. Sexual effects and side effects of heroin and methadone. In *Proceedings of the Third National Conference on Methadone Treatment, New York, 1970.* Washington, D.C.: U.S. Government Printing Office, 1970. Pp. 50–53.

16

Aging and Sexuality

Eugene M. Dagon

It is common to hear a physician state, "I do not see many sexual problems in my practice," or, should an older person broach a sexual problem, hear him greeted with the rejoinder, "What do you expect for your age?" These examples reflect the physician's attitude as part of a larger, frequently ageist and sexist society.

Burnap and Golden (1967) indicated that two-thirds of the physicians who obtain sexual histories from patients note significant dysfunctions in at least half of them, whereas those physicians who did not routinely inquire about sexual practices estimated that less than 10% of their patients had sexual problems. This study indicates that when the physician took the initiative to ask about sexual behavior problems were uncovered. Masters and Johnson (1970) verified these data, noting that at least 50% of married couples in their studies reported some sexual dysfunction. Leif and Ebert (1975) reporting on a survey conducted by the Center for the Study of Sex Education in Medicine at the University of Pennsylvania School of Medicine noted that 68% of the medical sex educators felt that attitude modification was the most significant need of their students. This suggests that the attitudes and interests of the physician are important determinants in eliciting a sexual history. It is certainly predictable that few patients will express sexual concerns spontaneously.

In a recent gerontological conference, Libow (1978) reiterated that "ageist" attitudes on the part of the clinicians are prime determinants in limiting care to the elderly.

Cultural Myths and Individual Attitudes

Part of the skills of the clinician involves an awareness of how prevailing cultural mythologies affect the attitudes of both him/herself and the patient. Greene (1975)

Eugene M. Dagon • Department of Psychiatry, College of Medicine, University of South Florida, Tampa, Florida.

notes two periods of extremely rapid change in sexual attitudes in this century—the period from 1915 to 1920 and again in the mid-1960s. He indicates that they were "high-water marks" of change followed by periods of consolidation in changing sexual values. He reports that premarital nonvirginity rates of females doubled in the period from 1915 to 1920 from 25 to 50%, and, in the second period (1960s), it rose to 75% and that there was a concomitant rise in marital orgasm rates for females during these periods.

Chronology Myth

One of the most common myths is the chronology myth, that is, that as an individual ages, "sexuality" diminishes. Thus, an individual is arbitrarily assigned as "old," having passed an arbitrary age (e.g., over 35, over 40, over 50, or whatever is viewed as old by the particular clinician), and is expected to experience decreasing sexual activity. Presumably this process culminates when one becomes a blissful, asexual "golden ager" at 65 or 70. This attitude is largely enculturated. Bengston et al. (1977) in a recent study comparing Chicano, black, and white attitudes noted "old" as being in the fifties, sixties, and seventies, respectively.

What accounts for this self-fulfilling prophecy? Pfeiffer (1974) suggests that it is fueled by an unconscious process of desexualizing individuals whose traits are similar to our parents. To demythologize, the following facts are offered by Pfeiffer: At age 68, about 70% of the men still were sexually active, and even at age 78 about 25% were sexually active. For men, the married state was not a necessary factor, whereas for the majority of women, the availability of a sanctioned sexual partner was essential to continual coital activity.

Myth of Aging as Disease

Physicians often prescribe sexual abstinence for a number of *acute* illnesses, including myocardial infarcts, urinary tract infections, low back pain, and even emotional disorders. Although this may be useful, and even necessary for some acute problems, many clinicians fail to recognize that sexual needs reemerge after the acute phase of an illness.

With regard to chronic illnesses, 50% of the over-60 age group and 80% of the over-70 age group have chronic health problems. Physicians often erroneously assume that the individuals are "too ill" to care about sex or that when it becomes important the person will ask. Unfortunately, this often leads to a "conspiracy of silence." Spouses also will not broach the subject for fear of further upsetting or exacerbating an illness in their partners. Another corollary myth suggested that menopause for the woman is similar to castration for the male and that sexual feelings cease with the coming of aging. The insidious nature of these myths is that sexuality is only for the young. Culturally, this can be stated as the bias that old bodies are less beautiful than young bodies. In a youth-oriented culture, this would deny the affirmation or desirability and self-worth of an individual as they aged. Butler and Lewis (1976) note the need to expand the "aesthetic narrowness" of the definition of beauty to include "those individual traits that a person has made of themselves, their uniqueness, character, intelligence, expressiveness, knowledge, achievement, disposition, warmth, style, social skills, posture, and bearing."

Guilt and Shame Myth

Very often shame is associated with sexuality. This myth has been stated as "nice girls don't; women must submit to men's pleasure, but do not take pleasure in such things themselves." There was also something called a *frugality myth* in which sexuality was assumed to be of a limited quantity, and those individuals who "sowed wild oats, spending their sexual favors early and foolishly, would end up sorry." Ironically, these individuals, unaware of nature's dictum of disuse atrophy, became victims of not using it and lost it.

Another very potent attitudinal myth arose from the emphasis on sex for procreation, with deemphasis of the part it played in mutual pleasure and bonding. Thus, sex was seen as a woman's duty, and intercourse was passive, painful, or even disgusting. As these women aged, for some it was a release from disturbing passions, whereas others continued to have sexual feelings that often were associated with a deep sense of guilt.

Myth of Aging as Second-Class Status

Butler (1969) has used the term *ageism* to denote the collection of negative societal attitudes toward the elderly. He defines it as "an irrational prejudice with the application of stereotypes to older people sheerly on the basis of their chronological age." Ageism deprives the elderly of power and productive roles. The personhood of the elderly individual is often assaulted by loss of role and status with mandatory retirement, fixed income, the losses of companions, friends, and spouses, and the stress of adjustment to changes in physical appearance, vigor, and health. When the elderly become devalued and viewed as "useless" and without a role, they are viewed as an economic liability and become second-class citizens.

This second-class status is perhaps one of the most insidious aspects of aging! It obscures the view of aging as a developmental phase and precludes the possibility of successful aging. It stirs in clinicians unconscious fears regarding their own aging, lest they become as devalued as their patients and risk the scorn of their colleagues. Failure to cure chronic disorders may also be a threat to the physician's sense of competence and lead him/her to avoid elderly patients. The elderly, by their proximity to the end of life, often stimulate unconscious fears of death, thus stimulating avoidance and denial. The ultimate irony is, of course, that the clinician eventually becomes the object of his own irrational prejudices.

The psychiatric consultant must not only possess cognitive knowledge of geriatrics/gerontology, sexual assessment, and treatment skills but also be sensitive to his/her own attitudes and those of the consultees as they reflect the culture at large.

Normal Sexuality

What are the sexual facts behind these myths? Masters and Johnson concur with the data of Kinsey et al. (1948, 1953) that men experience a peak in sexual responsiveness in the late teens and thereafter show a steady decline. Women attain their sexual peak in their late thirties or early forties. They subsequently experience a decline, but at a slower rate, and the decline appears to be affected much more by psychosocial influences, whereas for the men the decline appears to have a greater biologic component.

Let us examine some important male and female changes that accomany aging. Masters and Johnson (1966) described the human sexual response as composed of four phases: excitement, plateau, orgasm, and resolution. How are these affected over time?

Excitement Phase

Some men recall their adolescence as a "perpetual erection" with a daily mental preoccupation with sexual gratification. It is often this awareness of decreasing libido that causes anxiety in some men in their late forties or fifties. The excitement phase, as one now becomes older, takes on a slower pace. In men, it may take much greater direct stimulation, extended foreplay, and the use of fantasy to achieve an erection than it did previously. The erections may also not be as "hard" as in younger years. The female equivalent of an erection is vaginal lubrication. It appears that women, too, take longer to become aroused. Vaginal lubrication in aging diminishes slowly with time if there is continued sexual activity whether by coitus or by masturbation. Here, a cultural factor appears to be operative between younger and older women. The present generation of young women are more likely to masturbate than their mothers or grandmothers. Although almost all males masturbate, only 40% of women report doing so, although this figure appears higher in succeeding generations. (If there has been a sexual revolution at all, it would appear to have affected females, with their patterns approaching male patterns.)

Plateau Phase

The plateau phase is an intensification of the excitement phase. The penis is at its maximum size, while, in women, the breasts and labia swell. The pleasurable sensation associated with this stage does not decrease with age; however, the firmness of an erection or the fullness of the labial folds will be less. For men, the plateau phase is lengthened and could allow for longer pleasuring and better control of ejaculation.

Orgasm Phase

Orgasm is shorter in duration and less intense in older men and women. The sensation of ejaculatory inevitability disappears in many men, and the force and volume of seminal fluid decreases. Women, with aging, experience fewer uterine contractions. Women past the childbearing age are released from the worry over pregnancy and often experience an increased sense of abandonment to sensuality and increased pleasure.

Resolution Phase

It is, at this point, that aging men and women experience their major change in sexual response. The male, following an orgasm, has a refractory period during which he is unable to achieve another erection. The female, on the other hand, does not have a refractory period and hence is potentially capable of multiple orgasms with appropriate stimulation. Aging men experience a prolongation of the refractory period from minutes to hours or days. For some men, there also occurs a "paradoxical" refractory period. That is, an erection may be lost during the plateau period, and the individual, even though there was no orgasm, will enter a refractory period and have neither the desire nor capacity for an erection. Although a fairly common occurrence, this little-appreciated fact causes a good deal of disturbance.

The Components of Sexual Dysfunction

Adolph Meyer conceptualized the whole person in action in his environment as his focus of study. His theory of psychobiology emphasized the importance of a longitudinal biographical study. This took the form of the life chart in which multiple factors, such as constitution, development, and environment, could be seen to be operative at any cross-sectional moment in an individual's life span. The model implied to Meyer a method of history taking and a system of treatment that integrated many diverse, simultaneous, and eclectic approaches. Meyer's often unappreciated contribution is an important legacy that may serve as a lens with which to observe sexual functioning and dysfunction in the elderly. The child-centered bias of earlier personality theorists has left midlife and late life as a poorly conceptualized area that has only recently begun to gain the attention of researchers.

I would like to suggest a model in which the person is represented as a cylinder with different circumferential bandwidths representing various time periods in the life span. If the center is viewed as optimal functioning, then the circumference can represent dysfunction as displaced by various stresses. At any cross-sectional moment in time, an individual's behavior coping mechanism may be seen as a result of past history, present adaptation, and future expectations. The cross-sectional adaptation may be separated out into biopsychosocial components.

The various factors may, for expositional purposes, be listed in columns as in Table 1. However, it is important to note that items are not exclusively operative in a single area and are interrelated. For example, religion may have a profound influence on the behavioral expression of an individual's sexuality but has obvious predominant modes of action through psychodynamic and sociodynamic factors.

Various disciplines have tended to develop a predominant single-factor approach

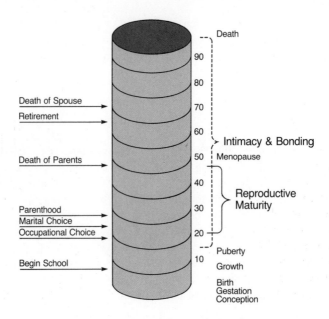

Figure 1 Life-span sexual development by decades with approximate impact of life stress units.

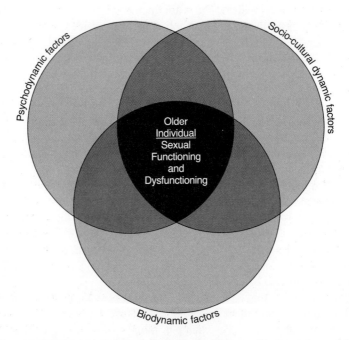

Figure 2 Cross-sectional moment along an individual's life span. The area of sexual functioning has been separated into biopsychosociocultural components.

Table 1 Biopsychosocial Parameters of Function

Biodynamic factors	Psychodynamic factors	Sociocultural dynamic factors
Anatomic and physiologic changes of aging	Intrapsychic and interpersonal changes accompanying aging	Environmental changes
Genetic	Personality type	Socioeconomic status: income, poverty, housing
Environmental	Intelligence, creative abilities	Ethnic and racial background
Surgical	Defenses and coping styles	Cultural values
Traumatic	Object losses, e.g., death of spouse, divorce, marital sepa-	Family support systems
Infectious	ration, status role, income	Community networks
Toxic	Dyadic relations: marital,	Shame-vs.-guilt cultures
Metabolic	parent–child	Culture age-graded for male and female roles
Endocrine	Family support system	

to problems while giving "lip service" acknowledgment to the other factors. One only has to do a little empirical observation to realize how pervasive is the single schism approach. Medical, mental, and social services are generally offered through separate systems, facilities, and staff, and woe to the individual who needs a coordinated effort at one time.

There does appear to be a growing appreciation that these factors are *not* mutually exclusive and are, in fact, interrelated. A change in one set of factors has major ripple effects in the others. It is important to remember that various factor approaches are but intellectual conveniences to assimilate the information explosion.

To illustrate the growing awareness of the interrelatedness of these factors, Holmes and Rahe (1967) have devised a social readjustment rating scale (SSRQ) that quantified various stress factors that impacted on individuals. Holmes has shown that the accumulation of more than 150 points in a year on the social readjustment scale would significantly increase the incidence of such diverse diseases as peptic ulcer, myocardial infarction, infections, and emotional disorders. He further stated that the more changes a person has, the more likely he is to become sick. Of those people with over 300 life change units for the past year, almost 80% developed a physical or emotional illness within a year; with 150 to 299 life change units, about 50% developed an illness; and with less than 150 life change units, only about 30% became ill.

The social readjustment rating scale's most potent life event change was the loss of a spouse, whether through death, divorce, or separation. Parkes et al. (1969, 1970) found that elderly widowers had a higher death rate in the first 6 months' bereavement and had more medical problems than widows. The relationships of stress and losses to the onset of disease among the elderly remains one of the most intriguing research questions.

The role of the psychiatrist in dealing with the elderly who present with sexual dysfunction is critical. The elderly may, with changes of aging and multiple physical and psychosocial losses, present for the first time with a sexual dysfunction. A compre-

Table 2   The Social Readjustment Rating Scale[a]

Life event	Mean value
1. Death of spouse	100
2. Divorce	73
3. Marital separation from mate	65
4. Detention in jail or other institution	63
5. Death of close family member	63
6. Major personal injury or illness	53
7. Marriage	50
8. Being fired at work	47
9. Marital reconciliation with mate	45
10. Retirement from work	45
11. Major change in the health or behavior of family member	44
12. Pregnancy	40
13. Sexual difficulties	39
14. Gaining a new family member (e.g., through birth, adoption, oldster moving in, etc.)	39
15. Major business readjustment (e.g., merger, reorganization, bankruptcy, etc.)	39
16. Major change in financial state (e.g., a lot worse off or a lot better off than usual)	38
17. Death of a close friend	37
18. Changing to a different line of work	36
19. Major change in the number of arguments with spouse (e.g., either a lot more or a lot less than usual regarding child-rearing, personal habits, etc.)	35
20. Taking on mortgage greater than $10,000 (e.g., purchasing a home, business, etc.)	31
21. Foreclosure on a mortgage or loan	50
22. Major change in responsibilities at work (e.g., promotion, demotion, lateral transfer)	29
23. Son or daughter leaving home (e.g., marriage, attending college, etc.)	29
24. In-law troubles	29
25. Outstanding personal achievement	28
26. Wife beginning or ceasing work outside the home	26
27. Beginning or ceasing formal schooling	26
28. Major change in living conditions (e.g., building a new home, remodeling, deterioration of home or neighborhood)	25
29. Revision of personal habits (dress, manners, associations, etc.)	24
30. Troubles with boss	23
31. Major change in working hours or conditions	20
32. Change in residence	20
33. Changing to a new school	20
34. Major change in usual type and/or amount of recreation	19
35. Major change in church activities (e.g., a lot more or a lot less than usual)	19
36. Major change in social activities (e.g., clubs, dancing, movies, visiting, etc.)	18
37. Taking on a mortgage or loan less than $10,000 (e.g., purchasing a car, TV, freezer, etc.)	17
38. Major change in sleeping habits (a lot more or a lot less sleep, or change in part of day when asleep)	16
39. Major change in number of family get-togethers (e.g., a lot more or a lot less than usual)	15
40. Major change in eating habits (a lot more or a lot less food intake or very different meal hours or surroundings)	15
41. Vacation	13
42. Christmas	12
43. Minor violations of the law (e.g., traffic tickets for jaywalking, disturbing the peace, etc.)	11

[a]Source: Holmes and Rahe (1967).

hensive approach to assessment and treatment is indicated. Let us examine a case as referred by a family physician and note the perceptual and decision-making process.

> Mrs. T. was a 59-year-old, devout, Polish-American, Catholic housewife, who was married for 42 years to a blue collar worker. Mrs. T. was referred by her family physician for evaluation and treatment of a depression that was not responding to medications.
>
> The patient's chief complains were: "I'm a mess. I'm afraid my husband doesn't love me any more. Dr. B. has tried everything and nothing seems to work. I think my family would be better off without me."
>
> Dr. B's referral noted the patient's several-month history of worsening symptoms of insomnia, poor appetite, 5-pound weight loss, crying spells "for no reason," and an inability to perform her usual household chores. There was no overt suicidal ideation, and there was no previous history of depressive episodes or family history of affective disorders. Dr. B felt the patient had a depressive syndrome and prescribed tricyclic antidepressant therapy.
>
> There was only a minimal improvement of symptoms after 6 weeks of medication at up to 150 mg q.d. Another trial period of 6 weeks of another tricyclic medication was also unsuccessful and eventuated in a psychiatric referral.
>
> Dr. B. described the patient as hardworking and always neat and cheerful although a somewhat anxious woman. She had reared five children in spite of difficulties with chronic rheumatoid arthritis. The arthritis was presently quiescent due to conservative management of rest and aspirin. The patient had residual deformity and subluxation of the small joints of the hands and feet. This resulted in a weakened grasp and impaired gait. He also described a several-year history of labile, mild, essential hypertension for which he prescribed hydrochlorthiazide. Blood pressure had been around 140–130/90–85. Menopause had occurred prior to the patient's 50th birthday.
>
> The family physician, in diagnosing and treating this woman, had utilized predominantly a biomedical model. Her problem was visualized as a depressive syndrome perhaps caused by catecholamine depletion correlated with endocrine changes of the involutional period.

Engel (1977, 1980) has criticized the biomedical model for its reductionism to phyiscal or chemical underlying principles as sufficient cause and suggested a need for a biopsychosocial model. The crippling flaw as he saw it was that the biomedical model did not include the patient and his attributes as a person. Lazare (1973) has described a hypothetical case and showed how observers using disciplinary perceptual screens from medical, psychological, behavioral, and social sciences each described the case and focused on somewhat different data, appreciated a different facet, and drew different conclusions about etiology and implications for therapy. The psychiatrist as a clinician with background in both biological and behavioral social services plays a key role in attempting to bridge in a pragmatic way these somewhat overlapping views to bring services together to meet this unique person's need. Yager (1977), in conceptualizing these issues, noted "pluralism is necessary in psychiatry to compensate for the errors and biases characteristic of our perceptual cognitive apparatus . . . and that clinical 'reality' is skewed by the data we notice based on past assumptions and formulations, and consequently, those views are reinforced by our perceptions.''

Let us reexamine the chief complaints of Mrs. T. in the previous example. An old aphorism in psychiatry comes to mind ''frequently the patient will tell you the diagnosis and the treatment, if you will only listen.''

''I'm a mess'' was explored with the patient. Initially, she began to describe her back and hip pain and her increasing difficulty getting up and down stairs. Mrs. T. had been a meticulous housewife who had previously derived a good deal of esteem from working and keeping her home and family ''just so.'' A work ethic was strongly imprinted in her family. She recalled that praise was almost nonexistent from her strict Catholic, immigrant parents. Self-esteem was contingent on doing rather than being. Earlier in her life she could secretly congratulate herself for getting her laundry on the line before her neighbor. Advancing age and disability had slowed Mrs. T. so that she could no longer keep up with her self-imposed standards. She thought of her illness as possible a punishment from God and blamed herself for letting things get so much out of control. On further questioning, Mrs. T. noted a worsening of her situation when her youngest daughter and last child residing at home had moved to attend school in a nearby city. Mrs. T. had tended to use this daughter as a confidante and lately had depended on her for transportation. Although Mrs. T. had been able to drive many years ago, her dependency on her family and her arthritis had allowed her driving skill to atrophy.

The patient's second complaint was that she was afraid her husband didn't love her any longer. This complaint was initially explored with her and then jointly with the husband. Mrs. T. had come to this conclusion after her husband had had several episodes of erectile failure a year previously followed by her husband's complete avoidance of any sexual activity or intimacy. Both she and her husband had mutually enjoyed fairly frequent intercourse in the past, and Mrs. T. now had concluded that her deformities and age had rendered her unlovable and so entered into a conspiracy of silence with her husband. She assumed her sex life was now over.

Mr. T. was a 62-year-old factory worker. He initially appeared embarrassed but relieved to be able to talk over the impotence problem. He denied loss of affection for his wife but admitted to frustration over the boring routine of their sex life. He recalled that his wife was raised a very strict Catholic and was ashamed of sexual feelings. He recalled how, for the first 15 years of their marriage, she insisted on undressing in the closet and insisted on sexual activity only at bedtime in the dark with little foreplay and only a conventional position. He was very disturbed by the first episode of impotence in his experience. Subsequent attempts engendered such anxiety that he was unable to perform sexually and eventually led to his decision to suppress any sexual thoughts or activities. His wife's recent complaints of dyspareunia and difficulty with pain from the arthritis left him feeling guilty over what he felt was only pleasurable for him.

Both of them were surprised and reassured when they found they were sexually desirable to each other. It was pointed out that sexual activity was but one form of communication. Their competitiveness in their relationship and their separate but parallel lives had led to a lifetime of little communication and avoided intimacy.

Mrs. T.'s third complaint ''Dr. B. has tried everything and nothing seems to work'' was now seen as premature closure in diagnosis and treatment because of Mrs. T.'s reticence to discuss the sexual problems. Mrs. T. was immediately referred back to Dr. B. for a genital exam. It was noted that there were no major problems and that dyspareunia was a result of estrogen-deficient vaginitis and was readily remedied by local creams.

As therapy progressed, it was noted that the arthritis pain was minimal after a night's rest, aspirin, and a warm bath. Sex was now possible without difficulty; however, this required permission and information to engage in pleasuring techniques, in the daylight, and utilizing various positions for comfort and enjoyment. Some specific suggestions were made of genital pleasuring by self and through partner with orgasm specifically avoided. This was followed by squeeze technique and eventually vaginal containment and finally pelvic thrusting. Over time, the prohibition against intercourse was lifted as more effective forms of sexual behavior were added to the couple's repertoire. Mr. and Mrs. T. responded quite well to sex therapy and communications therapy that eventually merged into family therapy that eventually precluded the relevance of Mrs. T.'s fourth complaint.

Medicine often focuses primarily on biological underpinnings as causal in the production of disease, whereas other disciplines involved in the treatment of sexual dysfunctions, notably psychologists, social workers, and ministers, usually have little training in biological underpinnings of sexual dysfunctions. Thus, the perspective of each may be polarized and the psychiatrist has a particular important integrating role.

Training in psychosocial areas is crucial in understanding sexual dysfunctions. Anatomic and physiologic factors as prime etiologic agents account for only 3 to 20% of sexual dysfunctions (Kaplan, 1974). The recognition of this has led to the expansion and acknowledged efficacy of behavioral, social learning models and integrated treatment of sexual dysfunctions over strictly biomedical or psychoanalytic treatments.

It becomes obvious that there is no single linear causality model that explains all of the phenomena inovlved in sexual dysfunctions and various therapy approaches. Hogan (1978) has suggested an interactional systems approach in which current factors, such as illness, lack of sexual knowledge and/or skill, misinformation, anxiety, and depression, have feedback loops with historical factors, such as religious orthodoxy, homosexuality, marital problems, and sexual trauma. These factors may result in acute sexual failure, which, when combined with performance anxiety, could lead to the vicious circle of communication breakdowns, withdrawal, hostility, and subsequent chronic sexual dysfunction. The conceptualization of these patterns in a system implies intervention points and also, partially, explains why varied treatment approaches have been successful. The system approach lends itself to a better understanding of the quantum increase in life change units that may adversely affect previously successful patterns of sexual behavior in the elderly.

Models of Assessment and Intervention

Older individuals, because of respect for perceived professional values, expertise, and authority, have relied on physicians for problem definition and solution. This established pattern of consumer preference places physicians in a critical early fulcrum position. Often their training has been inadequate and they will seek psychiatric consultation.

People in their fifties and sixties, if understood to represent a "biological elite," have survived innumerable stresses, made many decisions, and experienced their consequences. Many of these individuals may, for the first time in their lives, experience vaginismus, male or female dyspareunia, inhibited desire, impotence, or premature or delayed ejaculations. These individuals, at this point, require an assessment that covers biopsychosocial factors. To dismiss inquiry into a sexual area as irrelevant because of ageist attitude or, on the other hand, adopt a policy of uncritical referral, is to abdicate responsibility inherent in the patient–physician relationship.

Annon (1976) has proposed a rational continuum of increasingly skilled treatment interventions that allow each professional to select his own level of intervention based on training and experience. The model had four levels of intervention: P–LI–SS–IT (P, permission giving; LI, limited information; SS, specific suggestions; IT, intensive therapy). Theoretically, all physicians could function in the earlier levels of intervention and see the largest number of individuals. These individuals require careful evaluation and diagnosis and then, as Annon points out, simply need reassurance and permission that they are not abnormal. Then, if permission is not sufficient to resolve the continued concern, the clinician, depending on interest and training, will proceed to levels requiring more knowledge. This model would have the cost and care-effective theoretical possibility of trying to resolve sexual problems with brief therapy before involving patients in long-term treatment programs and allow the clinician to decide at which point intensive therapy is advantageous. Annon, in his work, describes graded assessment and treatment strategies for the various levels. The challenge to the psychiatrist in applying the principles of this model to an elderly clientele is the biopsychosociocultural assessment.

The assessment process in the elderly is similar to that used with younger patients; however, the genital and the general physical examination become increasingly important. The critical difference in treating older people is the importance of recognizing normal changes of aging and differentiating the presence of multiple-system disease states affecting an individual with less resiliency to stress. Although aging itself is not a disease, 80% of elderly individuals suffer from one or more chronic diseases. The most commonly reported physical disorders in order of frequency are arthritis, heart disease, hypertension, hypotension, asthma and hay fever, diabetes, peptic disease, severe visual and hearing impairments, and neurological motor disorders. About half of all over-65-year-old people are impaired by these chronic conditions, and 15% are unable to carry out major activities of daily living. It is, however, mistakenly assumed that these disorders are the reasons to forego sexual activity. Many elderly people silently give up sexual activity because of lack of permission or information to successfully accommodate to changes. Permanent sexual dysfunction may be the outcome of a transient problem.

An excellent prognosis can be expected with brief treatment techniques of such disorders as secondary impotence, erectile failures, premature ejaculation, difficulty with lubrication, or secondary orgasmic dysfunction in the absence of severe marital problems. The best prognosis results when the dysfunction is of short or recent duration, the couple is heterosexual and is motivated and cooperative in therapy, and the partners are committed to their relationship. It is the ease of treatment that has led many allied health personnel to embark upon treatment before obtaining a thorough assessment, particularly genital and physical examinations.

Medications and Sexual Functioning

Elderly patients with chronic disease conditions are frequently taking medications. Older Americans receive, on the average, 13 prescriptions annually, including renewals. Medications frequently have untoward effects on sexuality and may cause decreased libido, difficulty lubricating, or erectile failures. Other medication side effects in the elderly may go undetected because of their insidious ability to mimic stereotypic conditions associated with old age, such as absentmindedness, confusion, and anxiety. Table 3 illustrates some of the most common medications that may decrease libido or interfere with sexual response. Alcohol deserves special mention as it very frequently is the beginning step of a "sexual dysfunction, marital breakdown pattern" that is so common as to be classified as a syndrome. A common pattern is seen when a man, anxious over changes of aging, begins to consume large quantities of alcohol to relieve anxiety. This eventually leads to erectile failure, which leads to marital stress and increasing anxiety with future attempts at intercourse. Some men, at the point of erectile failure, performance anxiety, marital stress, and displaced anger will then sometimes seek out an extramarital affair. Often these men, after experiencing the reassurance of their desirability, have decreased anxiety and are then able to successfully have intercourse. They erroneously conclude that their nagging, no-waisted, gray-haired, sagging-breasted wife is the cause of the sexual dysfunction and a good reason to drink.

Table 3 Drugs That May Interfere with Sexual Responses

CNS depressants	*Antidepressants*
Alcohol	Tricyclics
Sedatives–Hypnotics	MAO inhibitors
Barbiturates	*Antihypertensives*
Glutethimide	Commonly affect sexuality
Methaqualone	Ganglionic blockers
Fluorazepam	Pentolinium tartrate
Antianxiety agents	Guanethidine
Chlordiazepoxide	Rauwolfia alkaloids
Diazepam	Less likely to affect sexuality
Oxazepam.	Methyldopa
Meprobamate	Thiazide–diuretic
Narcotics-Codeine	Least likely to affect sexuality
Neuroleptics	Propanolol
Phenothiazines	*Stimulants*
Butyrophenones	Caffeine
Thioxanthenes	Methylphenidate
Dihydroindolones	Amphetamines
Dibenzoxazepines	Ephedrine

Mr. M. was a 56-year-old, married appliance salesman. He had become increasingly preoccupied with financial problems, failing career aspirations, and future retirement goals. He felt "old and useless" with the promotion of younger men in his department over him.

He has a moderate history of social drinking in the past, but presently began a pattern of anxiety-reducing relief drinking. His absence from the family and drinking became a focus for marital strife. It was at this point that Mr. M. experienced his first erectile failure. Performance anxiety led him to withdraw completely from sexual activity with his wife. Mrs. M. became increasingly angry and bitter. Eventually Mr. M. sought out an extramarital affair with his secretary who made him "feel young" again. Mr. M. was torn between his love for his wife and family and the woman who reaffirmed his "lost youth" and presumed worth.

This affair came to the attention of the wife and resulted in a stormy confrontation and a visit to their pastor. The alcohol problem by this time had become a fairly entrenched pattern of addiction. On the advice of the pastor, the couple sought out psychiatric consultation.

When the full syndrome is developed, the couple is then a candidate for psychotherapy and alcohol counseling, as well as sexual therapy. Early identification and treatment of sexual problems associated with aging can prevent the full syndrome from developing.

Disease States That Affect Sexual Functioning in the Elderly

Of the diseases associated with sexual dysfunction, the most common are diseases of the genitourinary tract and reproductive systems and diseases of the secondary sexual organs. The most common general disorders affecting sexual functioning are, of course, cardiovascular disease, respiratory disease, and endocrine disease.

Over one-half of older men develop benign prostatic hypertrophy. When bladder neck obstruction is developing, the physician probably will recommend surgery. This is the time for critical counseling intervention. Almost invariably, men fear that surgery will be the prelude to the end of sexuality. The physician has an important role in educating, listening, and reassuring the patient. The role of the prostate gland and how sexual functioning will be affected postsurgery should be explained in detail. It is important to clarify that transurethral resection of the prostate, retropubic and suprapubic prostatectomy, can produce some degree of incompetence at the bladder neck with retrograde ejaculation of semen into the bladder. Although this obviously interferes with fertility, it does not interfere with erection or physical sensations of pleasure. Damage to the innervation of the erectile system does occur sometimes with perineal approaches to the prostate. The latter procedure is considered "safer" for some cancer resections or for men whom the physician judges debilitated and "too old to care about sex." The physician or psychiatric consultant should be careful not to make this assumption regardless of the patient's age without discussing with the patient his knowledge and feelings of sexual functioning. To underscore this point, it is important

to note that the majority of instances of postsurgical erectile failures following prostatectomy procedures are psychogenic. A period of bereavement for the perceived loss
is usual and requires continued support and treatment.

The most common disorders affecting aging women are the changes associated
with target organs because of decreased production of estrogen. Two important estrogen targets are local genitourinary changes and calcium resorbtion from bone.
Thinning of the vaginal mucosa secondary to estrogen deficiency predisposes to infection with bleeding and itching and is a common cause for dyspareunia and vaginismus.
The clinician should not use the older pejorative term *senile vaginitis* and may profit
from the experience of one angry woman who refused to see her former physician
when she was informed that her "vagina was senile."

The loss of tissue support also predisposes to cystitis and stress incontinence.
Since the publication in the literature of the higher risk of endometrial cancers with
hormone replacement, more women have been taken off systemic estrogens and are
likely to develop sexual complaints. Women are particularly susceptible to cultural
influences. Married women tend to be younger than and live longer than their husbands
and are more likely to stop coital activity after separation or divorce or after illness or
death of their spouse. Self-stimulation is effective in preserving tone and lubricating
ability, as well as serving as an effective measure of relieving anxiety. However, older
women are less likely to masturbate than their grandchildren. Older women, particularly, need permission and information. When there are religious strictures against
masturbating, it is important to differentiate information from advice and to correct
some of the myths and misconceptions that continue to surround the issue of masturbation, if possible. Local vaginal use of estrogen creams and suppositories may alleviate
some of the atrophic vaginal changes.

Many women have had hysterectomies and need information regarding hormone
replacement. Progestational compounds often decrease sexual desire and may cause
mood disturbances. Since sexual desire and arousal are dependent in both male and
females on testosterone, no alteration in sexual interest in females can be expected
from somatic origin secondary to hysterectomy and oophorectomy. Although surgery
may alter body image and can be experienced as a psychological loss, testosterone is
produced by the adrenal gland in women and will not be altered by such surgery. It is
important then to reassure women that a total hysterectomy (including bilateral
oophorectomy) will not alter sexual desire on a hormonal basis. As with any surgical
loss of symbolic significance, a period of bereavement usually follows and will require
clarification, continued information, and empathic support. Many authors (Drellich
1967; Nadelson, 1977) have noted that the uterus is viewed by women as a symbol of
their femininity. For many of these women, the loss of the uterus is equated with loss
of sexual identity as women and its association with youth and attractiveness.

Mastectomy, a visible, mutilating surgery, can be symbolically more traumatic
than the loss of a uterus (Polivz, 1974). Nadelson and Notman (1977) have pointed out
that there are several issues raised by mastectomy. They are confrontation with a life-
threatening illness, loss of a body part, and specific concerns related to the breast as an
important component of femininity combining nutrient maternal potential and sexual
attractiveness. Surgeons (generally males) will often focus predominantly on the life-
threatening illness aspect and pay lip service to other aspects. Psychiatrists as consultants play a crucial role in expanding treatment beyond the biological to include

psychosocial aspects. Ervin (1973) describes a program of supportive therapy that actively involves the husband in reassurance and sharing of feelings, as well as participation in rehabilitation (e.g., dressing changes, exercise, and massage). This type of support has facilitated bereavement of the loss and the return to normal sexual functioning.

Disease of the heart and blood vessels now account for more than half of all deaths in the United States, whereas they accounted for less than 20% in 1900 (Bureau of Census, U. S. Department of Commerce). The development of heart disease by an individual is often viewed as a major insult to the self-image and initiates a period of bereavement or depression with decreased libido.

Many elderly, postcoronary males fail to resume coital activity even though they are physiologically capable of intercourse. There is a psychologic stress reaction whereby some men feel betrayed by their bodies and out of control. They become withdrawn and often give up, stating "nothing can be done." Many of these men become overly dependent on their spouses and may develop a frank depressive syndrome. The psychiatrist should be prepared to work with men whose self-image is injured. Separating their self-image from the heart that is injured is an important starting point. Returning, as soon as possible, to normal activities, especially sexuality, is essential to rehabilitation. Hackett and Cassem (1973) has shown that exercise conditioning programs enhance self-image and allow the early return of sexual expression.

Hellerstein and Friedman (1970) have shown that heart rates in males with postmyocardial infarctions rarely exceed 125 beats/min during coitus with an accustomed partner. This is approximately the same effort and oxygen consumption as in walking up two flights of stairs and is easily tolerated. If there is no marked angina or congestive heart failure, a couple can usually resume intercourse within 4 to 6 weeks of an acute myocardial infarction.

Although some physicians do talk to patients about sexual concerns, few approach the patient's spouse with the same concerns. Often a wife, fearful of "precipitating a heart attack" in her husband, will simply remain silent and even harbor guilt over her own sexual feelings that eventually becomes unacknowledged resentment. The "conspiracy of silence" is best treated by early intervention with counseling of both husband and wife.

> Mr. R. was a 67-year-old, married, retired accountant who had had a seemingly uncomplicated convalescence from a coronary 1 year previously. After the anniversary of his coronary, Mr. R. had become irritable and depressed and sought psychiatric consultation.
>
> In reviewing his history, it was noted that the internist had prescribed nitroglycerine, progressive exercises, and had given permission to resume sexual activity after 2 months. Additionally, he suggested to the patient the possibility of a nitroglycerine prior to intercourse for angina. Mrs. R. accompanied her husband on his follow-up visits but did not take part in the discussions. Mr. R. informed his wife that the internist stated it was permissible to have sex when he could walk several blocks without pain.
>
> Although Mr. R. was free from angina while walking, he thought the advice to take a nitroglycerine prior to sex implied that the doctor thought

sex was risky, if not potentially fatal. His anxiety over a repeat coronary caused him to avoid sexual activity. His wife, feeling guilty over her sexual needs and a fantasy of coital death, also entered into the conspiracy of silence. It was only after Mr. R. became depressed that the sexual problem came to light.

Widowhood and Sexuality

Females in the United States live, on the average, 7 years longer than males. In addition, women tend to marry men 3 years older, which ensures the average American women 10 years of widowhood (U.S. Department of Health and Human Services, NIH, 1980). Culturally, mores conspire against female sexuality. The taboo of older women dating younger men is considerably stronger than the reverse. There are also prolonged cultural pressures of enforced passivity (Gerber, 1975), e.g., the widow who is suddenly faced with financial affairs of which she has little understanding. Sexually expressed, the male is responsible for the woman's sexuality. The male is the initiator of sex. The sudden shock of widowhood leaves many women with sexual feelings, survival guilt, and learned passivity.

The clinician should be aware of vague complaints involving headache, backache, and, particularly, genitourinary complaints that defy physical assessment or treatment. These may represent blocked grief reactions and/or unacknowledged sexual feelings. The clinician can pursue with the patient how sexual needs are being satisfied since the loss. If there appears to be a relationship, assurance that such feelings are natural and expected will often elicit relief. Whether the patient prefers abstinence, masturbation, or a new sexual partner, the psychiatrist can be in a key area to assess and treat the problem.

Aging, Sexuality, and Institutionalization

There are a number of mistaken attitudes concerning institutionalization of the elderly. There is the myth that most elderly will eventually become "senile" and institutionalized. The fact is that on any one day, only 5% of the over-65-year-old age group are institutionalized. This 5%, however, does represent over 1 million Americans. In recent years nursing home costs have soared and depleted the savings of elderly. Public funds now account for $2 out of every $3 in nursing home revenues.

What has been the impact on those individuals who take the "pauper's oath" for medical reimbursement? One should recall that the historical roots of today's nursing homes have been the alms houses, work houses, and county poor homes of an earlier era. There remains today a residual puritan ethic, particularly among older Americans, that poverty and illness are punishment for sin. This stigma attached to nursing home care can be an assault on the identity of an older individual. It is because one's self-concept is so closely related with sexual identity that assaults upon the personal identity are often translated into suppression of sexual behaviors. The few nursing home studies that have looked at sexuality have tended to define sexuality in a very narrow sense, that is, coital activity, fantasy, or masturbation. Sexual behavior may be sublimated and expressed as handholding, touching, hugging, kissing, or even as a need to feel feminine or masculine by simply adopting cultural stereotypic behaviors (e.g., knitting versus leather-working in activity therapy). Sexuality may also be expressed negatively. Kassel (1976) feels that a significant portion of disturbed behavior, as seen in elderly nursing home patients, is from unresolved sexual needs, which are forbidden expressions. Nursing homes, as total institutions, vary tremendously in their "tolerance" of sexual behavior. Some seemingly tolerant staff reactions to patients' sexual behaviors take the form of voyeuristic manipulations (e.g., petting rooms or nursing reports that detail and supervise the "cute, puppy love crushes" of the elderly residents). Although the intent may be benign, its outcome is to infantilize the resident under the eye of a controlling parent. It is important to remember that nursing homes are very matriarchal cultures. On the national average, female residents outnumber males 3 to 1, and the daily staff contact is almost entirely female. Other overtly negative staff attitudes view any sexual behavior in older persons as inappropriate and disgusting. Masturbation may be dealt with by hand restraints, gerichairs, or drugs, to the point of stupor. Administrators, anxious over public reputation or scrutiny by visiting relatives, may promulgate and support policies of sexual suppression out of expediency. Even handholding among female residents may be discouraged.

> The nurse ran into the administrator's office and blurted out that she had just walked into Mr. B.'s room, an 82-year-old widower, to give him his medication and "he was doing it with a female visitor." The administrator delayed long enough to allow Mr. B. and his "guest" to finish and for her to leave. Later discussion by the administrator with Mr. B. disclosed that his guest was a "hooker" with whom he had had an ongoing relationship for several years prior to coming to the nursing home. Mr. B. was advised that this was upsetting to the staff and he should be more discreet and conduct his "business" elsewhere.

This example questions the identity of the nursing home as an extension of an individual's private home or as an extension of the hospital and the right of an individual versus the responsibility of staff. Many aspects of the institution are assaults on the identity and worth of the elderly individual.

What is needed for elderly residents is a sense of mastery over aspects of their lives in the face of a total institution. Pfeiffer (1974) commented that if privacy is assured, then opportunity for sexual expression, if desired, is also assured. A further question is "Can sexual expression be promoted rather than tolerated?" Would we wish less autonomy for ourselves?

References

Annon, J.S. *The behavioral treatment of sexual problems: Brief therapy.* New York: Harper & Row, 1976.
Bengston, V.L., Cuellar, J.B., and Ragan, P.K. Contrasts and similarities in attitudes toward death by race, age, social class, and sex. *Journal of Gerontology,* 1977, *32,* 204–216.

Burnap, D.W., and Golden, J.S. Sexual problems in medical practice. *Medical Education,* 1967, *42,* 673–680.

Butler, R.N. The effects of medical and economic aspects of the life cycle. *Industrial Gerontology,* 1969, *1,* 1–9.

Butler, R.N., and Lewis, M.I. *Sex after sixty,* A guide for men and women for their later years. New York: Harper & Row, 1976.

Drellich, M.G. Sex after hysterectomy. *Medical Aspects of Human Sex,* 1967, *11,* 62–64.

Engel, G.L. The need for a new medical model: A challenge for biomedicine. *Science,* 1977, *196,* 129–136.

Engel, G.L. The clinical application of the biopsychosocial model, *American Journal of Psychiatry,* May 1980, *137,* 5.

Ervin, E.V. Psychological adjustment to mastectomy. *Medical Aspects of Human Sex,* 1973, *7,* 42.

Gerber, I., Rusalem, R., Hannon, N., Battin, D., and Arkin, A. Anticipatory grief and aged widows and widowers, *Journal of Gerontology,* 1975, *30,* 325–329.

Greene, R. *Human Sexuality, A Health Practitioner's Text.* Baltimore, Md.: Williams & Wilkins, 1975.

Hackett, T.P., and Cassem, N.H. Psychologic adaptation to convalescence in myocardial infarction patients. In J.P. Naughton and H.K. Hellerstein (Eds.), *Exercise testing and exercise training in coronary heart disease.* New York: Academic Press, 1973.

Hellerstein, H.K., and Friedman, E.H. Sexual activity and the post-coronary patient. *Archives of Internal Medicine,* 1970, *125,* 987.

Hogan, D.R. The effectiveness of sex therapy. In LoPiccolo and LoPiccolo (Eds.), *Handbook of sex therapy.* New York: Plenum Press, 1978.

Holmes, T.H., and Rahe, R.H. The social readjustment rating scale. *Journal of Psychosomatic Research,* 1967, *11,* 213–218.

Kaplan, H.S. *The new sex therapy.* New York: Brunner/Mazel, 1974.

Kassel, V. Sex in nursing homes. *Medical Aspects of Human Sexuality,* 1976, *10*(3).

Kinsey, A.C., Pomeroy, W.B., and Martin, C.E. *Sexual behavior in the human male.* Philadelphia: Saunders, 1948.

Kinsey, A.C., Pomeroy, W.B., Martin, C.E., and Gebhard, P.H. *Sexual behavior in the human female.* Philadelphia: Saunders, 1953.

Leif, H.I., and Ebert, R.K. Sexual knowledge, attitudes, and behavior of medical students: Implications for medical practice. In D.W. Abse and L.M.R. Louder (Eds.), *Marital and sexual counseling in medical practice.* New York: Harper & Row, 1974.

Libow, L. Address at Gerontological Society Annual Meeting, Dallas, 1978.

Masters, V., and Johnson, W. *Human sexual response.* Boston: Little, Brown, 1966.

Masters, V., and Johnson, W. *Human sexual inadequacy.* Boston: Little, Brown, 1970.

Moss, F.E., and Halamandaris, V.J. *Too old, too sick, too bad: Nursing homes in America.* Germantown, Md.: Aspen Systems, 1977.

Nadelson, C., and Notman, M. Emotional aspects of the symptoms, functions and disorders of women. In Usdin G. (Ed.), *Psychiatric medicine.* New York: Brunner/Mazel, 1977.

National Institutes of Health. *Publication No. 89-969,* Epidemiology of Aging. Washington, D.C.: July, 1980.

Parkes, C.M., Benjamin, B., and Fitzgerald, R.G. Broken heart: a statistical study of increased mortality among widowers. *British Medical Journal,* 1969, *1,* 740–745.

Pfeiffer, E. Sexuality in the aging individual. *Journal of the American Geriatric Society,* 1974, *12*(11).

Polivz, J. Psychological reaction to hysterectomy: A critical review. *American Journal of Obstetrics— Gynecology,* 1974, *118,* 417–426.

U.S. Department of Health, Education, and Welfare. *Public policy and the frail elderly* (Publication No. OHDS-79-20959) Washington, D.C.: U.S. Government Printing Office, 1978.

Yager, J. Psychiatric eclecticism: A cognitive view. *American Journal of Psychiatry,* 1977, *134*(7).

The Marital Relationship: Adapting an Old Model to Contemporary Needs

Eugenia L. Gullick

The subjects of marriage and marital relationships have long escaped rigorous scientific inquiry. Considered by many to be too "soft" a topic to study empirically, marriage had most often been dealt with through case studies and anecdotal descriptions. In recent decades, however, the marital relationship has received increased cultural and societal attention; consequently social scientists have become more curious *and* rigorous in their investigation of the salient issues (Gurman and Kniskern, 1979; Jacobson, 1978).

Recent societal and cultural changes have had an impact on many aspects of life, including marital relationships. During the last half-century, we have witnessed and documented major changes in family roles, as well as career roles. The increased urbanization in our country has led to a shift in marital goals, values, and expectations. In a more agrarian culture, marriage provides a clear distinction of roles for the spouses; it offers economic security, opportunity for "legitimate" sexual expression and procreation, and clear division of labor. Our highly industrialized culture has led to changes in roles for the sexes and, thus, has called to question many of the traditional marital values.

Scientific, technologic achievements heralded by the "space race" of the 1950s led to an increased national concern about academic achievement. For both sexes there has been a greater emphasis on higher education and professional expression for women as well as men. For the first time in American history, the "typical wife" may be pursuing her own professional career rather than working as a primary homemaker. The emergence of the assertiveness ethic in the late 1960s has further emphasized the importance of personal needs for expression and development. It has introduced the notion that each individual must assume responsibility for his/her own satisfaction; it has granted permission and encouragement for individuals to make their own needs and

Eugenia L. Gullick • Salem Psychiatric Associates, Winston-Salem, North Carolina.

satisfaction top priority items; and has led some to label the 1970s as the "me" decade. At any rate, the expectation has been created that individual need, fulfillment, and personal development are worthy and legitimate goals for one's adult life.

The "sexual renaissance" (Hunt, 1974) of the 1960s and 1970s has been accompanied by drastic alterations in sexual attitudes and behaviors. Many old taboos have been reexamined and redefined. Following a philosophy reminiscent of the assertiveness ethic, sexual "normality," and culturally sanctioned behavior have come to be defined in terms of the individual satisfaction and fulfillment provided for each partner. Consequently, various forms of premarital, extramarital, and nonmarital sexual activity are now widely accepted and frequently practiced. The feasibility and appeal of sexual freedom and activity outside of marriage have certainly been enhanced by the introduction of relatively safe and effective oral contraceptives, the development and legalization of abortion procedures, and the perfection of sterilization technology.

Although granting permission and encouragement for the pursuit of personal development and individual fulfillment, the assertiveness ethic and the sexual renaissance have heralded a critical reexamination of the traditional marriage and its capacity for the individual development of its partners. This critical review has led many scientists in the field to conclude that traditional marital styles provide an inadequate framework for achievement of individual growth. Mace and Mace (1974) describe conventional marriage as paternalistic, ritualistic, rigid, and destructive. Bernard (1972) cites studies suggesting that marriage has primarily benefited men at the expense of their female partners. She states that marriage has been found to produce a decrease in self-esteem, self-development, and assertiveness in wives, whereas *increasing* those qualities in husbands. Certainly the male-dominated traditional style of marriage is appropriate and functional in an agrarian culture where physical prowess and leadership of the male are critical for the survival of the family unit. Our industrialized society with its emphasis on and opportunity for personal development and individual growth seems to have outgrown conventional marriage styles. Prochaska and Prochaska (1978, p. 5) state:

> The twentieth century has witnessed a cultural lag phenomenon in which the traditional marriage continued dominant even though it remained tied to the waning agricultural society. Many modern marriages have been caught in a cultural bind between the emerging egalitarianism of the industrial society and a family socialization process that prepared the spouses for a traditional marriage.

The ease of divorce as well as the availability and acceptability of a number of alternative lifestyles have led many to a rejection of conventional marital styles. Since the 1960s, increasing numbers of individuals have chosen singlehood or cohabitation as attractive alternatives to marriage (Mace and Mace, 1974). The introduction of the no-fault divorce makes it unnecessary for couples to remain in an unfulfilling union. Recent statistics give the United States the highest divorce rate of any country in the world (Glick, 1975). This lends statistical credence to the rejection of traditionalism, which has been documented by many (Bernard, 1972; Glick, 1975; Kaplan, 1974; Lederer and Jackson, 1968; Mace and Mace, 1974; Prochaska and Prochaska, 1978).

Mace and Mace (1974) conclude that traditional marriage has given birth to the companionship marriage, which is more egalitarian and democratic than its predecessor. It is characterized by mutual respect, empathic understanding, and friendship

(Burgess and Locke, 1945; Prochaska and Prochaska, 1978). Jacobson (1977) claims that this evolution has resulted in the emergence of "more fastidious marital partners," expecting and demanding more intimacy, companionship, and individual self-development than economic security and parenthood. Unfortunately most of those making such demands have been socialized and prepared to live within a traditional marriage. Scanzoni (1972) demonstrates that attempts to transform conventional marriages into companionship ones lead to considerable conflict and tension. This is due in large part to the fact that partners have not learned some of the basic relationship skills involved in egalitarian communication. Weiss (1978, p. 190) points out that

> the less a relationship is governed by clearly stated rules (traditional vs. egalitarian), the greater the potential for idiosyncratic solutions, and eventual discord. Relationships based on egalitarian ideologies require considerable accommodation without benefit of seasoned rules.

In spite of the abundance of scientific and popular literature emphasizing the importance of effective marital communication (Azrin et al., 1973; Bach and Wyden, 1969; Birchler et al., 1975; Lederer and Jackson, 1968; Stuart, 1969), most individuals enter the marital endeavor with no education or training regarding effective methodology for the development of such communication (Gottman et al., 1976).

The growing societal concern regarding marital disillusionment and inadequacy has led to much scientific inquiry and has resulted in the development of several models of marital discord and marital therapy. In a recent review of marital therapy research, Weiss (1978) concluded that the dynamic behavioral model that incorporates training in communication skills into dynamic therapeutic experiences emerges as one of the more successful models. It is this model that will serve as the focus of this chapter. It should be pointed out that rigid theoretical models rarely are followed in effective clinical practice, rather the skilled clinician borrows from each as he needs to develop sensitive and effective intervention techniques.

A Dynamic Behavioral Communication Model of Marital Discord

Weiss (1978) states that a dynamic behavioral communications approach to marital discord draws heavily on theories of social exchange (Birchler et al., 1975; Gottman et al., 1976; Patterson et al., 1976), reciprocity (Patterson et al., 1976; Stuart, 1969) and interpersonal communication (Gottman et al., 1976; Jacobson and Margolin, 1979). A marital relationship resembles other types of contractual arrangements in its appearance; however, Weiss (1978, p. 191) states that marriage has three unique characteristics that distinguish it from all other relationships.

> In a marriage, behaviors are exchanged in a relatively closed system where producer and consumer are mutually dependent upon one another for repeat business. With the exception of the telephone company, most business can be taken elsewhere if dissatisfied. While it may be good business sense to aim for the short-term gain—make a killing and leave—marriages, like the corner store, cannot afford this zero sum game tactic. If there is to be an exchange of commodities of value, the closed system limits the extent to which one can maximize individual gains. Furthermore, marriage is

characterized by pervasiveness of exchange which is not apparent in other contractual arrangements. The same person with whom one struggles over finances, plans for vacations, helps with one's infirmed parents, keeps the child from becoming a neighborhood menace, is also the source of sexual satisfaction and understanding comfort!

Finally, marital transactions (behavioral exchanges between partners) have relevance to self-values. The importance of equitable exchanges between partners is clear; one must also remember the importance of the symbolic meaning of the behaviors exchanged. Certain behaviors or exchanges may relate to the self-esteem of an individual partner. Furthermore, partners frequently interpret the behaviors of their spouse and draw conclusions about causality and intent.

> For example, failing to get gas for the car or calling to announce one's lateness are not just simple omissions which require remediation; they are commissions having to do with love, consideration, or caring. "It is because you don't care enough about me. . . ." (Weiss, 1978, p. 193)

The uniqueness of the marital relationship has led many to the conclusion that marriage provides each partner with an opportunity to develop high levels of interpersonal intimacy (Askham, 1976; Mace and Mace, 1975; Nadelson, 1978; Rogers, 1972; Sager, 1974). Marital intimacy is said to result from sexual satisfaction (Kaplan, 1974; Lederer and Jackson, 1968; Masters and Johnson, 1970) and a climate of trust between partners (Lederer and Jackson, 1968); its development requires mutual openness and the willingness to risk genuine encounters in areas that are important to either partner (Satir, 1967). It is characterized by each individual's respect of his partner's need for periods of solitude (Satir, 1967) and by the capacity of each partner to bear and express anger (Kuten, 1976). Its development requires adaptive and sensitive management of different personal issues that are particularly salient at particular points in the life cycle (Nadelson et al., 1979). Finally, intimacy between partners is enhanced through their individual fulfillment of two needs: the need for personal identity and development and the need for a stable home environment (Askham, 1976; Rogers, 1972).

Any discussion of intimacy development is incomplete without an examination of the impact of partner communication styles on such development. Clearly, openness, risk taking, individual need fulfillment, and warmth are attainable only if partners can communicate their needs and approval of one another in a sensitive and effective manner (Gottman et al., 1976; Lederer and Jackson, 1968; Mace and Mace, 1975; Rogers, 1972). It is the purpose of this chapter to (1) examine common communication deficits and their impact on marital intimacy; and (2) discuss some effective methods of therapeutic intervention that might be used with patients requiring relationship enhancement or improvement.

Types of Communication Deficits

Use of Aversive Control

Weiss (1978) has conceptualized that relationhips striving for egalitarianism attempt to follow a behavior exchange or give–get model (Weiss, 1978, p. 197). If the marital system is in balance, each partner feels that he/she is receiving benefits from the relationship that are at least equivalent to the "gifts" or compromises he/she has invested in it. When a partner feels he/she is giving more than he/she is receiving, the balance is in disequilibrium for that partner, and he/she experiences a need to return it to equilibrium. This is accomplished through behavior change. Unfortunately, most partners report that they regain balance through negative behavior control, such as complaining, criticizing, nagging, crying, and guilting. It is rare to hear a partner report that imbalances are corrected by making positive, nonblaming assertive statements about individual needs or requests. It seems that in the absence of appropriate and positive communication skills, partners quite rapidly learn methods of aversive or negative control (Patterson and Reid, 1970; Stuart, 1969; Weiss, 1978).

Low Rate of Positive Behavior between Partners

Gottman et al. (1976) examined communication patterns within a group of maritally distressed (clinical) couples and compared them to patterns exhibited by a group of nondistressed (nonclinical) couples. Their work indicates that distressed couples exhibit lower rates of positive behavior (behavior defined by the spouse as pleasant) and higher rates of negative behavior (behavior defined by the spouse as unpleasant) than nondistressed couples. For example, distressed couples exhibit significantly fewer warm, sharing conversations of the type often enjoyed during courtship; most verbal exchanges are either task-oriented (e.g., discussion of which private school children should attend) or argumentative in nature (e.g., quarrel over Mrs. S.'s management of household finances) (Stuart, 1969). Furthermore, partners from nondistressed marriages demonstrate more rewarding and effective listening techniques with one another than do distressed partners (Gottman et al., 1976).

Nonconcordance of Intent and Impact

Effective marital communication is further characterized by positive correlations between the intent and impact of messages (Gottman et al., 1976), that is, messages sent from a speaker to his partner are received as the speaker intended; they have the desired impact on the partner. Clear and precisely received messages are most easily communicated when (1) the speaker takes responsibility for stating his ideas exactly, he does not expect or require his partner to mind read, and (2) the listener assumes responsibility for making certain he understands the message, if unclear, he attempts to improve his understanding by asking clarifying questions of the speaker. When the message is not interpreted as the speaker intended, it is said that intent does not equal impact. Predictably, this deficit produces misunderstandings and eventual conflict and discord between partners.

Intent will not be equivalent to impact if the speaker's manner of delivering the message is inconsistent with his intent. For example,

> Mr. J. may be quite irritable one afternoon due to a number of the problems that arose at work. He returns home, unaware of the fact that his irritability is still apparent. He actually is looking forward to a quiet evening over one of his wife's delicious meals.

> In an effort to make conversation (intent) he asks, "Have you started dinner yet?"
> Mr. J. asks this in an irritated tone of voice, and his wife feels he is reprimanding her
> (impact). She becomes angry, and their evening is off to an unpleasant start. (Gullick,
> 1978, p. 103)

Intent may not equal impact if the listener fails to hear the message the way it was delivered. For example,

> Mrs. R. has been distressed the last week; she feels worthless to herself and her
> family. She dreads attending this evening's party at Mr. R.'s employer's home.
> Nevertheless, she dons her cocktail dress and is trying to fix her hair to her satisfac-
> tion, when Mr. R. says warmly, "Leona, you look lovely this evening." Mrs. R.
> becomes incensed at his "phoniness," convinced that he simply is trying to lift her
> spirits so that she will be more sociable. (Gullick, 1978, p. 103)

Gottman et al. (1976) found that distressed couples did not differ from non-distressed couples in the usual intent of their messages; however, distressed couples had less positive impact on their spouses than they intended.

Deficient Conflict-Resolution Skills

A frequent cause of marital discord is the inability of couples to solve problems in an efficient and mutually satisfying manner (Gottman et al., 1976; Stuart, 1969; Winter et al., 1973). Gottman et al. (1976) demonstrate that the manner in which problems are discussed by partners distinguishes between distressed and nondistressed couples. When a distressed partner complains, he is more likely to make his complaint a personal attack on the character of his partner (i.e., "You have always been a lazy person"), than to keep it behavior specific (i.e., "When you forget to take out the trash when it's full, I feel angry") (Gullick, 1978).

Requirements for Effective Communication and Relationship Satisfaction

Partner's Acceptance of Responsibility for His Own Satisfaction

In spite of the pessimism many feel toward the institution of marriage, most have been socialized and seduced by cultural messages that lead them to see marriage as an ideal solution to a number of problems. Many marry with the hope and expectation that the new relationship will bring an end to the loneliness of singlehood; they believe marriage has an inherent capacity for producing effortless fulfillment for each partner. Marital mythology holds that the agent through which marital happiness is realized is the spouse. This belief suggests that the partner, because he loves and desires to please his spouse, is attributed with nearly "supernatural" powers; he is expected to know intuitively what his partner needs, desires, and feels. Any imprecision in accomplishing that goal may be interpreted as an indication that he does *not* love the partner as he says or that he is insensitive to the partner's needs.

Bearing the entire responsibility for a partner's happiness is far too burdensome for any individual. The most loving and sensitive spouse may need some assistance in *learning* about the preferences and needs of his partner. Mutual satisfaction is more attainable when each individual assumes responsibility for his *own* happiness. Each must attempt to identify his needs and communicate these in a straightforward, yet sensitive, manner (Gullick, 1978).

Objectification

Weiss (1978) concludes that effective and fulfilling relationships require that partners demonstrate and practice the ability to objectify. That is, each partner must be able to describe his complaint (or compliment) in an objective, behavioral manner, clearly identifying antecedents and consequences of the particular behavioral event. Requests or complaints are easier to receive if behavioral rather than descriptive terms are used in the problem definition. Partners who demonstrate the ability to objectify generally avoid the use of labels and personal assaults (Gottman et al., 1976). Gottman et al. (1976) provide a model for objectifying between partners:

> A "distressed" wife who is frustrated because her husband prefers to read the newspaper rather than discuss current events with her on a particular evening may say, "You *never* want to discuss relevant issues going on in the world! I don't know what possessed me to marry such an uninformed, apathetic man!" (Gullick, 1978, p. 107)

A more objective and less offensive manner of handling the same problem would be to say, "John, when you say you'd prefer to read the newspaper rather than talk with me, I feel rejected and hurt." This behavior-specific method of stating a complaint is more effective because it clarifies the relationship between the "offender's" behavior and the "complainant's" emotional reactions. Consequently, the "offender" may understand the impact of his behavior on his partner and then may choose to modify his behavior if he desires. Another obvious advantage of this—"When you do X in situation Y, I feel Z" (Gottman et al., 1976)—type of statement is that the couple is spared the destructive and disruptive effects of the character attack obvious in the previous example.

A second critical component of objectification is the ability to state requests in an open, direct, but nonthreatening way. For example, a partner requesting more affection from his spouse may be disappointed, even if the spouse attempts to comply; the two partners simply may have different ideas of what constitutes affection. The request is more likely to be granted if the partner says, "I would like you to be more affectionate with me; for example, I would enjoy a kiss when you come, and I enjoy holding hands when we are in public."

One of the most common hindrances to clear objective communication between partners is the presence of inconsistency between one's verbal and nonverbal messages (Gottman et al., 1976; Lederer and Jackson, 1968). This phenomenon in a nonmarital situation is exemplified by the following example of the ''double bind'' phenomenon (Bateson et al., 1956).

> Mrs. J. went to visit her son, whom she had not seen for several months. When he hugged his mother, the son noticed her body grow stiff; as he withdrew from her, she asked, ''What's the matter? Aren't you glad to see your mother?''

In this situation, the son is presented with a confusing, inconsistent message about his mother's pleasure at seeing him. The *content* of her verbal message indicates she is pleased, but her nonverbal cues contradict this. The son must decide which message he must attend and respond to. Such a decision necessitates that he ignore *one* of the messages and, therefore, creates for him an insoluble dilemma.

In a couple's situation, one spouse may feel pressure to give his/her consent to a decision which he/she is unenthusiastic about; consequently, he/she may give confusing and inconsistent messages to his/her partner. For example,

> Mr. B. calls home during the afternoon and tells his wife he has a very important business meeting that evening, which will cause him to arrive home later than he had expected. It had been planned earlier that he would take Mrs. B. and the children to a movie, but he tells his wife that his employer has indicated that his attendance at the meeting is quite important. Mrs. B. tells her husband that she would not mind postponing their evening until next week. This reassurance may not reflect her real feelings; when her husband returns home he may find her very distant, perhaps not even speaking to him. She may be sending non-verbal cues indicating that the postponement was *not* acceptable to her. At this point the husband finds himself in a situation where he cannot possibly win. He has been straightforward and honest in his questions, and she has given him an answer which does not accurately reflect her feelings. He regrets ever having asked for her opinion. Her position is that she did not want him to work late, but felt guilty for feeling that way; she did not feel she had the right to insist that an evening movie take precedence over an important business meeting. Mrs. B. might have handled this situation more successfully for herself and her husband if she simply had said, 'I understand the demands that are being placed on you at work. I don't like changing our plans and the children aren't going to like it, but I understand, and I think this meeting is probably more important than the movie. I appreciate you asking me before changing the plans.' (Gullick, 1978, p. 105)

The husband who is concerned about effective communication will remember this concession and hopefully will make an effort to reciprocate at some future time.

Development of Support/Understanding Skills

An important component of effective communication involves being attended to, listened to, understood, and supported by one's partner (Gottman et al. 1976; Gullick, 1978; Lederer and Jackson, 1968; Rogers, 1972). Success in this type of communication results in the development of companionship, comforting, and ''understanding'' behaviors (Weiss, 1978). The importance of describing events and feelings in a clear, direct, objective manner has been demonstrated; however, the ability to do so does not ensure that partners can communicate acceptance, support, and understanding of one another. Development of these later skills requires that each spouse emphasize the give end of Weiss' (1978) give–get relationship. The therapist concerned with client difficulties in this area may use three structures "exercises" as he works with the couple toward improvement: (1) the listening exercise, (2) talk time, and (3) love days.

A partner is more inclined to feel understood and supported when he/she recognizes that his/her spouse is actually listening. *Active* listening requires that a partner *communicate* his attention to and understanding of his/her spouse's message, without digressing into a discussion of his/her own ideas and opinions on the matter being discussed. It must be remembered that understanding does not imply agreement. When active listening is a pattern between partners it can reduce significantly the tension level often accompanying difficult discussions, thus, allowing spouses to engage in more comfortable and effective problem solving. The introduction of active listening to a couple's communication repertoire frequently begins a self-perpetuating contagion of effective support and understanding skills. The speaker may feel, for the first time, that his partner understands how he (the speaker) feels and that he supports the speaker's right to feel that way. This encourages active listening when the roles are reversed. Once established as a routine practice within a couple, active listening provides a mechanism by which disagreements and decisions may be handled with relative ease and a minimum of frustration.

The development of active listening skills can be enhanced by the therapeutic suggestion that the couple learn and practice the "listening exercises." The instructions for this exercise require that spouses alternate listening to one another as nonargumentative topics are discussed. (Choice of a nonargumentative topic ensures that partners will focus more on the *process* of listening than on their individual needs to express their opinions.) The speaker is to choose a topic of interest and talk for 5 min about his ideas, opinions, thoughts, and feelings on the topic. Meanwhile, the listener attempts to understand the ideas and feelings described and to communicate this understanding to the speaker. This can be accomplished (1) through the use of summarization and paraphrasing statements and (2) by checking with the speaker to make certain that he (the listener) has received the message accurately. For example, after listening for a few moments, Mr. T. might say,

> From what you're saying it sounds like the main thing you dislike about your job is the amount of work they require each day [paraphrasing]. Is that right? Am I hearing you correctly? [checking accuracy].

When using the listening exercise, the listener is not to mention his ideas or opinions regarding the topic being discussed. Furthermore, he must *assume* nothing about the speaker's ideas or feelings; all assumptions must be checked out by questioning the speaker as in the earlier example.

As listening skills are being taught, the therapist should suggest practicing the listening exercise once a day, with partners reversing roles within each exercise so that each may listen as well as speak. Due to its tension-reduction capacity, the listening exercise may be an especially effective beginning exercise for the therapist to introduce to partners who have established a disruptively tenacious pattern of aversive control. Intervention with such couples requires that *some* reduction of tension and negativism occur before the salient relationship issues can be examined and discussed.

Although the listening exercise focuses on the *process* of couples' conversations, other techniques must be adopted to deal with issues of *content*. It has been mentioned earlier that conversations within distressed couples generally are task-oriented or argumentative in nature; there are few sharing conversations of the type often enjoyed during courtship (Stuart, 1969). Although effective administrative decision making is a valuable activity for marital partners, it does not necessarily lead to the development of companionship. Certainly, if a couple communicates only to make household decisions or to argue, they may find themselves relating as business partners rather than as intimate companions.

Feelings of companionship, support, and understanding between partners can be enhanced through a conscious attempt to reinstitute warm sharing conversations within the couple. Therapeutic application of the "talk time" technique is helpful in accomplishing this improvement. The use of this technique requires that the couple have a specified period of time daily (15–30 min) that is set aside for an uninterrupted conversation. During this talk time, partners are to avoid task-oriented, administrative topics, as well as those that predictably might lead to an argument. The therapist should encourage partners to discuss topics of mutual interest, much as they did during courtship. The talk time must be respected and treated as a priority event by both partners; it should occur without interruption from children, telephone, or television. Couples may need encouragement and clear "permission" from the therapist to make this activity a high priority, since they may have treated is as a luxury in their daily schedules. The tendency to avoid such companionship times when faced with multitudinous tasks and time demands should be discussed with the couple; the therapist may feel the need to emphasize the importance of measured selfishness in the development and maintenance of marital intimacy. Though apparently a quite simple technique, talk time will assist in maintaining a feeling of intimate companionship in the face of numerous, disruptive problems, which may routinely occur during the course of a marriage.

Finally, the development of support/understanding/companionship experiences can be enhanced if each partner can devote some time and energy to the give portion of the give–get model (Weiss, 1978). For distressed spouses, this will require a certain amount of risk taking and trust. It may effectively interrupt the cycle of aversive interactions between partners, which is characteristic of many distressed couples (Stuart, 1969; Weiss, 1978). For many couples, such an interruption will be sufficient for the effective resolution of relationship difficulties; for others it will demonstrate (1) there *is* a capacity within the relationship for enjoyable, pleasing experiences; and (2) the potent, beneficial, healing impact of each partner's willingness to provide substantial increases in the give portion of the give–get relationship (Weiss, 1978). The therapist can assist partners in such accomplishment by suggesting that they engage in "love days" (Weiss, 1978). Such a suggestion requires that each partner set aside 1 day or partial day during the week as his spouse's love day. On that day, the partner planning the love day provides for his/her spouse a number of experiences, surprises, activities, or gifts which he/she predicts will be pleasing to the partner. The planning partner may enlist the help and input of the "receiver" in choosing the activities for the love day; however, the planner should stay focused entirely on the task of giving and pleasing his partner. During the week there should be 2 love days; the roles should be reversed so that each spouse can experience giving as well as receiving.

Commitment to Participate in Appropriate Conflict Resolution

Although the aforementioned three areas of relationship accomplishment focus on *process* and *content* of marital communications, effective problem solving requires that the couple develop the capacity for being *outcome*-oriented from time to time. Obviously, achievement in the previous three areas will prevent many conflicts and problems. However, all couples should have an effective mechanism for dealing with disagreements and interspouse problems. Evidence suggests that conflicts may be dealt with most comfortably and effectively if they are approached with an attitude of partner trust (Satir, 1964), handled quickly rather than avoided (Gottman et al., 1976), and if each partner refrains from personal attacks on the character of his spouse (Gottman et al., 1976). The couple demonstrating accomplishment in objectification and support/ understanding skills will assuredly find conflict–resolution and problem solving a more manageable process than the couple lacking these skills; consequently, skillfulness in the previously described areas of relationship accomplishment is a prerequisite for success in this area.

One of the most threatening components of the problem-solving process for couples is the implicit assumption that it frequently requires one or both partners to change his/her behavior. Remembering Weiss' (1978) give–get model reminds the therapist of the occasional need felt by one or both partners for behavior change before they have had an opportunity to develop more appropriate methods; too frequently, behavior change follows on the heels of a crisis in which one partner has decided his gifts to the relationship have grossly excelled his benefits from it. In frustration, desperation, and anger, he/she implements an aversive method of behavior change (complaint, criticism, sulking, withdrawal, etc.). Effectively negotiated behavior change requires that the couple avoid crisis management of problems and that positive rather than negative methods of control (change) prevail.

The development of effective problem solving skills usually depends upon accomplishment at each of the three preceding levels followed by an understanding and practice of negotiation and contracting skills. Just as methods of aversive control tend to be self-perpetuating and follow the rules of reciprocity, so do those of positive and sensitive negotiation. Therefore, an important goal for the therapist is to assist in establishing comfortable, positive methods of problem solving (Gottman et al., 1976; Lederer and Jackson, 1978; Jacobson and Margolin, 1979; Weiss, 1978). The dynamic behavioral communication approach to marital intervention has introduced the technique of behavioral contracting and has demonstrated its effectiveness with couples (Azrin et al., 1973; Gullick, 1973; Harrell and Guerney, 1976; Rappaport, 1976; Sager, 1976; Stuart, 1969; Weiss, 1978; Weiss et al., 1974). The scientific literature offers examples of several types of contracts between partners. The *quid pro quo* type (Weiss et al., 1974) is the oldest documented form of marital contracting. Though it represents contracting in its most simple form (Stuart, 1969), its effectiveness is unsurpassed by newer, more elegant types (Jacobson, 1978). It is based upon principles of reciprocal behavior exchange and involves the direct, simultaneous exchange of behaviors between partners. In the negotiation process each partner alters some aspect of his behavior in accordance with his partner's wishes; consequently, each partner's behavior change is reinforced (rewarded) by the other's behavior change. Jacobson and Margolin (1979) provide the following example of a *quid pro quo* contract between partners. The contract is designed to deal with Holly's complaint that her husband (Jim) usually appeared disinterested in her workday, and Jim's concern that his wife avoided playing recreational games with him in the evening. Their contract was written in the following manner:

> (a) Jim agrees to spend between 10–15 minutes each week night, between 5:00–6:00 p.m., discussing Holly's day at work. During this period, he will ask her at least five questions about her day, based on what she says. He will not make derogatory remarks during this period (e.g., "big deal"). Holly will be the judge of whether or not a remark is derogatory, based on the impact of the remark on her.
>
> b) Holly agrees to play a board game of Jim's choice on Tuesday and Thursday evenings between 9:00–11:00 p.m. If Jim complies with his end of the contract on Friday, Monday, and Tuesday, Holly must agree to her end of the contract on that Tuesday evening.
>
> If Jim complies with his agreement on Wednesday and Thursday, Holly must agree to her end on that Thursday evening.
>
> If Holly fails to participate in the game suggested by Jim on days when he has earned it, the work conversation is automatically suspended until the next scheduled game, at which time the work conversation will resume, as long as Holly participates in the game which Jim chooses for that evening. (Jacobson and Margolin, 1979, p. 265)

Although the above is a *clear* example of a behavioral contract, it is stated more formally than other equally effective agreements. The sensitive clinician will adapt and modify the contracting process to fit his individual style and the needs of his patients. The types of contracts established by experienced clinicians range from simple to complex, verbal to written, etc., depending upon the clinical judgment of the therapist. Regardless of the type of contract used, the following guidelines for establishing a couple's behavioral contract should help insure its success.

The contract must be:

1. Stated clearly and deal with only *observable* behaviors rather than with traits or attitudes
2. Stated as positively as possible
3. Focused on increasing positive behaviors rather than decreasing negative ones
4. As simple as possible, dealing with only one or two behavioral requests per partner

Behavioral contracting provides a mechanism for clear negotiation of needs, requests, and compromises. Its usefulness for the egalitarian relationship is striking; as it offers partners an opportunity to discuss openly evolving partner roles, it ensures that the negotiation of those requests, needs, and roles need not be unduly demanding of either partner. Through the use of such contracting, a relationship can maintain the fluidity and flexibility required to endure the many changes required by contemporary partners of marriage.

Clearly, successful conflict resolution requires accomplishment in all areas of communication that have been discussed. As Weiss (1978) has mentioned, the areas are hierarchially ordered, each depending upon successful accomplishment of the previous one. Therapeutic marital intervention generally focuses on skill development at each of the four levels. To support this notion, Rappaport (1976) has indicated that a didactic approach to training couples in communication skills results in a significant increase in self-reported marital happiness in trained couples. Similarly, Jacobson (1978) indicates that structured communication training emerges as the single therapeutic component common to all marital interventions of demonstrated effectiveness. It must be remembered that the development of dyadic problems is multidetermined and usually results from a combination of intrapsychic, environmental, and family systems etiological variables; however, research indicates that the most effective and efficient methods for therapeutic amelioration of these problems are the provision of education and training in communication skills within a therapeutic relationship. The following example illustrates a typical marital problem which may present to the therapist. It includes suggested guidelines for intervention by the therapist using a number of the techniques discussed earlier.

> Jim and Carol had been married for 1 year and had no children when they sought marital–sexual therapy. The decision to enter therapy was precipitated by several episodes of anger that erupted in their relationship. Jim, a 33-year-old attorney of Irish extraction, was in the habit of leaving their apartment for several hours to "cool off" when he became angry. Carol, a 29-year-old nurse of German heritage, would perceive his departure as abandonment and a personal assault on her as a female.
>
> Jim and Carol reported a relatively common sexual problem. Their "routine" was for Jim to engage in cursory sexual activity (foreplay) prior to intercourse and ejaculate seconds after penetration. After several months, Carol became secondarily nonorgasmic with Jim due to the short duration of their sexual activity (5–10 min).
>
> When first seen by the therapist, Carol reported being angry that Jim had left the previous evening for several hours. Jim was contrite and apologetic during the therapy hour; however, he appeared to avoid Carol by looking away from her and appealing to the cotherapists to calm her down. Carol began the session by stating, "Jim *always* does this; he is an escapist when it comes to tough decisions. He never listens or understands me" (lack of objectification, labeling, personal assault).
>
> After a few minutes, one therapist intervened to state, "I can understand that you are angry and frustrated, but it would help if you could be very specific about your annoyance, and avoid using labels, the words 'never' or 'always'." As Carol reframed her complaints of the night before, Jim responded by attending to her as she listed her concerns.
>
> After a few minutes, Jim interrupted Carol to clarify for the therapists her perspective of their current struggles. "We see eye-to-eye on many things, Doc. We're usually pretty responsive to each other. We always have been" (lack of objectification). At this point, careful intervention must focus on Jim's method of communication for the couple through the prevailing use of "we" statements rather than "I" statements. It was explained that a couple is composed of two *individuals;* although Jim may be correct in his assumptions about his wife's feelings, effective therapy requires that he speak for *himself* rather than for both ("I think" rather than "we think").

Although puzzled by the request, he began once more describing his perspective of their relationship but would glance occasionally at Carol as he
expressed his observations.

It became apparent to the therapists that Jim had grown to feel responsible for the relationship; yet he felt helpless when Carol expressed disapproval. He would immediately attempt to solve "her problem" rather than
listen effectively to her concerns. Typically, when Carol would mention
complaints or show anger or frustration, Jim interrupted her and attempted to
"talk her out of" her opinions by showing that she was not being logical or
considering all sides of the respective issue. When this occurred, Carol's
anger and frustration grew and an argument usually followed.

The cotherapists intervened over the next week by explaining the *listening exercise* and giving a "prescription" for its daily occurrence. The exercise was introduced by the therapists by telling Jim that his skill in rational
problem solving was highly developed and obviously quite adaptive for his
legal profession; however, that expertise is counterproductive in the marital
relationship.

As a result of the listening exercise, Carol saw some change in Jim's
willingness to let her speak and state her opinions without argument. She
stated that she was greatly relieved and encouraged about their relationship.

Carol had spent some of the therapy time discussing her work at the
hospital. She reported particular difficulty in speaking to a physician on her
ward who was imposing and aggressive in his demeanor, she described him
as "almost imperial." Jim had difficulty listening to her frustration without
interrupting to suggest more successful strategies for her discussion with this
physician.

As the session developed, Carol began to list complaints about Jim's
various activities. She stated that he was late frequently and that he did not
call her when delayed at the office. She continued to list his shortcomings
until the cotherapists intervened to request that she state clearly the *impact* of
his behavior on her. For example, she might state to Jim, "When you don't
call and let me know that you will be late, I become angry and resentful"
(objectification behavior, specific complaint). Then the therapists asked her
to state her request positively and clearly, without using blaming statements.
Carol then requested that he call when he knew he would be late. He agreed
and requested, in return, that she not respond with anger or frustration. She
agreed that she would not respond with an angry message about his delay but
felt that she still might be disappointed (simple behavioral contract).

These interventions set the stage for specific communications skills that
the couple needed to be able to focus on highly charged areas of concern. As
such they prepared them for the comfortable discussion of their sexual
difficulty. Though not surprising, their general relationship was reflected in
their sexual behavior. Carol demonstrated a nonassertive pattern and in-
wardly blamed Jim for his lack of intuitive knowledge about her own sexual
desires and preferences. Jim had grown to feel overresponsible for their
sexual enjoyment as a couple, and he was intolerant of Carol's disappointment.

During the next several weeks, they were instructed to begin sensate
focus exercises, coupled with specific behavioral assignments designed to
help Carol develop more awareness and knowledge of her sexual fantasies

and bodily responses. She quickly developed an interest in erotic magazines and learned to use imagery to help her initiate sexual activity.

The interventions in their communication styles were influential in altering sexual and nonsexual components of their relationship. Treatment was aimed at helping them develop more clear methods of communication, alter their styles of responding, and develop a better balance of self-responsibility during therapy.

Contemporary Trends in Marital Intervention

Certainly, marriage emerges as a topic about which scientists and the public ponder, puzzle, write, and study. Though the Biblical image of marriage as the merging of two individuals to become "one flesh" has been rejected by many contemporary couples, it appears that, as a popular life-style, marriage continues to exist, if not thrive. The contrast between the rising divorce rate and the relatively stable remarriage rate suggests that most marital cynicism and dissatisfaction is associated with specific relationships rather than the institution itself (Carter and Glick, 1970; Weiss, 1978). Couples continue to marry, even though provided with a number of alternative lifestyles that enjoy some degree of social sanction. The cultural changes evidenced in this country in the last century—increased urbanization, higher levels of education, elective parenthood, sexual renaissance, and focus on individual development—appear to have continued and perhaps heightened individuals' needs for companionship and interpersonal intimacy. More than any other relationship, marriage is expected to help fulfill these needs for its partners—and yet the traditional model of marriage falls short in its capacity for companionship and intimacy development.

It is predictable then that contemporary couples, equipped with their capacity for openness and assertiveness will be more vocal and numerous in their search for professional help with marital dissatisfaction. The task of the therapist then becomes critical and quite different from that of his predecessors 25 years ago. He will be called upon to help fit an old relationship model to contemporary needs, expectations, and life-styles. His patients may appear to be more uncomfortable and less patient with the bad fit than those of his older colleagues. How does the sensitive and conscientious clinician deal with this predictable problem? Weiss (1978, p. 190) wisely advises

> The concerns of professionals in this area should be with prevention and not curing—prevention of the destructiveness that spouses can wreak upon one another, not of marriage. An effective theory of intimate relationships should point the way to providing individuals with relationship skills prior to the time that they have acquired skillfulness in aversive control.

As the contemporary clinician attempts to help couples struggle with cultural change, he/she will deal with conflicts that have resulted from our country's massive cultural changes. He/she will find himself/herself with "new" clinical problems. Such "new" problems as spouse abuse, second marriages (Visher and Visher, 1979), dual-career marriages (Nadelson et al., 1979), conflicts of independence vs. affiliation, depression and its relationship to marital maladjustment (Coleman and Miller, 1975;

Johnson and Lobitz, 1974), and others. The effective and conscientious therapist will develop an acute sense of prgamatism. He/she will borrow from the psychoanalytic, behavioral and systems theories as he strives to evaluate and understand his couples' struggles; he/she will recognize the need for intensive and, above all, rapid ameliora- tion of the marital conflicts; he/she will become interested in teaching couples *skills* in marital communication, that they may learn to alter their prevailing *process,* as well as current problem. Finally, the sensitive clinician will learn to value and teach skills to facilitate the flexibility and fluidity required to contemporary marital relationships.

References

Ashkam, J. Identity and stability within the marriage relationship. *Journal of Marriage and the Family,* 1976, *38,* 535–547.

Azrin, N.H., Naster, B.M., and Jones, R. Reciprocity counseling: A rapid learning-based procedure for marital counseling. *Behavior Research and Therapy,* 1973, *11,* 365–382.

Bach, G.R., and Wyden, P. *The intimate enemy: How to fight fair in love and marriage.* New York: Avon Books, 1969.

Bateson, G., Jackson, D.D., Haley, J., and Weakland, J. Toward a theory of schezophrenia. *Behavioral Science,* 1956, *1,* 251–264.

Bernard, J. *The future of marriage* New York: Bantam, 1972.

Birchler, G.R., Weiss, R.L., and Vincent, J.P. Multimethod analysis of social reinforcement exchange between maritally distressed and non-distressed spouse and stranger dyads. *Journal of Personality and Social Psychology,* 1975, *31,* 349–360.

Burgess, E., and Locke, H. *The family: From institution to companionship.* New York: American Book Co., 1945.

Carter, H., and Glick, P.C. *Marriage and divorce: A social and economic study.* Cambridge: Harvard, 1970.

Coleman, R.E., and Miller, A.G. The relationship between depression and marital maladjustment in a clinic population: A multi-trait, multimethod study. *Journal of Consulting and Clinical Psychology,* 1975, *43,* 647–651.

Glick, P.C. A demographer looks at American families. *Journal of Marriage and the Family,* 1975, *37,* 15–26.

Gottman, J., Notarius, C., Gonso, J., and Markham, H. *A couple's guide to communication.* Champaign, Ill.: Research Press, 1976.

Gullick, E.L. *Behavioral contracting: A controlled study.* Unpublished doctoral dissertation, 1973.

Gullick, E.L. Marital intimacy and the communication process. In E.L. Gullick and S.F. Peed (Eds.), *The role of the health practitioner in family relationships: Marital and sexual issues.* New Haven: Westport Technomics, 1978,

Gurman, A.S., and Kniskern, D.P. Research on marital and family therapy: Progress, perspective, and prospect. In S.L. Garfield and A.E. Bergin (Eds.), *Handbook of psychotherapy and behavior change: An empirical analysis.* New York: Wiley, 1979.

Harrell, J., and Guerney, B. Training married couples in conflict negotiation skills. In D.H.L. Olson (Ed.), *Treating Relationships.* Lake Mills, Iowa: Graphic Press, 1976.

Hunt, M. *Sexual behavior in the 70's.* Chicago: Playboy Press, 1974.

Jacobson, N.S. Problem solving and contingency contracting in the treatment of marital discord. *Journal of Consulting and Clinical Psychology,* 1977, *45,* 92–100.

Jacobson, N.S. A review of the research on the effectiveness of marital therapy. In T.J. Paolino and B.S. McCrady (Eds.), *Marriage and marital therapy: Psychoanalytic, behavioral and systems theory per- spectives.* New York: Brunner/Mazel, 1978. Pp. 395–444.

Jacobson, N.S., and Margolin, G. *Marital therapy: Strategies based on social learning and behavior exchange principles.* New York: Brunner/Mazel, 1979.

Johnson, S.M., and Lobitz, G.K. The personal and marital adjustment of parents as related to observed child deviance and parenting behaviors. *Journal of Abnormal Child Psychology,* 1974, *2,* 193–207.

Kaplan, H.S. *The new sex therapy: Active treatment of sexual dysfunctions.* New York: Brunner/Mazel, 1974.

Knox, D. *Marriage happiness.* Champaign, Ill.: Research Press, 1971.

Kuten, J. Anger, sexuality, and the growth of the ego. *Journal of Sex and Marital Therapy,* 1976, *2,* 289–296.

Lederer, W.J., and Jackson, D.D. *The mirages of marriage.* New York: Norton, 1968.

Mace, D., and Mace, V. *We can have better marriages.* Nashville, Tenn.: Abingdon, 1974.

Mace, D., and Mace, V. The joy of human sexuality in marriage. *Journal of Sex Education and Therapy,* 1975, *2,* 35–41.

Masters, W.H., and Johnson, V.E. *Human sexual inadequacy.* Boston: Little, Brown, 1970.

Nadelson, C. Marital therapy from a psychoanalytic perspective. In T.J. Paolino and B.S. McCrady (Eds.), *Marriage and marital therapy: Psychoanalytic, behavioral and systems theory perspectives.* New York: Brunner/Mazel, 1978. Pp. 89–165.

Nadelson, C., Polonsky, D.C., and Matthews, M.A. Marriage and midlife: The impact of social change. *Journal of Clinical Psychiatry,* 1979, *40*(7), 15–24.

Patterson, G.R., and Reid, J.B. Reciprocity and coercion: Two facets of social systems. In C. Neuringer and J.L. Michael (Eds.), *Behavior modification in clinical psychology.* New York: Appleton– Century–Crofts, 1970.

Patterson, G.R., Weiss, R.L., and Hops, H. Training of marital skills: Some problems and concepts. In H. Leitenburg (Ed.), *Handbook of behavior modification.* New York: Appleton–Century–Crofts, 1976.

Prochaska, J., and Prochaska, J. Twentieth century trends in marriage and marital therapy. In T.J. Paolino and B.S. McCrady (Eds.), *Marriage and marital therapy: Psychoanalytic, behavioral and systems theory perspectives.* New York: Brunner/Mazel, 1978. Pp. 1–25.

Rappaport, A.F. Conjugal relationship enhancement program. In D.H.L. Olson (Ed.), *Treating relationships.* Lake Mills, Iowa: Graphic Press, 1976.

Rogers, C. *Becoming partners: Marriage and its alternatives.* New York: Dell, 1972.

Sager, C. *Marriage contracts and couples' therapy.* New York: Brunner/Mazel, 1976.

Sager, C.J. Sexual dysfunctions and marital discord. In H. Kaplan (Ed.), *The new sex therapy: Active treatment for sexual dysfunctions.* New York: Brunner/Mazel, 1974. Pp. 501–516.

Satir, V. *Conjoint family therapy.* Palo Alto, Calif.: Science and Behavioral Books, 1967.

Scanzoni, J. *Sexual bargaining: Power politics in the American marriage.* New York: Prentice–Hall, 1972.

Stuart, R.B. Operant interpersonal treatment for marital discord. *Journal of Consulting and Clinical Psychology,* 1969, *33,* 675–682.

Visher, E.B., and Visher, J.S. *Step-families: A guide to working with stepparents and stepchildren.* New York: Brunner/Mazel, 1979.

Weiss, R.L. The conceptualization of marriage from a behavioral perspective. In T.J. Paolino and B.S. McCrady (Eds.), *Marriage and marital therapy: Psychoanalytic, behavioral and systems theory perspectives.* New York: Brunner/Mazel, 1978. Pp. 165–239.

Weiss, R.L., Birchler, G.R., and Vincent, J.P. Contractual models for negotiation training in marital dyads. *Journal of Marriage and the Family,* 1974, *36,* 321–331.

Winter, W.D., Ferreira, A.J., and Bowers, M. Decision-making in married and unrelated couples. *Family Process,* 1973, *12,* 83–94.

Gay Patients in the Medical Setting

Nanette Gartrell

Introduction

Approximately 20 million people in this country are predominantly homosexual for some part of their lives.[1,2] An even larger number engage in homosexual activity from time to time. Although the average physician may not be aware of the sexual orientation of most patients, he can expect that about 5%–10% of patients are homosexual. This chapter examines the special needs and problems of the gay patient in seeking health care from non-gay physicians.

The sexual problems of gay people are not essentially different from those of heterosexual men and women. However, gay people often have terrible anxieties about seeing physicians for sex-related problems—especially when it is necessary to reveal their sexual orientation. They fear that physicians will disapprove of their lifestyle and consequently provide less-than-adequate medical care. Unfortunately, surveys of gay patients and non-gay physicians indicate that these fears are not unrealistic.

Over 50% of patients in one survey at Boston's Homophile Community Health Service reported previous negative experiences with non-gay health professionals.[3] Furthermore, 74% of nearly 1000 Oregon physicians acknowledged that negative attitudes toward male homosexual patients could adversely affect their medical management.[4] Clearly, homosexuals risk receiving inadequate medical treatment if their sexual orientation is disclosed.

The principal task of the physician is to accept and appreciate every patient as a unique human being, regardless of the patient's sexual orientation. The physician must make every effort to replace cultural stereotypes of homosexuals—which are largely negative—with an understanding of the diversified life experiences of gay people. Medical ethics require that physicians demonstrate the same care and concern for homosexuals who have sexual problems as for heterosexuals with similar complaints.

The physician should be able to take a careful, nonjudgmental medical and sexual history as indicated by the patient's complaint, and to have an understanding of the

Nanette Gartrell • Departments of Psychiatry, Harvard Medical School and Beth Israel Hospital, Boston, Massachusetts wide range of sexual behaviors and lifestyles that occur in gay people, so that a correct assessment of potential problems is possible. The physician, ideally, will help the patient to develop objective attitudes about homosexuality; this should facilitate referral of patients who present with sex-related problems outside the physician's area of expertise.

Myths and Facts

The physician must be able to separate myth from fact when seeking information on any topic related to human sexuality. Myths about homosexuality are prevalent in our society and they pervade much of the clinical and experimental research reported to date. A number of these myths are listed below:

1. Most gay men are effeminate and most lesbians are masculine in appearance and behavior.
2. Most gay couples adopt male/female (active/passive) roles in their relationships.
3. All gay men are sexually promiscuous.
4. Gay men believe that they are women in men's bodies and gay women believe that they are men in women's bodies.
5. Most gay people would have a sex change operation if they could afford it.
6. Most gay people are child molesters.
7. People choose to become homosexual.
8. Most gay people are unhappy with their sexual orientation and seek therapy to convert to heterosexuality.
9. Therapists report high success rates in converting homosexuals to heterosexuals.
10. Most gay people are easily identifiable by their dress and mannerisms.
11. Homosexual behavior is unnatural because it does not occur in other species.
12. Homosexuality is the result of an hereditary defect.
13. Homosexuals have hormone abnormalities.
14. All homosexual males have dominant, overbearing mothers and weak, passive fathers.
15. Homosexuality threatens the continuity of the species.
16. All male hairdressers, interior decorators and ballet dancers are homosexuals.
17. Homosexuality is an illness which can be cured.

In fact, new data from the Kinsey Institute indicate that there are as many different kinds of homosexuals as heterosexuals, and that it is impossible to predict a person's appearance, personality, occupation, ethnic background, sexual functioning, or social adjustment on the basis of sexual orientation.[5] At present, researchers have very little information about the etiology of homosexuality, bisexuality or heterosexuality. Presumably, all forms of sexual behavior are to some degree biologically, constitutionally, environmentally, and socially determined.

Definitions of homosexuality vary considerably. Men and women who are attracted to persons of the same sex are not necessarily homosexual; they may be homosexual, bisexual, heterosexual, or even asexual. Although an estimated 46% of the population engages in homosexual behavior during adult life,[1,2] a much smaller percentage defines itself as homosexual. Kinsey viewed sexual behavior as a continuum ranging from exclusive heterosexuality at one extreme to exclusive homosexuality at the other, with various proportions of each behavior in between. Unfortunately, his classification system did not account for the possible divergence of emotion and behavior in some individuals. For example, there are women who are sexually active only with men but define themselves as homosexual because they find it easier to become emotionally involved with women. Likewise, there are men whose most stimulating and exciting regular sexual contacts are other men, but who define themselves as heterosexual because they are married.[6] Because it is possible for a person to be exclusively heterosexual in behavior, yet exclusively homosexual in feeling (or vice versa), both aspects of a person's erotic experiences must be included in any definition of sexual orientation.

Researchers have found that nonclinical populations of homosexuals show insignificant differences from heterosexuals in psychological adjustment,[5–11] and in 1973, the American Psychiatric Association removed "homosexuality" from its list of mental disorders. Although the difficulty of being gay in a society hostile to this sexual orientation leads some homosexuals to psychiatric treatment, they are generally looking for ways to combat external and internal stereotypes of homosexuals rather than "treatment" of their homosexuality *per se*. Today, relatively few homosexuals seek treatment to change their sexual orientation. Indeed, all forms of therapy (psychoanalysis, behavior modification, shock therapy, etc.) have been remarkably unsuccessful in their attempts to provide homosexuals with long-term conversions to heterosexuality.[12]

Stereotypes of homosexuals as child molesters and social/genetic/endocrinologic misfits have little basis in fact. Police statistics indicate that child molestation is almost exclusively (> 90%) a heterosexual crime.[a] Endocrine studies fail to demonstrate significant hormone abnormalities when comparing healthy homosexuals to heterosexuals,[13–16] and there is no evidence that homosexuality has ever threatened the continuity of the species. Since approximately 50% of the human population and most other mammalian species engage in homosexual activity, it has been impossible to demonstrate that homosexuality is a genetically-determined behavior.

---

[a]Information on child molestation is available in the following publications: *Regional Resource Center for Child Abuse Report,* Boise, Idaho, 1976; *San Francisco Police Report,* 1972; *American Humane Society Report,* Children's Division, Denver, Colorado, 1969.

The Clinical Interview

The evaluation of any patient with a sex-related problem must include a comprehensive sexual and developmental history. Since gay patients are likely to be much more anxious than heterosexual patients when consulting physicians for sexual problems, the physician must make every effort to solicit information from these patients in a nonjudgmental manner. Confidentiality of patient records is particularly important to gay people because of potential legal, employment and social discrimination against them.

Most physicians prefer to take the initial sexual history in person. Because one has no way of knowing which patients may be homosexual, it is very important to ask questions in a way which does not offend particular patients. The physician should *not* begin a general sexual history with questions about contraception. Such questions convey the physician's assumption that all patients are heterosexual, and gay patients may consequently feel that the physician is insensitive to alternative sexual preferences.[17] General questions about the patient's sexual experiences since puberty (i.e., questions which are *least* sensitive for both patient and physician) should be followed by more specific questions about the patient's current sexual practices. Having the patient describe his or her sexual experiences chronologically from puberty to the present gives the physician an opportunity to assess variations in the patient's sexual experiences over time. If the patient does not specify the sex of the current sexual partner (gay patients often do not), the physician can then ask, "Do you relate sexually to men, women or both?" This type of question communicates an objective attitude toward various sexual preferences and allows the patient to describe his or her sexual preferences along the Kinsey spectrum. The physician can then proceed to ask appropriate questions about sexual activity, sexual problems and related social experiences.

The physician must understand that it may be extremely anxiety-provoking for some homosexuals to reveal their sexual orientation to non-gay health professionals. Homosexuality is not sanctioned by our society (any sexual activity other than "missionary-position" heterosexual intercourse is illegal in most states), and gay people are often unreasonably subjected to social, religious and institutional discrimination. Overt homosexuals risk police harassment, assault by gangs, dishonorable discharge from the military, loss of children in custody cases, and loss of employment as pediatricians, teachers, and child psychiatrists. "Closeted"[b] gays are frequently blackmailed with threats of disclosure to family, friends or employers. Some "closeted" gay or bisexual patients have so much to lose that they will not reveal their sexual orientation to a non-gay physician, regardless of the physician's attitude toward homosexuality and assurances of confidentiality.

Although the physician's private attitudes may favor one sexual orientation over another, the clinical interview must be conducted in an objective, professional manner. A relatively simple way of communicating acceptance and understanding to any patient

---

[b]"Closeted" or "in the closet" refers to gay people who conceal their sexual orientation from all but close friends or intimate acquaintances.

with a sexual problem is to adopt the patient's vocabulary—insofar as one feels comfortable with it—during the clinical interview. Some gay people dislike the term "homosexual," because it exaggerates the sexual component of their lives; they (and most major homophile organizations) prefer the term "gay," which connotes a more general psycho-sociocultural way of life. These people interpret the physician's use of the word "homosexual" after being informed by the patient that he or she is "gay" as a subtle form of rejection. Negative body language—tenseness or raised eyebrows when a person discloses his or her sexual orientation—is likewise viewed pejoratively.

Anecdotes demonstrating the physician's liberal sexual attitudes, excessive curiosity about irrelevant details of the patient's sex life, and immediate psychiatric referrals for all gay patients constitute poor clinical judgment. The physician must not assume that every gay patient with a sex-related problem is suffering from an identity crisis. Many gay people are very happy with their relationships and lifestyles. Inappropriate psychiatric referral communicates to the patient that the physician considers homosexuality a mental illness. As previously discussed, this attitude is the result of personal bias rather than clinical fact.

Sexual Behaviors

Gay people engage in the same variety of sexual activities as heterosexuals, with the obvious exception of penile-vaginal intercourse. It is difficult to generalize about the techniques of homosexual lovemaking because of the wide variation in individual sexual practices. Only the most common sexual practices of gay men and women will be discussed, and should refer physicians who are interested in more detailed descriptions to books listed in the Reference section at the end of this chapter.

Foreplay is very important in lovemaking between women. The degree of sexual arousal in women is enhanced by mutual kissing, holding, touching, stroking and fondling. Women take turns stimulating their partners' breasts and nipples with fingers, lips and tongues. Oral–genital stimulation (cunnilingus) and manual-genital stimulation are the two most common methods of inducing orgasm in women. Simultaneous stimulation of the clitoris, vagina and anus (orally and manually) is one of many variations in sexual technique. Although mechanical devices (vibrators for clitoral stimulation) are increasing in popularity, the use of dildos for vaginal penetration is relatively uncommon in gay women.

Sexual behavior in gay men includes foreplay as well as genital and anal (prostate) stimulation to orgasm. Oral–genital (fellatio), oral–anal (analingus or "rimming"), manual–genital, genital–anal (anal intercourse) and manual–anal stimulation are common sexual practices in men. Rubbing one's penis against another man's body or between his thighs is sufficient to induce orgasm in some men. A variety of mechanical devices ("cock rings" for sustaining erections, vibrators for anal penetration, etc.) are also utilized by some men to increase stimulation, sustain erection, and prolong ejaculation.

The physician should avoid making assumptions about the sexual practices of gay male and female patients prior to taking a sexual history. Individual sexual practices are as diversified as the personalities of the participants. For example, not all gay women engage in oral sex, nor do all gay men engage in anal intercourse. Mechanical devices may be highly stimulating to one person and unappealing to another. Even though gay men tend toward multiple sexual relationships and gay women toward monogamy, there are enough gay men and women in unconventional relationships (i.e., strictly monogamous gay men, nonmonogamous gay women, and celibate gay men and women) to warrant specific questions about the quality and quantity of relationships in any clinical interview.

Sexual and Sex-Related Problems[c]

Gay people have become as concerned as heterosexuals about sexual conquest and performance. Mass-media accounts of the "ultimate sexual experience" have inundated homosexual and heterosexual communities alike. More people than ever before have begun to look outside themselves for definitions of what is sexually acceptable and pleasurable. As a result, both homosexuals and heterosexuals are becoming increasingly insecure about the quality of their sexual experiences.

Etiologies of sexual dysfunction in gay men and women are numerous. Medical illness, congenital abnormalities, anger, anxiety, depression, intrapsychic conflict, and drug abuse are some of the many factors which can affect sexual function. Relationship problems which inhibit sexual performance include sexual inhibitions, failures of communication, unrealistic expectations, restrictive lovemaking patterns, sexual ignorance, and general sexual dysfunction.[18] Ambivalence about homosexual orientation can also produce sexual dysfunction. In addition to the problem of post-Victorian guilt and anxiety about sexuality *per se*, gay men and women have the added burden of engaging in socially unacceptable sexual relationships. It is often difficult for gays to ignore public allegations that homosexual liaisons are "anti-God, anti-Nature and anti-Life."[19] Hostile social attitudes, as well as religious censure, can produce sexual problems in some gay people.

The most common sexual problem in gay women (as in heterosexual women) is orgasmic dysfunction. Less frequent complaints include dislike of oral sex, loss of interest in sex, and dissatisfaction with the quality or quantity of sexual experiences. Vaginismus occurs very infrequently in gay women, probably due to the fact that lesbian lovemaking does not require the insertion of large objects into the vagina.

Gay men report problems with impotence and premature ejaculation. The time-pressured sexual encounter in a public place (bars, baths, etc.) may produce premature ejaculation in more relaxed environments. Rectal pain during anal intercourse is also a complaint in gay men whose rectal sphincters have not dilated sufficiently to allow insertion of the penis.

---

[c]This section was prepared with the assistance of Carol Ribner, M.D., who served as medical director at Fenway Community Health Center, a predominantly gay medical clinic in Boston, from 1976 to 1978.

The physician should be prepared to discuss the psychological and social ramifications of sexual problems in gay patients. As stated previously, the physician should not assume that difficulties in gay sexual relationships represent dissatisfaction with homosexual orientation unless this is indicated by the sexual history.

Although venereal disease among exclusively gay women is very uncommon, isolated cases of pharyngeal gonorrhea in the female partner of a bisexual woman have been reported. Genital infections that may be transmitted by sexual contact between women include monilia, trichomonas, nonspecific vaginitis, and herpes. Nonspecific vaginitis in gay women may be caused by colonization of the vagina with organisms that are usually found in the oral cavity. Infections of the bowel or related structures (bacterial, viral, and parasitic diarrhea, as well as hepatitis) can be transmitted to any sexual partner via oral sex; this problem is not unique to gay women. Condyloma, which are commonly found in heterosexuals and gay men, are only rarely seen in gay women.[d]

The incidence of venereal disease among sexually active gay men has reached epidemic proportions in recent years. Although the incidence of venereal disease has increased in the population as a whole, the sexual practices of many gay men (i.e., numerous brief sexual encounters in bars, baths, etc.) and the lack of proper medical treatment probably account for the prevalence of disease in this community. Among the many diseases potentially transmissible during sexual contact are the following thirteen which are frequently encountered in gay male clinic populations:

1. Syphilis
2. Gonorrhea
3. Nonspecific, nongonococcal urethritis
4. Viral hepatitis—Hepatitis A and B
5. Venereal warts—condyloma acuminata
6. Candida
7. Herpes
8. Amebiasis
9. Shigellosis
10. Giardiasis
11. Lice and mites
12. Molluscum contagiosum
13. Pinworms

Practitioners interested in specific information about venereal disease symptomatology in gay men should consult the references at the end of this chapter.[21–28]

Sexual injury occurs almost exclusively in gay males who engage in anal intercourse. Sexual injury is caused by inadequate dilation of the rectal sphincter or inadequate lubrication of the anus. Just as the heterosexual woman learns to control her vaginal muscles to allow insertion of the penis, the homosexual man must learn to relax

---

[d]Information on female genital infections is derived from Dr. Ribner's clinical experiences at Fenway Community Health Center, as well as the work of H. Joan Waitkevicz, M.D., at St. Mark's Clinic in New York (see Reference 20).

his rectal sphincter to allow anal intercourse. However, unlike the vagina, which is self-lubricating, the anus has no natural lubrication. Gay men must utilize saliva or lubricating jellies to facilitate insertion of the penis through the anus. Some commercial lubricants contain irritant chemicals (perfumes, etc.) which may produce proctitis or cryptitis in susceptible males.

Sex-related injuries of the anus and rectum include fissures (with or without associated infection), hemorrhoid thrombosis, rectal prolapse, contusion or laceration of the bowel wall (usually as a result of fist fornication) and traumatic prostatitis. Although fecal incontinence may develop after surgical repair of fissures and fistulas or surgical removal of widespread condyloma, incontinence as a result of frequent anal intercourse is rare.

Because homosexuality is viewed so negatively in our culture, adolescents and young adults frequently consult physicians when they become concerned about homosexual feelings. Children in this country are taught to ridicule homosexuals and to identify them as "perverts." The prospect of "becoming"[e] a homosexual is consequently quite frightening to most young people. The physician who is consulted during this time of crisis can help these young patients to develop objective attitudes about homosexuality.

Parents of gays who have recently learned of their son's or daughter's sexual orientation may also turn to the family physician for support. Some insist that their child be evaluated by the physician in order to be referred for psychiatric "cure." Others blame themselves for their child's homosexuality and experience moderate to severe depression as a result. Still others seek more information about homosexuality than the public libraries provide. The physician should evaluate the parents' complaint so that appropriate interventions may be utilized.

Interventions

The physician should make every effort to include the patient's partner in the evaluation and treatment of any sex-related problem. Inclusion of the partner in treatment planning is as important to the gay patient as inclusion of the spouse (or significant other) is to the heterosexual patient. Sexual problems invariably affect both partners in an intimate relationship.

Treatment of sexual dysfunction in gay men and women usually requires referral to a qualified sex therapist. Unfortunately, it is sometimes difficult to locate sex therapists who have experience treating gay patients with sexual dysfunctions. Since the sexual problems of homosexuals and heterosexuals are similar, a capable and

[e]Clinical evidence favors the theory that sexual orientation is fixed at an early age rather than "chosen" in later life.[29,30] It is hypothesized that children are homosexual, bisexual or heterosexual by the time they reach adolescence and that subsequent sexual experimentation generally confirms previously determined preferences. Consequently, it is thought that an adolescent does *not* have a choice of "becoming" a homosexual, only about whether or not to act on homosexual feelings.

imaginative sex therapist should be able to adapt heterosexual therapy techniques[18] to the problems of gay patients. For example, the "squeeze technique" has been very successful in treating premature ejaculation in male homosexual couples. Likewise, vibrators can be utilized in lovemaking between gay women to increase clitoral stimulation for the inorgasmic woman. A detailed discussion of treatment for sexual dysfunction has already been presented in Chapter 2. If a relationship problem appears to be the primary etiology of the dysfunction, referral to a general psychotherapist is probably the first order of business. This therapist can then refer the patient to a sex therapist at a later time if indicated. The importance of referring gay patients to therapists who offer objective therapeutic interventions is discussed in the Referrals section which follows.

Interventions for patients who present with sexually transmitted diseases fall into three basic categories: 1. diagnosis; 2. patient education; and 3. medical and surgical treatment. Information on the differential diagnoses of venereal disease in gay men can be obtained from the references at the end of this chapter. Gay patients who present with genital infections should also be educated about the potential for disease transmission during sexual contact. Since the medical or surgical treatment of venereal disease does not vary according to the patient's sexual orientation, a discussion of specific treatment will not be included in this chapter. Protocols for the treatment of venereal diseases are changing rapidly, however, and therefore physicians should contact a State Health Department or the Venereal Disease Control Division of the Center for Disease Control for information on the most up-to-date treatments.

Case 1

Mr. A. was a 28-year-old gay graduate student in biochemistry who sought treatment at a State V.D. Clinic after a male student with whom he had been sexually involved developed urethral gonorrhea. Mr. A. was informed at this clinic that he did not need a V.D. workup or treatment because he was asymptomatic. During the next several months, two other men informed Mr. A. that they had developed gonorrhea after sexual contact with him. Mr. A. then consulted a second state V.D. clinic, as well as two private physicians, from whom he received the same information—he did not need a workup or treatment unless he developed symptoms. He was told that his male sexual contacts must have erroneously assumed that he had been infectious. Mr. A. subsequently became involved in a monogamous sexual relationship with another man. When his lover developed urethral gonorrhea, Mr. A. concluded that he was the source of infection and that the site of infection was probably his rectum.

He did not return to a State V.D. clinic, because he had previously been denied proper treatment. He was concerned about seeking treatment from the University Health Clinic, because rectal gonorrhea would identify him as a homosexual. Students could be expelled from his university for engaging in homosexual activity. After much deliberation, he decided to inoculate his urethra with fecal matter until he developed a urethral discharge. He then went to his University Health Service for diagnosis and treatment.

This case demonstrates the importance of taking a comprehensive sexual history and culturing all potential sources of infection—especially in patients who are too anxious to spontaneously provide a detailed history.

Young adults who are concerned about homosexual feelings or experiences may consult a physician to determine whether they are indeed "homosexual." They may ask the physician to explain "what a homosexual is" and to identify "symptoms" characteristic of homosexuality.[17] Questions such as these require open-ended responses that allow the patient to explore his or her own feelings and concerns. Without condoning or condemning homosexuality, the physician can point out that sexual attraction between persons of the same sex is common in many young adults. The physician may also explain that it may take some time for the patient to determine which sexual experiences (with males, females, or both) are most satisfying. The physician should not describe homosexuality as a "transient adolescent phase"; this explanation is neither accurate nor reassuring, particularly to those who fail to "grow out of it." It is *rarely* appropriate to refer this kind of patient to a psychiatrist after the initial visit—even if the patient requests such a referral. The physician demonstrates much more understanding and acceptance of the patient's concerns by offering him or her one or more follow-up appointments to discuss the matter further.

Case 2

Mr. C., a 16-year-old male, was seen by his family physician for a pre-football physical. During the physical, the physician asked routine questions about his school and social life. Mr. C. stated that he was doing well in school, but that his social life was "not so great." He said that status among the guys was based on "how many girls we make it with," and he said that "they think you're queer if you don't make it with a girl at least once a week." The physician asked several open-ended questions that allowed Mr. C. to elaborate his feelings. Mr. C. reported that sometimes he worried that he was less interested in girls than some of the other guys, and that he was also concerned about having erections in the locker room. He asked if these were symptoms of homosexuality. The physician explained that adolescents are often confused about sexual feelings. He said that it might take time for Mr. C. to sort out his various feelings to determine whether he was attracted to girls, guys, or both. He also explained that adolescent males often had erections in embarrassing situations and that the patient would have better control over his erections as he got older. The physician asked Mr. C. if he had other specific questions. Mr. C. asked, "What if I am one of the people who does become homosexual?" The physician encouraged Mr. C. to discuss his fears of "becoming" a homosexual. The physician then explained that even though it was difficult to be homosexual in our society, one did not have to lead one's life as a social outcast. He pointed out that over 20 million people in this country are homosexual, that many of them lead very happy, ordinary lives. He also mentioned that many famous people—including football players like David Kopay—were homosexuals. Mr. C. appeared visibly relieved by this information. The physician said he would be happy to discuss Mr. C's concerns further during another appointment. Mr. C.

declined this offer and said he would call if he wanted to talk about it again. When the physician saw Mr. C. one year later, Mr. C. was happily involved in a steady relationship with a 17-year-old girl.

People who have recently identified themselves as homosexual and feel lonely or isolated as a result may turn to their physicians for assistance. These patients often have negative stereotypes of homosexuals which contribute to their feelings of isolation and depression. In addition to facilitating the patient's expression of these concerns, the physician can function as a resource for more objective information about homosexuality. For example, the physician can explain that most homosexuals lead healthy, productive lives. He or she can also inform the patient that homosexuality is more common than most people assume—that approximately 10% of the population is homosexual. The physician may provide books and articles for the patient to read, and suggest homophile organizations for the patient to contact (see Resource section at the end of this chapter). Psychiatric referrals are discussed in the Referrals section.

Case 3

Mrs. B., a 33-year-old mother of two children, was seen by her gynecologist for her annual GYN exam and pap smear. The sexual history revealed that Mrs. B. had experienced sexual problems with her husband for approximately eight months. She was inorgasmic and she had lost interest in sex. On further questioning, she reported that her husband was extremely dedicated to his professional work but that he rarely had time for her or their children. Although she was a professional woman herself, she worked only part-time and was devoted to her children. The gynecologist suggested that Mrs. B. and her husband consider some form of couples and/or sex therapy for their marital and sexual problems. Mrs. B. told the gynecologist that she would think about it, but that her husband would never consider therapy.

Several months later, Mrs. B. was seen by her internist for complaints of loss of interest in work and loss of energy. Mrs. B. also informed the physician that she was extremely dissatisfied with her marital relationship. The physician took a relationship- and sexual history, which included a question about the importance of any other person—man or woman—in her present life. Mrs. B. began to cry and said that she had been involved in a relationship with a woman for the previous two years. The physician's nonjudgmental attitude allowed Mrs. B. to discuss the conflict she felt between the two relationships. She described her relationship with Ms. R. in very positive terms—sexually and emotionally—and said that she felt a strong desire to take her two children and move in with Ms. R. However, she was terrified that her husband would find out that she was a lesbian and then sue for custody of the children. Despite the fact that she was a good mother, she knew that as a lesbian she was unlikely to win a custody case. She asked the physician not to include any information in her medical record about her relationship with Ms. R., and the physician assured her of complete confidentiality. He then offered her a list of several organizations that provided counseling and legal services to gay parents (e.g., Lesbian Mothers Legal Defense Fund, Gay Parents Custody and Visitation Center, Homophile

Community Health Service). She gratefully accepted this information and
that day made appointments for counseling and legal assistance.

Parents of gays are often quite upset when they learn of their child's homosexuality. They commonly turn to a family physician for support and/or assistance at this time of crisis. Some parents insist that the physician talk to their child in order to "straighten him or her out." The physician can agree to be available, but should explain that it is not helpful to force the child to talk to a physician, particularly if the child is not experiencing a conflict about being gay. Parents should be encouraged to express their own feelings and conflicts about homosexuality in the presence of the physician. Most parents want to know if they are responsible for their child's homosexuality. The physician can explain that researchers do not know what "causes" homosexuality or heterosexuality, although scientists suspect that no single factor (such as parental influence) is responsible. Physicians may also serve as objective resources for information about homosexuality, as discussed previously. There is an organization called Parents of Gays which offers support groups for parents in various parts of the country. Physicians should provide information about this organization and the location of the nearest chapter to any parents who are having difficulty adjusting to their child's homosexuality. Referral to a psychotherapist who has experience in dealing with these problems may also be indicated for some severely troubled parents.

Case 4

Mr. and Mrs. D. consulted their family physician after Mr. D's 22-year-old daughter (L.D.) by a former marriage informed them that she was gay. L.D. came with them to see the physician. After taking a brief history from the parents in the daughter's presence, the physician elected to discuss the matter with daughter and parents separately.

L.D., who was seen first, reported that she had been involved in a lesbian relationship for two years and that she was very happy in this relationship. She had decided to inform her father and stepmother of her sexual orientation because she was tired of concealing such an important part of her life from them. Since she was not experiencing any psychological conflict, she saw no need for psychotherapy. She gave the physician permission to discuss her feelings with Mr. and Mrs. D.

Mr. and Mrs. D. were quite distressed about L.D.'s lesbianism. They assured the physician that they would pay for any treatment which might be able to "cure L.D. of this illness." Mrs. D. also expressed a concern about leaving L.D. home alone with Mrs. D.'s two young daughters (ages nine and eleven). The physician very tactfully explained that homosexuality was not an illness and that physicians did not know what "caused" homosexuality or heterosexuality. She also said that the so-called "treatments" for homosexuality were generally unsuccessful—particularly when the person, as in L.D.'s case, was unwilling to consider therapy. The physician explained that homosexuals molested children far less frequently than the media suggested—and less frequently than heterosexuals—and she informed Mrs. D. that there was no reason to be concerned about L.D.'s sexual interest in Mrs. D.'s daughters. (L.D. had been babysitting her stepsisters for ten years, had known she was a lesbian for five years, and had never been sexually interested in children.) The physician commented on the fact that Mr. and Mrs. D. were much more alarmed about L.D.'s lifestyle than L.D. herself. She suggested that it might help them to talk with someone who had experience in counseling parents with concerns similar to theirs. They agreed that this would be useful. The physician gave them the name of a family counselor who specialized in helping parents and siblings adjust to a child/sibling's homosexuality. The physician also informed Mr. and Mrs. D. about the local Parents of Gays group, and she provided phone numbers of the group leaders.

Referrals

The physician should refer gay patients to a medical or psychiatric colleague if any of the following situations exist:

1. The physician's personal attitudes about homosexuality make it impossible for him or her to respect the patient and to approach the patient in an objective, professional manner.
2. The patient demonstrates significant psychiatric symptomatology (depression, anxiety, psychosis, etc.) which is interfering with his or her ability to function.
3. The patient presents with a sexual or sex-related problem outside the physician's area of expertise.
4. The patient is severely distressed by some problem related to his or her homosexuality (relationship difficulty, family rejection, employment discrimination, child custody case, etc.) and would like an opportunity to discuss the problem at length with a competent therapist.

The physician should be confident of the qualifications of any colleague to whom gay patients are referred. The colleague must have prior experience treating gay patients and must demonstrate objective attitudes toward homosexuality. We recommend that every physician contact a local or national homophile organization (or women's center) annually to obtain a list of psychiatrists and other physicians who are known to provide objective treatment for gay people. (See Resource section.)

Conclusion

This chapter provides information for physicians on the evaluation and treatment of sexual and sex-related problems in gay patients. Any physician who attempts treatment of gay sexual problems should be able to take a comprehensive sexual and developmental history in a nonjudgmental manner. In order to do so, the physician must have an understanding of the wide variety of sexual and life experiences of gay people. The physician should have access to information and organizations that can help gays and their families develop positive attitudes about homosexuality. In addition, the physician should be able to make referrals to other physicians and therapists who offer objective treatment to homosexuals. The physician who understands the special needs and problems of gay patients and their families is able to provide more effective medical care.

Resources

Books and Publications

On Women:

> *Our right to love,* Vida, G. (ed), 1978
> *Rubyfruit jungle,* Brown, R. M., 1973
> *Woman plus woman: Attitudes toward lesbianism,* Klaich, D., 1974
> *Lesbian/Woman,* Martin, D. & Lyon, P., 1972
> *The joy of lesbian sex,* Sisley, E. & Harris, B., 1977

On Men:

> *The homosexual and his society,* Cory, D. & LeRoy, L., 1973
> *Familiar faces, hidden lives: The story of homosexual men in America today,* Brown, H., 1976
> *The David Kopay story,* Kopay, D., 1976
> *The joy of gay sex,* Silverstein, C. & White, E., 1977

On Women and Men:

> *Homosexualities,* Bell, A. & Weinberg, M., 1978
> *The homosexual matrix,* Tripp, C.A., 1975
> *Gay: What you should know about homosexuality,* Hunt, M., 1977
> What we don't know about homosexuality, *The New York Times Magazine,* Gould, R., 1974
> *The Journal of Homosexuality*
> *Homosexuality in perspective,* Masters, W. & Johnson, V., 1979

For Parents:

> "Letter to an American Mother," Freud, S. In Ruitenbeak, H. (ed), *The problem of homosexuality in modern society,* 1963
> *Consenting adult,* Hobson, L., 1975
> *A family matter: A parents' guide to homosexuality,* Silverstein, C., 1977

Organizations and Hotlines:

National Gay Task Force, 50 Fifth Avenue, New York 10011: Telephone: 212-741-1010. Clearinghouse for any information related to homosexuality.

Operation Venus: toll-free number, 800-272-2577 (from Pennsylvania, 800-462-4966). Provides information to any caller on sexually transmitted diseases.

Local women's centers or chapters of the National Organization for Women (N.O.W.): Most major cities and college campuses have organizations such as these that can provide information on local homophile organizations.

Local homophile organizations: e.g., Daughters of Bilitis, Mattachine Society, Gay Student Union, Gay People in Medicine, Gay Nurses Alliance, Metropolitan Community Church, Homophile Community Health Service. These groups have names of physicians and therapists who provide nonjudgmental treatment for gay people.

References

1. Kinsey, A. C., Pomeroy, W. B., & Martin, C. E. *Sexual behavior in the human male.* Philadelphia: Saunders, 1948.
2. Kinsey, A. C., Pomeroy, W. B., Martin, C. E., & Gebhard, P. H. *Sexual behavior in the human female.* Philadelphia: Saunders, 1953.
3. Lawrence, J. C. Homosexuals, hospitalization and the nurse. *Nursing Forum,* 1975, *14*(3):305–317.
4. Pauly, I., & Goldstein, S. Physicians' attitudes in treating male homosexuals. *Medical Aspects of Human Sexuality,* 1970, *4*:22–45.
5. Bell, A. P., & Weinberg, M. S. *Homosexualities.* New York: Simon and Schuster, 1978.
6. Bell, A. P. The homosexual as patient. In Green, R. (ed), *Human sexuality.* Baltimore: Williams and Wilkins, 1975.
7. Saghir, M. T., & Robins, E. *Male and female homosexuality.* Baltimore: Williams and Wilkins, 1973.
8. Siegelman, M. Adjustment of homosexual and heterosexual women. *British Journal of Psychiatry,* 1972, *120*:477–481.
9. Siegelman, M. Adjustment of male homosexuals and heterosexuals. *Archives of Sexual Behavior,* 1972, *2*(1):9–25.
10. Freedman, M. J. Homosexuality among women and psychological adjustment. *Dissertation Abstracts International,* 1971, *38*:347–350.
11. Hart, M., Roback, H., Tittle, B., Weitz, L., Walston, B., & McKee, E. Psychological adjustment of non-patient homosexuals: Critical review of research literature. *Journal of Clinical Psychiatry,* 1978, *39*:604–608.
12. Freund, K. Should homosexuality arouse therapeutic concern? *Journal of Homosexuality,* 1977, *2*(4):235–240.
13. Brodie, H. K. H., Gartrell, N. K., Doering, C., & Kraemer, H. Plasma testosterone levels in heterosexual and homosexual men. *American Journal of Psychiatry,* 1974, *131*(1):82–83.
14. Gartrell, N. K., Loriaux, D. L., & Chase, T. N. Plasma testosterone in homosexual and heterosexual women. *American Journal of Psychiatry,* 1977, *134*(10):1117–1119.

15. Meyer-Bahlburg, H. F. L. Sex hormones and male homosexuality in comparative perspective. *Archives of Sexual Behavior,* 1977, *6*(4):297–325.
16. Meyer-Bahlburg, H. F. L. Sex hormones and female homosexuality: A critical examination. *Archives of Sexual Behavior,* 1979, *8*(2):101–119.
17. Hornstein, A., & Cook, C. Counseling patients with sexual identity stresses. *Interaction,* 1978, *2*(2):1–12.
18. Kaplan, H. *The new sex therapy.* New York: Quadrangle, 1974.
19. Toder, N. Sexual problems of lesbians. In Vida, G. (ed). *Our right to love.* Englewood Cliffs, N.J.: Prentice-Hall, 1978.
20. Vida, G. (ed): *Our right to love.* Englewood Cliffs, N.J.: Prentice-Hall, 1978.
21. Carr, G., & William, D. Anal warts in a population of gay men in New York City. *Sexually Transmitted Disease,* 1977, *4*(2):56–57.
22. Felman, Y. M., & Morrison, J. M. Examining the homosexual male for sexually transmitted disease. *JAMA,* 1977, *238*(19):2046–2047.
23. Henderson, R. H. Improving sexually transmitted disease health services for gays: A national prospective. *Sexually Transmitted Disease,* 1977, *4*(2):58–62.
24. Judson, F. N., Miller, K. G., & Schaffnit, T. R. Screening for gonorrhea and syphilis in the gay baths—Denver, Colorado. *American Journal of Public Health,* 1977, *67*(8):740–742.
25. Merino, H., & Richards, J. An innovative program for venereal disease: Case finding, treatment and education for a population of gay men. *Sexually Transmitted Disease,* 1977, *4*(2):50–52.
26. Ostrow, D., & Shaskey, D. The experience of the Howard Brown Memorial Clinic of Chicago with sexually transmitted disease. *Sexually Transmitted Disease,* 1977, *4*(2):53–55.
27. Sohn, N., Robilotti, J. G. The gay bowel syndrome. *American Journal of Gastroenterology,* 1977, *67*(5):478–484.
28. Smuzness, W., Much, M. L., & Prince, A. M. On the role of sexual behavior in the spread of Hepatitis B infection. *Annals of Internal Medicine,* 1975, *83*:489–495.
29. Money, J., & Russo, A. Establishment of homosexual gender identity/role: Longitudinal follow-up of gender identity/role in childhood. Paper presented to 2nd International Congress of Sexology, Montreal, 1977.
30. Money, J., & Schwartz, M. Dating, romantic and nonromantic friendships, and sexuality in 17 early-treated adrenogenital females, aged 16–25. In Lee, P. A. (ed). *Congenital adrenal hyperplasia.* Baltimore: University Park Press, 1977.

Parent Patient Management Problem

James P. Held and David B. Marcotte

Instructions

The following patient management problem (PMP) is designed to simulate a physician/patient interaction in order to test your clinical judgment and provide feedback concerning your management of this patient.

First read the initial description of the setting and the preliminary general history; then follow the directions at the beginning of each frame. You will be asked to make management decisions throughout the PMP. The consequences of each decision and further interactions are revealed. This problem will be most valuable if you approach it not as a test or examination but rather as a learning experience where you react as you would in the actual situation.

When you have completed the problem, you may wish to read the discussion by the authors and the scoring instructions at the end. The authors' discussion outlines the optimal solutions and discusses the crucial management issues raised in this problem.

Setting

You are a psychiatric consultant to a primary-care clinic in a town of 4,000 whose economy is agriculturally based. You have access to an office equipped with an X-ray machine and a minor surgical room. There is a hospital in a larger community 40 miles away.

Preliminary General History

A patient, Mr. Al Brett, has been scheduled for you. He has been treated for

The Patient Management Problems are available in audiovisual form: Department of Continuing Education, University of Minnesota Medical School, Mayo Bldg., Minneapolis MN 55455. © 1976, University of Minnesota.

several minor illnesses, the latest of which was a urinary tract infection in 1973. He has heard of you and always spoke well of you in the town where he owns a Ford dealership. He is prominent in town and currently holds a position on the Town Council. He also is a member of the School Board, the Board of Public Safety, and the Veterans of Foreign Wars. Mr. Brett is married to Lillian. They have two children, Louise and Henry, 16 and 17 years old, respectively. Yesterday Mr. Brett scheduled an appointment and asked to be seen by you right away.
GO TO FRAME A

Frame A

Introductory pleasantries about the car the doctor owns; other familiarities. The patient is agitated, restless, taps his feet, folds his arms, gets up, moves the chair he is sitting in. He asks distracting questions about the *female* doctor's children, how are they liking the town, the house, etc. He finally states, in an embarrassed way, that he has made the appointment to discuss his son. He reveals that his son locks the bathroom door for a long time at night and even during the day. The doctor says, "You're concerned." The patient says, "Frankly, I'm worried he . . . uh . . . you know, 'jerks off' too much."

At this point you would:
   1.   Tell Mr. Brett that most children pleasure themselves, especially males, and say "Don't worry about it; it's just normal development."
   2.   Say, "It is usual for children to stimulate themselves. Tell me more about your concern."
   3.   Say, "It is usual for children to stimulate themselves; what can you tell me about your own sexual activity during adolescence?"

Frame B

Mr. Brett asks a direct question of the doctor: "Is it usual for males to masturbate daily?" The doctor says, "Yes, it is quite common. Tell me more about your concern." The patient is uneasy, hesitant, and shifts about in his chair. The patient states that yesterday Lillian discovered some pornographic magazines (he looks disgusted) in his son's closet.

At this point you would:
   1.   Tell Mr. Brett that Henry's masturbation and its frequency are common and say, "You seem concerned. Tell me more about that concern."
   2.   Mention that, in addition to the commonness of masturbation, frequent use of pornography is exceedingly common, especially among males.
   3.   Tell Mr. Brett that Henry's masturbation and its frequency are quite common. Urge him to have a discussion with his son about sex, assuring him that this will help.

Frame C

Mr. Brett says that yes, he did stimulate himself beginning at 12 years of age, once or twice a week. He thought of girls at school or used Esquire magazine or the Sears and Roebuck catalogue when masturbating. He is not embarrassed as he discusses this.

At this point you would say:

1. "You see how natural and normal it is for children to stimulate themselves. About 95% of all males do, and almost two-thirds of females do. It is our attitude about it that makes us ashamed."

2. "Well, now do you see how normal such behavior is? I wouldn't worry about it if I were you."

3. "I would like to know more about your concern about Henry."

Frame D

The patient says, "Well, I know about what you've said, and maybe I shouldn't worry about it so much. Perhaps he'll outgrow it." Mr. Brett looks away from the doctor. He indicates that he wishes to leave by edging further forward on his chair and putting his coat on. He crosses his arms in front of him with his fists clenched.

At this point you would say:

1. "I'm concerned that things aren't settled. What else can you tell me?"

2. "Well, you seem ready to leave. Is there anything else I can do for you today?"

3. "It seems like I haven't really dealt with what you're concerned about. Is there anything more that has you worried that you'd be willing to tell me?"

4. "You say that, and yet I sense that you don't really mean it. What really has you concerned?"

Frame E

Mr. Brett finally reveals being quite ashamed and has difficulty in mentioning that the magazines he and his wife have found are filled with pictures of nude males, some performing "sodomy."

At this point you would say:

1. "No wonder you were concerned. Actually, most males experience same-sex contact during adolescence. It's quite normal and really no cause to be alarmed to that degree."

2. "I can see that you are upset about this. What does your concern center on,

the question of whether Henry is homosexual? Many parents can be quite alarmed with that possibility.''

3. ''How do you feel about homosexuality, Mr. Brett?''

Frame F

Mr. Brett is visibly anxious and uncomfortable. He reveals that he was brought up in a strict Lutheran background where ''we knew right from wrong. I can understand a young man sowing wild oats and accept that, but I can't stand to be around any pansies or queers. We had some at the University when I was a student and you could always tell them. You know what I mean, Doc!'' He is still visibly upset and begs you to help him with this problem.

At this point you would say:

1. ''No wonder you were concerned. Actually, most males experience same-sex contact during adolescence. It's quite normal and really no cause to be alarmed to that degree.''

2. ''I can see that you are upset about this. What does your concern center on, the question of whether Henry is homosexual? Many parents can be quite alarmed with that possibility!''

3. ''How do you feel about homosexuality, Mr. Brett.''

Frame G

Mr. Brett appears surprised and angered by your comments and says that he never experienced any homosexual contact, and he is certain that none of his boyhood friends did either. He expresses his trust in you and once more begs you to help them, saying, ''I'll do what you say is best, Doc.''

At this point you would:

1. Explain to Mr. Brett that that is a serious concern and suggest that the family contact their minister.

2. Say, ''I can see that you are upset about this. What does your concern center on, the question of whether Henry is homosexual? Many parents can be quite alarmed with that possibility!''

3. Explain to Mr. Brett that many adolescents pass through a phase of same-sex attraction so Henry's behavior doesn't necessarily mean that he is homosexual. Suggest that he discuss this with Henry alone.

4. Say, ''No wonder you were concerned. Actually, most males experience same-sex contact during adolescence. It's quite normal and really no cause to be alarmed to that degree.''

5. Explain to Mr. Brett that many adolescents pass through a phase same-sex attraction so Henry's behavior doesn't necessarily mean that he is homosexual.

Suggest counseling with a minister you know in town who does a very competent work with sex-related problems.

6.   Explain to Mr. Brett that most adolescents pass through a phase of same-sex attraction. Reassure him that most will outgrow the phase and they should treat Henry normally.

Frame H

Henry enters your office and is somewhat shy and appears frightened of you. You reassure him that what is said will be in confidence. Henry appears more relaxed. A sex history reveals that he has masturbated since 11 years of age. His thoughts during masturbation include both males and females. He has used pornography featuring both males and females. He indicates that his father, who was a guard for the University of Minnesota Gophers, pressures him to play football. Also, Mr. Brett keeps talking about Henry taking over the Ford dealership when Henry finishes school. Henry has successfully competed for the lead in his high school play. He shows visible pleasure in describing his part and then indicates that his parents tease him about being in the play and question him about going to rehearsals in the evening.

At this point you would:
1.   Refer Henry to a mental health specialist whom you know well for individual and/or family counseling and notify Mr. Brett of your recommendation. Then contact the specialist and acquaint him/her with the situation.
2.   Recommend to Henry that you would like to see the entire family to further explore the family's conflict.

Frame I

The family enters your office. Henry holds his head down, walks slowly, and sits down. Mr. and Mrs. Brett sit opposite Henry with Louise between them. The parents ask what can be done about Henry. Lillian indicates that he only goes out with boyfriends. Louise adds that her classmates call Henry a wierdo and a fag. She cries while saying this. Henry is visibly uncomfortable, taps his feet, squirms in his chair. He fails to respond to your supportive remarks. At this point Mr. Brett asks, "What are you going to do, Doc?"

At this point you would:
1.   Recommend family therapy and give Mr. Brett names of three counselors you trust.
2.   Recommend family therapy, suggesting several therapists and ask permission to contact one. The Bretts agree to have you call the therapist and give information about them.

3.   Recommend that the family stop forcing Henry to do things that the father and mother think are indicated. Suggest a family vacation to take some pressure off, as soon as school is out. Don't make an issue of the sexual behavior.

4.   Begin the family therapy yourself.

Answer Key

A-1

> Mr. Brett responds, "Well, if you say so, Doc." He invites you to look at the new car he has purchased at the garage.
>
> Your premature reassurance is unlikely to help Mr. Brett. His degree of shame and embarrassment will not be relieved by the simple statement, "Don't worry about it." Mr. Brett is agitated and concerned; explore these feelings. Your failure to explore the complaint fully leads to premature closure. Note Mr. Brett's nonverbal expressions of dissatisfaction. MAKE ANOTHER CHOICE.

A-2

> GO TO FRAME B.

A-3

> GO TO FRAME C.

B-1

> GO TO FRAME E.

B-2

> GO TO FRAME D.

B-3

> GO TO FRAME D.

C-1

> GO TO FRAME D.

C-2

Mr. Brett changes the subject.

Your premature reassurance is not likely to help. Mr. Brett's degree of shame and embarrassment will not be relieved by the simple statement, "Don't worry about it." Mr. Brett is agitated and concerned; explore these feelings. Your failure to explore the complaint fully leads to premature closure. Note Mr. Brett's nonverbal expressions of dissatisfaction. MAKE ANOTHER CHOICE.

C-3

GO TO FRAME B.

D-1

GO TO FRAME E.

D-2

Mr. Brett leaves. No return visit is scheduled.

Your premature reassurance is not likely to help. Mr. Brett's degree of shame and embarrassment will not be relieved by the simple statement, "Don't worry about it." Mr. Brett is agitated and concerned; explore these feelings. Your failure to explore the complaint fully leads to premature closure. Note Mr. Brett's nonverbal expressions of dissatisfaction. MAKE ANOTHER CHOICE.

D-3

GO TO FRAME E.

D-4

GO TO FRAME E.

E-1

Mr. Brett responds with an icy "Well, thank you, Doctor" and leaves. One month later the Medical Society forwards a copy of an angry letter about immoral young physicians.

Even though reassurance may be indicated, you have failed to explore Mr. Brett's concerns. Also, your reassurance is stated in a way that puts Mr. Brett down for his concern. MAKE ANOTHER CHOICE.

E-2

GO TO FRAME F.

E-3   GO TO FRAME F.

F-1   An appointment is made. Mr. Brett is visibly relieved and says,
           "Thanks. I knew you would help." GO TO FRAME H.

F-2   The appointment is made. Mr. Brett hesitates about Louise's coming
           but says they will be there. GO TO FRAME I.

F-3   GO TO FRAME G.

G-1   You seem to be passing the buck to the family minister. Is the minister
           competent to handle sex-related problems? How do you know? Perhaps
           your discomfort with homosexuality is interfering with your being ef-
           fective. MAKE ANOTHER CHOICE.

G-2   The appointment is made. Mr. Brett hesitates about Louise's coming
           but says they will be there. GO TO FRAME I.

G-3   It is unlikely that Mr. Brett could discuss the issue alone with his son.
           Your own attitudes about homosexuality may be related to premature
           closure of the problem. MAKE ANOTHER CHOICE.

G-4   An appointment is made. Mr. Brett is visibly relieved and says,
           "Thanks. I knew you would help." GO TO FRAME H.

G-5   The minister calls and thanks you for the referral. The family is in
           counseling.

           This is the minimum pass performance level of the Patient Management
           Problem. If you wish to continue, GO TO J-1 IN THE ANSWER KEY.

G-6

It is impossible for them to treat Henry "normally." The family is in crisis. They will convey to Henry their discomfort with their situation. Your attitude about homosexuality may be generating a "simple" solution. MAKE ANOTHER CHOICE.

H-1

Two weeks later you receive a phone call from the Mental Health Center. The Brett family is in family counseling and treatment is going well.

This is the minimum pass performance level of the Patient Management Problem. If you wish to continue, GO TO J-1 IN THE ANSWER KEY.

H-2

Henry is somewhat reluctant but agrees to be present with his family for the appointment. GO TO FRAME I.

I-1

Three weeks later, the counselor calls to tell you that therapy is going well with the Bretts, and Henry is being supported by his father.

This is the minimum pass performance level of the Patient Management Problem. If you wish to continue, GO TO J-1 IN THE ANSWER KEY.

I-2

GO TO J-1 IN THE ANSWER KEY.

I-3

Six months later, Mr. Brett worriedly brings his son in to see you. Henry appears listless and tired. He stares blankly at you, and then begins to sob. "I can't take it any more. . . I just can't. I feel so terrible. My dad is so good to me. What should I do?"

You seem to be missing the family interaction. The parents are clearly lined up against the son. The son has no support in the family. Your attitudes about family dynamics, perhaps based on those in your own family, may be interfering with your decisions. MAKE ANOTHER CHOICE.

J-1

Write a treatment plan for your follow-up. Use the questions on the following page.

Patient Follow-up

1. What potential problem areas do you expect to see on follow-up?
   A.
   B.
   C.
2. How would you manage each problem area?
   A.
   B.
   C.
3. What would be the expected outcome in each problem area?
   A.
   B.
   C.

END OF PARENT PMP

Critical Decision Points

Frames A & B   Mr. Brett is visibly anxious and agitated. He attempts to control the interview and interviewer in the same way that he controls his family. Early in the problem, continued focus on his concerns is essential. Early reassurance will not be effective with his degree of anxiety and agitation nor will urging Mr. Brett to talk to his son.

Frame C   Again, premature reassurance will not be effective and sends you into Frame D. It is critical to get some information about his fears.

Frame D   Mr. Brett is now angry and has not been reassured by your comments. Now it becomes critical to ask him further open-ended questions.

Frame E   Premature reassurance again is unhelpful.

Frame F   A real choice point here is whether to see Henry alone or with the family. Some experts feel that seeing Henry alone singles Henry out as "the problem." Others believe that seeing Henry alone can be supportive. One choice is to see the whole family for assessment, not necessarily for definitive treatment. Most experts agree that this is an optimal choice since the family is in crisis.

Frame G   Again, similar choices exist to those in Frame F. Additionally, leaving Mr. Brett to deal with Henry alone is a poor choice. Competent referral is an acceptable option in this frame.

Frame H   Same as above

Frame I   It is critical to facilitate the family referral or to treat the family yourself; do not assume they will follow up without your help.

Discussion

Potential Problem Areas

A.   There may be continued lack of support for Henry because he does not fulfill his father's expectations.

B.   There may be increased suspicion of Henry's activities outside of the home.

C.   Henry may possibly comply with the family and withdraw from his activities.

D.   Increased suspicion of Henry at home may cause parental invasion of his privacy by checking out his books, closets, etc.

E.   His father may attempt to control Henry by financial withholding or restrictive rules.

Management

A.   Call more attention in sessions to worries that the parents may have in other areas.

B.   Search for an ally for Henry and ask them both to assist in joining forces against the father.

C.   Increase sex education for the family.

D.   Explore the parents' relationship and control and power issues with others in the family besides Henry.

E.   Suggest that the mother explore all drawers of everyone's room for contraband (paradox intention).

F.   See Henry alone and advise to be less revealing to his parents.

Outcomes

A.   There could be increased resistance initially by the father's seeing the therapist as a powerful figure (might quit therapy).

B.   There could be possible increased tension with other members besides Henry in the family.

C.   There may be a gradual decline in interest with Henry's sexual activity.

D.   There is potential for the women to challenge the father's power and control.

Scoring Instructions

The scoring sheet gives the weighted and unweighted scoring values for each possible response of a PMP. The unweighted values are on a 4+ to 4− rating system giving the relative merit of each possible response for that particular frame considering the situation in that frame. The weighted values also take into account the pathway to that frame and, therefore, may seem at odds with the unweighted values. They are necessarily quite different in some cases in order to avoid scoring errors, such as giving someone credit for taking all the best choices on a loop or sidetrack that came out of a relatively neutral or slightly negative choice, that is, to avoid giving credit for running in circles.

The unweighted values, therefore, are provided for your information about a particular frame, not for scoring. The weighted values are to be used in all scoring procedures. The following are instructions for deriving several different types of scores from your responses on the PMP and a brief description of the meaning of each.

$$\text{Proficiency Index} = \frac{\text{sum of the weighted value of all responses}}{\text{maximum score for this PMP}} \times 100.$$

The Proficiency Index is the best overall indicator of how well one completed the PMP relative to the optimal. This measure both rewards better choices while penalizing negative ones. It doesn't, however, consider neutral choices.

$$\text{Errors of Omission} = \frac{\text{sum of all positive choices}}{\text{maximum score for this PMP}} \times 100.$$

The Errors of Omission score gives an indication of how likely you are to hesitate to do things that are beneficial or desirable, perhaps out of concern that you might make an error.

$$\text{Errors of Commission} = \frac{\text{sum of all negative choices}}{\text{maximum score for this PMP}} \times 100.$$

The Errors of Commission score gives an indication of how likely you are to do too much or make mistakes by doing rather than not doing. The ''shotgun approach'' to laboratory testing, for example, will generate a high Errors of Commission score.

$$\text{Efficiency Index} = \frac{\text{the number (not sum) of positive choices}}{\text{the number of } all \text{ choices made by you}} \times 100.$$

The Efficiency Index is the best indicator of how well you proceeded through the problem in terms of economy of time and effort. It does include an indication of the effect of neutral as well as negative and positive choices. It is not the best measure of overall performance, however, since it is possible to proceed efficiently through the problem to a much less than optimal solution by making many Errors of Omission.

These scores are designed to be considered as a group in order to get the most information about your approach to this type of problem and how it might be improved. For example, given a low Proficiency Index, one may look to the Errors of Omission and Errors of Commission to determine if your approach should be more bold or more cautious in the future. If the Proficiency Index is fairly high but the

Efficiency Index is low, you may consider where in the problem you may have been led off onto a fairly neutral but unproductive sidetrack and how you might have avoided it.

Scoring values

Maximum score (sum of weighted values from optimal path) = 32.5.

Frame	Response number	Unweighted value	Weighted value
A	1	−2.0	−4.0
	2	2.5	6.5
	3	1.7	1.0
B	1	2.5	6.5
	2	1.0	1.0
	3	−3.0	−8.0
C	1	1.0	1.0
	2	−2.5	−6.5
	3	1.7	3.2
D	1	2.3	3.0
	2	−2.7	−6.5
	3	3.0	4.0
	4	2.0	2.0
E	1	−2.0	−4.0
	2	2.5	6.5
	3	0.0	0.0
F	1	2.0	4.0
	2	2.0	5.0
	3	1.0	1.0
G	1	−3.0	−8.0
	2	3.0	2.0
	3	−2.5	−6.5
	4	3.0	2.0
	5	3.0	6.0
	6	−2.3	−4.9
H	1	0.6	0.6
	2	2.6	0.0
I	1	0.0	0.0
	2	3.0	8.0
	3	−1.3	−2.5
	4	2.0	4.0

Spinal Cord Patient Management Problem

David B. Marcotte and James P. Held

Instructions

The following patient management problem (PMP) is designed to stimulate a physician–patient interaction in order to test your clinical judgment and provide feedback concerning your management of this patient.

First read the initial description of the setting and the preliminary general history, then follow the directions at the beginning of each frame. You will be asked to make management decisions throughout the PMP. The consequences of each decision and further interactions are revealed. This problem will be most valuable if you approach it not as a test or examination but rather as a learning experience where you react as you would in the actual situation.

When you have completed the problem, you may wish to read the discussion by the authors and the scoring instructions at the end of this booklet. The authors' discussion outlines the optimal solutions and discusses the crucial management issues raised in this problem.

Setting

You are a psychiatrist in a metropolis (population 500,000). You have a busy practice, which includes liaison to General Hospital. Dr. Meldor, a family-physician colleague, has asked you to stop in to see Mrs. Jones, who is about to be discharged.

Preliminary General History

Mrs. Jones, a 28-year-old female has been a patient since she was admitted 4 months ago with a cervical spinal fracture sustained in a collision of her auto. She was returning home alone from a bridge club meeting when another auto ran a stoplight and collided with the left front of her auto. She was thrown into the steering column, sustaining minor lacerations of her scalp and she noted that she was unable to loosen her seat belt. She was taken to General Hospital where X-rays revealed a fractured C-6 vertebra with compression of the cord. Surgery was performed; however, Mrs. Jones has a permanent, complete spastic paralysis of the lower extremities and partial paralysis of her uper extremeties. She has received physical and occupational therapy and has been cheerful and optimistic about returning to her work as a junior high school teacher, and the nursing staff has remarked on her positive attitude and their respect for her. Her husband, Ralph Jones, visits her regularly and brings their two children, Ralph Jr. and Barney (ages 4 and 2), to visit on Sundays. You stop in to see her on the afternoon prior to her discharge.

GO TO FRAME A

Frame A

Mrs. Jones is seated by her bed in a wheelchair. She greets you cheerfully. She talks at length about her job as a teacher. She wants to see her students again and misses contacts with them and with her friends. When you indicate her impending discharge, she doesn't smile. Instead, she looks down, and with a great deal of hesitation asks if she will need birth control now.

At this point you would:
  1. Refer her to Dr. Storey, a trusted GYN colleague to whom you have referred patients previously.
  2. Tell her that she has made excellent progress, which all the staff have noted, and that she will not have to worry about birth control.
  3. Tell her that she needs to continue using birth control and ask her about her prior use of contraceptives.
  4. Suggest that it is too early for her to be concerned about birth control and that she should concentrate on the activities of daily living that she learned while in the hospital.

Frame B

At this point you would:
  1. Recommend use of an IUD and explain its advantages and risks.
  2. Recommend use of an oral contraceptive and explain its advantages and risks.

3. Recommend that she continue use of the same contraceptive devices, explaining their advantages and risks; they worked so well in the past.

4. Recommend that she have a tubal ligation, explaining the advantages and risks of this procedure. It will be so much trouble for her to handle two children and a job from a wheelchair.

5. Recommend the use of a condom and explain its advantages and risks.

6. Recommend the rhythm method and explain its advantages and risks.

Frame C

Mrs. Jones starts to weep, putting her head down and covering her eyes as best she can with her arm. Between sobs, she speaks of her fear that her life as a wife is over. She asks, "What good am I? I feel so down. We had such a good life together and now it's all ruined."

At this point you would:

1. Inquire about suicidal thoughts, since she is so distraught.

2. Tell her, "Everybody has that concern. There really won't be much of a problem. You have done well here."

3. State that many patients are concerned about their sexual adjustment following a severe injury; that they may have to alter sex positions, e.g., oral sex, but most still receive pleasure.

4. Ask her what she is so concerned about.

5. Say that many people are concerned about changes in sexual function and how the change will affect their relationship. Ask if she is concerned about that.

6. Postpone her discharge for several days and observe her.

Frame D

Mrs. Jones reports some casually considered suicidal thoughts. However, since the accident, she has no plan to carry out such thoughts. You ask about weight loss and sleep. She has lost 12 pounds since the accident, and she sleeps well according to the nursing report. She has had no sexual contact since her injury.

At this point you would: *

1. Take a thorough psychiatric history. The purpose would be to evaluate the patient's depression.

2. Say that many people are concerned about changes in sexual function and how the changes will affect their relationship and ask if she is concerned about that.

3. Ask her what she is so concerned about.

4.   Tell her, "Everybody has that concern. There really won't be much of a problem. You have done well here.

5.   State that many patients are concerned about their sexual adjustment following a severe injury; they may have to alter sex positions, e.g., oral sex, but most still receive pleasure.

Frame E

Mrs. Jones expresses concern about her body: the muscle wasting, her protuberant belly, her spastic legs, and her inability to move her hips. She talks of her fear that Ralph will not like her and wonders whether they will be able to have sexual intercourse. Mrs. Jones is concerned about positions of lovemaking and oral sexuality. You reassure her that she needs to talk about her concerns with Ralph and that she and Ralph will need to experiment to find out exactly what they can do sexually.

After she has aired her concerns, Mrs. Jones recovers her bright appearance.

At this point you would:
1.   Tell her that things will go well for her and suggest that she call if she has further trouble.
2.   Schedule her to be seen alone in your office in a week.
3.   Schedule her to be seen with her husband in your office in a week.

Frame F

Mrs. Jones states, "I'm the one who is paralyzed, Doctor, not you. It's easy for you to say it will work out okay, but you're not paralyzed!" Her teeth are clenched and her eyebrows wrinkled.

At this point you would:
1.   Say, "I understand you are upset. That is typical of people who have accidents such as yours. I know many people with similar reactions."
2.   Say, "I'm really not thinking today. I missed the point you were making. What is on your mind?"
3.   Consider psychiatric hospitalization.
4.   Say, "I deal with patients with similar injuries every day. Most tend to feel sorry for themselves and improve only when they acknowledge it."
5.   Say, "I know this is hard on you, but you really have done so well in the hospital, and you should continue to do well when you get home and begin teaching once more."
6.   Say, "I can see you're upset. Tell me more about it."
7.   Say, "That was insensitive of me to say. Can you go on?"

Frame G

Mrs. Jones returns alone to your office. She makes a point of opening the door and refuses assistance. She tells you that she has resumed intercourse with her husband and he seems pleased that she is home. She has not had oral sex with him yet. She spends some time talking about her job and how it is so different now that she has to ride the elevator at school rather than walk.

She asks for another appointment, and you schedule her to be seen again in 2 weeks.

GO TO G-1 IN THE ANSWER KEY.

Frame H

Two weeks later, you are called by General Hospital Emergency Room, Mrs. Jones is in with severe pain of the cervico-occipital area. It starts in the post-spinal column and radiates up to the occiput. The ER physician describes it as constant, excruciating, unrelieved by aspirin and Darvon, and of 36 hr duration. Her vital signs are normal, and her P.E. and neurological exam are unchanged from time of discharge. The ER physician suggests admission and orders cervical spine films. The wet reading of the X-rays reveals a well-healed fracture of the C-6 with no displacement or change from the predischarge film. She has been given Darvon (65 mg) and ASA (600 mg) by the staff doctor. After admission you schedule her to be seen on rounds.

At this point you would:
1. Ask her to tell you how she is doing at home and about her relationship with Ralph.
2. Request a consult from Dr. Baker, a sensitive and concerned orthopedic specialist who managed the patient during the acute phase of her injury.
3. Do a CBC.
4. Do a sedimentation rate.
5. Do a spinal tap.
6. Refer her to Dr. Angelo, the neurologist who consulted while she was hospitalized.
7. Treat her with analgesics and observe 48 hr.

Frame I

Mrs. Jones once more talks with her head down, weeping at the same time. She expresses fear of her life as a wife ending. She is worried and concerned.

At this point you would:
1. Ask her what she is so concerned about.

2.   State that many patients are concerned about their sexual adjustment following a severe injury; they may have to alter sex positions, e.g., oral sex, but most
still receive pleasure.

3.   Say that many people are concerned about changes in sexual function and
how the changes will affect their relationship and ask if she is concerned about
that.

4.   Inquire about suicidal thoughts, since she is so distraught.

Frame J

Mrs. Jones once more talks with her head down, weeping at the same time. She
expresses fear of her life as a wife ending. She is worried and concerned.

At this point you would:

1.   State that many patients are concerned about their sexual adjustments following a severe injury; they may have to alter sex positions, e.g., oral sex, but most
still receive pleasure.

2.   Inquire about suicidal thoughts, since she is so distraught.

3.   Tell her, "Everybody has that concern. There really won't be much of a
problem. You have done well here."

4.   Say that many people are concerned about changes in sexual function and
how the changes will affect their relationship. Ask her if she is concerned about
that.

5.   Ask her what she is so concerned about.

Frame K

Mr. and Mrs. Jones come in as scheduled. He is a well-dressed postal inspector
who is solicitous toward his wife and anxious to talk to his wife about their sexual life.
You inquire about *his* concerns and learn that he is worried that his wife's neck may be
reinjured during his orgasm or with oral sex. You assure him that the fracture is healed
and he need not be concerned about extension of the paralysis. You ask Mrs. Jones to
tell her husband what sex activity currently is more comfortable, and she responds with
a smile as she describes intercourse with her on top. You ask her if she would like to try
any other sexual activity, and she responds by saying yes, she would like to "blow"
Ralph but wonders whether she would gag from the ejaculation now that she is
paralyzed. You tell her that she is able to move her head and neck, and so as long as
she is comfortable and free to move, gagging shouldn't be a problem.

Mr. and Mrs. Jones spend additional time showing you pictures of the new
camper they have purchased so that they can still enjoy their vacation.

GO TO K-1 IN THE ANSWER KEY.

Answer Key

A-1
> Report: Patient is fertile; oral contraceptives recommended. Additionally, cord injury may predispose to thrombophlebitis. When you ask Mrs. Jones about her previous use of contraceptives, she reports having used foam and a diaphragm. GO TO FRAME B.

A-2
> Fertility is not affected by spinal cord lesions in women. A major concern of patients with spinal cord injuries is sexual function. You are shaping the content of the interview away from sexuality. MAKE ANOTHER CHOICE.

A-3
> When you ask Mrs. Jones about her previous use of contraceptives, she reports having used foam and a diaphragm in the past. GO TO FRAME B.

A-4
> Fertility is not affected by spinal cord lesions in women. A major concern of patients with spinal cord injuries is sexual function. You are shaping the content of the interview away from sexuality. MAKE ANOTHER CHOICE.

B-1
> Risks include perforation of the uterus. Also, loss of pain appreciation may predispose to complications. Follow closely. After Mrs. Jones thanks you, she again hesitantly begins to discuss fears that she has had following her injury. You ask her what fears she has. GO TO FRAME C.

B-2
> Spinal cord injury plus oral contraceptives may predispose patients to thrombophlebitis. Follow carefully. After Mrs. Jones thanks you, she again hesitantly begins to discuss fears that she has had following her injury. You ask her what fears she has. GO TO FRAME C.

B-3
> Mrs. Jones shrugs and fumbles with a glass of water. She is physically unable to button her dress alone. She says she will have difficulty with your suggestion. MAKE ANOTHER CHOICE.

B-4

> Your attitudes about spinal cord injured patients and their abilities may be interfering in Mrs. Jones' decision about family planning. She may perceive your comment as a negative view of herself and her abilities. MAKE ANOTHER CHOICE.

B-5

> A good choice! You will need to assess Ralph's agreement to this possibility. After Mrs. Jones thanks you, she again hesitantly begins to discuss fears she has had since her injury. You ask her what fears she has. GO TO FRAME C.

B-6

> Thermoregulation may be unstable in quadriplegia, invalidating this method. MAKE ANOTHER CHOICE.

C-1

> GO TO FRAME D.

C-2

> GO TO FRAME F.

C-3

> GO TO FRAME E.

C-4

> Mrs. Jones changes the subject to her diet. She asks if she can eat everything or if she will have to watch certain foods. She talks about her protuberant belly and how awful she looks now. Your statement may be considered condescending and pejorative by the patient. MAKE ANOTHER CHOICE.

C-5

> Mrs. Jones responds, "Yes! How am I ever going to satisfy Ralph? Will he ever turn on to me now? Will I be able to enjoy it?" GO TO FRAME E.

C-6

> Nurses report no change in her behavior. She repeats her concerns once more when her discharge date approaches. MAKE ANOTHER CHOICE.

D-1

There is no previous psychiatric illness in the patient or family.
1. Her stress level relates to a marked change in her life subsequent to her injury.
2. It is not unusual for people to consider suicide.
3. No sleep loss is noted, and she is cheerful and responsive in most settings.
4. Weight loss is due to muscle atrophy—her appetite is good.
5. She is fearful of her *role* as a wife ending and not of her life's ending.
MAKE ANOTHER CHOICE.

D-2

Mrs. Jones responds, "Yes! How am I ever going to satisfy Ralph? Will he ever turn on to me now? Will I be able to enjoy it?" GO TO FRAME E.

D-3

Mrs. Jones changes the subject to her diet. She asks if she can eat everything or if she will have to watch certain foods. She talks about her protuberant belly and how awful she looks now. Your statement may be considered as condescending and pejoratively by the patient. MAKE ANOTHER CHOICE.

D-4

GO TO FRAME F.

D-5

GO TO FRAME E.

E-1

GO TO FRAME H.

E-2

GO TO FRAME G.

E-3

GO TO FRAME K.

F-1

Your response here will likely be perceived as condescending and of little help to Mrs. Jones. She wants to tell you her story, not to hear generalized comments about others. A power struggle exists for control of the interview. Allow *her* to define the problem. MAKE ANOTHER CHOICE.

F-2

GO TO FRAME I.

F-3

The patient refuses to discuss prolonging her hospitalization.
1.   She is reacting to the stress of a marked change in her life.
2.   She is concerned about her role as a wife ending.
MAKE ANOTHER CHOICE.

F-4

Your response will likely be perceived as condescending and of little help to the patient. Mrs. Jones wants to tell you her story, not to hear generalized comments about others. A power struggle exists for control of the interview. Allow *her* to define the problem. MAKE ANOTHER CHOICE.

F-5

Your response is evasive. She is still concerned bout her relationship while you proceed to talk about recovery. MAKE ANOTHER CHOICE.

F-6

Mrs. Jones. retorts, "Well, I don't like doctors telling me how things are going to be when I don't even know that myself." GO TO FRAME I.

F-7

GO TO FRAME I.

G-1

This is the Minimum Pass performance level of the Spinal Cord PMP. If you would like to continue working with the problem, GO TO L-1 IN THE ANSWER KEY.

H-1

> GO TO FRAME J.

H-2

> Mrs. Jones may be expressing a conflict symbolically. There are no objective signs of change since her discharge. Normal blood pressure confirms that her headaches are not related to autonomic hyperflexia. Your decision is costly and may sidetrack Mrs. Jones into expensive treatments. MAKE ANOTHER CHOICE.

H-3

> 6000 leukocytes: 65% neutrophils, 25% lymphocytes, 3% eosinophils 7% monocytes. MAKE ANOTHER CHOICE.

H-4

> 0–20 ml. MAKE ANOTHER CHOICE.

H-5

> Opening pressure 100 mm/H_2O; closing pressure 75 mm/H_2O. Clear fluid obtained. No cells in centrifugant. Prot. sug. nl., 40 mg protein/dl. sugar mg/dl. Culture pending. MAKE ANOTHER CHOICE.

H-6

> Results of neurologic examination remain unchanged from previous hospitalization. MAKE ANOTHER CHOICE.

H-7

> After 48 hr Mrs. Jones' pain subsides. You stop by to discharge her. GO TO FRAME J.

I-1

> Mrs. Jones changes the subject to her diet. She asks if she can eat everything or if she will have to watch certain foods. She talks about her protuberant belly and how awful she looks. MAKE ANOTHER CHOICE.

I-2

> GO TO FRAME E.

I-3

Mrs. Jones responds, "Yes! How am I ever going to satisfy Ralph? Will he ever turn on to me now? Will I ever be able to enjoy it?" GO TO FRAME E.

I-4

GO TO FRAME D.

J-1

GO TO FRAME E.

J-2

GO TO FRAME D.

J-3

GO TO FRAME F.

J-4

Mrs. Jones responds, "Yes! How am I ever going to satisfy Ralph? Will he ever turn on to me now? Will I ever be able to enjoy it?" GO TO FRAME E.

J-5

Mrs. Jones changes the subject to her diet. She asks if she can eat everything or if she will have to watch certain foods. She talks about her protuberant belly and how awful she looks. MAKE ANOTHER CHOICE.

K-1

If you want to continue with the Spinal Cord PMP, GO TO L-1 IN THE ANSWER KEY.

L-1

If you scheduled follow-up visits and want to proceed, write a treatment plan for your follow-up. Use the form on the following page.

Patient Follow-up

1. What potential problem areas do you expect to see on follow-up?
   A.
   B.
   C.
2. How would you manage each problem area?
   A.
   B.
   C.
3. What would be the expected outcome in each problem area?
   A.
   B.
   C.

END OF SPINAL CORD PMP

Critical Discussion Points

Frame A   Injury to the cord interferes with fertility in the male but not the female. It is critical to explore her prior use of contraceptives and her thoughts and feelings about it.

Frame B   Each choice of a contraceptive has a risk and this increases with the disability of the patient. Alteration of her physical ability will affect the choice (foam and diaphram). The only contraindicated answer is B-4, where attitudes about spinal cord injured people are dictating the choice the patient might make.

Frame C   Here the patient reveals she is concerned about her future. Choices 3 and 5 are deemed optimal while 4 is perjorative in that the patient may hear *so* concerned and increase her alarm. It is critical to respond that her reaction is common and ask her to tell you more. Choice 2 shuts off her revealing and prematurely reassures her.

Frame D   This repeats previous choices after additional history from choice 1 from Frame C. The same comments from Frame C apply. Choice D-1 might be thorough but costly.

Frame E   The critical decision in this frame is to *schedule* her to return. Do not leave her to *have* trouble in order to return. She is making a marked adjustment in her relationship and all other areas of her life. She will need support.

Frame F   This frame is entered from C-2 or D-4. The patient is annoyed and angry with your shutting her off. We believe it best to acknowledge your hasty reassurance and allow her to shape the interview further.

Frame H   The patient is expressing her adjustment reaction symbolically. There is no change from previous hospitalization. In order to see you, she now develops "trouble." Explore what is happening at home with Ralph.

Frame I   This frame is entered from F-2 and F-7. The patient now continues with her concern. It is important to reassure her about the commonness of the problem but do not suggest that there is nothing to worry about.

Frame J   This frame is entered from H-1 and H-7. She once more reveals her concerns. It is important to reassure her about the commonness of the problem but do not suggest that there is nothing to worry about.

Discussion

The authors list potential problem areas and management problem solutions give the expected outcomes of further work. All possibilities cannot be covered. You may elucidate unique or common concerns that we have overlooked or develop an imaginative management technique.

Potential Problem Areas

A.   There could be possible complications of birth control.

B.   If seen alone, she could continue to avoid adjustment to her relationship.

C.   Increasing self-doubt may arise at points of adjustment in her relationship of a "real" mother.

E.   There might be separation and possible divorce, which is common after a disabling injury.

F.   She might withdraw and depend increasingly on her husband and physician (secondary gain).

G.   The husband might tend to overprotect his wife in his concern for her.

Management

A.   Alter birth control use and involve the husband in the decision-making process.

B.   Bring in the husband if she avoids the relationship.

C.   Reassure her about the progress of adjustment and that concerns about her relationship will continue to occur for some time.

D.   Give her group counseling with other para- or quadraplegic persons.

E.   Involve her in social groups of persons with spinal cord injuries.

F.   Give her relationship counseling with her husband to help them arrive at a decision about the marriage.

G.   For her withdrawal and dependency, it is imperative to counsel both wife and husband to help discontinue overprotection on his part.

H.   Have individual sessions with the husband if he is the instigator of overprotection.

Scoring Instructions

The scoring sheet gives the weighted and unweighted scoring values for each possible response of a PMP. The unweighted values are on a 4+ to 4− rating system giving the relative merit of each possible response for that particular frame considering the situation in that frame. The weighted values also take into account the pathway to that frame and, therefore, may seem at odds with the unweighted values. They are necessarily quite different in some cases in order to avoid scoring errors, such as giving someone credit for taking all the best choices on a loop or sidetrack that came out of a relatively neutral or slightly negative choice, that is, to avoid giving credit for running in circles.

The unweighted values, therefore, are provided for your information about a particular frame, not for scoring. The weighted values are to be used in all scoring procedures. The following are instructions for deriving several different types of scores from your responses on the PMP, and a brief description of the meaning of each.

$$\text{Proficiency Index} = \frac{\text{sum of the weighted value of all responses}}{\text{maximum score for this PMP}} \times 100.$$

The Proficiency Index is the best overall indicator of how well one completed the PMP relative to the optimal. This measure both rewards better choices while penalizing negative ones. It doesn't, however, consider neutral choices.

$$\text{Errors of Omission} = \frac{\text{sum of all positive choices}}{\text{maximum score for this PMP}} \times 100.$$

The Errors of Omission score gives an indication of how likely you are to hesitate to do things that are beneficial or desirable, perhaps out of concern that you might make an error.

$$\text{Errors of Commission} = \frac{\text{sum of all negative choices}}{\text{maximum score for this PMP}} \times 100.$$

The Errors of Commission score gives an indication of how likely you are to do too much or make mistakes by doing rather than not doing. The "shotgun approach" to lab testing, for example, will generate a high Errors of Commission score.

$$\text{Efficiency Index} = \frac{\text{the number (not sum) of positive choices}}{\text{the number of }all\text{ choices made by you}} \times 100.$$

The Efficiency Index is the best indicator of how well you proceeded through the problem in terms of economy of time and effort. It does include an indication of the effect of neutral as well as negative and positive choices. It is not the best measure of overall performance, however, since it is possible to proceed efficiently through the problem to a much less than optimal solution by making many Errors of Omission.

These scores are designed to be considered as a group in order to get the most information about your approach to this type of problem and how it might be improved. For example, given a low Proficiency Index, one may look to the Errors of Omission and Errors of Commission to determine if your approach should be more bold or more cautious in the future. If the Proficiency Index is fairly high but the Efficiency Index is low, you may consider where in the problem you may have been led off onto a fairly neutral but unproductive sidetrack and how you might have avoided it.

Scoring Values

Maximum score (sum of weighted values from optimal path) = 40.0.

Frame	Response Number	Unweighted Values	Weighted Values
A	1	2.0	4.0
	2	−2.0	−4.0
	3	3.0	8.0
	4	−1.5	−2.8
B	1	3.0	8.0
	2	3.0	8.0
	3	−2.0	−4.0
	4	−3.5	−12.1
	5	3.0	8.0
	6	−2.0	−4.0
C	1	0.0	0.0
	2	−1.5	−13.6
	3	3.0	8.0
	4	−2.0	−4.0
	5	3.0	8.0
	6	−2.0	−4.0
D	1	−2.0	−4.0
	2	3.0	8.0
	3	−2.0	−4.0
	4	−1.5	−2.8
	5	3.0	8.0
E	1	−1.0	−13.0
	2	2.5	6.1
	3	4.0	16.0
F	1	−2.0	−4.0
	2	2.0	−2.8

Frame	Response Number	Unweighted Values	Weighted Values
	3	−3.0	−8.0
	4	−3.0	−8.0
	5	−1.0	−1.0
	6	1.0	1.0
	7	4.0	2.8
G		No choices	
H	1	2.0	−4.0
	2	−2.0	−4.0
	3	−1.0	−1.0
	4	−1.0	−1.0
	5	−4.0	−16.0
	6	−2.0	−4.0
	7	−1.0	−1.0

Appendix C

Nursing-Home Patient Management Problem

James P. Held and David B. Marcotte

Instructions

The following patient management problem (PMP) is designed to simulate a physician/ patient interaction in order to test your clinical judgment and provide feedback concerning your management of this patient.

First read the initial description of the setting and the preliminary general history, then follow the directions at the beginning of each frame. You will be asked to make management decisions throughout the PMP. The consequences of each decision and further interactions are revealed. This problem will be most valuable if you approach it not as a test or examination but rather as a learning experience where you react as you would in the actual situation.

When you have completed the problem, you may wish to read the discussion by the authors and the scoring instructions at the end. The authors' discussion outlines the optimal solutions and discusses the crucial management issues raised in this problem.

Setting

You are a general psychiatrist in Portville, a city of 50,000. You have a busy practice; however, half a day per week you consult at the Sunny Acres Nursing Home. You are employed in a consultant basis to manage medical–psychiatric problems and to educate nursing personnel on an "inservice" program at the nursing home. Mr. Anderson, nursing home director, called yesterday and scheduled a patient, Mrs. Goldberg, from the home to see you.

Preliminary General History

Nursing reports indicate that she is frequently excited and struck an attendant with her purse last week. She complains about "everything," and supportive concern hasn't helped. She accused the head nurse of stealing $2 from her purse, and she just isn't adjusting well since entering the Sunny Acres home 1 month ago. She was admitted after a fx hip injury and was unable to manage her own home with physical limitations secondary to the fracture.

GO TO FRAME A

Frame A

Mrs. Goldberg is an elderly woman appearing to be about 75 years of age, who is poorly dressed and clutches her purse. She questions who you are and appears angry and suspicious, squinting her eyes. She talks about the nurses not taking care of her and asks, "Are you going to report me to them?" She complains about the food and states that they tie her in bed at night. She then describes her former house and how she managed before and how well she liked her neighbors. She waxes on, visibly relaxing, and talks about her grandchildren. Then she says, "I just don't have any privacy anymore," and becomes angry again.

At this point you would:
1.   Acknowledge Mrs. Goldberg's anger and ask her about it.
2.   End the interview with Mrs. Goldberg and call the nursing home for further information about her.
3.   Since she is garrulous and petulant with reported assault, prescribe ataractic (major tranquilizer) in low doses and call Mr. Anderson suggesting that she will take some time to adjust.
4.   Report back to Mr. Anderson that she is not impaired organically but will require some additional counseling to make an adjustment in the home.

Frame B

Mr. Anderson reports that she has been so unappreciative of her care, argues with the staff, and tells them to get out and leave her alone. She constantly complains. She does not socialize well with others. She does some knitting, but no contact exists between patient and staff that is not negative.

At this point you would:
1.   Ask for more information and have it sent to your office.
2.   Since she is garrulous and petulant, with purported assault, prescribe an

ataractic (major tranquilizer) in low doses, and tell Mr. Anderson that she will take some time to adjust.

3. Schedule an interview with Mrs. Goldberg for one week later.

4. Ask Mr. Anderson for additional specific details about her behavior.

5. Report back to Mr. Anderson that she is not impaired organically but will require additional counseling to make an adjustment in the home.

6. Tell Mr. Anderson that she misses her family and suggest that he pressure them to visit more frequently.

Frame C

Mr. Anderson asks for a minute to get the report. He cites that Mrs. Goldberg pushed an attendant who was trying to get her to join a sing-along patient activity. She swore at another staff member who was simply wanting to hold her purse while she was taking a bath. Yesterday she threw her plate on the floor at lunch and complained. Last night she tried to caress one of the attendants who was making bed check.

At this point you would:

1. Since she exhibits signs and symptoms of organic brain syndrome, decide that the best course of action would be to begin ataractic medications (major tranquilizers) in low doses (25 mg Mellaril q.i.d.).

2. Request an appointment with Mr. Anderson, the nursing home administrator, on your next scheduled inservice education day at the Sunny Acres Nursing Home.

3. Refer her to Dr. Bell, a noted mental-health counselor whom you trust.

4. Reschedule another interview with the patient in 1 week.

Frame D

Mrs. Goldberg enters your office and immediately begins by asking, "What in blazes is going on? There's nothing wrong with me, Doctor. If you ask me, you should spend your time talking to the head nurse at the home, Mrs. Pritchett." You tell Mrs. Goldberg that you want to know more about her, and she talks once more about her grandchildren. She is less garrulous than on the previous visit but still suspicious of you.

At this point you would.

1. Reassure her of the difficulty of her adjusting to a nursing home and suggest that she make a better effort to get along with the staff since they are trying to help her.

2. Take a sex history from her.

3. Ask Mrs. Goldberg what it's been like for her to adjust to the nursing home.

Frame E

Mrs. Goldberg blanches visibly and with her head tilted up says, "Why, that's none of your business! Land sakes! What ever would you want to know about that for?"

At this point you would:
1.   Reassure Mrs. Goldberg that information about her sexual life is important to you as her physician. You need to know how her life has changed since she has been in the nursing home.
2.   Apologize, then reassure her of the difficulty of adjusting to a nursing home and suggest that she make a better effort to get along with the staff since they are trying to help her.
3.   Tell Mrs. Goldberg you are sorry you have upset her and reschedule another visit when she can be more composed.
4.   Prescribe a minor tranquilizer (chlordiazepoxide, Valium) for her anxiety and moderate hostility. Tell her this is a mild drug that will help her in the home.

Frame F

Mrs. Goldberg talks about how difficult it is to give up her belongings and her furniture and how pictures of the children were lost in the move. She describes that things haven't been the same since Abe died 2 years ago. "He was such a fine man." She then mentions the regimentation of the home; they don't have Saturday services or keep Kosher. They are always watching out for her and babying her. "I know when they try to cheer me up. I'm so alone." She covers her face with her hands and weeps.

At this point you would:
1.   Ask Mrs. Goldberg about how she feels about missing an intimate relationship and what that means to her now in relation to her sexual life.
2.   Tell her it's tough to lose so much in such a short time. Suggest that she socialize more in the nursing home.
3.   Ask her more about her feelings about the nursing staff.
4.   Call in another consulting psychiatrist, especially one who is familiar with geriatric problems. She is depressed and you need to know the extent of her depression.

Frame G

Mrs. Goldberg talks about how difficult it is to give up her belongings and her furniture and how pictures of the children were lost in the move. She describes that things haven't been the same since Abe died 2 years ago. "He was such a fine man." She then mentions the regimentation of the home; they don't have Saturday services or keep Kosher. They are always watching out for her and babying her. ''I know when they try to cheer me up. I'm so alone.'' She covers her face with her hands and weeps.

At this point you would:
1. Call in a consulting psychiatrist, especially one who is familiar with geriatric problems. She is depressed and you need to know the extent of her depression.
2. Tell her it's tough to lose so much in such a short time. Suggest that she socialize more in the nursing home.
3. Reassure Mrs. Goldberg that it is very difficult to adjust to some place new, especially after being on her own for so long. Confront her with specific reports from the nursing home.
4. Ask her about how she feels about missing an intimate relationship and what that means to her now in relation to her sexual life.

Frame H

Mrs. Goldberg says that she has tried to socialize but they keep her away from the others in the nursing home. ''What would you do with that head nurse breathing down your neck, Doctor?''

At this point you would:
1. Call the nursing home and schedule an informal ward conference about Mrs. Goldberg.
2. Ask Mrs. Goldberg how she feels about missing an intimate relationship and what that means for her now in relation to her sexual life.
3. Ask her how she sees the staff interfering with her friendships.
4. Tell her you understand how difficult it is but that she should keep trying anyway.

Frame I

Mrs. Goldberg states that she has been so lonely since Abe died. She wishes she could just talk to a man without everyone jumping to conclusions. ''You can't imagine, Doctor, how that stuff is. Well, actually, I have started playing with myself again once in a while. I like this one man at home, Sam. He's funny and bright and from a fine family.''

At this point you would:
1. Ask her if she has acted on her feelings toward Sam.
2. Suggest that Mrs. Goldberg marry someone that she likes.
3. Suggest to Mrs. Goldberg that she follow through with her feelings about Sam.
4. Ask Mrs. Goldberg how she felt when she acted on her feelings toward Sam.

Frame J

The staff has assembled for the ward conference at the nursing home. The staff knows you have asked for a discussion about Mrs. Goldberg. The chief nurse, Mrs. Pritchett, introduces you and says that you have come today to help them out with Mrs. Goldberg and tell them what to do. Several members of the staff voice complaints about her as a crochety, unappreciative woman. They state that they have done their best.

At this point you would:

1. Suggest that the staff encourage more socialization with others, mentioning her many losses in the last month.

2. Suggest to the staff that their attitudes are causing Mrs. Goldberg to react to them. They should emphasize her positive attributes and reward her behavior between outbursts.

3. Ask the staff more about the incidents and what they notice as a problem.

Frame K

At this point you would:

1. Arrange to meet with the staff of the Sunny Acres Nursing Home at your next inservice program, mentioning that you would like to talk about Mrs. Goldberg.

2. Refer her to a mental-health counselor. Call and arrange the apointment and tell the counselor what you have found out about Mrs. Goldberg after asking her if it's okay.

3. Tell Mrs. Goldberg that it's okay to act on her feelings, that it's only natural and normal behavior. Arrange to meet with the staff of the Sunny Acres Nursing Home at your next inservice program, mentioning that you would like to talk about Mrs. Goldberg.

4. End the interview and call the nursing home for further information. Ask Mr. Anderson, the director, for specific details of Mrs. Goldberg's behavior.

Frame L

Mrs. Pritchett, the chief nurse, calls you and states that the staff is concerned and puzzled about the conference. They were looking forward to a presentation on decubitus ulcers and air-bed treatment. She agrees that the staff will be there nevertheless. At the meeting Mrs. Pritchett introduces you and says that you have come to help them out with Mrs. Goldberg and tell them what to do. Several members of the staff voice complaints about her as a crochety, unappreciative woman. They state that they have done their best.

At this point you would:

1.   Suggest to the staff that she is acting out her loneliness and loss of family, especially her husband. She needs their support to enable her to form a relationship in the home.

2.   Ask the staff more about the incidents and what they notice as a problem.

3.   Suggest to the staff that their attitudes are causing Mrs. Goldberg to react to them. They should emphasize her positive attributes and reward her behavior between outbursts.

Frame M

Several of the staff appear disgusted. Mrs. Pritchett interrupts to mention that you have received every nursing incident written, if you had only looked in the record. Several staff members mention that Mrs. Goldberg is a born troublemaker.

At this point you would:

1.   Probe the staff for more details of specific difficulties with Mrs. Goldberg.

2.   Reschedule an appointment with Mrs. Goldberg.

3.   Mention to the staff that although she is troublesome, she is acting out her loneliness and loss of family, especially her husband. She needs their support to enable her to form a relationship in the home.

Frame N

One staff member responds with "What do you mean by her intimacy needs? How far should we allow her to act in the home, Doctor?" Several more staff members mention that they have seen her masturbating in the bathroom.

At this point you would:

1.   Advise the staff that many persons remain active sexually in later life, and a great difficulty is that they have lost their privacy, especially in an institution. Relate her attraction to Sam, a fellow patient, and remind them that there is no danger of pregnancy. Schedule a follow-up meeting with the staff.

2.   Advise the staff that many persons remain active sexually in later life, and a great difficulty is that they have lost their privacy, especially in an institution. Relate her attraction to Sam, a fellow patient, and remind them that there is no danger of pregnancy.

3.   Advise the staff that many persons remain active sexually in later life, and a great difficulty is that they have lost their privacy, especially in any institution. Relate her attraction to Sam, a fellow patient, and remind them that there is no danger of pregnancy. Schedule a follow-up meeting with the staff. Suggest that Mrs. Goldberg be seen by a counselor you know and trust after Mrs. Goldberg agrees and you have personally contacted the counselor.

Frame O

Mrs. Goldberg comes in for an additional interview complaining about the staff, saying that it's gotten much worse. They watch her all the time, especially the head nurse. They took away her knitting needles. "They think I'm going to kill someone. I sure would like to sometimes."

At this point you would:
1. Since she is garrulous and petulant with reported assault, prescribe an atarac-tic (major tranquilizer) in low doses and call Mr. Anderson suggesting that she will take some time to adjust.
2. Ask Mrs. Goldberg what differences in her sexuality she notes with her loss of privacy.
3. Report back to Mr. Anderson that she is not impaired organically but will require additional counseling to make an adjustment in the home. Suggest referral to Dr. Bell, a well-respected, mental-health counselor.
4. Call the nursing home for further information about Mrs. Goldberg.
5. Suggest that she try socializing more in the nursing home.

Answer Key

A-1

> GO TO FRAME F.

A-2

> GO TO FRAME B.

A-3

> The nursing home reports that the patient is doing fine. Six months later her daughter calls you to complain that she is apathetic and non-talkative.
>
> You are failing to explore symbolic problems. Although suspicious and hostile at times, she has recently been admitted. Look for conflicts behind the behavior. Medication here will control her garrulousness but will blunt her faculties and additionally cause side effects. Although medications may at times be indicated for organic brain syndrome, frequently they increase confusion. Minor tranquilizers produce tachy-phylaxis and offer only a temporary solution or avoidance of solution.
> SELECT ANOTHER CHOICE PLEASE.

A-4

No additional contact from nursing home.

The patient responds well with affective modulation during the interview. Explore her concerns. Many symbolic references exist in the problem. Check again. SELECT ANOTHER CHOICE PLEASE.

B-1

One week later, a 300-page Xerox copy of her medical records from previous hospitals and the current nursing home arrives. SELECT ANOTHER CHOICE PLEASE.

B-2

Nursing reports indicate that the patient is doing fine. No further patient contact.

You are failing to explore symbolic problems. Although suspicious and hostile at times, she has recently been admitted. Look for conflicts behind the behavior. Medication here will control her garrulousness but will blunt her faculties and additionally cause side effects. Although medications may at times be indicated for organic brain syndrome, frequently they increase confusion. Minor tranquilizers produce tachyphylaxis and offer only a temporary solution or avoidance of solution. SELECT ANOTHER CHOICE PLEASE.

B-3

GO TO FRAME O.

B-4

GO TO FRAME C.

B-5

No further patient contact.

The patient responds well during the interview. Explore her concerns. Many symbolic references exist in the problem. Check again. SELECT ANOTHER CHOICE PLEASE.

B-6

Six months later the patient is re-referred to you. GO TO FRAME O.

C-1

The nursing home reports that all is going well. A peer review board asks to meet with you regarding your use of drugs in this case.

You are failing to explore symbolic problems. Although suspicious and hostile at times, she has recently been admitted. Look for conflicts behind the behavior. Medication here will control her garrulousness but will blunt her faculties and additionally cause side effects. Although medications may at times be indicated for organic brain syndrome, frequently they increase confusion. Minor tranquilizers produce tachyphylaxis and offer a temporary solution or avoidance of solution. SELECT ANOTHER CHOICE PLEASE.

C-2

Mr. Anderson will be on vacation and can't see you then; the earliest time would be in 6 weeks. SELECT ANOTHER CHOICE PLEASE.

C-3

No more is heard of Mrs. Goldberg.

The patient responds well with affective modulation. Explore her concerns. Many symbolic references exist in the problem. Check again. START AT FRAME A ONCE AGAIN.

C-4

GO TO FRAME D.

D-1

Six months later Mrs. Goldberg is referred again. Same complaint. GO TO FRAME O.

D-2

GO TO FRAME E.

D-3

GO TO FRAME G.

E-1

GO TO FRAME I.

E-2

> Six months later Mrs. Goldberg is referred again. Same complaint. GO TO FRAME O.

E-3

> GO TO FRAME O.

E-4

> Nursing home reports no change in her behavior.
>
> You are failing to explore symbolic problems. Although suspicious and hostile at times, she has recently been admitted. Look for conflicts behind the behavior. Medication here will control her garrulousness but will blunt her faculties and additionally cause side effects. Although medications may at times be indicated for organic brain syndrome, frequently they increase confusion. Minor tranquilizers produce tachyphylaxis and offer only a temporary solution or avoidance of solution. SELECT ANOTHER CHOICE PLEASE.

F-1

> GO TO FRAME I.

F-2

> GO TO FRAME H.

F-3

> The patient responds, "Doctor, they treat me like I'm bonkers or that I don't have any sense at all." SELECT ANOTHER CHOICE PLEASE.

F-4

> The report from the consulting psychiatrist states that she is experiencing a mild grief reaction; recommendations are that you follow her for a month and monitor progress in her adjustment to the nursing home. SELECT ANOTHER CHOICE PLEASE.

G-1

> The report from the consulting psychiatrist states that she is experiencing a mild grief reaction and he recommends that you follow her for a month and monitor progress in adjustment to the nursing home. SELECT ANOTHER CHOICE PLEASE.

G-2   GO TO FRAME H.

G-3   Mrs. Goldberg responds by mentioning that the report is hogwash. She does remember waking up one night from a dream and touching an attendant. SELECT ANOTHER CHOICE PLEASE.

G-4   GO TO FRAME I.

H-1   GO TO FRAME J.

H-2   GO TO FRAME I.

H-3   The patient responds, "They keep separating me from other people, especially the men." GO TO FRAME K.

H-4   Mrs. Goldberg says, "Fine, Doctor." One week later Mrs. Pritchett calls you to say that Mrs. Goldberg is impossible; she's worse than ever.

You're missing her needs. Also, the job indicates that you are a consultant to the staff. Could be this is a "systems problem." Why not check it out? You must attend to staff needs as well. It is critical to understand the staff and their reactions. SELECT ANOTHER CHOICE PLEASE.

I-1   Mrs. Goldberg responds, "Of course, Doctor. I wasn't born yesterday. What do you think that the nurses are upset about anyway?" GO TO FRAME K.

I-2   She responds laughingly with, "You've got to be kidding, Doctor."

Your attitudes are interfering with your being an effective helper. Why do you presume sex behavior only within marriage for other people? SELECT ANOTHER CHOICE PLEASE.

I-3

Mrs. Goldberg says, "Really." One week later Mrs. Pritchett, the chief nurse, calls to tell you that Mrs. Goldberg is "impossible" and much worse than before.

You're missing her needs. Also, the job indicates that you are a consultant to the staff. Could be this is a "systems problem." Why not check it out? You must attend to staff needs as well. It is critical to understand the staff and their reactions. SELECT ANOTHER CHOICE PLEASE.

I-4

She answers, "Well, I feel O.K., maybe a little scared, but the nurses really think I'm nuts." GO TO FRAME K.

J-1

Five staff members speak at once, assuring you that they have tried everything from bingo to sing-along, and she still is angry and sullen. SELECT ANOTHER CHOICE PLEASE.

J-2

Several staff members grumble without direct comment. Mrs. Pritchett thanks you for coming and being so helpful. Mrs. Goldberg is not seen again.

You're missing her needs. Also, the job indicates that you are a consultant to the staff. Could be this is a "systems problem." Why not check it out? You must attend to staff needs as well. It is critical to understand the staff and their reactions. SELECT ANOTHER CHOICE PLEASE.

J-3

GO TO FRAME M.

K-1

GO TO FRAME L.

K-2

Counselor reports that she is doing very well. Nursing home reports no progress or change in her behavior.

You're missing her needs. Also, the job indicates that you are a consultant to the staff. Could be this is a "systems problem." Why not check it out? You must attend to staff needs as well. It is critical to understand the staff and their reactions. SELECT ANOTHER CHOICE PLEASE.

K-3 | GO TO FRAME L.

K-4 | He cites that Mrs. Goldberg pushed an attendant, swore at another staff member, threw her plate on the floor and complained, and tried to caress one of the attendants who was making bed check. SELECT ANOTHER CHOICE PLEASE.

L-1 | GO TO FRAME N.

L-2 | Mrs. Pritchett cites that Mrs. Goldberg pushed an attendant, swore at another staff member, threw her plate on the floor and complained, and tried to caress one of the attendants who was making bed check. SELECT ANOTHER CHOICE PLEASE.

L-3 | GO TO FRAME M.

M-1 | Mrs. Pritchett appears startled and asks, "What *are* you looking for, Doctor?"

The staff is defensive with you; you are probably coming across too heavy with them. Give them information on the patient as well as ask for information. SELECT ANOTHER CHOICE PLEASE.

M-2 | GO TO FRAME D.

M-3 | GO TO FRAME N.

N-1 | Several members ask you if it's okay to let her spend private time with Sam. You support them in their decisions. At the next staff meeting reports from the staff indicate a marked improvement in Mrs. Goldberg's behavior and attitude. *END OF PATIENT MANAGEMENT PROBLEM.

N-2

You do not hear about Mrs. Goldberg, and at the next meeting you discuss decubitis ulcers.

The attitudes of the staff are central. You need follow-up with the staff to support their change in policy! SELECT ANOTHER CHOICE PLEASE.

N-3

Mrs. Pritchett calls to thank you for your help with Mrs. Goldberg who is doing just beautifully. The counselor reports excellent progress with Mrs. Goldberg. *END OF PATIENT MANAGEMENT PROBLEM.

O-1

The nursing home reports that the patient is doing fine. Six months later her daughter calls you to complain that she is apathetic and untalkative.

You are failing to explore symbolic problems. Although suspicious and hostile at times, she has recently been admitted. Look for conflicts behind the behavior. Medication here will control her garrulousness but will blunt her faculties and additionally cause side effects. Although medications may at times be indicated for organic brain syndrome, frequently they increase confusion. Minor tranquilizers produce tachyphylaxis and offer only a temporary solution or avoidance of solution. SELECT ANOTHER CHOICE PLEASE.

O-2

GO TO FRAME E.

O-3

No additional contact from nursing home.

The patient responds well in the interview. Explore her concerns. Many symbolic references exist in the problem. SELECT ANOTHER CHOICE.

O-4

GO TO FRAME B.

O-5

GO TO FRAME H.

Patient Follow-up

1. What potential problem areas do you expect to see on follow-up?
   A.
   B.
   C.
2. How would you manage each problem area?
   A.
   B.
   C.
3. What would be the expected outcome in each problem area?
   A.
   B.
   C.

END OF NURSING HOME PMP

Critical Discussion Points

Frame A   Mrs. Goldberg is adjusting to a new setting. She is angry and frightened of your intentions. You must explore her anger and concern. Referral or medications will avoid her problem.

Frame B   It is important to continue contact with Mrs. Goldberg in order to explore her concerns. Other options only avoid her crisis in the home.

Frame C   The conflict is evident between staff and patient. You have followed the staff's concern but must also attend to Mrs. Goldberg.

Frame D   You must explore her concerns further. A sex history is premature unless the setting for your interest is explained.

Frame E   You need to explain your interest in her sexual behavior and the importance of that information.

Frame F   The patient has alluded to loss throughout her story. It is worthwhile to explore her current intimate relationships or feelings about intimacy. Redirecting the interview to nursing staff will bring up "more of the same battle."

Frame G   Same as Frame F.

Frame H   You can elucidate a "systems" problem as the basis for the staff/patient conflict. As a consultant, you must attend to both staff and patient.

Frame I   The data indicate that her sexual behavior may be the concern of the staff and is also a concern to Mrs. Goldberg. To what extent has the sexual activity proceeded? Choices 1 and 4 are preferred by the authors.

Frame J   In this frame you are being set up by the staff as the expert. They will attempt to find information to convince you she is "sick" and needs to be removed. Addressing your comments to the patient is the preferred choice. Choice 2 makes the conference a power struggle and choice 3 will result in "more of the same" comments by staff.

Frame K   In this frame you have the opportunity of reassuring Mrs. Goldberg but must follow-up with the consultation with the staff to help with the systems problem. Without follow-up, Mrs. Goldberg will be "scapegoated."

Frame L   Repeat Frame J. Exception: choice 3 makes the conference a power struggle. Choice 2 results in "more of the same" comments by the staff.

Frame M   The preferred choice here is choice 3 where you explain what Mrs. Goldberg is dealing with and then look for staff who will support her. Remember you must deal with the staff's anxiety.

Frame N   It is critical to follow-up on the staff; they need support in the management of Mrs. Goldberg. Also Mrs. Goldberg represents only one person in the institution and continued enforcement of the rules will produce other "problem" patients.

Frame O   The preferred choice is to explore the meaning of her loss of privacy. All other options shut off the patient and her concerns.

Scoring Instructions

The scoring sheet gives the weighted and unweighted scoring values for each possible response of a PMP. The unweighted values are on a 4+ to 4− rating system giving the relative merit of each possible response for that particular frame considering the situation in that frame. The weighted values also take into account the pathway to that frame and, therefore, may seem at odds with the unweighted values. They are necessarily quite different in some cases in order to avoid scoring errors, such as giving someone credit for taking all the best choices on a loop or sidetrack that came out of a relatively neutral or slightly negative choice, that is, to avoid giving credit for running in circles.

The unweighted values, therefore, are provided for your information about a particular frame, not for scoring. The weighted values are to be used in all scoring procedures. The following are instructions for deriving several different types of scores from your responses on the PMP and a brief description of the meaning of each.

$$\text{Proficiency Index} = \frac{\text{sum of the weighted value of all responses}}{\text{maximum score for this PMP}} \times 100.$$

The Proficiency Index is the best overall indicator of how well one completed the PMP relative to the optimal. This measure both rewards better choices while penalizing negative ones. It doesn't, however, consider neutral choices.

$$\text{Errors of Omission} = \frac{\text{sum of all positive choices}}{\text{maximum score for this PMP}} \times 100.$$

The Errors of Omission score gives an indication of how likely you are to hesitate to do things that are beneficial or desirable, perhaps out of concern that you might make an error.

$$\text{Errors of Commission} = \frac{\text{sum of all negative choices}}{\text{maximum score for this PMP}} \times 100.$$

The Errors of Commission score gives an indication of how likely you are to do too much or make mistakes by doing rather than not doing. The "shotgun approach" to laboratory testing, for example, will generate a high Errors of Commission score.

$$\text{Efficiency Index} = \frac{\text{the number (not sum) of positive choices}}{\text{the number of } \textit{all} \text{ choices made by you}} \times 100.$$

The Efficiency Index is the best indicator of how well you proceeded through the problem in terms of economy of time and effort. It does include an indication of the effect of neutral as well as negative and positive choices. It is not the best measure of overall performance, however, since it is possible to proceed efficiently through the problem to a much less than optimal solution by making many Errors of Omission.

These scores are designed to be considered as a group in order to get the most information about your approach to this type of problem and how it might be improved. For example, given a low Proficiency Index, one may look to the Errors of Omission and Errors of Commission to determine if your approach should be more bold or more cautious in the future. If the Proficiency Index is fairly high but the Efficiency Index is low, you may consider where in the problem you may have been led off onto a fairly neutral but unproductive sidetrack and how you might have avoided it.

Scoring values

Maximum score (sum of weighted values from optimal path) = 36.2.

Frame	Response number	Unweighted values	Weighted values
A	1	3.0	8.0
	2	1.0	−7.0
	3	−1.0	−1.0
	4	−1.5	−2.8
B	1	−1.5	−2.8
	2	−2.0	−4.0
	3	1.5	2.8
	4	2.0	4.0
	5	−1.5	−2.8
	6	−1.5	−2.8
C	1	−2.5	−6.1
	2	−0.5	−0.5
	3	1.5	−3.3
	4	0.0	0.0

Frame	Response number	Unweighted values	Weighted values
D	1	−1.5	−2.8
	2	0.5	0.5
	3	2.5	6.1
E	1	2.5	6.1
	2	−1.0	−1.0
	3	−2.0	−4.0
	4	−0.5	−0.5
F	1	2.5	6.1
	2	−1.0	−1.0
	3	0.0	0.0
	4	−1.0	−1
G	1	−2.5	−6.1
	2	−1.5	−2.8
	3	1.0	1.0
	4	2.5	6.1
H	1	1.0	1.0
	2	2.5	6.1
	3	1.5	2.8
	4	−1.5	−2.8
I	1	1.5	2.8
	2	−1.5	−2.8
	3	−2.5	−6.1
	4	2.0	4.0
J	1	−2.0	−4.0
	2	−2.5	−6.1
	3	2.5	6.1
K	1	2.5	6.1
	2	−1.0	−1.0
	3	1.0	1.0
	4	−1.0	−1.0
L	1	2.0	4.0
	2	0.0	0.0
	3	−2.5	−6.1
M	1	0.0	0.0
	2	−2.0	−2.8
	3	2.0	4.0
N	1	3.0	8.0
	2	−0.5	−0.5
	3	1.5	2.8
O	1	−2.0	−4.0
	2	2.0	−8.5
	3	−1.5	−2.8
	4	1.0	−5.1
	5	0.0	−11.5

Prostatitis Patient Management Problem

David B. Marcotte, James P. Held, and Howard Dichter

Instructions

The following patient management problem (PMP) is designed to simulate a physician/ patient interaction in order to test your clinical judgment and provide feedback concerning your management of this patient.

First read the initial description of the setting and the preliminary general history; then follow the directions at the beginning of each frame. You will be asked to make management decisions throughout the PMP. The consequences of each decision and further interactions are revealed. This problem will be most valuable if you approach it not as a test or examination but rather as a learning experience where you react as you would in the actual situation.

When you have completed the problem, you may wish to read the authors' discussion and the scoring instructions at the end. The authors' discussion outlines the optimal solutions and discusses the crucial management issues raised in this problem.

Setting

You are a general psychiatrist practicing in Mellville, a city of 100,000 people. In addition, you are on the staff of Samaritan Hospital where you have admitting privileges.

Preliminary General History

A patient of yours, Mr. Urban, is an engineer at a large electronics firm. He has been married for 24 years and has two children ages 22 and 20; both are attending State University. Mrs. Urban operates a small dress shop in town.

Mr. Urban was treated by you as an outpatient 1½ years ago and was referred to Alcoholics Anonymous. He comes in with the complaint of a burning pain during urination and an occasional clear serous discharge from his penis. You inquire if he has ever had venereal disease. He states that he couldn't have because he has never had any extramarital intercourse. He is bright and verbal but keeps his head down and avoids eye contact during history taking. You note in his records that he began drinking heavily 5 years ago but has been sober for 3 years. He has come to see you because you previously had helped him with his alcohol problem.

GO TO FRAME A

Frame A

At this point you would:
1. Do a physical examination.
2. Proceed to take a sexual history, having ruled out the necessity of a physical examination.

Frame B

After considering the results of the physical examination you would:
1. Order laboratory data.
2. Order no laboratory data but obtain additional history.

Frame C

The laboratory tests you would order at this point include:
1. Urinalysis
2. CBC
3. Microscopic examination of serous discharge
4. Culture of discharge
5. Sedimentation rate
6. Urine culture
7. Lower abdominal X ray
8. Hematocrit
9. Prostatic acid phosphatase

After you look at the results of the laboratory tests you ordered, GO TO FRAME D.

Frame D

At this point you would:
1. Explain to the patient the results of the examination and that the culture reports are pending and make a referral to a urologist for consultation.
2. Reassure the patient that it is most probably nonspecific prostatitis and say that you would like to see him again in 2 weeks when you will have the laboratory results back. Treat with force fluids and a urinary antibiotic.
3. Reassure the patient that it is most probably nonspecific prostatitis. Tell him that there are no abnormalities so far in the physicial or laboratory data, with culture reports pending. Inquire more about sexual function.

Frame E

Mr. Urban haltingly describes "not being what he used to be." You ask him in what way. He says that he "can't get it up anymore" and hasn't been able to for the last year. During a 5-year period before that, he occasionally experienced impotence, but now he has no erection whatsoever. He denies masturbating or having morning erections. He states his wife doesn't seem to care. First he attacks her, and then he defends her. He describes her as involved in her business and preoccupied with social events. He states that it isn't the same as when they were young. He quickly interjects "that she is really a fine woman."

At this point you would (you may pick more than one):
1. Suggest that the wife come in for an appointment with or without her husband.
2. Suggest that the patient needs a full-scale work-up at Med U. Hospital, and call Dr. Broder, a noted internist, to refer your patient to her.
3. Inquire about similar experiences with erection difficulties.
4. Explain that since he has no morning erections and doesn't masturbate, he is likely to have organic impotence. Explain to him about the new penile implant and how successful it can be. Refer him to Dr. Reed who specializes in penile implants.
5. Inquire about bladder and bowel incontinence.
6. Take a family history.
7. Order FBS.
8. Order a glucose tolerance test.
9. Inquire about present medications.

Frame F

Mr. Urban calls you on the phone. In a loud voice barely in control he states, "Doc! Dr. Broder charged me $200, and the lab bill came to $550. I can't afford that! Why did you do it? And besides, everything was normal."

At this point you would:

    1.   Tell him that you are his doctor and must in all good conscience decide these matters.

    2.   Tell him that it is extremely important to rule out possible underlying causes, and because Med U. Hospital is the finest one around, costs are higher.

    3.   Mention that you were perhaps hasty in making the referral, and you can understand his annoyance. Invite him to come in and discuss it with you.

    4.   Tell him that it is important to rule out organic cause, but that you had expected Dr. Broder to be more concerned with finances. You are sorry that the costs were too high.

    5.   Suggest the Minnesota Multiphasic Inventory (MMPI) and projective testing and refer Mr. Urban to Dr. Slawson, a psychologist.

Frame G

Mr. Urban reveals that actually he has masturbated several times, but he is worried because for the last 2 months, he has been unable to have an erection while masturbating. He is shy and inhibited as he reveals this. When asked by you about extramarital relationships, he haltingly says that yes, he has had a relationship with a co-worker during the past year. He meets her for lunch and they stimulate each other in his car. There is no full erection and no penetration involved in these encounters. He is ashamed of himself.

At this point you would:

    1.   Refer the patient to a mental-health clinician who deals with sex and marital problems.

    2.   Request that the patient's wife come in.

    3.   Tell him that this is common and inquire about what he wants to do.

    4.   Suggest a divorce.

    5.   Tell him that nothing can be done until he gives up extramarital sex.

    6.   Tell him that he must tell his wife about his affair and bring her in for an appointment. This course of action will be the best for all.

Frame H

The patient looks down and signs. He describes his job as a dead-end job and says that it's dull at home. He is worried about his lover, his daughters at school, and the high cost of living. He doesn't know what to do.

At this point you would:

    1.   Tell the patient he must decide between his lover and his wife.

2. Refer him to a known clinician who deals with sexual and marital problems.
3. Recommend beginning sensate focus treatment with his wife and assign them some sexual homework, such as mutual massage.
4. Recommend sensate focus treatment with his lover and ask him to bring her in which him for another appointment.
5. Recommend a job change.

Frame I

Write a treatment plan for your follow-up on Mr. Urban if you decide to treat him at this point.

1. What potential problems do you expect to see with this patient?
   A.
   B.
   C.
2. How would you manage each of the above problems?
   A.
   B.
   C.
3. What would be the expected outcome for each of the above?
   A.
   B.
   C.

Answer Key

A-1

Results of physical examination:
Well-developed, well-nourished, white male. Blood pressure, $^{130}/_{85}$; pulse, 78 regular; respiration, 16; temperature, 98.4°F.
HEENT: PERLA: slight anisocoria. Fundi clear. Hearing grossly nl. bilaterally. ENT clear.
Chest: Good expansion—R.S.R. No cardiomegaly.
Abdomen: No hepatosplenomegaly.
Extremities: Good pulses bilaterally.
Neuro: Slight resting tremor. No diminished vibratory perception. No ataxia or disturbance in gait or station.
Genitorectal: Penis; no evidence of scarring or lesion. Rectal prostate soft and boggy, not enlarged. Serous discharge obtained.
GO TO FRAME B.

A-2

Mr. Urban is angry that you have not examined him. The history indicates a possibility of infection, e.g., trichomonas. Your decision to rule out a physical is inappropriate. MAKE ANOTHER CHOICE.

B-1

GO TO FRAME C.

B-2

History indicates the possibility of infection. Your decision to order no laboratory data is inappropriate. MAKE ANOTHER CHOICE.

C-1

Appearance: clear   Glucose: trace
Specific gravity: 1.015 (n1)   Ketones: negative
pH: 6   Blood: negative
Protein: trace   Bile: negative
Spun sediment: 8–10 WBC?HPR

A GOOD CHOICE FOR SCREENING.

C-2

6000 Leukocytes: 65% neutrophils, 25% lymphocytes, 3% eosinophils, 7% monocytes. A GOOD CHOICE FOR SCREENING.

C-3

Negative for gram-negative diplocci. EXCELLENT.

C-4

Done, report pending. NECESSARY.

C-5

5 (0–9 nl). NOT ESSENTIAL AND WILL NOT HELP WITH SPECIFICS.

C-6

Done, report pending. GOOD CHOICE.

C-7

n1. UNNECESSARY, PULSES EQUAL AND ACTIVE ANEURYSM RARELY INTERFERES WITH SEX FUNCTIONING.

C-8

47.2 (47.0 ± 0.7 n1) UNNECESSARY.

C-9

L.T. 0.2 BLB units. GOOD CHOICE FOR DETERMINING ENDOCRINE STATUS BUT TOO EARLY IN PROBLEM.

D-1

The patient fails to keep his appointment with the urologist.

Why a urologist when there were no specific physical findings? You are avoiding follow-up with the patient. Most sexual problems present themselves as physical complaints. MAKE ANOTHER CHOICE.

D-2

Two weeks later, Mr. Urban returns as scheduled and reports no change in his symptoms. He has taken the medication and drank copious fluids. You report to him that the laboratory data are normal and without any evidence of infection. GO TO FRAME E.

D-3

GO TO FRAME E.

E-1

Mr. Urban fails to keep his appointment, and his wife does not come in.

The patient is ambivalent about his wife. Explore his feelings about her more before you suggest her involvement. Also, though the patient has denied extramarital sexual intercourse, you could inquire about sexual contact outside of marriage that does not involve intercourse. MAKE ANOTHER CHOICE.

E-2

Med U. Hospital Report

Dear Dr. Primary:

Thank you for your recent referral, Mr. Urban. We performed many tests, the results of which you will find below. We were unable to pinpoint the cause of his secondary impotence, and he seemed rather put out and angry with us. We would recommend an MMPI and counseling for this man who has obvious deep-seated conflicts.

Blood glucose: 90 mg/100 ml   (60–100 mg/ml nl)
Oral glucose tolerance test: 1 hr   150 mg/100 ml
                                 1.5 hr   135 mg/100 ml
                                 2 hr   100 mg/100 ml
4-hr ACTH test: fasting cortisol 20 mg%; 4 hr, 50 mg%
                          (nl fasting cortisol, 3–26 mg%; 4 hr, 32–
                          55 mg%).
Soffer Garbrilove modification of the Robinson–Power–Kepler
    water test: excretion of 75% of administered load (excretion
    greater than 60% nl)
CAT scan: nl
Visual fields: nl
Skull X ray: nl
              Thyroxine (T_4):   2.0 ng%   (1.0–2.3 ng% nl)
              Blood level FSH: 10 mIU/ml   (4–25 mIU/ml nl)
          CSF protein: 45 mg/100 ml   (30–45 mg/100 ml nl)
          CSF glucose: 55 mg/dl
CSF electrophoresis: 7   0 gamma globulin   (7.2 ± 1.1 gamma
    globulin nl)
EMG conduction velocity of the median nerve: 35/msec (nl)

                                         Sincerely yours,

Summary of costs to patient for full-scale work-up:

Blood glucose	5.00
Oral glucose tolerance test	5.00
4-hr ACTH test	5.00
Soffer Garbrilove modification of the Robin-son–Power–Kepler water test	6.00
CAT scan	200.00
Visual fields	120.00
Skull X ray	112.80
Thyroxine (T_4)	16.00
Blood level FSH	18.30
Spinal tap	4.00
CSF protein	9.60
CSF electrophoresis	12.20
EMG conduction velocity of the median nerve	35.00
Total costs	$549.40

GO TO FRAME F.

E-3

GO TO FRAME G.

E-4

Your failure to explore sex history and relationship issues results in your premature closure. Let Mr. Urban define the problem further. MAKE ANOTHER CHOICE.

E-5

He reports none. MAKE ANOTHER CHOICE.

E-6

There is no history of diabetes or neurologic impairment. MAKE ANOTHER CHOICE.

E-7

FBS, 90 mg%.

E-8

1 hr   140 mg/100 ml
1.5 hr   125 mg/100 ml
2 hr   100 mg/100 ml
MAKE ANOTHER CHOICE.

E-9

Patient reports he is using none.

F1

Defensiveness on the part of the physician rarely helps. Apologize—it's okay to do so. Medical practice is a contract, not a controlling relationship. Discuss the situation with the patient. Don't shut him off. MAKE ANOTHER CHOICE.

F-2

Defensiveness on the part of the physician rarely helps. Apologize—it's okay to do so. Medical practice is a contract, not a controlling relationship. Discuss the situation with the patient. Don't shut him off. MAKE ANOTHER CHOICE.

F-3
> Mr. Urban comes in at your suggestion and accepts your apology in regard to the expenses. With that issue resolved, you inquire further about his original concerns. GO TO FRAME G.

F-4
> Mr. Urban replies, "I've already spent more money than I can afford, and there is still no help in sight for my problem. Why should I spend more money to see you?" MAKE ANOTHER CHOICE.

F-5
> Mr. Urban fails to make the appointment because of the additional expense involved. MAKE ANOTHER CHOICE.

G-1
> The counselor reports that Mr. Urban has begun treatment. GO TO FRAME I.

G-2
> Mr. Urban refuses this request but continues to talk. GO TO FRAME H.

G-3
> GO TO FRAME H.

G-4
> Mr. Urban is shocked at your suggestion. Your attitudes are potentially interfering with the patient's decision. Your suggestion is a premature closure on what the patient wants to talk about. MAKE ANOTHER CHOICE.

G-5
> The patient clams up. Your attitudes are potentially interfering with the patient's decision. Your suggestion is a premature closure on what the patient wants to talk about. MAKE ANOTHER CHOICE.

G-6
> Mr. Urban leaves and complains to the Medical Society. Your attitudes are potentially interfering with the patient's decision. Your suggestion is a premature closure on what the patient wants to talk about. MAKE ANOTHER CHOICE.

H-1

Your need for the patient to decide is not shared by him. Attitudes you hold interfere with how he potentially can resolve his conflict. MAKE ANOTHER CHOICE.

H-2

The counselor reports that the patient has entered treatment. GO TO FRAME I.

H-3

Mr. Urban resists and fails to return. He is ambivalent not only about sex but about his wife, his marriage, his job, his children, his finances, and his lover. A simple behavioral approach will not suffice. MAKE ANOTHER CHOICE.

H-4

Mr. Urban and his lover resist, and he fails to return. He is ambivalent not only about sex but about his wife, his marriage, his job, his children, his finances, and his lover. A simple behavioral approach will not suffice. Also, there are potential legal and ethical implications involved in a decision to see the patient together with his lover. MAKE ANOTHER CHOICE.

H-5

Mr. Urban resists and fails to return. He is ambivalent not only about his wife, but about his marriage, his job, his children, his finances, and his lover. A job change is too simple an answer. MAKE ANOTHER CHOICE.

Patient Follow-up

1. What potential problem areas do you expect to see on follow-up?
   A.
   B.
   C.
2. How would you manage each problem area?
   A.
   B.
   C.

3. What would be the expected outcome in each problem area?
   A.
   B.
   C.

END OF PROSTATITIS PMP

Critical Discussion Points

Frame A   It is critical to perform a physical examination. One might continue on with the history taking as a suitable alternative at this point. In the opinion of experts, we suggest a physical to rule out acute infectious disease.

Frame B   Ordering laboratory data is a requirement to continue to rule out infectious disease. Mr. Urban has come to you because he is worried and concerned about symptoms that could be secondary to venereal disease.

Frame C   Experts select laboratory data that includes urinalysis, microscopic examination culture of discharge, and CBC.

Frame D   Since Mr. Urban is married, it is unlikely that he will give you all the details of his sex history initially. Our experts agree that once you have ruled out venereal disease, inquiry about his sexual function is the best choice. Referral is considered inappropriate.

Frame E   A decision to involve the wife at this point is premature. Consultation is costly and not warranted yet without further knowledge about his endocrine status. Referral for penile transplant is contraindicated unless much more information about neurologic deficit is available as well as further information about sexual activity. Inquiry into bowel and bladder incontinence, family history of diabetes, and present medications are all useful data. Also FBS and glucose tolerance test are indicated to rule out diabetes. Experts agree that further inquiry into his erection difficulties and/or sex history is indicated.

Frame F   Mr. Urban is angry, and decisions to defend yourself and the institution or to refer Mr. Urban will result in continued hostile behavior on his part. It is best to encourage him to deal with you directly and be open about your hasty decision to refer.

Frame G   Mr. Urban is ashamed and anxious. An acceptable solution would be to refer Mr. Urban to a sex and marital therapist. It is too premature to "solve" his problem; further exploration of his values, reactions, and what he wants to do is necessary. Any other choices are seen as allowing your attitude to interfere in his solution.

Frame H   Mr. Urban is discouraged and is in a midlife crisis. Simple sex therapy with either wife or lover will likely be ineffective until he makes a commitment to one relationship. A job change will not likely be effective. Referral gives you an acceptable management choice.

Discussion

The authors outline their potential problems and list management and expected outcomes of further contact with Mr. Urban. Not all problem areas or management can be explored. You may select some unique problem and/or innovative management technique.

Potential Problem Areas

A. He will have continued ambivalence about home, job, and marriage.

B. He may make a precipitous decision to end his marriage and/or leave his work.

C. He could make a sudden decision to cut off his extramarital relationship and confess to his wife.

D. Mr. Urban may withdraw from all pleasures and increase self-criticism.

E. He could fail to return for a follow-up because of shame and embarrassment.

F. He may make a precipitous job change.

Management

A. You may explore his goals and objectives where he feels inadequate as well as explore his family of origin attitudes and ideals.

B. You could confront him with not making a decision right now but discuss his options further.

C. His increasing self-critical ideas along with appearance of negativism and signs of depression could be managed with a tricyclic antidepressant.

D. You could contact him at work if he fails to return and invite him in to discuss his termination and goals.

E. You could confront him about sudden decisions that have not been well worked out.

F. You can recommend sex therapy on one relationship after he makes a well-thought-out decision.

Outcomes

A. A possible resolution of self-doubt and increased energy to enjoy his life.

B. Possible intensive therapy if no resolution occurs in five sessions to explore his early development.

C. Recommend crisis marital therapy if he confesses to his wife.

D. Gradually withdraw antidepressants medication after 6 months of treatment.

E. Mr. Urban may have a return of sex functioning with commitment and diminished anxiety about sexual performance.

F. He may decide not to work in therapy at this time.

Scoring Instructions

The scoring sheet gives the weighted and unweighted scoring values for each possible response of a PMP. The unweighted values are on a $4+$ to $4-$ rating system giving the relative merit of each possible response for that particular frame considering the situation in that frame. The weighted values also take into account the pathway to that frame and, therefore, may seem at odds with the unweighted values. They are necessarily quite different in some cases in order to avoid scoring errors, such as giving someone credit for taking all the best choices on a loop or sidetrack that came out of a relatively neutral or slightly negative choice, that is, to avoid giving credit for running in circles.

The unweighted values, therefore, are provided for your information about a particular frame, not for scoring. The weighted values are to be used in all scoring procedures. The following are instructions for deriving several different types of scores from your responses on the PMP, and a brief description of the meaning of each.

$$\text{Proficiency Index} = \frac{\text{sum of the weighted value of all responses}}{\text{maximum score for this PMP}} \times 100.$$

The Proficiency Index is the best overall indicator of how well one completed the PMP relative to the optimal. This measure both rewards better choices while penalizing negative ones. It doesn't, however, consider neutral choices.

$$\text{Errors of Omission} = \frac{\text{sum of all positive choices}}{\text{maximum score for this PMP}} \times 100.$$

The Errors of Omission score gives an indication of how likely you are to hesitate to do things that are beneficial or desirable, perhaps out of concern that you might make an error.

$$\text{Errors of Commission} = \frac{\text{sum of all negative choices}}{\text{maximum score for this PMP}} \times 100.$$

The Errors of Commission score gives an indication of how likely you are to do too much or make mistakes by doing rather than not doing. The ''shotgun approach'' to laboratory testing, for example, will generate a high Errors of Commission score.

$$\text{Efficiency Index} = \frac{\text{the number (not sum) of positive choices}}{\text{the number of \textit{all} choices made by you}} \times 100.$$

The Efficiency Index is the best indicator of how well you proceeded through the problem in terms of economy of time and effort. It does include an indication of the effect of neutral as well as negative and positive choices. It is not the best measure of overall performance, however, since it is possible to proceed efficiently through the problem to a much less than optimal solution by making many Errors of Ommission.

These scores are designed to be considered as a group in order to get the most information about your approach to this type of problem and how it might be improved. For example, given a low Proficiency Index, one may look to the Errors of Omission and Errors of Commission to determine if your approach should be more bold or more cautious in the future. If the Proficiency Index is fairly high but the Efficiency Index is low, you may consider where in the problem you may have been led off onto a fairly neutral but unproductive sidetrack and how you might have avoided it.

Scoring values*

Maximum score (sum of weighted values on optimal path) = 186.00.

Frame	Response number	Unweighted values	Weighted values
A	1	4.0	16.0
	2	−1.5	−2.8
B	1	4.0	16.0
	2	−3.0	−8.0
C	1	4.0	16.0
	2	1.0	1.0
	3	4.0	16.0
	4	4.0	16.0
	5	0.0	0.0
	6	3.0	8.0
	7	−3.0	−8.0
	8	−2.0	−4.0
	9	−2.0	−4.0
D	1	−2.0	−4.0
	2	−1.5	−2.8
	3	4.0	16.0
E	1	1.5	0
	2	−1.0	−1.0
	3	3.0	8.0
	4	−4.0	−16.0
	5	2.0	4.0
	6	2.0	4.0
	7	2.0	4.0
	8	1.0	1.0
	9	4.0	16.0
F	1	−4.0	−16.0
	2	−1.5	−2.8
	3	3.0	8.0

Frame	Response number	Unweighted values	Weighted values
	4	2.0	4.0
	5	−4.0	−16.0
G	1	4.0	16.0
	2	2.0	−4.0
	3	1.5	−6.1
	4	−4.0	−16.0
	5	−2.5	−6.1
	6	−3.0	−8.0
H	1	−2.5	−6.1
	2	4.0	16.0
	3	0.0	0.0
	4	−1.5	−2.8
	5	0.0	0.0

Index